ANNUAL REVIEW OF PUBLIC HEALTH

EDITORIAL COMMITTEE (1991)

ANNUAL REVIEW OF PUBLIC HEALTH

VOLUME 12, 1991

GILBERT S. OMENN, *Editor*

University of Washington

JONATHAN E. FIELDING, *Associate Editor*

University of California at Los Angeles

LESTER B. LAVE, *Associate Editor*

Carnegie Mellon University

ANNUAL REVIEWS INC.   4139 EL CAMINO WAY   P.O. BOX 10139   PALO ALTO. CALIFORNIA 94303-0897

Annual Review of Public Health
Volume 12, 1991

CONTENTS

vi   CONTENTS   (continued)

SOME RELATED ARTICLES IN OTHER *ANNUAL REVIEWS*

From the *Annual Review of Genetics*, Volume 24 (1990):

Genetics of Atherosclerosis, C. F. Sing and P. P. Moll
In Vivo Somatic Mutations in Humans: Measurement and Analysis, Richard J. Albertini, Janice A. Nicklas, J. Patrick O'Neill, and Steven H. Robison
The Comparative Radiation Genetics of Humans and Mice, James V. Neel and Susan E. Lewis
Human Tumor Suppressive Genes, Eric Stanbridge

From the *Annual Review of Medicine*, Volume 42 (1991):

Long-Term Results of Coronary Balloon Angioplasty, B. Meier
Cardiac Complications of Cocaine Abuse, Jeffrey M. Isner and Saurabh K. Chokshi
Anabolic Steroids in the Athlete, Richard H. Strauss and Charles E. Yesalis
Infectious Diarrhea, Mitchell J. Rubinoff and Michael Field
Transfusion Practice in the 1990s, Jay E. Menitove
Prevention and Treatment of Cytomegalovirus Infection, Joel D. Meyers
Prevention and Treatment of Pneumocystis carinii *Pneumonia*, Walter T. Hughes
Epidemiology and Outcome of Child Abuse, Donna A. Rosenberg and Richard D. Krugman
Organic Bases of Depression in the Elderly, K. Ranga Rama Krishnan
Tuberculosis in Elderly Persons, William W Stead and Asim K. Dutt
Long-Term Results of Cardiac Transplantation, Sharon Hunt and Margaret Billingham

From the *Annual Review of Nutrition*, Volume 11 (1991):

Should There Be Intervention to Alter Serum Lipids in Children?, Alvin M. Mauer
Fluorides and Osteoporosis, Michael Kleerekoper and Raffaella Balena
Dietary Regulation of Cytochrome P450, Karl E. Anderson and Attallah Kappas
Nutritional Consequences of Vegetarianism, Johanna T. Dwyer

From the *Annual Review of Psychology*, Volume 42 (1991):

Human Behavioral Genetics, Robert Plomin and Richard Rende
Psychological Perspectives on Nuclear Deterrence, Philip E. Tetlock, Charles B. McGuire, and Gregory Mitchell
The Classroom as a Social Context for Learning, Carol Simon Weinstein

(*continued*)

Annu. Rev. Publ. Health 1991. 12:1–15

RECENT DEVELOPMENTS IN MENTAL HEALTH: PERSPECTIVES AND SERVICES

David Mechanic

Institute for Health, Health Care Policy, and Aging Research, Rutgers University, New Brunswick, New Jersey 08903

KEY WORDS: deinstitutionalization, community mental health care, schizophrenia, mental
            health policy, mental illness

Observers of the history of mental health policy note recurrent cycles reflecting changing perceptions of treatment opportunities and altered willingness to invest public resources. These historical trends are a product of social ideologies, changing public opinion, fiscal conditions, new technologies, and changes in political dialogue. In the 30 years following World War II, major changes in concepts of mental health and provision of mental health services have been apparent, but the US is again ambivalent. Whether this period is simply one of readjustment in a long-range trend or a major discontinuity and realignment of priorities relevant to community-based systems of mental health care remains unclear. I take as my point of departure developments in the past ten years; however, to put these in perspective, a brief review of long-term mental health trends is helpful.

POST–WORLD WAR II MENTAL HEALTH POLICY

A confluence of social, economic, and technological influences transformed mental health services in the post–World War II period. These already have been reviewed in detail (8, 23, 26), but we need some general observations to put current public policy in its proper context. Experience in the selective

1

0163-7525/91/0501-0001$02.00

service system and in the management of psychiatric casualties during wartime impressed policymakers with the magnitude of mental health needs. They saw the requirement for broad approaches that could be responsive without enlarging already overcrowded public hospital systems, which were a burden to the states. Drawing on evolving social conceptions about the nature of mental illness and society, advocates built support for a widely accepted ideology about preventive community intervention and the social management of mental illness.

In the 1950s, the introduction of neuroleptic drugs in large mental hospitals helped control the most bizarre manifestations of psychotic illness. The drugs also gave administrators, families, and communities confidence to experiment with new hospital and community arrangements. These arrangements were facilitated further by a strong critique of mental hospitalization and its noxious effects on the coping capacities and social adaptations of patients. Though the ideological conditions were ripe for deinstitutionalization, hospitals found great difficulty in appropriately resettling patients in the community and supporting their subsistence. Deinstitutionalization became more feasible with the broad expansion of social programs in the middle 1960s, which enhanced housing opportunities, medical care, and disability subsistence (22, 23). Large-scale reduction of the number of public mental hospital beds only became possible with these developments, and the rate of deinstitutionalization between 1966 and 1980 was almost five times that of the previous decade (9, 26).

In the society at large, the rapid expansion of health insurance (particularly the growth of insured mental health benefits), the commitment of the federal government to support community mental health centers, and the growing acceptance of mental health care among the general public transformed the scope and configuration of the mental health care system. Between 1955 and 1983, the number of mental illness episodes treated in organized mental health settings increased from 1.7 to 7 million. The voluntary general hospital became the central site for acute inpatient psychiatric care. And, the number of public mental hospital beds decreased to 115,000. The locus of care shifted dramatically from inpatient to ambulatory settings, and the mentally ill and demented elderly were relocated to nursing homes that expanded in the mid-1960s, stimulated by Medicare and Medicaid. During the Kennedy and Johnson presidencies, the initiatives for mental health policy shifted to the federal government. The trend away from traditional, involuntary hospitalization and toward community care was reinforced by vigorous legal advocacy that made it more difficult to use state police powers to treat the mentally ill.

The momentum that developed in building a community mental health system parallel to and independent of the state programs progressed rapidly into the 1970s, when fiscal constraints and the hostility of the Nixon Administration slowed the momentum of the emerging infrastructure. It also became clear that the new community mental health centers (CMHCs) had attracted many new clients, and the boundaries of mental health care were expanded. However, the CMHCs had substantially neglected the most disadvantaged and seriously mentally ill.

During the Carter Administration, the establishment of a Presidential Commission on mental health and the interests of Rosalyn Carter set the stage for a reexamination of mental health policy and strong advocacy for a range of interested constituencies. The Commission's efforts, however, underscored the conflicting conceptions of mental health and system priorities and the competing viewpoints about the role of government, constituency groups, and mental health services, such as treatment, rehabilitation, or prevention activities (6). Moreover, the reality of fiscal constraint was becoming abundantly clear. Not prepared to adjudicate these conflicts, the Commission recommended something for everyone, with no clear priorities, and served primarily as a platform for mental health advocacy.

The tougher task came in passing comprehensive legislation. After much contentiousness and compromise, Congress passed the Mental Health Systems Act of 1980, resolving few of the real conceptual difficulties. This legislation supported enhancement of community mental health and programming for the chronically mentally ill. It also supported a variety of other groups (children, the elderly) and functions (prevention, advocacy). Despite its defects, the legislation represented a new federal commitment. Parallel to these efforts, the Department of Health and Human Services put together a useful strategy for identifying and coordinating federal resources and programs to design a comprehensive service system for the most critically and chronically ill (36).

With the Reagan Administration, and the introduction of a "new federalism" philosophy, the mental health systems legislation was never implemented. It was superseded by a program to distribute mental health services funds to states in block grants at reduced expenditure levels. Initiative for mental health policy was returned to the states, and the National Institute of Mental Health (NIMH), stripped of its service and policy functions, became substantially a research funding institute.

The Reagan Administration's efforts to reduce the role of federal government and to cut health and welfare programs affected the fate of the seriously mentally ill far more than the reductions in categorical mental health funding and the failure to implement the Systems Act. In the 1980s, the social and welfare programs that made deinstitutionalization possible were substantially reduced (e.g. housing and Social Security Disability Insurance/Supplemental Security Income) or failed to keep pace with the growth of the poverty population (Medicaid). Many chronically ill, who in earlier times would have been hospitalized, were in the community. They had neither adequate subsistence and life supports nor an adequate infrastructure of essential community mental health services. Many persons with serious mental illness became part of the homeless population (13); however, the major cause was the erosion of the safety net, not deinstitutionalization policies. In the total context of efforts to restrain government expenditures and health care costs, reduce the federal deficit, and resist increased taxes, the chronically mentally ill occupied a low position in the nation's priorities.

The problems associated with welfare reductions would have been acute in any case, but they are substantially exacerbated by the changing demography of the American population. As the baby boom generations have reached young adulthood, the period of life in which schizophrenia has its highest incidence, the aggregate numbers of seriously mentally ill persons in the community have increased substantially. Similarly, the oldest-old population, the age segment at highest risk of dementia and incapacity, is growing more rapidly than any other subgroup, which places large burdens on long-term care assistance. In the absence of a coherent long-term care policy, Medicaid is by default the nation's long-term care program, and the elderly in nursing homes account for almost half of total Medicaid expenditures. The growing burden of disability, combined with the government's unwillingness to tackle these issues in fear of the potential cost, contributes to the chaos characterizing these policy areas.

The problems of severe mental illness are compounded by the increasingly prevalent pattern of drug and alcohol abuse, which presents a challenge for conventional mental health services. Patients with dual diagnoses are an increasing proportion of the psychiatric caseload; however, these patients are particularly difficult, and many facilities and programs refuse to treat them. At a broader level, drug abuse and the AIDS epidemic are overloading already strained crisis facilities in some of the nation's largest cities.

One serious consequence of these trends is the growing gap between private and public mental health services. The more affluent employed population has attained increased mental health insurance coverage, provided fully or partially by employers (2). This expansion in recent decades has encouraged the growth of private psychiatric hospitals and clinics and fee-for-service personnel from a variety of professional groups. Similarly, the availability of insurance has motivated nonprofit hospitals to develop specialized psychiatric units and expand their mental health services. In contrast, constrained public budgets, the enlargement of the uninsured population to 35–40 million persons, and the decreased willingness of the nongovernmental sector to provide indigent care have put extraordinary pressures on public institutions (21). Long-term, chronically ill patients typically become indigent and reliant on the public sector; however, this sector is underfinanced, fragmented, disorganized, and incapable of responding to the magnitude of need.

As the states have come to play a larger role in financing CMHCs, these centers now more commonly treat the seriously ill and long-term chronic patients. But, as these centers face budgetary difficulties, they substitute other, lower paid professionals for psychiatrists and use the latter in more restrictive roles, such as approving medication. The numbers of psychiatrists employed in CMHCs has diminished, and psychiatric responsibility for patient care has eroded substantially in many localities (5). It is ironic that even as the community centers have begun to deal with the more seriously disabled, in cases often involving complicated medical co-morbidity, they have had to cut back on the professional staff and other resources needed to treat those very patients.

DIRECTIONS IN MENTAL HEALTH SERVICES RESEARCH

With impressive developments in molecular biology, the neurosciences, and imaging technology, psychiatry has moved toward a more biological and medical emphasis. Although these fields hold great promise, efforts must proceed in a balanced way to provide high quality management for those currently ill while seeking more powerful technologies for the future. The history of mental health care attests to how endorsement of organic viewpoints and the professionalization of psychiatry, when it had little specific to offer in any immediate terms, undermined constructive and humane efforts for patient management and rehabilitation (7). Hopefully, we will retain a broad perspective in the management of illness concomitant with the pursuit of increased biological understanding.

As psychiatry has moved away from psychoanalytic formulations, which treat diagnosis as a subsidiary task, it has focused attention on more careful classification and differential diagnosis, which contribute to clearer communication and more specific treatments. The DSM-III, despite lacking a theoretical basis and depending on an arbitrary system of classification, has improved the overall clarity and uniformity of psychiatric practice and research design. The diagnostic awareness required in using DSM-III will continue to bring improved research and practice. Like many tools, however, it can be abused when insurers, attorneys, and others treat its arbitrary classifications as realities.

There has been an impressive movement in psychiatry away from simple unicausal theories to complex conceptions of multiple causality at all levels of research. As Kety puts it in a discussion of brain processes, ". . . we now regard the synapses of the brain as constituting a great orchestra which creates its changing moods by an interplay between the strings, woodwinds, and brasses rather than by a sequence of solo voices" (15). Virtually everyone now regards the etiology of schizophrenia as unknown, a consequence of complex but inadequately understood interactions between genetic predisposition, brain processes, and psychosocial events. Much of the dogma of earlier periods that interfered with necessary inquiry has been replaced by sophisticated conceptions of etiology and course, which demonstrate awareness of our limited knowledge.

Longitudinal studies of schizophrenia, completed in different countries, have demonstrated that the perception of the condition as one with a course of continuing deterioration and a pessimistic future is exaggerated (10). Long-term studies demonstrate a variety of outcomes with many patients either having a single episode or returning to a reasonable level of function after several episodes. Shepherd (32), for example, in one five-year follow-up, classifies patients into four groups: one episode with no impairment (13%); several episodes with little or no impairment (30%); impairment following the first episode associated with occasional exacerbations of symptoms or failure to return to normality (10%); and impairment increasing with each episode (47%). Other studies show improvements in function after as many as 30 to 40 years of illness and disability (1).

It is not clear why clinicians have commonly perceived schizophrenia as a hopeless condition. One hypothesis is that they are influenced less by the epidemiological picture than by the subset of schizophrenic patients who are treatment failures. These patients return to clinical care repeatedly over the years and show successive increments of deterioration. They are the basis for the exaggerated pessimism that forms much of professional opinion.

Some clinicians dismiss the recurrent observations on the more favorable course of the condition by maintaining that patients who have a single episode are not schizophrenic. In some centers, a diagnosis is not made until there are repeated episodes, which results in a classification system that makes an unfavorable prognosis a criterion for diagnosis. The sampling and classification issues are central to understanding prognosis, but a World Health Organization (WHO) collaborative study (39) suggests that the results of recent longitudinal studies cannot be explained simply on this basis.

In the late 1960s, the WHO, using a standardized diagnostic approach, carried out a collaborative study of 1202 schizophrenia patients in nine countries (39). One of the remarkable findings was a less favorable prognosis in developed as compared with developing nations. Some observers explained these differences in terms of family and social networks, labeling processes, and processes of inclusion and exclusion of the disabled; others were more skeptical and argued that patients from varying nations were not comparable. Thus, in a second study (30), efforts were made to obtain representative samples of new schizophrenic patients in ten countries. Sartorius et al monitored defined populations over a two-year period to identify first contact with a helping agency because of psychotic symptoms, and they carefully identified patients in different cultures by the same criteria. Subsequent analysis showed that the symptom profiles of schizophrenic patients in varying samples were similar. Again, the investigators found that the two-year pattern of schizophrenia was more favorable in developing countries. In such countries, 56% of schizophrenic patients had a mild course over the two-year period, whereas only 39% in the developed nations had comparable outcomes. The reasons for this remain highly speculative.

For those involved with community care for chronic schizophrenic patients, these results are not particularly surprising. Many of the disabilities associated with long-term illness can be contained by good community management. In a recent review, Kiesler & Sibulkin (16) identify 14 experimental studies, most with random assignment, that compare community care with hospital treatment. They find such alternatives to be more effective than hospitalization across a wide range of patient populations and treatment strategies. Perhaps best known of these alternatives is Stein & Test's "Training in Community Living" model, which combines aggressive psychiatric community care with case-management and psychosocial skills training (34). In the 1970s, this model was demonstrated to be highly effective in Dane County, Wisconsin, the location of the major state university.

Although replicated either totally or partially in a variety of communities, skepticism persisted as to whether the Dane County model could be translated to larger, more complex urban communities. In 1979–1981, the model was replicated in a randomized experimental trial in Sydney, Australia, with comparably good results (28). Particularly significant was that the approach was highly successful and favored by patients and their families over hospital care, despite the patients being maintained with a much lower level of staff intensity than in Dane County. The optimal and most cost-effective level of staffing for such programs is still uncertain. It is likely to depend on the array of community resources already in place, the mix of patients, and the complexity of the community.

Many of the newly developed community care programs have been pragmatic and oriented to patients' basic needs for medical and psychiatric care, subsistence and housing, basic living skills, and social support. Much more emphasis is given to working with other patient caretakers, by teaching them about mental illness and helping them cope with its uncertainties and burdens. From a theoretical perspective, the work on expressed emotion in families has helped focus some of the most impressive community care trials and has provided a more useful basis for working with families than unstructured therapies have had in the past (18).

Given the success of some community programs, why have they not diffused more widely over the past decade? The structure of financing and the lack of incentives are most commonly cited and are certainly of importance.

"Training in Community Living" has prospered in part because mental health financing in Wisconsin allows local programs to use savings from reduced hospital admissions to support their base. The state system of financing allows dollars to "follow the patient" and gives local program personnel the opportunity to balance community care against hospital care (33). That most counties in Wisconsin, despite its financing system and unique history of county mental health services, lack the programs so highly regarded in Dane County suggests that financing incentives are only a part of a more complex constellation. If providing counties with the funds and authority for decision-making is so crucial, why is the California system in such major disarray? In 1985, Wisconsin expended less per capita on its mental health agencies than the US average and only ranked in the middle among states (27); yet it seems to have maintained a reasonably high standard of care.

Financing provides the framework, but the success of community care also depends on professional leadership, interagency communication and cooperation, and a supportive community environment. There are no substantial professional rewards for community care efforts, and managing the care of schizophrenic patients brings neither high income nor prestige among one's colleagues. In addition, there is great potential for blame when patients get into trouble. For many professionals, resistance and inertia is a comfortable stance. Few professional schools, whether of psychology, social work, or nursing, specifically train students to work with the chronically ill; thus, special burdens are placed on innovative programs for on-the-job training. An advantage of the longevity of the Dane County program is its accessibility to mental health professional students who learn to feel comfortable with this model of care. Over time, the effective institutionalization of community care depends on its effective integration with professional training and recruitment.

THE CHANGING LEGAL CONTEXT OF MENTAL HEALTH CARE

Since the late 1960s public interest lawyers socialized in the civil rights movement directed their energies to the mental health arena, particularly to civil commitment procedures. Efforts were also made on many other fronts, such as "right to treatment" and "right to refuse treatment." Mental health lawyers had great expectations about the potentials of legal reform. In retrospect, despite significant gains in extending mental patients' rights and protections, the hope that litigation could fundamentally shape the system of community services seems naive. By directing attention to particular deficiencies, legal advocates could induce service improvement, but often at the cost of neglecting other problems or discharging patients from the protection of service systems. The strategy behind much of the litigation was premised on the use of coercive powers by the state; thus, the remedies did not apply to those in noncoercive settings. More recently, legal efforts have been made in some jurisdictions to require government to provide an acceptable minimum of care, but the degree to which courts can direct state allocation of funds among competing priorities remains unclear.

Despite the attention given to civil commitment, great dissatisfaction and divisiveness remain. To many mental health professionals, the law has gone too far in protecting the freedoms of persons at high risk who are incapable of making reasonable judgments about their needs. Others, however, resist any erosion of hard-won liberty interests. There is great heat but not much useful dialogue between these two groups.

Although much acrimony is focused on commitment procedures, the key issue is the integrity and responsiveness of community care services. Many states are now experimenting with outpatient commitment, a less restrictive intervention than traditional civil commitment. Such commitments provide a mechanism to deal with the persistent failure to maintain essential drug treatment and the subsequent relapse within a less restrictive approach than coercive hospitalization. Studies in North Carolina indicate that the success of outpatient commitment depends on the responsiveness of the community mental health services system and the willingness to cooperate with the courts (12). When the services system and the courts work together, outpatient commitment appears to manage many troublesome problems. There is disillusionment and frustration with commitment statutes. It is increasingly difficult to provide treatment to uncooperative and psychotic patients who are not imminently dangerous. These problems and the increasing demands for more extensive involuntary hospitalization make exploration of such mechanisms as outpatient commitment particularly prudent (3).

THE RESEARCH ARENA

While research in mental health focuses on biology and the neurosciences, the desperate need for deeper knowledge of population, organizational, and behavioral factors and the functioning of mental health services systems continues. Research in the brain sciences is more dramatic, but we have made some significant gains in these other research areas, as well. In the past ten years, we have learned a great deal about the successful application of methods of behavior control and ways to manage illness to reduce disability. We have also seen advances in epidemiology and health services research, as the following examples illustrate.

Fifteen years ago, psychiatric epidemiology was in the doldrums. A large gap existed between psychiatric conditions as measured in community epidemiological studies and clinical psychiatric practice. With the development of the Diagnostic Interview Survey (DIS) based on DSM-III criteria, the gap was substantially closed, and the Epidemiological Catchment Area Program gave new vitality to epidemiological questions (4). Although many questions remain about the validity and applicability of the DIS to clinical efforts, it is a flexible instrument, allowing a wide range of investigatory approaches, that helps explore a broad range of substantive and methodological concerns.

With the encouragement of the NIMH, mental health services research has also advanced with increasing sophistication in organization and financing (35a). Some of the experimental work on models of care for the severely ill and on expressed emotion have already been noted, but such work as the RAND Health Insurance Experiment (HIE) also merits special attention. This controlled trial randomized 6970 respondents into insurance plans with varying coinsurance requirements, including one setting at Group Health Insurance in Seattle, a health maintenance organization (HMO) (29). This experiment has been a fund of information for health services research in general. It has also substantially contributed to our understanding of how insurance and health care organization affect the provision of mental health services. A few findings will be illustrative.

Cost-sharing has important effects on the use of general ambulatory care, but even larger effects on mental health services. In the HIE there was a fourfold variation between extreme coinsurance groups. Those with 50% coinsurance and no limits on cost-sharing spent two fifths as much as those who were not required to share costs (14). Coinsurance primarily affected the number of episodes of treatment, but once a person entered care the duration and intensity varied less.

The experiment made it possible to study how patients randomized to prepaid care used services differently than those in plans with no coinsurance, an equivalent group in terms of out-of-pocket expenditure risk. Prepaid enrollees actually used more mental health services, but they were provided much less intensively. Patients with prepaid insurance were more likely to receive services from a general medical provider, and overall mental health expenditures were only one third that of the comparable group with no coinsurance. When prepaid enrollees saw a mental health provider, they had only one third the number of mental health visits as patients in the general fee-for-service sector. The HMO relied more on social workers than on psychiatrists or psychologists and less on individual than on group or family therapies (19, 20).

Most patients who receive formal care for psychiatric disorders are managed exclusively by general physicians, typically within the context of overall medical care (31). The most severely and persistently mentally ill eventually enter specialty care, but a large proportion of patients with all diagnoses do not. These patients commonly receive no treatment at all (17). Affective disorders are most prevalent, but at least half are probably not recognized in general medical practice (37). Such conditions, however, are extremely distressing and disabling. The Medical Outcomes Study, involving more than 11,000 patients in varying outpatient settings, found that patients with a diagnosis of clinical depression, or depressive symptoms short of a clinical diagnosis, were equally or more disabled than patients with such major chronic conditions as gastrointestinal problems, diabetes, back problems, and angina. Only the patients with advanced coronary artery disease were more disabled. Depressed patients had the worst social and role functioning and had more days in bed than any group except the coronary artery disease group (38).

THE IMPORTANCE OF MENTAL HEALTH ADVOCACY

Mental health care has been transformed substantially in recent decades, and the availability and acceptability of services have grown. But with constraints on public funding, the gap has widened between insured persons and the uninsured or underinsured groups, which include the majority of long-term patients with persistent disabilities. In some sense, those who were traditional clients of public institutions may be worse off than ever before. They lost the refuge of the mental hospital, but are also excluded from the richness of community service options that have been developed for the insured.

The process of defining health needs is largely political, a product of interest group activity. The ability to draw attention to need, and evoke sympathy for patients and their families, depends substantially on the mobilization and skill of advocacy groups. Traditionally, mental health advocacy has been weak for a variety of reasons. With mental health almost exclusively a public responsibility of the individual states, it has been difficult to form a strong national constituency. Moreover, the severely mentally ill have neither the personal resources nor the credibility to compete successfully with other disease constituencies. Their families often avoid public identification because of stigma, which limits vigorous public participation. Although powerful advocates occasionally came forward, as in the case of Dorothea Dix, Clifford Beers, and Mike Gorman, and later those associated with the growing mental health professions and the establishment of the NIMH, there has never been the kind of sustained advocacy characteristic of other health lobbies.

Mental health advocacy has also been crippled by bitter contentiousness. Advocates are highly fragmented and encourage competing and conflicting agendas: the severely mentally ill versus mental health education and prevention; children versus adults; mental illness versus developmental disabilities; civil liberties versus tougher commitment laws; community care versus revitalizing public hospitals; social work versus psychology; psychology versus psychiatry; biological psychiatry versus social psychiatry; drugs versus psychotherapy, and so on. Many of the controversies are important and relate to core issues of care, but the internal bickering among consumers and professionals has diminished effective advocacy. As a consequence, the sector has great difficulty setting priorities as evidenced by the products of the Carter Presidential Commission, the controversies over the Mental Health Systems Act, and the failures to understand the importance of mental health categorical issues relative to larger health policy issues that affect the mentally ill. Mental health advocates have too frequently misdirected their main efforts. They confuse symbolic issues with the health policy initiatives that shape the mental health sector.

More forceful advocacy, which holds real promise for elevating mental health interests, has recently emerged. The establishment and rapid growth of the National Alliance for the Mentally Ill has mobilized a large and potentially effective lobby at the local, state, and federal levels (11). The challenge facing the Alliance, which incorporates conflicting viewpoints, is to develop its data acquisition, policy strategies, and political skills and more astutely bring competing perspectives together. Through the Alliance and other groups, former mental patients and their families now come forward publicly to address relevant issues. Such participation by visible and influential figures is increasingly common. Increased influence could come by orchestrating these efforts relative to the media and the policy formulation process.

Efforts are also now being made to develop coalitions among competing mental health interests. A visible coalition has not emerged at the national level, but local advocacy groups representing consumers, professional groups, and mental health organizations are beginning to appreciate the value of a united front. An agenda that satisfies diverse organizations is not easy to build, but it is essential if the sector is to have equal access to the policy process.

CONCLUSION

Compared with previous decades, the past decade has been characterized by less rhetoric. We have seen greater appreciation of the tough realities of providing effective community care to seriously mentally ill persons. We understand better the complexities of finance and organization of service arrangements and their interconnections with housing, welfare, and medical and legal arrangements. Research technologies have advanced significantly, which promises major potential for the future. The nation has a vast pool of mental health professionals and facilities that can form the basis of a highly effective mental health care system. Mental health advocacy is also more sophisticated and active than ever before.

Despite these gains, all is not well in mental health services. The promises of deinstitutionalization are largely unfulfilled, and the neglected condition of many seriously mentally ill persons in the community has contributed to a bitter backlash. The public sector and public welfare, on which many of these patients depend, have suffered significant erosion, and public sector delivery systems are in considerable disarray. Problems are exacerbated by the increased population of seriously mentally ill, a consequence of the changing demography of the American population. Moreover, the federal deficit and the pressures on public budgets make it particularly difficult to attract significant new public monies for services.

Although public mental health services are significantly underfunded, present resources are substantial. These resources could be used more effectively by correcting the fragmentation, duplication, and disorganization of the services system and establishing clear priorities focused on the seriously and persistently mentally ill (13a, 35). Building an integrated system requires new financing and organizational strategies, such as continuous team case-management arrangements, the development of strong local mental health authorities, and mental health HMOs organized around capitation arrangements (24–26).

The crisis in mental health care is substantially affected by the lack of insurance and the erosion of welfare for the most seriously and persistently mentally ill, and many of these patients cannot get the necessary services. They are homeless, in part, because of the dearth of housing programs in the 1980s and the loss of low income housing stock. Any long-term solution will be a product of health and welfare policy and some reasonable response to the large un- or underinsured population. It is a sad commentary that a nation that spends more than a half trillion dollars on health each year and has such rich resources of manpower and facilities cannot do better for its most needy and disadvantaged citizens.

Literature Cited

1. Bleuler, M. 1978. *The Schizophrenic Disorders: Long-Term Patient and Family Studies*. Transl. S. M. Clemens. New Haven: Yale Univ. Press
2. Brady, J., Sharfstein, S. S., Muszynski, I. L. Jr. 1986. Trends in private insurance coverage for mental illness. *Am. J. Psychiatry* 143:1276–79
3. Brooks, A. D. 1987. Outpatient commitment for the chronic mentally ill: Law and policy. See Ref. 23a, pp. 117–28
4. Eaton, W. W., Kessler, L. G., eds. 1985. *Epidemiologic Field Methods in Psychiatry: The NIMH Epidemiologic Catchment Area Program*. Orlando, Fla: Academic
5. Faulkner, L. R., Bloom, J. D., Bray, J. D., Maricle, R. 1986. Medical services in community mental health programs. *Hosp. Community Psychiatry* 37:1045–47
6. Foley, H. A., Sharfstein, S. 1983. *Madness and Government: Who Cares for*

the Mentally Ill? Washington, DC: Am. Psychiatr. Press

7. Grob, G. N. 1966. *The State and the Mentally Ill: A History of Worcester State Hospital in Massachusetts, 1830–1920.* Chapel Hill: Univ. North Carolina Press

8. Grob, G. N. 1987. Mental health policy in post World War II America. See Ref. 23a, pp. 15–32

9. Gronfein, W. 1985. Incentives and intentions in mental health policy: A comparison of the medicaid and community mental health programs. *J. Health Soc. Behav.* 26:192–206

10. Harding, C. M., Zubin, J., Strauss, J. S. 1987. Chronicity in schizophrenia: Fact, partial facts or artifact? *Hosp. Community Psychiatry* 38:477–86

11. Hatfield, A., ed. 1987. *Families of the Mentally Ill: Meeting the Challenges.* New Dir. Ment. Health Serv. No. 34. San Francisco: Jossey-Bass

12. Hiday, V., Scheid-Cook, T. 1986. *The North Carolina experience with outpatient commitment: a critical appraisal.* Presented at Int. Congr. Law Psychiatry, Montreal

13. Inst. Medicine. 1988. *Homelessness, Health and Human Needs.* Washington, DC: Natl. Acad. Press

13a. Johnson, A. B. 1990. *Out of Bedlam: The Truth About Deinstitutionalization.* New York: Basic Books

14. Keeler, E. B., Wells, K. B., Manning, W. G., Rumpel, J. D., Hanley, J. M. 1986. *The Demand for Episodes of Mental Health Services* (R-3432-NIMH). Santa Monica, Calif: RAND Corp.

15. Kety, S. 1986. The interface between neuroscience and psychiatry. In *Psychiatry and Its Related Disciplines,* ed. R. Rosenberg, F. Schulsinger, E. Strömgren, p. 23. Cophenhagen: World Psychiatr. Assoc.

16. Kiesler, C. A., Sibulkin, A. E. 1987. *Mental Hospitalization: Myths and Facts About a National Crisis.* Newbury Park, Calif: Sage

17. Leaf, P. J., Livingston, M. M., Tischler, G. L., Weissman, M. M., Holzer, C. E., Myers, J. K. 1985. Contact with health professionals for the treatment of psychiatric and emotional problems. *Med. Care* 23:1302–37

18. Leff, J., Vaughn, C. 1985. *Expressed Emotion in Families.* New York: Guilford

19. Manning, W. G., Wells, K. B. 1986. Preliminary results of a controlled trial of the effect of a prepaid group practice on the outpatient use of mental health services. *J. Hum. Resour.* 21:293–320

20. Manning, W. G., Wells, K. B., Benjamin, B. 1986. *Use of Outpatient Mental Health Care: Trial of a Prepaid Group Practice Versus Fee-For-Service* (R-3277-NIMH). Santa Monica, Calif: RAND Corp.

21. Mechanic, D. 1986. *From Advocacy to Allocation: The Evolving American Health Care System.* New York: Free Press

22. Mechanic, D. 1987. Correcting misconceptions in mental health policy: Strategies for improved care of the seriously mentally ill. *Milbank Fund Q.* 65:203–30

23. Mechanic, D. 1989. *Mental Health and Social Policy.* Englewood Cliffs, NJ: Prentice-Hall. 3rd ed.

23a. Mechanic, D., ed. 1987. *Improving Mental Health Services: What the Social Sciences Can Tell Us.* New Dir. Ment. Health Serv. No. 36 (Winter): 117–28. San Francisco: Jossey-Bass

24. Mechanic, D., Aiken, L. 1987. Improving the care of patients with chronic mental illness. *N. Engl. J. Med.* 317:1634–38

25. Mechanic, D., Aiken, L., eds. 1989. *Paying for Services: Promises and Pitfalls of Capitation.* New Directions Ser. 43. San Francisco: Jossey-Bass

26. Mechanic, D., Rochefort, D. A. 1990. Deinstitutionalization: An appraisal of reform. *Annu. Rev. Sociol.* 16:301–27

27. Natl. Inst. Mental Health. 1987. *Mental Health, United States, 1987,* ed. R. W. Manderscheid, S. A. Barrett. DHHS Publ. No. (ADM) 87-1518. Washington, DC: GPO

28. New South Wales, Dep. Health. 1983. *Psychiatric Hospital Versus Community Treatment: A Controlled Study.* (HSR 83-046), Sydney, Australia

29. Newhouse, J. 1974. A design for a health insurance experiment. *Inquiry* 11:5–27

30. Sartorius, N., Jablensky, A., Korten, A., Ernberg, A., Anker, M., et al. 1986. Early manifestations and first-contact incidence of schizophrenia in different cultures. *Psychol. Med.* 16:909–28

31. Shapiro, S., Skinner, E. A., Kramer, M., Steinwachs, D. M., Regier, D. A. 1985. Measuring need for mental health services in a general population. *Med. Care* 23:1033–43

32. Shepherd, M. 1987. Formulation of new research strategies on schizophrenia. In *Search for the Causes of Schizophrenia,* ed. H. Hafner, W. F. Gattaz, W. Janzarik, pp. 29–38. Berlin: Springer-Verlag

33. Stein, L. I., Ganser, L. J. 1983. Wisconsin system for funding mental health services. In *New Directions for Mental Health Services: Unified Mental Health System,* ed. J. Talbott, pp. 25–32. San Francisco: Jossey-Bass

34. Stein, L. I., Test, M. A., eds. 1985. *The Training in Community Living Model: A Decade of Experience.* New Dir. Ment. Health Serv. No. 26. San Francisco: Jossey-Bass

35. Torrey, E. F. 1988. *Nowhere to Go: The Tragic Odyssey of the Homeless Mentally Ill.* New York: Harper & Row

35a. Taube, C. A., Mechanic, D., Hohmann, A. A., eds. 1989. *The Future of Mental Health Services Research.* DHHS Publ. No. (ADM) 89-1600. Washington, DC: US Print. Off.

36. US DHHS. 1980. *Toward a National Plan for the Chronically Mentally Ill, Report to the Secretary—1980.* Publ. No. ADM 81-1077. Rockville, Md: DHHS

37. Wells, K. B. 1985. Depression as a tracer condition for the national study of medical care outcomes: Background review. *3293-RWJ-HJK RAND Corp.* Santa Monica, Calif: RAND Corp.

38. Wells, K. B., Stewart, A., Hays, R. D., Burnam, M. A., Rogers, W., et al. 1989. The functioning and well-being of depressed patients: Results from the medical outcomes study. *J. Am. Med. Assoc.* 262:914–19

39. WHO. 1979. *Schizophrenia: An International Follow-up Study.* Geneva, NY: Wiley

Annu. Rev. Puble. Health 1991. 12:17–40

THE EPIDEMIOLOGIC BASIS FOR THE PREVENTION OF FIREARM INJURIES[1]

Arthur L. Kellermann

Division of Emergency Medicine, Department of Medicine, University of Tennessee, Memphis, Tennessee 38103

Roberta K. Lee

University of Texas School of Nursing, University of Texas Medical Branch, Galveston, Texas 77550

James A. Mercy

Division of Injury Control, Center for Environmental Health and Injury Control, Centers for Disease Control. Public Health Service, US Department of Health and Human Services, Atlanta, Georgia 30333

Joyce Banton

Division of Emergency Medicine, Department of Medicine, University of Tennessee, Memphis, Tennessee 38103

KEY WORDS: suicide, homicide, injury prevention, accidental death

---

INTRODUCTION

In the United States, more than 1 million people died because of firearm injuries (72, 78) between 1933 and 1987. In 1986, firearms were second only to motor vehicles as a cause of fatal injury and ranked seventh among all

---

[1]The views expressed are those of the authors and do not necessarily reflect those of the University of Tennessee, the University of Texas, or the Centers for Disease Control. The US Government has the right to retain a nonexclusive, royalty-free license in and to any copyright covering this paper.

causes of death (28). During 1986 and 1987, the last two years for which data are available, the number of people who died from firearm injuries in the United States (50, 72) was greater than the number of casualties during the entire 8½-year Vietnam conflict. In a recent report on the cost of injury in the United States (57), investigators estimated that firearm injuries imposed a $14.4 billion economic burden in 1985. These statistics highlight the magnitude of what is one of the most serious public health problems facing the United States. Unfortunately, it is also one that has not yet received sufficient scientific attention.

Firearm injuries result from three general circumstances: interpersonal conflicts, suicidal behavior, and unintentional discharge of weapons. Traditionally, these types of firearm injury have been addressed separately. Criminal firearm injuries and gunshot injuries due to interpersonal violence are largely considered a "crime" problem; firearm suicides are considered a "mental health" problem. Unintentional firearm injuries, however, have long been dismissed as "accidents," which creates the impression that these are random events resulting from misfortune or fate and are, therefore, not preventable. Fortunately, the 1985 report *Injury in America* (21) stimulated broad interest in viewing injuries, including firearm injuries, from a public health perspective.

In this article we summarize the epidemiology of firearm injuries and describe the magnitude of firearm injury as a public health problem in the United States. We also review the public health approach towards understanding the etiology of firearm injury and use this approach to suggest strategies for prevention. Finally, we identify a research agenda for establishing a scientific basis for prevention. The key to this approach is to view these injuries, regardless of their medicolegal circumstances, as having one common factor—the discharge of a firearm.

THE CONCEPT OF INJURY CONTROL

At the beginning of the 19th century, we were largely ignorant of the physical, chemical, and biological hazards in our environment. Disease, injury, and death were regarded as matters of fate or divine intervention. Since then, we have made great progress in our understanding and control of infectious and chronic diseases. Only recently, however, have we begun to explore and define the physical and chemical hazards that kill or injure hundreds of thousands of Americans each year (79). Injuries cause the loss of more working years of life than heart disease and cancer combined (21).

Injuries result from the transfer of energy to humans in amounts that exceed the body's ability to tolerate such transfers without damage. This excess energy (in epidemiologic terms, the *agent* of injury), is most often mechani-

Table 1 Public health models of pathogenesis

	Disease model	Injury model
Agent	Microbe, toxin, or carcinogen	Energy (mechanical, thermal, or chemical)
Host	Human (patient)	Human (victim)
Vehicles	Poisoned or contaminated water, air, or food	Firearms, power lines, motor vehicles
Vectors	Mosquitoes, ticks, snails	Guard dogs, hornets, poisonous plants
Environment	Natural	Physical/societal

cal; it can also be thermal, electrical, or chemical (34, 35). For injury to occur, this excess energy must be conveyed to the victim (the *host*) through inanimate objects or living organisms (Table 1). Moving objects, such as bullets, speeding cars, or falling rocks, are *vehicles* of injury. Injuries can also be caused by stationary vehicles, such as electric power lines or hot irons. Living organisms, such as poisonous plants or animals that sting, bite, or kick, are *vectors* of injury. These agents, hosts, vehicles, and vectors interact in a given physical or social *environment*, the nature of which can independently affect the probability or severity of a given injury event (35).

By viewing injuries as the result of a complex dynamic, we can analyze their occurrence etiologically and formulate strategies for their prevention (35, 75). This injury control model was conceived as a conceptual framework to identify ways to prevent or limit the severity of unintentional injuries. If we include an additional dimension—the assailant—the model can be applied to intentional injuries, as well. By subdividing injury events into a temporal sequence of three phases (pre-event, event, and post-event), we can identify and specifically target different aspects of the injury dynamic for intervention (Table 2).

The most cost-effective way to control a disease is usually to prevent its occurrence. Experience with other public health interventions has shown that prevention is best accomplished by first identifying, then breaking, the chain of disease causation at its weakest link. This weak link may not always be obvious or proximate to the illness or injury.

Safety programs, such as firearm education, focus on modifying human behavior in the pre-event phase. However, educational interventions of this sort are often expensive and rarely result in lasting behavioral change. Some educational interventions, as Robertson has noted, may actually increase the probability of injury (58). In general, measures that modify the potential vehicle of injury or the environment in which the injury occurs have proven

Table 2 Injury control schematic: Illustrative approaches to the prevention and control of injuries

Injury factors	Pre-events	Events	Post-events
		Injury event phases	
Host	Drivers education Alcohol and drug avoidance	Fire retardant clothing Protective eye wear Child restraints	Citizen first-aid training Specialized trauma care Trained emergency medical technicians
Vehicle	Safe motor vehicle design Childproof drug packaging Self-extinguishing cigarettes	Soft playground surfaces Reset water heater thermostats down- ward	911 emergency number Special equipment for emergency medical service providers
Environment	Divided highways Pedestrian overpasses	Lower speed limits Mandatory helmet laws	Trauma centers Helicopter transport Rehabilitation centers
Assailant[a]	Anger management training Emergency psychiatric commitment	Case worker visits to detect ongoing child abuse Police intervention	Incarceration Post-event counseling of offenders

[a] Dimension relevant only to the control of intentional injuries. In the case of suicide or self-inflicted injuries, assailant and victim are same.

more successful. More crash-protective automobiles, lower speed limits, and improved engineering of highways, bridge abutments, and road surfaces have had a far greater impact on our rate of traffic-related deaths than driver education classes have had (76). Passive countermeasures, which exert their beneficial effect without the need for any specific human action or cooperation, are usually much more effective than active measures, which require cooperation to be effective. For example, air bags and automatic seat belts almost always exert their protective effects. Manual seat belts, however, can only work if the occupants of the car buckle them. In states lacking a mandatory seat belt law, 80% of occupants do not buckle up (76).

Building on the injury control model, Haddon devised ten generic strategies to prevent or control the rate and severity of injuries by breaking the chain of injury causation at various points (34). Although Haddon proposed these countermeasures as ways to prevent unintentional injuries, all have value as potential strategies for the prevention of firearm deaths and injuries, as well. Successful implementation of measures to prevent firearm deaths depends, however, on a clear understanding of the epidemiology of firearm injuries, the evidence linking firearm injuries to gun availability, the biomechanics of gunshot wounds, and relevant aspects of emergency and rehabilitative services.

EPIDEMIOLOGY OF FIREARM INJURIES

Surveillance

The National Center for Health Statistics collects death certificates from the 50 states and Washington, DC. This data base includes International Classification of Disease (ICD9) external cause of death codes (ICD9-E-codes), which permit analysis of mortality according to the cause (72), and provides relatively complete information regarding age, race, sex, and medicolegal classification of the incident (Table 3). However, these records are too incomplete to reliably determine the person's occupation, whether the injury occurred at work or home, and the type of firearm involved (rifle, shotgun, handgun, or other weapon). Most local police departments file reports on all incidents involving a firearm injury, but these are often difficult to retrieve. Data from the National Crime Survey (70) can be used to estimate the number of crimes committed with a firearm. However, these data provide little information about the incidence of serious but nonfatal firearm injuries. The most recent data of any sort regarding nonfatal cases were collected in 1972 for the National Health Interview Survey (73). That survey suggests that the ratio of fatal to nonfatal firearm injuries is 1:5. The collection of reliable national data regarding nonfatal firearm injury is essential to characterize these injuries. Recently, Sniezek et al (65) suggested adding E-codes to the

Table 3 United States firearm deaths and rates per 100,000 by age and medicolegal classification, 1987 (69, 72)

Age	Homicide		Suicide		Unintentional		Total firearm	
	No.	Rate	No.	Rate	No.	Rate	No.	Rate
0–4	49	0.3	0	0.0	37	0.2	85	0.5
5–9	55	0.3	1	0.0	66	0.4	126	0.7
10–14	173	1.1	151	0.9	144	0.9	485	2.9
15–19	1,298	7.0	1,129	6.1	220	1.2	2,720	14.7
20–24	2,452	12.4	1,795	9.1	213	1.1	4,561	23.0
25–29	2,327	10.6	1,900	8.6	160	0.7	4,504	20.5
30–34	1,867	8.8	1,729	8.1	131	0.6	3,822	17.9
35–39	1,439	7.7	1,494	8.0	102	0.5	3,108	16.6
40–44	887	5.7	1,245	8.0	70	0.5	2,233	14.3
45–49	609	4.9	1,085	8.8	57	0.5	1,780	14.4
50–54	417	3.8	1,032	9.5	51	0.5	1,519	13.9
55–59	341	3.1	1,131	10.2	48	0.4	1,542	13.9
60–64	243	2.2	1,151	10.6	45	0.4	1,463	13.5
65–69	194	2.0	1,177	11.9	22	0.2	1,406	14.2
70–74	116	1.5	1,148	14.8	28	0.4	1,302	16.7
75–79	78	1.4	1,003	17.4	25	0.4	1,113	19.3
80–84	59	1.7	612	17.4	12	0.3	691	19.7
85+	31	1.1	354	12.4	8	0.3	397	13.9
Total	**12,635**	**5.2**	**18,139**	**7.5**	**1,440**	**0.6**	**32,895**	**13.5**

National Hospital Discharge Survey data. Although this would improve our understanding of the epidemiology of severe firearm injuries, these data would not include people treated in emergency departments and released.

Overall Incidence of Firearm Mortality

In 1987, firearms accounted for 61% of homicides, 59% of suicides, and less than 2% of unintentional injury deaths (72). Males experience a rate of firearm mortality more than five times that of females. White males commit suicide with firearms at roughly twice the rate of black males, but black males are murdered by a firearm at roughly seven times the rate of white males. The cumulative incidence rate for black men is 5%, which suggests that firearm injuries cause one in 20 deaths.

Although our understanding is far from complete, the evidence to date suggests that relatively few suicides and homicides occur spontaneously. Many assailants and victims of violent death have previously been involved in nonfatal violent episodes (60). The case for the repetitive nature of violent behavior is strengthened by evidence that people who were victimized as children, or who even witnessed family violence, are more likely than the general population to commit similar acts of violence later in life (77). According to the results of a recently completed cohort study (61), violent trauma is associated with a recurrence rate of 44% and a five-year mortality rate of 20%. Give the evidence that many homicide and suicide victims have been intentionally injured in the past or have been repeatedly exposed to violence, persons seeking treatment for intentional injuries should be considered at high risk for violent deaths and should receive follow-up care and attention (52).

Firearm Suicide

Each year, more than 29,000 deaths in the United States are classified as suicides, making suicide the nation's eighth leading cause of death and the fifth leading cause of years of potential life lost before age 65 (16). Whites commit suicide at rates almost twice as high as blacks, and males commit suicide at rates almost three times as high as females. Certain Native American tribes and Eskimos have the highest suicide rates of all, probably because of the effects of poverty, alcoholism, and social disruption. The highest suicide rates among males are in the oldest age group (65+ years), and the highest rates of suicide in females occur in midlife (age 45 to 54). For all race and sex groups, married persons have the lowest rates, followed by singles; divorced and widowed persons have the highest rates (16).

Since 1953, the number of suicides in the United States has increased by more than 44%. This increase has been due to a marked rise in the rate of suicide involving firearms (Figure 1). During this same time period, the rate of suicide in the US by other means actually decreased (5, 9). The largest rate of increase in firearm suicides recently has been among 15- to 24-year-olds; that rate has doubled since 1968 (16).

Classifying suicides by method is important because the method is highly related to the likelihood that a suicide attempt will end in death. For example, in the US self-inflicted lacerations account for 15% of all nonfatal suicide attempts but only 1% of all suicides (4). Although less than 12% of all suicides involve poisons or drugs, ingestions account for 70% of all nonfatal suicide attempts. With modern medical treatment, relatively few of these people die. Nonfatal, self-inflicted gunshot wounds, on the other hand, are relatively uncommon, but three fifths of all US suicides involve firearms (Figure 1).

Weapon characteristics may also affect the chances that a given firearm will be chosen for a suicide attempt. In a recent study conducted in Sacramento County, California, researchers found that handguns are used to commit suicide more than twice as often as shotguns and rifles combined. Ready availability in the home and the likelihood that the weapon is kept loaded for protection may explain this fact (80).

Although women attempt suicide two to three times more often than men, men actually kill themselves three times more often than women. Women usually choose less effective means of attempting suicide, such as drug overdose; men are much more apt to use a firearm. Female patterns of suicide

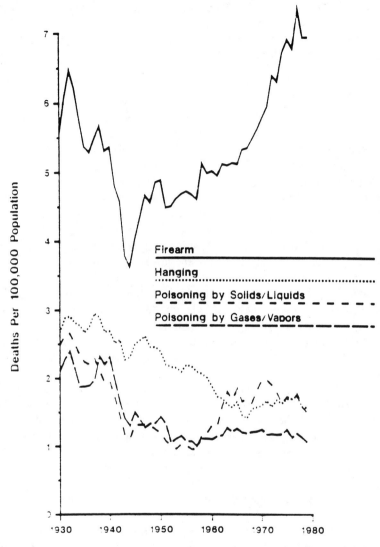

Figure 1   United States death rates from suicide by year and method, 1930–1979. Reprinted from Baker, S. P., O'Neill, B., Karpf, R. S. 1984. *The Injury Fact Book*. Lexington, Mass: Lexington Books, with permission of the author and publisher.

are changing, however. In response to the marketing of small handguns as effective protection for women, rates of gun ownership among women are increasing (39). Although the higher rates of gun ownership by women have not been shown to decrease rates of victimization, the proportion of female suicides involving guns has increased. In 1970, poisoning by solids or liquids was the suicide method most commonly used by women. Now, like men, women most often kill themselves with firearms (16).

Teen suicide has received increasing attention in recent years. Suicide is rare before age 15, but in the 15- to 34-year age groups, suicide is the third leading cause of death. The view that teen suicides are often impulsive is supported by reports of clusters of adolescent suicides (13). Given the apparently impulsive nature of teen suicide, the recent rise in the number of adolescents attempting suicide with firearms is particularly concerning, as guns provide little chance for salvage or rescue (16).

Firearm Homicide

Since 1900, the proportion of total mortality in the US attributable to homicide has increased twentyfold (51). Although this increase has been largely because of dramatic declines in rates of death from infectious diseases, the rates of deaths due to homicide have also risen sharply in absolute terms. In contrast to the gains we have made in public health, criminal justice agencies have long acknowledged that homicide and assault are societal problems over which law enforcement has little or no control (71).

According to both the Federal Bureau of Investigation (FBI) and the Centers for Disease Control (CDC), 85% to 90% of all homicide victims are killed by assailants of the same race (14, 68), i.e. whites kill whites, blacks kill blacks, and so forth. Because black men are more frequently murdered by firearms than white men, some might conclude from this observation that blacks are more likely to commit homicide. Evidence suggests, however, that most (if not all) of this difference can be explained on the basis of socioeconomic status not race (18, 46).

Between 1960 and 1980, the rate of homicide in the United States doubled (Figure 2). Homicides involving knives and other dangerous weapons increased by 60%, whereas homicides involving firearms have increased by 150% (4). As with suicide, the type of weapon employed substantially affects the probability that a given attack will end in death. Hospital statistics indicate that more people are injured by knives and other sharp instruments than by firearms, but gunshot wounds are more than five times more likely than knife wounds to result in death (74, 85, 87).

Although homicide has long been regarded as primarily a "crime" problem, fewer than 20% of homicides occur during the commission of another felony, such as robbery. In well over half of cases, the victim knows the assailant, and the homicide occurs during the course of an argument or some other nonfelonious circumstance (15, 71). In the United States, one of every six homicides involves members of the same family (51). Women are most often killed by their spouse or another family member, whereas men are most often killed by a friend or some other nonfamily acquaintance (66, 68, 71). Firearms are the weapon most commonly used to kill persons of either sex.

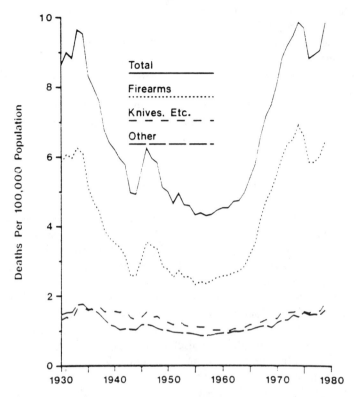

Figure 2   United States death rates from homicide by year and method, 1930–1979. Reprinted from Baker, S. P., O'Neill, B., Karpf, R. S. 1984. *The Injury Fact Book.* Lexington, Mass: Lexington Books, with permission of the author and publisher.

Drug and alcohol consumption are also associated with violent death. An increased willingness to take risks and a decreased ability to avoid harm are often a consequence of alcohol intoxication (12, 31). In a CDC sponsored study of homicides in Los Angeles, researchers found that more than half of victims killed during fights had been drinking (26). The explosive growth of illegal drugs in the United States has recently added yet another dimension to the homicide problem. In a 1981 study of 573 homicides in New York City, researchers found that approximately one third of male victims died in drug-related incidents (67). A majority of recent firearm homicides in Washington, DC, are suspected to be drug-related (55).

Unintentional Firearm Deaths

Although only 5% of firearm fatalities each year are considered unintentional, these incidents claim the lives of roughly 1400 people and disproportionately affect young males. In North Carolina (20), the firearm mortality rate associated with hunting was 0.6 per 100,000 population. No comparable data currently exist for the United States as a whole.

Most unintentional firearm deaths occur in or around the home and most involve handguns (56, 59, 81). Self-inflicted injuries are most often related to play, whereas injuries inflicted by someone else are associated with hunting or with play among small children (17). Although unintentional gunshot wounds cause a relatively small number of firearm deaths, they probably account for a much larger proportion of nonfatal, but potentially serious and disabling firearm injuries. Product design measures focused on better engineering to prevent inadvertent discharge by children and adults may have a greater impact than years of firearm safety training (34, 35). Adequate injury surveillance data by type and class of weapon are urgently needed.

READILY AVAILABLE HANDGUNS: PROTECTION OR PERIL?

Ironically, although only a minority of homicides are felony related and few involve an intruder, survey results show that the single most common reason handgun owners give for keeping a gun in the home is self-defense (84). The home can be a dangerous place, but evidence suggests that this danger comes most often from within. A recent study of gunshot deaths that occurred in homes in King County, Washington, found that guns kept in homes are far more often involved in the deaths of friends, neighbors, and household members than they are used to kill in self-defense. More than half of all fatal shootings that occurred in King County during the 6-year study took place in homes in which the firearm involved was kept. Nine (2.3%) involved the shooting of intruders or assailants in self-defense. During this same time frame, guns kept in homes were involved in 12 unintentional deaths, 41 criminal homicides, and 333 suicides. Even after excluding the suicides, researchers noted that guns kept in homes were involved in the death of a household member 18 times more often than in the death of an intruder (40).

Firearms that are readily available for self-protection are also readily available to children. Researchers studying the case histories of 88 California children, aged 0 to 14 years, who were fatally shot by other children or themselves between 1977 and 1983 found that most of these incidents occurred while the children were playing with loaded guns that they had found. Handguns were involved in 58% of these cases. Under the age of 8, many children cannot reliably distinguish a real gun from a toy (83).

Several investigators report a strong association between population-based rates of gun ownership and rates of firearm violence. Markush & Bartolucci correlated regional rates of firearm suicide with survey-based estimates of firearm prevalence (48). Boyd draws similar conclusions from increases in

US rates of gun ownership and suicide over time (9). Baker observed that rates of firearm suicide are highest in the mountain states and the Southeast, where rates of firearm ownership are high (4). Cook noted that high rates of firearm ownership in a community have little effect on overall rates of robbery, but are strongly associated to high rates of robbery murder (23). Alexander et al observed that South Carolina counties with high rates of gun ownership have higher than expected firearm death rates, whereas counties with lower rates of gun ownership have lower than expected firearm death rates (2).

International data are often cited to support both sides of the gun control issue, but these comparisons are often selected purposefully, to suit the political views of the authors (84). Gun control advocates like to compare the United States, where rates of gun ownership and homicide are high, with Great Britain, Canada, and Denmark, where rates of gun ownership and homicide are low. Opponents of gun control counter with statistics from Israel and Switzerland, where rates of homicide are low despite rates of home firearm ownership that are at least as high as those noted in the US. Japanese suicide rates are as high or higher than those noted in the US despite very low rates of gun ownership.

Unfortunately, few conclusions can be drawn from these studies because of the many social, cultural, and economic differences that characterize national groups. To better control for potentially confounding variables, Sloan et al (62, 63) studied rates of crime, assaults, homicide, and suicide in Seattle, Washington, and Vancouver, British Columbia, over a seven-year period (1980–1986). Both are large port cities in the Pacific Northwest, virtually identical in terms of population, median income, mean years of education, and other socioeconomic characteristics. However, these two cities differ markedly in their approach to gun control. In Seattle, handguns can be obtained with little difficulty. In Vancouver, the purchase of handguns is subject to significant restrictions. Although the rates of burglary, robbery, simple assault, and aggravated assault during the study interval were similar in these two communities, the investigators found that the risk of homicide in Seattle was more than 60% higher than that noted in Vancouver. This difference was largely due to a more than fivefold higher rate of firearm homicide in Seattle (Figure 3).

When Sloan et al (62) conducted a subsequent study to discern the relationship between gun control, weapons availability, and community rates of suicide, a somewhat different picture emerged. Their reference population was expanded to include the metropolitan areas of both communities, and the study interval was shifted to 1985–1987. However, their methods and analyses were otherwise identical to those of the homicide study. Not surprisingly, the rate of firearm suicides overall and the rate of handgun suicides in particular were substantially higher in King County, Washington, which

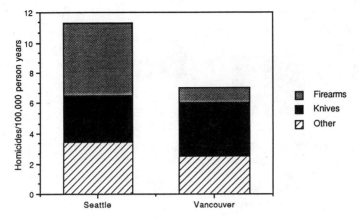

Figure 3 Annual homicide rate by mechanism of death (1980–1986): Seattle, Wash. vs. Vancouver, B.C.

includes Seattle, than in the Vancouver metropolitan area (relative risks were 2.3 and 5.7, respectively). However, King County's excess risk of firearm suicides was entirely offset by a 1.5-fold higher rate of nonfirearm suicides in the Vancouver metropolitan area (Figure 4). This finding suggests that most persons who were intent on committing suicide in Vancouver simply substituted another method with equal results. Among King County teenagers and persons in their early twenties (an age group thought to be more impulsive), ready access to firearms was associated with a moderately higher overall risk of suicide. This difference was due almost entirely to a 9.6-fold higher rate of handgun suicide compared with their counterparts in Vancouver. This difference is not entirely offset by higher rates of suicide by other methods in Vancouver (63).

Although population-based research, such as the Seattle-Vancouver studies, suggest an association between firearm availability and violent death, case control and cohort studies are needed to more precisely analyze the relationship between firearm availability and other individual factors (32). Many analysts believe that suicides and homicides frequently involve a combination of impulse and the close proximity of a firearm (1, 5, 10). Others argue that the choice of a firearm to attempt suicide or homicide simply reflects the strength of an individual's intent—the "guns don't kill people, people kill people" argument (24, 42). If the first hypothesis is true, and violent deaths involving guns are more often a product of ready availability than strength of intent, limiting access to firearms should ultimately decrease our high national rate of violent deaths. If the second argument is true, then persons intent on committing suicide or homicide will simply work harder to acquire a gun or kill by other means (84).

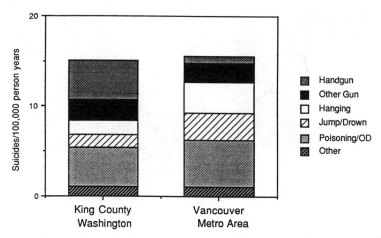

Figure 4   Annual suicide rate by mechanism of death (1985–1987): King County, Wash. vs. Vancouver, B. C., metro area.

THE BIOMECHANICS OF GUNSHOT WOUNDS

In general, the specific capacity of a firearm to cause injury depends on its accuracy, rate of fire, muzzle velocity, and specific characteristics of the projectile. Firearms are commonly categorized by major type, i.e. handguns, shotguns, and rifles, and are subdivided by action (single-shot weapons, which require manual reloading; semiautomatic weapons, which fire a single round with each squeeze of the trigger; and fully automatic weapons, which can fire a rapid succession of bullets with a single, sustained squeeze of the trigger.)

Because the kinetic energy of a moving object increases with the square of its velocity, weapons with high muzzle velocities, e.g. hunting rifles, generally cause greater tissue damage than weapons with lower muzzle velocities, e.g. handguns (45). However, the size, shape, and nature of the projectile also play a powerful role in determining the severity of the resultant injury. A nonfragmenting bullet traveling at high speed will penetrate and exit a body with little damage outside the bullet path. A slower bullet, designed to mushroom or fragment on impact (36), may damage a much larger amount of tissue through direct trauma, cavitation, and shock wave effects (26). Damage also increases in direct proportion to the mass of the projectile. Gunshot wounds caused by large caliber handguns are more than twice as likely to result in the death of the victim than wounds caused by small caliber handguns (86). The number of projectiles striking the body also influences the expected severity of injury. Shotguns fire a large number of independent and relatively slow moving pellets that are virtually harmless from a distance, but devastating at close range (25).

Although much is known about the specfic properties and characteristics of various firearms and their ammunition, little is known about the public health impact of specific classes or types of weapons. For example, considerable controversy has raged around proposals to ban semiautomatic "assault" rifles, but the relative burden of deaths and injuries due to these weapons is unknown. In the absence of reliable production or ownership data, it is impossible to tell whether one specific model of firearm is more or less likely to be used to kill than another. Epidemiologic data of this sort are essential, because many weapons can prove to be more dangerous than they might otherwise appear. Nonpowder firearms, for example, were once considered innocuous, but many of the pellet guns manufactured today have muzzle velocities that exceed those of some powder firearms (37). Several recent studies of children have shown that serious injuries and death can result (19, 54). The dangerousness of a weapon often depends on more than its intrinsic capacity to damage tissue. Although many handguns are of relatively small caliber and have low muzzle velocities, they are relatively inexpensive and easily concealed. They are often kept loaded in homes for self-defense, and few handguns have automatic safety catches or reliable loading indicators. As a result, this class of weapon, which comprises less than one third of all firearms in the United States, is used to kill more than twice as many citizens each year as shotguns and rifles combined (4).

ACUTE CARE AND REHABILITATION

Extensive literature has been devoted to the management of firearm injuries (7, 11, 41, 53). Emergency medical services systems, originally developed to reduce motor vehicle mortality (8), have also been used with great effect to treat and transport people with firearm-related trauma. Many important developments, such as helicopter transport to specialized trauma center care, grew out of the military's experience with victims of gunshot wounds during the Vietnam War. Surprisingly, the optimal prehospital management of patients with penetrating trauma is still highly controversial (64). Many maintain that rapid delivery of critical interventions in the field improves rates of survival; others argue that these measures simply delay patient access to definitive care in a trauma center. Some gunshot wounds are so extensive that survival is not possible given our current knowledge of treatment. Lee (44) found that 69% of people with fatal firearm injuries were declared dead at the scene or upon arrival at the hospital. Although Martin et al (49) note that 92% of persons hospitalized for firearm injuries survive to hospital discharge, this only includes those who survived long enough to be hospitalized. While the medical management debate continues, the field awaits carefully planned studies in controlled clinical trials to evaluate the relative value of these and other potential therapies. Basic data regarding the costs for care of these injuries are also needed.

Finally, many head (27) and spinal cord (43) injuries resulting in permanent disability are caused by firearms. In Detroit, 40% of all traumatic spinal cord injuries result from firearm wounds (33). Although the incidence of firearm-related injuries varies geographically, rural states, such as Arkansas and Oklahoma, have found that firearms cause between 8% and 9% of all spinal cord injuries (3; S. Mackintubee 1989, personal communication). Optimal strategies to speed the recovery of these patients is a topic in need of further research.

RESEARCH PRIORITIES

The development of a rational approach to prevention will depend on increased knowledge about the epidemiology of firearm injuries and the effectiveness of potential countermeasures. Although injuries account for more years of life lost before age 65 than cancer and heart disease combined, federal support for injury control research in the US is far less than that allocated to fight cancer, heart disease, and other health problems. Before the publication of *Injury in America,* little money was available to fund injury control research at any level (21).

Research funding for intentional injury and violent death prevention has been particularly limited. In 1983, the National Institutes of Health (NIH) awarded 19 research grants to study various aspects of five infectious diseases that, during the preceding year, caused only 17 cases of illness and nine fatalities in the United States. That same year, the NIH did not fund even one study of firearm deaths or injuries despite the involvement of guns in approximately 33,000 deaths and 198,000 injuries each year (38).

The prospects for research funding recently brightened when the Center for Environmental Health and Injury Control was created within the CDC. Since 1986, the CDC has funded more than 30 injury control research and demonstration projects and established six injury prevention centers (22). Total funding for CDC's grants program was increased in 1988, but support is still modest and declining with inflation. Further expansion of injury prevention work at the federal level will require direct Congressional appropriations. Several questions urgently need study:

Are particular types of firearms or classes of ammunition disproportionately involved in intentional deaths and injuries? Coroners' records and police files are needed to generate such statistics because death certificates rarely contain such information. The annual FBI Uniform Crime Reports bulletin categorizes homicides by major class of firearm or weapon, but not by caliber or manufacturer. At present, no reliable information is available about the manufacturer, type, and distribution of firearms in the United States. More precise data would be invaluable for examining the relationship between firearm injuries and the size and nature of the firearm supply, and could provide a basis for study of the biomechanical aspects of these injuries (50).

What is the economic and public health impact of firearm injuries? Currently, risk group assessment and computation of annual incidence rates of firearm injury have largely been confined to fatalities. Data on the costs of care for survivors of gunshot wounds are virtually nonexistent (49, 57). Few community-based firearm injury surveillance systems currently exist, and law enforcement data substantially underestimate rates of firearm injury (70, 73). Our understanding of firearm morbidity and mortality could be sustantially enhanced by development of a national fatal firearm injury reporting system, similar to the fatal motor vehicle accident reporting systems currently maintained by the National Highway Traffic Safety Administration.

Do particular behavioral or environmental factors make people safer or place them at greater risk of firearm death? Population-based studies cannot determine risk effects at the level of the individual. For example, no study has been published regarding the relative risk or benefit of keeping firearms in the home for protection. Comparing the number of intruders with the number of family members killed cannot identify cases in which would-be murderers or assailants were wounded or frightened away by the use or display of a firearm (40). Application of sophisticated epidemiologic techniques, such as cohort and case control methods, is needed to explore the effects of a family history of violence, current alcohol or drug use, a variety of home security measures (including firearm ownership), and other factors on an individual's risk of violent death (32, 50). Hopefully, information of this sort will lead to the identification of individual factors that may be modified or enhanced to prevent many suicides, homicides, and serious firearm injuries.

What is the optimal combination of acute and rehabilitative care for people with gunshot wounds? The magnitude of suffering and disability from these injuries is probably enormous, but essentially unknown. Studies are needed to identify more clearly the best approaches for providing emergency medical services, trauma care, and physical and psychological rehabilitation services. Long-term follow-up is also needed, as recent studies suggest these individuals are particularly prone to recurrent injury and death (61).

How effective are education programs to discourage firearm-related violence or to promote safe handling of firearms? Traditionally, educational programs to promote "safe behavior" have been emphasized by funding agencies despite their high cost and limited effectiveness (57). New, school-based curricula to decrease violence have been devised and need to be evaluated for evidence of impact. Firearm safety training programs have been advocated by the National Rifle Association (NRA) for many years, and some states recently added firearm safety training to their school-based curricula. In other states, completion of the NRA "safe hunter" program or equivalent training is a prerequisite to obtaining a hunting license. Studies evaluating the effectiveness of these programs for reducing rates of unintentional firearm injuries are urgently needed.

PREVENTING FIREARM INJURIES: A PUBLIC HEALTH APPROACH

Despite many gaps in our knowledge, a variety of strategies have been proposed or already implemented to reduce the number of firearm suicides, homicides, and unintentional injuries in the United States each year. All of these strategies fall under one or more of Haddon's ten generic strategies for breaking the chain of injury causation (Table 4). Some, such as installation of

Table 4 Options for the control of firearm injuries using Haddon's ten injury control strategies

Primary prevention (pre-injury phase)
1. Prevent the initial creation of the hazard.
    a. Prohibit manufacturing and importing of high risk firearms.
    b. Require firearms safety training and manadatory licensure in a manner analogous to use of automobiles.
    c. Encourage nonlethal home security measures to reduce perceived need to own weapons for protection.
    d. Require thorough background checks to restrict gun ownership by high risk persons.

2. Reduce the amount of hazard that is created.
    a. Restrict domestic manufacture or importing of high risk weapons and ammunition.
    b. Encourage police and others to use nonlethal weapons and techniques to control violent people.
    c. Prohibit manufacture or importation of specific calibers of ammunition used in high risk firearms.

3. Prevent release of a hazard that already exists.
    a. Require firearm safety training and a demonstration of proficiency before licensure of firearm owners.
    b. Provide community-based education to promote nonviolent resolution of arguments.
    c. Promote responsible alcohol consumption and ban weapons in establishments that serve alcohol.
    d. Store weapons at home in locked boxes.
    e. Require training in conflict resolution/anger management for known offenders.
    f. Require all new firearms to include a "child proof" automatic safety catch that remains engaged unless held in a disengaged position.
    g. Require loading indicators on all new firearms.
    h. Encourage installation of trigger locks on firearms kept in the home.
    i. Incarcerate repeat firearm offenders for longer periods of time (incapacitation).

Table 4   Options for the control of firearm injuries using Haddon's ten injury control strategies

Secondary prevention (injury phase)

4. Modify the rate of release or spatial distribution of the hazard from its source.
   a. Ban manufacture of weapons with metal content below the limit of current metal detectors.
   b. Require registration of firearms in a manner analogous to that used for automobile sales.
   c. Improve weapon "tracing" capabilities through new firearm labeling techniques and implement a national firearms tracking system.

5. Separate, in time or space, the hazard from persons to be protected.
   a. Establish a uniform national waiting period between application to purchase a firearm and sale.
   b. Require handguns to be transported in locked boxes in car trunks.
   c. Revise "circumstance" management procedures for law enforcement to require mandatory arrest of batterers in high risk domestic violence circumstances.
   d. Install weapon detection systems at the entrance to high risk establishments, e.g. airport gates, high schools, coliseums.
   e. Confiscate offender firearms following documented episodes of battering or assault.

6. Interpose a barrier between the hazard and person to be projected.
   a. Provide bullet proof vests to people in high risk occupations, e.g. law enforcement personnel.
   b. Provide bullet proof glass barriers for cabdrivers, convenience store clerks, and other high risk occupations.

7. Modify contact surfaces and structures to reduce injury.
   a. Redesign bullets to reduce injury severity.
   b. Redesign weapons to limit their rate of fire and/or muzzle velocity.
   c. Ban fragmenting or hollow point bullet in handguns and other high risk firearms.

8. Strengthen the resistance of persons who might be injured by the hazard.
   a. Institute measures to protect women from recurrent episodes of domestic violence.
   b. Provide training or counseling for persons with history of repeat victimization.
   c. Train persons in nonlethal means of self defense.
   d. Encourage nonlethal measures to increase home security, e.g. perimeter lights, better locks, and alarm systems.
   e. Promote use of nonlethal alternatives to firearms for self-defense, e.g. tear gas.

Tertiary prevention (post-injury phase)

9. Move rapidly to detect and limit damage that has occurred.
   a. Improve emergency medical and law enforcement responses at the scene.
   b. Improve access to acute trauma center care for gunshot victims.
   c. Assure prompt incarceration for firearm offenders.
   d. Provide helicopter and fixed wing air transport to trauma care for victims of gunshot wounds in rural and remote areas.

10. Initiate immediate and long-term reparative actions.
    a. Improve current approaches to the physical rehabilitation of gunshot victims.
    b. Develop counseling programs for persons who have been involved in firearm related violence.

bullet-proof booths for clerks at all-night gas stations, have already been implemented in some neighborhoods. Others are currently being debated: Several states have banned the sale of assault-type semiautomatic rifles. Maryland voters recently passed a referendum to restrict the manufacture or sale of "Saturday Night Special" handguns. In Florida on the other hand, the state legislature recently made permits to carry concealed weapons easier to obtain. Although many people believe that armed citizens effectively deter numerous cases of crime and violence (24, 42), others argue that strong gun control laws are needed to decrease rates of intentional firearm injuries and deaths (5).

Violence, by its very nature, is purposeful behavior. Often it follows actions, by the assailant or the person who is shot, that increase the potential for injury or death. In contrast to unintentional injuries, many measures intended to prevent violent injuries or deaths may be deliberately circumvented. Although restricting citizen access to guns or other means of intentional injury may decrease rates of death due to impulsive acts, the prevention of many other violent deaths and the vast majority of firearm injuries will require a better understanding of the etiology of violent behavior and the role of weapons in injury occurrence.

The rate of deaths due to firearm injury is not likely to remain static. The rise of cocaine has been linked to dramatic increases in rates of firearm homicide and drug-related violence in some cities (55). Firearms, the principal vehicles of serious intentional injury in the United States, are also becoming more dangerous. Since 1985, civilian purchases of semiautomatic assault rifles have soared, and drug dealers have found small caliber, fully automatic weapons easy to obtain (6). Of perhaps even greater concern, the technology now exists to mass produce handguns made almost entirely of plastic. In testimony before the US Congress, one industry representative stated that these guns can be made "dishwasher safe" (82). Under pressure from opponents of gun control, federal legislation to ban the production, sale, and importation of these remarkably dangerous weapons was defeated in the 101st session of Congress. Instead, a compromise bill requiring only 3.7 ounces of electromagnetically detectable material in each handgun was passed, a standard that will render most of the metal-detecting security devices now in use throughout the United States obsolete.

CONCLUSION

Rice et al (57) estimate that the average cost per person of a firearm fatality is $373,520 in 1985 dollars; this is the highest of any cause of injury. Although our economic costs related to firearm injuries exceeded $14.4 billion per year and our criminal justice expenditures exceeded $45 billion in 1985 (57, 68), the firearm mortality rates have not declined. From the perspective of public health policy, one might question why firearms have not received the level of attention given other dangerous consumer products.

For example, in March 1990, the United States Secretary of Health, Louis Sullivan, banned the sale of L-tryptophan because its use had been associated with 19 deaths and more than 1400 cases of eosinophilia-myalgia syndrome (29). In contrast to the small number of proponents of L-tryptophan, substantial economic and political forces in the United States encourage intense debate about potential approaches to prevention of firearm injuries. The intensity of this debate rivals that which occurred when cigarette smoking was first linked with lung cancer: Despite fierce resistance, the growing weight of scientific evidence led to incremental changes in public health policy.

The view that firearm injuries are an inevitable consequence of an industrialized society is being increasingly challenged. Many of the research methods and prevention strategies that have proven effective for the control of more traditional public health problems may be applicable to the problem of firearm injuries in America. Groups seeking to develop innovative strategies to prevent intentional injuries and deaths must be willing to view the problem from many perspectives. It is likely that the best approaches will ultimately arise from the collaboration of experts from disciplines with complementary resources and knowledge, e.g. criminology, behavioral science, mental health, and public health. Given the large number of suicides, homicides, and serious injuries that involve firearms in the United States, epidemiologic studies must continue if we are to learn how to deal effectively with the broader problems of intentional injury and violent death. Unfortunately, the politics of gun control have discouraged many researchers from applying their talents to these pressing social problems (30, 38). All scientists have a fundamental responsibility to produce research findings that are unbiased in nature and ultimately useful to society regardless of how the results will affect the political interests of any particular group. Firearm injuries are among the leading causes of death in the United States, and intentional injuries are a major cause of pain, suffering, and lifelong disability. With adequate knowledge and the will to act, many of these deaths and injuries may be prevented.

Literature Cited

1. Adelson, L. 1980. The gun and the sanctity of human life: Or the bullet as pathogen. *The Pharos* 43:15–25
2. Alexander, G. R., Massey, R. M., Gibbs, T., Alterkruse, J. 1985. Firearm related fatalities: An epidemiologic assessment of violent death. *Am. J. Public Health* 75:165–68
3. Arkansas Spinal Cord Commission. 1985. *Annual Report, 1985.* Little Rock, Ark: Arkansas Spinal Cord Commission
4. Baker, S., O'Neill, B., Karpf, R. S. 1984. *The Injury Fact Book.* Lexington, Mass: Lexington Books
5. Baker, S. 1985. Without guns, do people kill people? *Am. J. Public Health* 75:587–88
6. Beaty, J., Shannon, E., Woodbury, R. 1989. The other arms race. *Time* 6:20–26
6a. Becker, D. P., Povlishock, J. T., eds. 1985. *Central Nervous System Trauma*

Status Report—1985. Bethesda: Natl. Inst. Neurol. Commun. Disord. Stroke, Natl. Inst. Health

7. Bongard, F. S., Klein, S. R. 1989. The problem of vascular shotgun injuries: Diagnostic and management strategy. *Ann. Vasc. Surg.* 3:199–203

8. Boyd, D. R., Edlich, R. F., Micik, S. 1983. *Systems Approach to Emergency Medical Care*. Norwalk, Conn: Appleton-Century-Crofts

9. Boyd, J. 1983. The increasing role of suicide by firearms. *N. Engl. J. Med.* 308:872–74

10. Browning, C. 1986. Handguns and homicide: A public health problem. *J. Am. Med. Assoc.* 236:2198–2200

11. Brunner, R. G., Fallon, W. F. 1990. A prospective, randomized clinical trial of wound debridement versus conservative wound care in soft tissue injury from civilian gunshot wounds. *Am. Surg.* 56:104–7

12. Centers for Disease Control. 1984. Alcohol and violent death—Erie County, New York, 1973–1983. *Morbid. Mortal. Wkly. Rep.* 33:226–27

13. Centers for Disease Control. 1988. CDC recommendations for a community plan for the prevention and containment of suicide clusters. *Morbid. Mortal. Wkly. Rep.* 37(Suppl. S-6):1–12

14. Centers for Disease Control. September 1983. *Homicide surveillance, 1970–1978*. Atlanta: Cent. Dis. Control

15. Centers for Disease Control. November 1986. *Homicide surveillance: High risk racial and ethnic groups—blacks and Hispanics, 1970 to 1983*. Atlanta: Cent. Dis. Control

16. Centers for Disease Control. April 1985. *Suicide Surveillance, 1970–1980*. Atlanta: Centers for Disease Control

17. Centers for Disease Control. 1988. Unintentional firearm-related fatalities, 1970–1984. In CDC Surveillance Summaries, *Morbid. Mortal. Wkly. Rep.* 37(SS-1):47–52

18. Centerwall, B. 1984. Race, socioeconomic status and domestic homicide, Atlanta 1971–72. *Am. J. Public Health* 74:813–15

19. Christoffel, T., Christoffel, K. 1987. Nonpowder firearm injuries: Whose job is it to protect children? *Am. J. Public Health* 77:735–38

20. Cole, T. G., Patetta, M. J. 1988. Hunting firearm injuries, North Carolina. *Am. J. Public Health* 78:1585–86

21. Committee on Trauma Research. 1985. *Injury in America: A Continuing Public Health Problem*. Washington, DC: Natl. Acad. Press

22. Committee to Review the Status and Progress at the Centers for Disease Control. 1988. *Injury: A Review of the Status and Progress of the Injury Control Program at the Centers for Disease Control*. Washington, DC: Natl. Acad. Press

23. Cook, P. J. 1987. Robbery violence. *J. Crim. Law Criminol.* 78:357–76

24. Drooz, R. 1977. Handguns and hokum: A methodological problem. *J. Am. Med. Assoc.* 238:43–45

25. Fackler, M. L. 1986. Wound ballistics. In *Current Therapy of Trauma—2*, pp. 94–101, ed. D. D., Trunkey, F. R. Lewis, Toronto: Decker

26. Fackler, M. L. 1988. Wound ballistics: A review of common misconceptions. *J. Am. Med. Assoc.* 259:2730–36

27. Frankowski, R. F., Annegers, J. F., Whitman, S. 1985. Epidemiological and descriptive studies part I: Descriptive epidemiology of head trauma in the United States. See Ref. 6a, pp. 33–43

28. Frankowski, R. F., Lee, R. K. Contribution of firearms to brain injury in the United States. In *Penetrating Head Injuries*, ed. T. F. Dagi. Boston: Little, Brown. In press

29. Gladwell, M. 1990. All products containing L-tryptophan recalled. *Washington Post*, March 23

30. Goldsmith, M. 1989. Epidemiologists aim at new target: Health risk of handgun proliferation. *J. Am. Med. Assoc.* 261:675–76

31. Goodman, R. A., Mercy, J. A., Loya, F., Rosenberg, M. L., Smith, J. C., et al. 1986. Alcohol use and interpersonal violence: Alcohol detected in homicide victims. *Am. J. Public Health* 76:144–49

32. Goodman, R. A., Mercy, J. A., Layde, P. M., Thacker, S. B. 1988. Case-control studies: Design issues for criminological applications. *J. Quant. Criminol.* 4:71–84

33. Grahm, P. M., Weingarden, S. I. 1988. *Targeting teenagers in a spinal cord injury violence prevention program*. Presentation at 14th Annu. Sci. Meet. Am. Spinal Cord Injury Assoc., San Diego

34. Haddon, W. 1980. Advances in the epidemiology of injuries as a basis for public policy. *Public Health Rep.* 95:411–21

35. Haddon, W. 1968. The changing approach to the epidemiology, prevention, and amelioration of trauma: The transition to approaches etiologically rather than descriptively based. *Am. J. Public Health* 58:1431–38

36. Harrell, J. B. 1979. Hollowpoint ammu-

nition injuries: Experience in a police group. *J. Trauma* 19(2):115–16

37. Harris, W., Luterman, A., Curreri, P. W. 1983. BB and pellet guns—toys or deadly weapons? *J. Trauma* 23:566–69

38. Jagger, J., Dietz, P. 1988. Death and injury by firearms: Who cares? *J. Am. Med. Assoc.* 255:3143–44

39. Johnson, P. 1989. I feel more secure having a gun around. *USA Today*, March 1:1–2

40. Kellerman, A., Reay, D. 1986. Protection or peril? An analysis of firearm-related deaths in the home. *N. Engl. J. Med.* 314:1557–60

41. Kirkpatrick, J. B., DiMaio, V. 1978. Civilian gunshot wounds of the brain. *J. Neurosurg.* 49:185–98

42. Kleck, H. 1988. Crime control through the private use of armed force. *Soc. Probl.* 35:1–19

43. Kraus, J. F. 1985. Epidemiological aspects of acute spinal cord injury: A review of incidence, prevalence, causes, and outcome. See Ref. 6a, pp. 313–22

44. Lee, R. K. 1989. Incidence of fatal gunshot injuries among Galveston County residents, 1979–81. *Diss. Abstr. Int.* 50/4-B:1352(5004B)

45. Lindsey, D. 1980. The idolatry of velocity, or lies, damn lies, and ballistics. *J. Trauma* 20:1068–69

46. Lowry, P. W., Hassig, S. E., Gunn, R. A., Mathison, J. B. 1988. Homicide victims in New Orleans: Recent trends. *Am. J. Epidemiol.* 128:1130–36

47. Deleted in proof

48. Markush, R., Bartolucci, A. 1984. Firearms and suicide in the United States. *Am. J. Public Health* 64:123–27

49. Martin, M. J., Hunt, R. K., Hulley, S. B. 1988. The cost of hospitalization for firearm injuries. *J. Am. Med. Assoc.* 260:3048–50

50. Mercy, J. A., Houk, V. N. 1988. Firearm injuries: A call for science. *N. Engl. J. Med.* 319:1283–85

51. Mercy, J. A., O'Carroll, P. W. 1988. New directions in violence prediction: The public health arena. *Violence and Vict.* 3:285–301

52. McLeer, S. V., Anwar, R. A. H., Herman, S., Maquiling, K. 1989. Education is not enough: A systems failure in protecting battered women. *Ann. Emerg. Med.* 18:651–53

53. Miner, M. E., Ewing-Cobbs, L., Kopaniky, D. R., Cabrera, J., Kaufmann, P. 1990. Results of treatment of gunshot wounds to the brain in children. *Neurosurgery* 26:20–24

54. Morgan, J. C., Turner, C. S., Pennell, T. C. 1984. Air gun injuries of the abdo-

men in children. *Arch. Surg.* 119:1437–38

55. Morganthau, T., Miller, M., Sandza, R., Wingert, P. 1989. Murder wave in the capitol. *Newsweek* 13:16–19

56. Morrow, P. L., Hudson, P. 1986. Accidental firearm fatalities in North Carolina, 1976–80. *Am. J. Public Health* 76:1120–23

57. Rice, D. P., MacKenzie, E. J. & Associates 1989. *Cost of Injury in the United States: A Report to Congress.* San Francisco: Inst. Health and Aging, Univ. Calif. and Inj. Prevent. Ctr., Johns Hopkins Univ.

58. Robertson, L. S. 1983. *Injuries: Causes, Control Strategies, and Public Policy.* Lexington, Mass: Lexington Books

59. Rushforth, N. B., Hirsh, C. S., Ford, A B., Adelson, L. 1974. Accidental firearm fatalities in a metropolitan county (1958–1973). *Am. J. Epidemiol.* 100:499–505

60. Saltzman, L. E., Mercy, J. A., Rosenberg, M. L., Elsea, W. R., Napper, G., et al. 1990. Magnitude and patterns of family and intimate assault in Atlanta, Georgia, 1984. *Violence and Vict.* 5(1):5–21

61. Sims, D. W., Bivins, B. A., Farouck, N. O., Horst, H. M., Sorensen, V. J., Fath, J. J. 1989. Urban trauma: A chronic recurrent disease. *J. Trauma* 29:940–47

62. Sloan, J. H., Kellermann, A. L., Reay, D. T., Ferris, J. A., Koepsell, T., et al. 1988. Handgun regulations, crime, assaults and homicide: A tale of two cities. *N. Engl. J. Med.* 319:1256–62

63. Sloan, J. H., Rivara, F. P., Reay, D. T., Ferris, J. A., Kellermann, A. L. 1990. Firearm regulations and rates of suicide: A comparison of two metropolitan areas. *N. Engl. J. Med.* 322:369–73

64. Smith, J. P., Bodai, B. I., Hill, A. S., Frey, C. F. 1985. Prehospital stabilization of critically injured patients: A failed concept. *J. Trauma* 25:65–70

65. Sniezek, J. E., Finklea, J. F., Graitcer, P. L. 1989. Injury coding and hospital discharge data. *J. Am. Med. Assoc.* 262:2270–72

66. Deleted in proof

67. Tardiff, K., Gross, E., Messner, S. 1986. A study of homicides in Manhattan, 1981. *Am. J. Public Health* 76:139–43

68. Univ. Calif., Los Angeles, Centers for Disease Control. August 1985. *The Epidemiology of Homicide in the City of Los Angeles, 1970–79.* Dept. Health Hum. Serv., Public Health Serv., Cent. Dis. Control

69. US Bureau Census. 1987. 1987 Current Population Survey (Public use data tape)
70. US Dept. Justice. 1987. *Criminal Victimization in the United States, 1985: A National Crime Study Report.* Washington, DC: Natl. Acad. Press
71. US Dept. Justice. 1987. *Crime in the United States, 1986: Uniform Crime Reports for the United States.* Washington, DC: Fed. Bureau Invest.
72. US National Center for Health Statistics. 1988. United States Detailed Mortality Data, 1987 (Public use data tape)
73. US National Center for Health Statistics. 1976. *Persons Injured and Disability Days by Detailed Type and Class of Accident, United States—1971–72.* Vital and Health Stat., Ser. 10, No. 105. DHEW Publ. No. (HRA)76–1532. US Dept. Health Educ. Welfare
74. Vinson, T. 1974. Gun and knife attacks. *Aust. J. For. Sci.* 7:76–83
75. Waller, J. A. 1987. Injury: Conceptual shifts and preventive implications. *Annu. Rev. Public Health* 8:21–49
76. Waller, J. A. 1985. *Injury Control: A Guide to the Causes and Prevention of Trauma.* Lexington, Mass: Lexington Books/Heath
77. Widom, C. S. 1989. The intergenerational transmission of violence. In *Pathways to Criminal Violence,* ed. N. Weinger, M. Wolfgang, pp. 137–201. Newbury Park, Calif: Sage
78. Wintemute, G. J. 1987. Firearms as a cause of death in the United States, 1920–1982. *J. Trauma* 27:532–36
79. Wintemute, G. J. 1986. Prevention. In *Trauma Care Systems,* ed. R. Cales, R. Helig, pp. 39–48. Rockville, Md: Aspen
80. Wintemute, G. J., Teret, S. P., Kraus, J. F., Wright, M. W. 1988. The choice of weapons in firearm suicides. *Am. J. Public Health* 78:824–26
81. Wintemute, G. J., Kraus, J. F., Teret, S. P., Wright, M. A. 1989. Unintentional firearm deaths in California. *J. Trauma* 29:457–61
82. Wintemute, G. J., Teret, S. P., Kraus, J. F. 1988. Plastic handguns that resemble toy guns: New technology creates a uniquely hazardous product. *Pediatrics* 81:316–17
83. Wintemute, G. J., Teret, S. P., Kraus, J. F., Wright, M. A., Bradfield, G. 1987. When children shoot children: 88 unintended deaths in California. *J. Am. Med. Assoc.* 257:3107–9
84. Wright, J. D., Rossi, P., Daly, K., Weber-Burdin, E. 1981. *Weapons, Crime and Violence in America: A Literature Review and Research Agenda.* US Dept. Justice, Natl. Inst. Justice. Washington, DC: Govt. Print. Off.
85. Zimring, F. E. 1968. Is gun control likely to reduce violent killings? *Univ. Chicago Law Rev.* 35:721–37
86. Zimring, F. E. 1972. The medium is the message: Firearm caliber as a determinant of death from assaults. *J. Legal Stud.* 15:97–112
87. Zimring, F. E., Zuchl, J. 1986. Victim injury and death in urban robbery—a Chicago study. *J. Legal Stud.* 15:1–40

Annu. Rev. Publ. Health. 1991. 12:41–65

WORDS WITHOUT ACTION? THE PRODUCTION, DISSEMINATION, AND IMPACT OF CONSENSUS RECOMMENDATIONS

Jonathan Lomas

Centre for Health Economics and Policy Analysis, Department of Clinical Epidemiology and Biostatistics, Health Sciences Centre, McMaster University, Hamilton, Ontario, L8N 3Z5, Canada

KEY WORDS: practice guidelines, physician behavior, group judgment, technology assessment, evaluation studies

---

"Consensus means that lots of people say collectively what nobody believes individually"

Abba Eban

INTRODUCTION

The above quote from Israeli statesman Abba Eban voices a general concern about the increasing use of consensus processes as an imprimatur for certain practice patterns in medicine. Some critics fear that the implications of the consensus process will discourage physician autonomy or innovation. They point to the need to "protect the individual choices of each physician from the potential tyrannical domination of consensus and allow the process of development of new knowledge to continue" (61, p. 1077). Other critics claim that the methods used may overinterpret the available data and lead to conclusions based on "faith or zeal or alarm" (2, p. 1086). Finally, there are critics who, if correct, can assuage these fears, because they do not believe that consensus processes effect behavior change at all, but rather provide "primarily a dialogue among researchers . . . not a guide to action" (34, p. 2740).

41

0163-7525/91/0501-0041$02.00

Nevertheless, consensus processes as a means of information transfer are here to stay and will become even more popular. A recent *Directory on Technology Assessment* listed nearly 60 organizations in the United States with formal programs that are establishing hundreds of recommendations for practice. Nearly all of these organizations use some form of consensus in their deliberations (32). Formal consensus development programs now exist in Canada, Britain, Sweden, Norway, Finland, Denmark, Holland, and France (32). The programs use terms that differ across a spectrum of "consensus development conferences," "task force reports," "appropriateness ratings," "practice parameters or guidelines," or "technology assessment reports." However, they generally use varying degrees of formality to produce accessible and readily understandable consensus recommendations that summarize the implications of existing research evidence.

The need for such summaries is manifold: the burgeoning biomedical and social science literature, which increases awareness of the inadequacy of traditional journal articles as sources for direct adoption decisions (35, 93); evidence of uncertainty from medical practice variations on appropriate clinical policies (3); awareness that a significant proportion of care is inappropriately provided (10, 88); a shift from providing those services with expected benefit to only those with actual benefit (21); demands by third-party funding and quality monitoring agents for guidance on and succinct recommendations about appropriate practice (81); and pressure from the public for increased input to medical and technological decision-making (4).

The variety of catalysts produces variety among the specific aims, conduct, and output from each of the consensus processes. The target audience may be as narrow as a particular kind of practitioner or researcher (9, 39); as eclectic as politicians, administrators, clinicians, and planners (13, 86); or, as in Denmark, as diffuse as "public participation . . . for ensuring the democratic influence on decisions about medical technology" (4, p. 308).

The most common target is the practicing clinician, and the most common aim is to influence the clinician to improve the quality of care. Sometimes, the influence is indirect; it comes through funding or regulatory bodies. In this review, I focus largely on this specific purpose and target of consensus processes.

In the first section, I review some of the numerous methods for consensus production and the controversies surrounding them. I observe the lack of any recognized standards by which to judge the validity of the various approaches. One intent of the review is to begin assembling such a set of standards. This task can only be started here, however, because research comparing the effectiveness of different group judgment processes on "how best to put medical technologies to use, is not commensurate with the [research] effort and care devoted to developing these technologies" (37).

In the second section, I review the dissemination and impact of consensus by focusing on the apparently false assumption that dissemination is necessary and sufficient for behavior change. I review the methods used for dissemination and appraise the 19 studies identified in the literature that evaluate the impact of such dissemination on behavior. This appraisal yields a pessimistic conclusion—in most cases the words do not translate into action. I found some hope, however, in reviews of the impact of consensus on cognitive, rather than behavioral, outcomes, and the potential for combining the output of consensus with more active strategies for implementing changes in clinical practice.

I conclude with suggestions from recent work on how to improve the impact of the output. I also suggest a tentative set of standards by which to judge the validity of different consensus production methods.

I derived the materials for the review from a combination of sources:

1. Computerized searches of the US National Library of Medicine data base (MEDLINE) and the Educational Resources Information Clearinghouse (ERIC) for 1980 to the present, which use the search terms "consensus development," "guidelines," "standards," "official policy," "technology assessment," "evaluation studies," "epidemiologic methods," and "research";
2. Bibliographies on consensus methodology (26, 32a) and practice guidelines (75);
3. Citations in the articles retrieved;
4. Citations provided by colleagues; and
5. Personal files accumulated over the past eight years.

THE PRODUCTION OF CONSENSUS

A Framework for Evaluating Consensus Production

Ironically, the recognition standards routinely required of research studies are rarely found in the consensus reports that make the synthesis of such studies popularly available. The systematic and explicit description of the methods used is often partially or wholly missing. Thus, many consensus reports would fail the tests of replicability and defensibility: Based on the information given, could the methods in the exercise be replicated? Is the rationale for methodological choices provided?

The method and/or rationale for at least the following choices are desirable:

1. The topic selected;
2. The membership of the consensus group;
3. The nature and extent of background preparation;

4. The inclusion/exclusion criteria for information inputs;
5. The type of group process and definition of consensus;
6. The criteria for qualification as a recommendation; and
7. The preparation process and format of the report.

By making these choices and rationales explicit, the consensus group moves from "simply applying their intuitions and stating their beliefs, to reasoning through a problem step by step, and justifying the conclusions" (21).

There are some existing consensus programs that come close to meeting these rigorous standards of explication and justification, although some groups argue with the particular choices made by the programs (9, 14, 91). There are many other consensus exercises, however, that fail to make their choices explicit. These are often the "one-off" variety conducted by a disease-specific association or specialty group. Perhaps the most notable of these programs is the Consensus Development Conference (CDC) approach of the National Institutes of Health (NIH). This program has come in for much scrutiny and criticism, even from those involved in its organization (39).

At the same time, the NIH CDC program has been subject to more systematic evaluations, and consequent modification, than any of its competitors. Thus, it has spawned much valuable research information on the validity of different approaches to producing consensus (41, 46, 59, 99). Similarly, derivative CDC programs have also been evaluated in other countries, such as Sweden (13, 43), Holland (15, 89), and Canada (54, 55). There have even been cross-cultural comparisons of the processes and their outcomes (11, 79).

In the following sections, I use the results of these and other evaluations to review the explicit methodological and "political" choices needed for a consensus exercise to translate biomedical research into practical advice for clinical audiences.

Selecting a Topic

The topic can be either disease-based, e.g. prevention and treatment of breast cancer, or procedure-based, e.g. mammography (75). In the former, the focus is largely on the appropriate use of all alternatives for alleviating a particular burden of ill health. In the latter, the focus is on the particular indications for which an intervention should be used: it is generally termed technology assessment. Each focus brings particular advantages and disadvantages.

With disease-based topics, it is generally easier to maintain the focus of the exercise on the objective of improved patient or population health. Nevertheless, the task is more complex. It necessitates evaluation of different technologies for the same disease and questions which criteria are most appropriate for such comparisons. For instance, when attempting to reduce the morbidity and mortality of breast cancer, how do you weigh cost, convenience, effectiveness, labeling, and preference (patients' and providers') in comparing breast self-examination with mammography and dietary and reproductive behavior changes with lumpectomy?

With procedure-based topics, the task may be simplified. However, considerations of technical capabilities may override the criterion of actual health benefits. For example, should the threshold for routine screening for breast cancer be lowered to an age group at lower risk just because mammography now uses reduced levels of radiation? Futhermore, timing is an acute problem in technology assessments. If a new technology is appraised too soon there will not be an adequate base of scientific knowledge; if appraised too late, the technology will already have diffused across the system (25). Many persons argued that the 1984 NIH CDC on lowering blood cholesterol to prevent heart disease was undertaken too early; subsequent research made their recommendations highly suspect (2, 49, 60). In contrast, the 1979 CDC on surgery for primary breast cancer was clearly too late; the principal recommended change had already taken place (46).

Insofar as the target audience is the practicing clinician, diagnostic and surgical specialties may find procedure-based topics most relevant. Medical and public health professionals may have greater interest in disease- (or at least health problem-) based topics.

Even after the topic has been decided upon and justified, the topic area has to be specified. Many programs outline general criteria to assist them in setting priorities across competing topics. These usually include at least the following three general principles: importance (in terms of frequency, burden of morbidity/mortality, or resource-consumption grounds); reasonable base of existing scientific knowledge on effectiveness of intervention or alternatives; and resolvable on the basis of more than personal opinion and values (8, 69, 91). Although these are not unreasonable as criteria for topic selection, their focus is almost exclusively on the state of science in the potential topic area, not on the state of practice. This omission has been noted in the context of the potential objective to alter practice patterns (4, 46, 49a, 52, 74). An appraisal of existing practice provides information on both the extent (or even existence) of a problem and the nature of any changes that might be indicated. Such information is important to any decision on the need for a consensus on a particular topic—either because variations in practice demonstrate uncertainty regarding what is appropriate or because practice is uniformly not congruent with the message from current research evidence (52).

Consensus Group Membership

There are at least three distinct types of consensus group membership. Coronary artery bypass surgery is an interesting example because it has been subjected to each type. First, the RAND Corporation approach (and a

Canadian counterpart) used a panel of clinical experts on the area under consideration—cardiovascular surgeons and related specialists (9, 67). Second, a NIH CDC used a panel of scientific experts in both the clinical and related aspects of the topic—clinicians plus lawyers, epidemiologists, economists, and "expert consumers" (76). Third, a nonexpert or independent panel in the UK King's Fund conference included administrators, laymen, and providers, from a variety of specialty and disciplinary backgrounds (86).

These three panel types—clinical experts, scientific experts, and nonexperts—reflect the chosen focus and target audience of the consensus exercise. With clinical expert panels, the focus is almost entirely on the safety and effectiveness issues and on the target audience of the specialty physicians actually engaged in providing the care. Scientific expert panels have a broader mandate. They consider such additional issues as ethics, economics, or future research needs and they target an expanded audience of clinicians, scientists, and administrators. The nonexpert panels are less concerned with resolution of conflict and more with "broadening the debate among a wide range of professionals in health care and with the public about medical technologies" (86, p. 713).

The panel type is also influenced by the sponsor of the exercise. Medical specialty societies tend toward the clinical expert panel. Research council and university-based organizers favor the scientific expert panel. Public foundations or directly government-sponsored panels are more likely to be nonexpert.

Given an objective of influencing practitioners in the area under study, one concern in panel membership is that it be credible to this target audience. The difficulty of satisfying all potential audiences is illustrated by the results of one survey performed in conjunction with the above-mentioned King's Fund conference on coronary artery surgery. When questioned whether the panel and the proceedings were biased too strongly by the cardiac medical specialties, only 24% of the cardiac specialists surveyed replied yes, compared with 88% of community medicine specialists. This difference may have reflected the fact that those with a public health perspective are more favorably disposed to disease-based rather than procedure-based topics. Indeed, the community medicine specialists generally felt that the topic "was not presented in the whole context of the prevention and treatment of coronary heart disease" (86, p. 714). Nevertheless, the target audience for the actual performance of coronary surgery—cardiac specialists—was appropriately convinced by the credibility of the panel. Again, the attitude of the intended audience may be the most appropriate criterion to judge credibility. Had the topic been the prevention and treatment of coronary heart disease, then a panel and process less focused on cardiac specialists and more on public health personnel would likely have been more appropriate and credible to the intended audience.

Many consensus panels concentrate membership among academics, rather than community-based practitioners. Although this approach satisfies the apparent role of the consensus process in synthesizing research information, it can conflict with the credibility to a community practitioner audience. In other work, researchers found significant resistance among community practitioners to "ivory tower" medicine as espoused by academic consensus panels (35, 56). There is no obvious balance between these potentially competing demands on consensus group membership. However, if one purpose is for community practitioners to identify with and find credible the recommendations, it is advisable to at least ensure visible representation of their viewpoint.

Consensus group membership inherently has tension between the panelists' appeal to the intended audience and the necessary skills to adequately consider relevant viewpoints and appraise scientific evidence. However, the need to include at least an epidemiologist to bring both public health perspective and methodological skills to the process is increasingly recognized (46). Sometimes, an economist is also needed to evaluate opportunity costs and resource allocation matters (13, 86).

An ongoing debate surrounding the NIH CDC program concerns the panelists' ability to meet the "science court" and "judicial jury" requirement of not having strong, preexisting views on the topic under consideration (65). This is more of a concern for the expert than the nonexpert panel, given the likelihood that both expertise and opinions flow from involvement. The social psychology literature warns of the potential bias (57). Other evidence suggests that when methodologic quality is stressed as the criterion for decision-making, such preexisting views can be appropriately altered by the consensus process (56). Some groups have argued that at least the panel chairperson should be neutral toward the topic (42).

Overall, prior consensus exercises have not been explicit about the criteria used to select topics and/or members of the consensus group. Any existing criteria often have not been carefully related to the objectives of the exercise and the target audience. Wortman and his colleagues, after evaluating one consensus program, pointed out that the absence of clear criteria and procedures leads to "the potential for selection bias in the choice of conference topics, questions, and participants [which] poses a set of related problems that can undermine the credibility of the CD [consensus development] process" (99, p. 490). They point out that formalization of these selection processes can reduce the problems. They also suggest using the Delphi method (17) with relevant medical schools, researchers, and associations to "rapidly produce a list of questions, panelists, speakers, and relevant research literature in two or three rounds of mailed questionnaires" (99, p. 491). Whether such a formal process is used or not, it is advisable to describe the criteria and procedures used in selecting topics and participants, if only to clarify that they relate directly to the objectives of the consensus exercise.

Background Preparation

The broad areas of potential preparation for the panel are the state of science for the topic, the state of practice in the area, and the ground rules for operation of the group process.

Some consensus processes have provided none of this background; they prefer to rely on the existing knowledge of a clinical expert panel (e.g. 22, 27, 44). Nevertheless, the majority provide at least a bibliography of relevant literature for the state of science, if not an actual synthesis or summary. The most comprehensive exercises favor organization of a synthesis around the methodological quality of the various studies of interest (e.g. 9, 14, 71, 91). This approach has the advantage of orienting the panel away from clinical opinion and toward methodologically sound evidence, when it is available, as the adjudicator of controversy.

One former director of the NIH CDCs described the importance of the state of the science background preparation by bemoaning its sporadic availability for some 30 previous topics covered by the program:

> On the occasions when such a synthesis was prepared by the staff and accepted by the panel, evidence was well integrated into both the deliberations and the consensus statement . . . When a data synthesis was unavailable or was not used . . . the difficulty of coping was exacerbated. Probably as a result, some consensus statements show evidence of influence by panelists' assertions of common sense or knowledge of acceptable practices, without having been explicitly stated" (40, p. 3039).

I have already described the infrequent use but high value of background input on the state of practice. In the context of panel preparation, the value of this information is its ability to correct any "imbalance between the nature of the panel's task and the information it has available for accomplishing the task. . . . The consensus panel is supposed to translate biomedical research findings into clinically meaningful recommendations. To do its job well, the panel should be well-informed about both the current state of science and the current state of practice" (46, p. 242). If such background preparation had been included in many previous consensus processes, it may have saved time and effort by preventing mere "codification" recommendations that reflected practice patterns already diffused and in place (e.g. 36, 49a).

In countries such as Canada, where accessible data bases on practice patterns are routinely collected, background preparation can be completed easily (12). In countries such as the United States, where access to these data is more problematic, researchers can perform specific surveys, or even establish a routine collection, using a panel of "Neilsen hospitals," similar to the monitoring of families for television viewing patterns (46).

Information Inputs

In addition to background reviews before deliberations, there is the question of the source and nature of information inputs during deliberations. The source and, to some extent, the nature interact with how cloistered or how public is the conduct of the consensus process. At one end of the continuum are the most cloistered of the clinical expert panels; they operate behind closed doors and consider little besides the published literature and their own views on safety and effectiveness (e.g. 9, 14). At the other end are the highly public forums, common in Scandinavian countries, that solicit both information and views from various sources—the general public, administrators, politicians, patients, researchers, and care-givers—on numerous aspects of the topic (4, 90).

These differences reflect, in part, the extent to which some processes restrict deliberations to the results of experimental research, whereas others wish to synthesize values and other "normative" components with the "objective research." Some researchers argue that the former is not a valid approach because even the research information is not value-free: The choice of a more public process that takes "part of its format from a societal instrument, the jury/court, which deals with moral values, means the format provides a strong impetus to evaluate health technology from societal viewpoints rather than from that of scientific evidence" (90, p. 67).[1]

The choice of narrow inclusion criteria for information inputs by the cloistered exercises can be seen as the equivalent of the researcher's *ceteris paribus*—by excluding the overtly normative issues (ethics, economics, patient preferences) and their sponsoring sources (social scientists, economists, the public), control is better maintained over the outcome of the safety and effectiveness variables of interest. The exercise is more easily perceived as an objective one, even if it is less relevant to the world in which the decisions are actually being made.

The degree of relevance to public, or at least nonclinician, viewpoints is nevertheless central to many of the current consensus programs. Not coincidently, the most publicly oriented of all consensus programs, the Danish process, chose early detection of breast cancer in 1983 for its first exercise because "this was primarily a public-interest issue: Potentially it had a preventive impact, it certainly dealt with health care costs, but there was little

---

[1]Some of the difficulties encountered by the NIH CDC program might be attributable to ambiguity on this issue. They restrict consideration to matters of safety and efficacy, but also use an open format that allows input from numerous sources, including the general public (99).

basic scientific information available to answer the questions it raised, since controlled clinical trials had not yet been finalized at the time of the meeting" (90, p. 71).

For such public health topics, with ethical issues around screening and allocation, the importance of obtaining information inputs on values to integrate with clinical science may be greater than in some of the more restricted clinical areas where the demonstrations of benefit and cost-benefit may be relatively black and white. In particular, the central nature of patient preferences in determining many public health treatment or screening decisions is not easily considered by methods that ignore the importance of values (21). A few consensus exercises have, largely unsuccessfully, tried to incorporate this element using formal medical decision-making models (48, 73). Similar attempts to incorporate economic evaluations have met with somewhat more success (92).

Many researchers have expressed the "need for a more general technology to allow for the assimilation of a much wider variety of evidentiary material, including expert opinions, biological theories and supporting laboratory data, and evaluations of component pieces of the overall practice under review" (50). Some methodologies aimed at an objective assimilation of disparate evidence are being developed. There are, for instance, variations on meta-analysis (83), Bayesian meta-modeling (50), and even a science of designing practice policies (21). With the increasing popularity of evidence synthesis, we can expect more innovation.

The actual format of the information inputs is not crucial. However, many surveys of panelists, speakers, and audiences suggest that the use of "witnesses" giving oral presentations and engaging in debate of "testimony," is preferred to impersonal written submissions, at least from the perspective of the actual participants (13, 43, 86). One survey found that those groups exposed to such presentations and debate were the most likely to have taken actions based on the consensus report (43).

Type of Group Judgment Process

As described above, many formal methodologies are being developed for the kind of synthesis and integration demanded in consensus processes. These methodologies, however, are largely related to marshaling the appropriate information inputs into a manageable format for consideration by the consensus group. Setting the ground rules for interaction among participants and for definition of a consensus requires a separate process. Many excellent reviews of group judgment processes already exist (e.g. 18, 26, 30, 37, 64). There also has been much written about the science court approach (87) and the NIH CDC variant, which involves elements of judicial process, scientific conference, and the town hall meeting (65). Most, if not all, of the literature addresses three components: how to generate a common focus in a group, what criteria to use to resolve controversy, and how to define consensus.

The provision of comprehensive background materials and the opportunity for group members to have input can help generate and define a common focus. The two primary methods, however, have been the formulation of a few specific questions, whose answers form the actual consensus (70), and the development of a comprehensive set of scenarios for rating and/or discussing appropriate intervention strategies by the group (10, 67, 72).

Formulating questions is most amenable to processes that have face-to-face contact among group members. Although the practice has not been validated, no more than four to six questions should generally be posed to a group, and the questions should lead to concrete and unambiguous answers (45).

Constructing scenarios for rating is most valuable when a procedure-based topic is under consideration and when the main concerns are safety and effectiveness. Disease-based topics make it much more difficult to comprehensively describe all potential clinical situations. It is even more difficult to integrate the economic, ethical, or other social factors into the scenarios. Some researchers construct representative, rather than comprehensive, scenarios to overcome this difficulty. This approach, however, counteracts the potential advantage of being done by mail—in a manner similar to Delphi techniques (17)—because the group must come together to "fill the gaps" left by the representative scenarios. This hybrid method can, nevertheless, be valuable. The scenarios should generate a common focus and identify the areas of agreement and disagreement between panelists before the meeting. The focus can then be on initial disagreements in a face-to-face meeting that uses time more efficiently to address contentious areas in the form of pre-formulated questions (56).

Defining the criteria for resolution of conflict is perhaps the most difficult part of any group process. Most exercises have not made the criteria for resolution explicit, although many have pointed to the responsibility of the chairperson to ensure smooth operation of this aspect of group process (37, 42, 99). Many panels have an implicit hierarchy of criteria that place controlled trial research above other, less methodologically stringent research evidence, which in turn is valued more highly than clinical experience or personal opinion. Evidence and opinion criteria are less in competition and more complementary: When evidence is available, it is the preeminent determinant; when it is not, the credibility and experience of the various proponents of differing opinions will determine resolution. The ability of research evidence, rather than personal opinion, to better resolve disagreements among group members has been demonstrated in the literature (56, 63). In one exercise, when the above hierarchy of criteria was made explicit, disagreements among panelists before deliberations were resolved by the consensus process for 71% of situations when research evidence existed, but for only 24% when no research was available (56).

Related to the criteria for resolving disagreement is the mechanism used to define consensus, which may be quantitative or qualitative. With the quantitative mechanism, there is less concern over being explicit about the resolving criteria (and less discretion is left in the hands of the group's chairperson). However, the basis for the consensus may be left unclear. Many investigators have explored the properties of different quantitative definitions of consensus in the context of the ratings done on the scenarios (9, 67). No clear guidelines independent of the exercise's purpose have emerged, other than the relatively obvious conclusion that the stricter the criteria the more difficult it is to arrive at consensus. One author has arbitrarily proposed that "if agreement from at least two thirds of the participants can be reached . . . consensus is established" (26).

Although there has been much written to describe alternative group judgment methods, surprisingly little research has been performed to relate chosen options to the outcome. Hence, there is little information to assist prospective convenors of consensus processes in choosing among the alternative approaches. The field needs more systematic assessments of the various methods when they are used under different consensus circumstances. At present, "although we do quite well at assembling experts, we often provide them with inadequate, largely untested means for drawing upon their expertise and for organizing and weighing the evidence" (37).

Criteria for Qualification as a Recommendation

After an exhaustive evaluation of the NIH CDC program, Kanouse et al concluded that "the purposes of the program are better served if the panel approaches its task by asking, 'What meaningful guidance can we give to clinicians based on the current scientific evidence?' rather than 'What definitive recommendations will the biomedical literature support?' " (46). Herein lies probably the single most contentious issue in the debates surrounding choice of consensus approach: Is the purpose of recommendations from consensus processes to establish the best possible guidance for clinical care despite imperfect or incomplete evidence, or is it to promulgate science based only on watertight conclusions derived from methodologically incontestable studies?

The latter approach places great reliance on the randomized controlled trial (RCT). The RCT has been favored by both the Canadian and the American Task Forces on the Periodic Health Examination, and many epidemiologically based consensus conferences restricted to the safety and effectiveness of defined clinical interventions (e.g. 51, 66, 88). When the purpose of the exercise is entirely science-related, e.g. establishing future research requirements, the stringency of such a criterion is appropriate.

For the development of practice guidance, however, there are at least three problems with strict reliance on randomized controlled trial evidence as the only justification for a recommendation. First, such reliance significantly limits the areas of clinical practice in which consensus recommendations can be made. For instance, studies of causation in occupational health would be unethical when using a RCT. For many preventive medicine and public health issues, the length of time between intervention and potential outcome is so long as to make RCTs infeasible (8).

Second, RCTs alone are largely unable to consider economic, ethical, or other social considerations. Thus, a highly effective, but extremely expensive, drug may not warrant recommendation given the opportunity cost of its use. This is precisely the issue in the current debate of tissue plasminogen activator versus streptokinase for the treatment of thrombolysis.

Third, negative recommendations are sometimes appropriate because management options or technologies are being diffused too rapidly or too widely. For example, "the use of cesarean section is *not* indicated for women with an uncomplicated previous cesarean section" (71). Indeed, a major impetus for NIH CDC program was Congress' perception that there was widespread use of many technologies "without sufficient information about their health benefits, clinical risks, cost effectiveness, and societal side effects" (78). In this case, failure to provide a negative recommendation because of the absence of RCT evidence is placing the onus of proof on those trying to prevent unproven interventions from diffusing into practice.

Nevertheless, for strictly clinical effectiveness issues, reliance on methodologies other than the RCT, where it is feasible, can be severely misleading. Recalled experience of clinicians is a notoriously unreliable source of accurate effectiveness estimates. Such estimates tend to be overly optimistic for reasons such as recall bias, regression toward the mean, and placebo effects (20, 82). Even if the purpose of the consensus exercise is to provide guidance for practice, and not the strict promulgation of science, accuracy still requires a distinction between those recommendations supported by RCTs, and those supported by evidence of less certainty.

Many systems have been proposed for such grading of recommendations (14, 21, 82). One of the simplest systems reserves the term "recommendation" for a high level of certainty because of support from methodologically sound studies. The system uses some lesser term, such as "guideline" or "suggestion," for situations supported by less certain forms of evidence (54). The particular grading system is less important than the explicit recognition that different grades of recommendation do exist, based on the methodologic quality of the supporting evidence (40). Thus, consensus groups need not be prevented from producing conclusions that rely largely upon their experience or their interpretation of ethical and social considerations. They should, however, be clearly differentiated as "informed opinions," rather than given the imprimatur of "proven science."

Report Preparation and Format

Who prepares a report can vary from a single professional writer, through planning secretariat, to panel chairperson, and on to joint efforts of the entire consensus group. Many researchers have stressed the importance of a readily understandable and accessible report. They recommend that a professional writer should at least be involved with the final draft (39, 46, 99).

The time taken over report preparation has been the subject of much greater debate. Some panels are put under time pressure to increase their motivations for consensus, use the limited time of experts most efficiently, and capitalize on the attention generated by the group process of evidence consideration (if it has been public). This pressure has resulted in one strategy that has the consensus group drafting and finalizing the report over a period of 24 to 48 hours (39). The approach has been highly criticized because it leads to "lowest common denominator" recommendations on particularly difficult and controversial issues (99), or "is bound to lead to hurried conclusions" (68, p. 1088).

In contrast to this approach, lengthy iterative processes have been used that allow careful consideration of complex issues. It has been argued, however, that procedurally this is cumbersome, time-consuming, and expensive and fails to make maximum and efficient use of all the expert skills convened at one time for the consensus group.

These approaches are not, however, mutually exclusive. They can be combined to obtain the best of both and maximize the amount of input to the final product. After preparation of an initial draft under time pressure, circulation and feedback are undertaken; final drafting follows some weeks or months later (52, 68, 74).

The format of high quality and/or particularly influential reports has been the subject of two evaluations (45, 98). Conclusions from both are similar and, not surprisingly, suggest formats for consensus statements that "1. recommend concrete specific actions; 2. differentiate patients into subclasses when appropriate; and 3. offer didactic advice to the clinician on precise techniques that should be used" (46, p. 26).

These suggestions presume that the objective of the consensus exercise is to give guidance to clinical practice. Thus, they reflect the finding from other surveys that physicians desire "easy-to-read, short, authoritative articles giving the best medical judgment on the value and limitations of new scientific works" (16). In one recent survey of physicians' information preferences, only about one third wished to receive information in "complete form (with evidence)"; the others preferred it in "summary form (with references)." In the same survey, almost 100% had a preference for clinically rather than research-oriented information. Nevertheless, about 60% believed that reports in professional medical journals were very important when first hearing about or deciding to use a new procedure (46).

A credible and potentially influential format clearly demonstrates that a scholarly process has been carefully followed, but presents the guidance in a nonscholarly and easy-to-read manner. It should also provide references (74) and estimates of expected outcomes (21, 37). Finally, the future validation and development of consensus methodology can best be advanced by including explicit descriptions of the procedures and the choices made for each of the seven methodologic areas described in this section on the production of consensus. Without such descriptions, it is difficult to accurately judge the scholarly credibility of the consensus.

THE DISSEMINATION AND IMPACT OF CONSENSUS

Models of Diffusion

Words, whether credible or not, rarely flow automatically into action. Recommendations must be disseminated in ways that provide incentives for such action. Or, those to whom the words are directed must be remarkably receptive to, and already prepared to act on, the message.

Unfortunately, traditional diffusion models, which appear to have been the guide for the dissemination strategies of most previous consensus exercises, "have perhaps placed too much faith in the model of the rational, information-seeking, and probabilistic practitioner, expecting the mere availability of new information to lead to changes in his or her clinical policies" (56, p. 90). This model of the practitioner has been called into question by many recent reviews that point out that research information (synthesized or otherwise) is only one of many determinants of the policies adopted by practitioners.

This more recent work stresses the interaction between characteristics of the receiver, the source, the message and, the channel of the information. This work implies that publication without regard for such interactions is a very weak form of dissemination (5, 30). Furthermore, the process of behavior change requires a set of stages starting with predisposing or priming activities to trigger consideration of change, followed by enabling strategies to motivate and facilitate change, and concluding with reinforcing activities to sustain the change (28, 29, 33, 35, 47). Thus, dissemination should be directed not only at increasing awareness but also at influencing attitudes, knowledge, and, finally, behavior.

Dissemination Strategies

This more recent conception of practitioner behavior change has not, however, been reflected well in the dissemination strategies of most consensus exercises. The overwhelming strategy has been mere publication, sometimes distributed in booklets, sometimes in specialty journals, but most often in general medical journals. Some of the more high-profile programs also rely on the media for short-term dissemination via press conferences. The quality of this reporting, when assessed, has been judged as largely factual and balanced (94).

Multiple sources are identified by practitioners for where they became aware of a consensus statement. The three most frequently cited potential sources were professional medical journals (50%), printed materials such as booklets (30%), and the popular press (25%) (46, 55).

However, awareness of consensus statements among the entire relevant population of practitioners varies considerably. It has been as low as 20% with cardiac surgeons (46) and as high as 90–95% with obstetricians (55) and Swedish physicians (43). Usually, awareness is in the 30–60% range (1, 36, 46). For any specific statement, specialists are more likely to be aware of the recommendations than are general or family practitioners (43, 46).

Direct mailing of the statement to the relevant practitioner population does increase awareness, but even then awareness does not seem to exceed 40% (41, 55). This level of awareness can, however, be significantly increased by making the materials visually attractive and/or "staging" their delivery by dividing them into bite-sized chunks of information (6, 24). However, even this increased awareness may not be reflected in a consequent change in behavior.

The Impact of Dissemination

Methodologically, it is not easy to definitively evaluate the impact of consensus exercises. They are widely disseminated, which makes control groups impossible. It is difficult to insulate an experimentally defined portion of the relevant practitioners from exposure to the consensus. One possibility is to evaluate impact separately from those practitioners aware and those not aware of a particular consensus. Such evaluations have produced conflicting results. Sometimes those aware of the consensus were more likely to have made recent changes that conform to the recommendations (43, 46), but sometimes not (36).

The difficulty with this approach, however, is that the assessment is not representative of the target practitioner population. This is because the likelihood of awareness is correlated with other practitioner variables, such as degree of participation in continuing medical education or journal reading habits (46), which might equally well explain their greater propensity to change. Furthermore, the low levels of awareness for some consensus recommendations makes such an analysis of little relevance.

Thus, evaluations of impact in the entire relevant population require the use of representative chart reviews, analysis of administrative data, or surveys of self-reported behavior. The strongest conclusions about impact can be drawn from those studies that use actual practice data, rather than self-report, and take measurements both before and after the consensus (preferably with a time series to account for preexisting trends in behavior). Weaker, cross-sectional designs can provide impact information only if they require self-reported recall of prior behavior—an unreliable source of measurement. Such cross-sectional designs can, however, provide an estimate of the conformity of practice with the consensus recommendations at a point in time. If the point in time is subsequent to dissemination of a consensus, then we can measure how far the recommendations are falling short in achieving their goal, even if the degree of conformity is unrelated to impacts from the consensus.

Table 1 presents evaluations since 1980 that provide information on either the impact of consensus recommendations on practice behavior or the percent conformity with recommendations. Studies were identified from the sources described earlier. They were included if they measured impact on physician behavior, defined the consensus exercise from which recommendations were drawn, and provided enough description to adequately define the methods used. Nineteen studies met these criteria; they are divided according to whether they used actual practice data or self-reports of behavior.[2]

In the ten instances where impact was measured using actual practice data, six found no impact, two found minor impact, and two found major impact. Interestingly, three of the four studies showing any impact were from Europe [Fowkes & Roberts: UK (28); van Everdingen et al: Holland (88, 89)]. All six of the studies finding no impact were from North America. In the eight instances where an estimate of percent conformity with recommendations was possible, it was less than two thirds of potential for all but one. The one instance was, again, one of the Dutch studies. It was performed in a highly circumscribed practice area (reporting of Breslow thickness for the diagnosis of cutaneous melanoma) and was at a preconsensus conformity level of 83%.

The self-report studies are a less reliable indicator of impact. In the one study where both types of data were available, the percent conformity from the actual practice measure was less than half that of the self-reported estimate (27% versus 63%) (62). Nevertheless, even among these studies where impact is likely overestimated, only one of a possible four shows a major

---

[2]Two studies, McPhee et al (62) and Lomas et al (55), are reported twice because they used both actual practice data and physician self-report.

Table 1 Studies evaluating physicians' practices for impact of or conformity with consensus recommendations

Author	Topic	Method	Impact[a]	Outcome Percent conformity to recommendations[b]
Using Actual Practice Data				
Romm et al 1981	Cancer screening	Chart review, x-sectional	N/A	59
Dietrich & Goldberg 1984	Cancer screening	Chart review, x-sectional	N/A	49
Woo et al 1985	Periodic health exam tests	Chart review, x-sectional	N/A	<100[c]
McPhee et al 1986	Cancer screening	Chart review, x-sectional	N/A	27[d]
Lurie et al 1987	Preventive maneuvers	Claims data, x-sectional	N/A	47[e]
Retchin et al 1985	Coronary surgery	Chart review, x-sectional	N/A	<100[c]
Gleicher 1984	Cesarean section	Hospital discharge data, time series	0	N/A
Fowkes & Roberts 1984	Chest x-rays	Hospital records, time series	+	N/A
Van Everdingen et al 1988	Blood transfusion	Chart review, time series	(+)	N/A
Lomas et al 1989	Cesarean section	Hospital discharge data, time series	0	N/A
Ford et al 1987	Breast cancer	Chart review, before-after	0	33
	Lung cancer	Chart review, before-after	0	67

Kosecoff et al 1987	Coronary surgery	Chart review, time series	0	⎫
	Breast cancer	Chart review, time series	0	⎬ 57[f]
	Cesarean section	Chart review, time series	(+)	⎭
Van Everdingen et al 1989	Cancer pathology	Chart review, before-after	+	97
Using Physician Self Report				
Battista 1983	Periodic health exam	Survey, x-sectional	N/A	61[g]
Winkler et al 1989	8 NIH consensus topics[h]	Survey, x-sectional	N/A	51[j]
Abelson & Lomas 1990	Periodic health exam	Survey, x-sectional	N/A	24–85
McPhee et al 1986	Cancer screening	Survey, x-sectional	N/A	63[d]
Casparie et al 1987	Bed sores	Survey, x-sectional	+	N/A
Lomas et al 1989	Cesarean section	Survey, before-after	(+)	N/A
Hill et al 1988	Hypertension	Survey, before-after	0	73[k]
Johnsson 1988	4 Swedish topics[m]	Survey, x-sectional	0	61–83

[a] 0 = no impact, (+) = minor impact, + = major impact, N/A = not applicable.
[b] percents may represent physicians or cases; N/A = not applicable.
[c] results not reported in a way amenable to calculating mean percent conformity.
[d] mean across 5 screening tests (2 excluded because their expected compliance would be <100); range 13–39 for actual practice and 56–81 for self report.
[e] mean across 9 maneuvers (2 excluded because their expected compliance would be <100); range 1–93.
[f] median value across all 11 consensus recommendations for post recommendation period; range 16–97.
[g] mean across 8 screening tests; range 8–99.
[h] the 8 topics were: coronary surgery, thrombolysis, estrogen use in post menopausal women, pap smear, breast cancer (2), cesarean section, antenatal diagnosis.
[j] median value across all 49 consensus recommendations; range 7.4–98.8.
[k] mean value across 10 recommendations; range 31–96.
[m] the four topics were: hip joint replacement, myocardial infarction, depressive disorders, sight improving surgery.

impact of the consensus on practice (another Dutch study). Percent conformity in the five studies with this measure is still well below 100% in all cases.

These evaluations suggest that, in North America at least, most consensus recommendations have little impact on the behavior of the practitioners at which they are targeted, and leave actual practice far short of what is recommended. The topic areas vary from preventive and public health issues through medical diagnosis and therapy to surgery, but no major differences are discernible. Given the relatively passive dissemination strategies used by most of these consensus exercises, perhaps the results are not surprising.

In light of my earlier discussion of newer models of information diffusion and behavior change, the most that we might expect is that the consensus recommendations would predispose physicians toward change, even if the recommendations fail to motivate or enable the actual change to occur. There is some evidence to support this view of consensus recommendations as "catalysts for consideration of change" from assessments of attitudes toward them and of the changes in attitude that they bring about. In one survey, over 90% of respondents considered consensus recommendations to be usually or sometimes "realistic for clinical practice" (46). In another, nearly 90% of the relevant specialists (obstetricians) fully agreed with the recommendations of a consensus on cesarean birth; one third claimed to have changed practice, even though validating data showed that they were not translating it into action (55).

The future value of consensus exercises may well be in "softening up" practitioners to implement action based on the recommendations. On the basis of reviews elsewhere, the most successful of such behavior change strategies operate at a more local level, and with more careful targeting, than is feasible with a national or regional consensus exercise (23, 56, 84). There is, however, some indication that this "symbiotic" relationship with active strategies that enable and reinforce behavior change may be a potentially fruitful role for future consensus exercises and the recommendations they produce (28, 53).

SUMMARY

When existing evaluations find little or no evidence of consensus recommendations leading to action, one can justifiably ask why so much of this review was dedicated to analyzing alternative ways of producing such "words without action." There are, however, at least two reasons why consensus recommendations should be produced with care and attention to validity.

First, recommendations do sometimes have an impact on behavior as a consequence of mere dissemination activity—the Dutch program, for instance, was more successful than most. This success may occur when the target audience is already particularly receptive to change and the message is timely and delivered by a credible source in a clinically relevant way. Thus, although "such a conjunction of favorable conditions is probably the exception rather than the rule for consensus topics" (46, 240) it does happen.

Second, the output from consensus processes is increasingly a potential input to other processes. Consensus recommendations can be used as the criteria for evaluation and appraisal aimed at changing practice behavior, making administrative decisions on resource allocation, or defining research protocols. For instance, quality assurance activities, such as peer assessment, practitioner certification, or utilization review, are actively seeking criteria with which to make judgments and elicit changes in practice to improve the quality of care. Funding agencies are looking for information to help make reimbursement, capital expenditure, or fee-for-service decisions on cessation of insurance for particular procedures or approaches. These uses of the consensus criteria are potentially major and controversial.

Therefore, even if dissemination rarely leads to action, consensus processes should still be done carefully and with valid techniques. The use of their recommendations embedded within other activities may well lead to (forced) changes in behavior. On ethical grounds alone, we should be as sure as possible that the behavior changes being implied and encouraged are indeed advisable.

For these reasons, the review describes the decision points in the production process for consensus recommendations as a start on the development of a set of recognized standards. The review offers a critical appraisal of the various methodological choices available at each decision point. The seven decision points are selecting a topic, picking the consensus group, providing background preparation, identifying information inputs, choosing a group judgment process, defining the criteria for recommendations, and choosing a report preparation procedure and format.

At least two important points emerged from this review. First, the research is often not well enough developed to give clear indications for many of the choices on what is the "best" alternative. Second, there is often not a single and definitive best, because ultimately choices are most importantly determined by the chosen objective of the exercise. For instance, a scientific expert panel is likely most appropriate for defining future research needs, but a nonexpert panel is preferable when the aim is public participation in technology decisions. It is hoped, however, that the current popularity of consensus processes, the increasing use of their outputs, and the expanding body of research on their conduct will make more definitive conclusions about appropriate alternatives and valid methods possible in the future.

ACKNOWLEDGMENTS

The author receives personnel support as a Career Scientist from the Ontario Ministry of Health. Support for the preparation of this review, and much of the personal research reported in it, was provided by a grant from the National Health Research and Development Programme, Health and Welfare, Canada. For support, comments, and assistance with Table 1, I am grateful to B. J. Porter.

Literature Cited

1. Abelson, J., Lomas, J. 1990. Do health service organizations and community health centres have higher disease prevention and health promotion levels than fee-for-service practices? *Can. Med. Assoc. J.* 142:575–81
2. Ahrens, E. H. 1985. The diet-heart question in 1985: Has it really been settled? *Lancet* 1:1085–87
3. Andersen, T. F., Mooney, G., eds. 1990. *The Challenge of Medical Practice Variations.* London: Macmillan
4. Andreasen, P. B. 1988. Consensus conferences in different countries. Aims and perspectives. *Int. J. Technol. Assess. Health Care* 4:305–8
5. Asch, S. M., Lowe, C. U. 1984. The consensus development program: Theory, process, and critique. *Knowl. Creation Diffus. Util.* 5:369–85
6. Avorn, J., Soumerai, S. B. 1983. Improving drug-therapy decisions through educational outreach. A randomized trial of academically based "detailing." *N. Engl. J. Med.* 308:1457–63
7. Battista, R. N. 1983. Adult cancer prevention in primary care: Patterns of practice in Quebec. *Am. J. Public Health* 73:1036–39
8. Battista, R. N., Fletcher, S. W. 1988. Making recommendations on preventive practices: Methodological issues. *Am. J. Prev. Med.* 4(Suppl.):53–67
9. Brook, R. H., Chassin, M. R., Fink, A., Solomon, D. H., Kosecoff, J., et al. 1986. A method for the detailed assessment of the appropriateness of medical technologies. *Int. J. Technol. Assess. Health Care* 2:53–64
10. Brook, R. H., Lohr, K. 1985. Efficacy, effectiveness, variations, and quality: Boundary-crossing research. *Med. Care* 23:710–22
11. Brook, R. H., Park, R. E., Winslow, C. M., Kosecoff, J. B., Chassin, M. R., et al. 1988. Diagnosis and treatment of coronary disease: Comparison of doctors' attitudes in the USA and the UK. *Lancet* 1:750–53
12. Bunker, J. P., Roos, L. L., Fowles, J., Roos, N. P. 1985. Information systems and routine monitoring in the United States and Canada—with examples from surgical practice. In *Oxford Textbook of Public Health*, ed. L. Holland. Toronto: Oxford Univ. Press. pp. 77–86
13. Calltorp, J. 1988. Consensus development conferences in Sweden. Effects on health policy and administration. *Int. J. Technol. Assess. Health Care* 4:75–88
14. Canadian Task Force on the Periodic Health Examination. 1979. The periodic health examination. *Can. Med. Assoc. J.* 121:1194–1254
15. Casparie, A. F., Klazinga, N. S., van Everdingen, J. J., Touw, P. P. 1987. Health-care providers resolve clinical controversies: The Dutch consensus approach. *Aust. Clin. Rev.* 7:43–47
16. Comroe, J. H. 1978. The road from research to new diagnosis and therapy. *Science* 200:931–37
17. Dalkey, N. 1969. An experimental study of group opinion: the Delphi Method. *Futures* (September), pp. 408–26
18. Delbecq, A. L., Van de Ven, A., Gustafson, D. H. 1975. *Group Techniques for Program Planning.* Glenview, Ill: Scott, Foresman
19. Dietrich, A. J., Goldberg, H. 1984. Preventive content of adult primary care: Do generalists and subspecialists differ? *Am. J. Public Health* 74:223–27
20. Eddy, D. M. 1982. Clinical policies and the quality of clinical practice. *N. Engl. J. Med.* 307:343–47
21. Eddy, D. M. 1989. *A Manual for Assessing Health Practices and Designing Practice Policies (Draft, May 31).* Washington, DC: Counc. Med. Specialty Soc. Task Force Pract. Policies
22. Eichhorn, A. J., Cooper, J. B., Cullen, D. J., Maier, W. R., Philip, J. H., et al. 1986. Standards for patient monitoring

during anesthesia at Harvard Medical School. *J. Am. Med. Assoc.* 256:1017–20

23. Eisenberg, J. M. 1986. *Doctors' Decisions and the Costs of Medical Care.* Ann Arbor, Mich: Health Adm. Press

24. Evans, C. E., Haynes, R. B., Birkett, N. J. 1986. Does a mailed continuing education program improve physician performance? Results of a randomized tiral in antihypertensive care. *J. Am. Med. Assoc.* 255:501–4

25. Feeny, D., Guyatt, G., Tugwell, P., eds. 1986. *Health Care Technology: Effectiveness, Efficiency, and Public Policy.* Montreal: Inst. Res. Public Policy

26. Fink, A., Kosecoff, J., Chassin, M. R., Brook, R. H. 1984. Consensus methods: Characteristics and guidelines for use. *Am. J. Public Health* 74:979–83

27. Ford, L. G., Hunter, C. P., Diehr, P., Frelick, R. W., Yates, J. 1987. Effects of patient management guidelines on physician practice patterns: The community hospital oncology program experience. *J. Clin. Oncol.* 5:504–11

28. Fowkes, F. G., Roberts, C. J. 1984. Introducing guidelines into clinical practice. *Effect. Health Care* 1:313–23

29. Geertsma, R. H., Parker, R. C., Whitbourne, S. K. 1982. How physicians view the process of change in their practice behavior. *J. Med. Educ.* 57:752–61

30. Glaser, E. M. 1980. Using behavioral science strategies for defining the state-of-the-art. *J. Appl. Behav. Sci.* 16:79–92

31. Gleicher, N. 1984. Cesarean section rates in the United States: The short-term failure of the National Consensus Development Conference in 1980. *J. Am. Med. Assoc.* 252:3273–76

32. Goodman, C., ed. 1988. *Medical Technology Assessment Directory: A Pilot Reference to Organizations, Assessments, and Information Sources.* Washington, DC: Natl. Acad. Press

32a. Goodman, C., Baratz, S. R., eds. 1990. *Improving Consensus Development for Health Technology Assessment: An International Perspective.* Council Health Care Tech., Inst. Med., Washington, DC: Nat. Acad Press

33. Green, L. W., Eriksen, M. P. 1988. Behavioral determinants of preventive practices by physicians. *Am. J. Prev. Med.* 4(Suppl.):101–7

34. Greer, A. L. 1987. The two cultures of biomedicine: Can there be consensus? *J. Am. Med. Assoc.* 258:2739–40

35. Greer, A. L. 1988. The state of the art versus the state of the science: The diffu-

sion of new medical technologies into practice. *Int. J. Technol. Assess. Health Care* 4:5–26

36. Hill, M. N., Levine, D. M., Whelton, P. K. 1988. Awareness, use, and impact of the 1984 Joint National Committee consensus report on high blood pressure. *Am. J. Public Health* 78:1190–94

37. Inst. Medicine. 1985. *Assessing Medical Technologies.* Washington, DC: Natl. Acad. Press

38. Deleted in proof

39. Jacoby, I. 1985. The consensus development program of the National Institutes of Health. *Int. J. Technol. Assess. Health Care* 2:420–32

40. Jacoby, I. 1988. Evidence and consensus. *J. Am. Med. Assoc.* 259:3039

41. Jacoby, I., Clark, S. 1986. Direct mailing as a means of disseminating NIH consensus statements. *J. Am. Med. Assoc.* 255:1328–30

42. Jennett, B. 1985. First consensus development conference in United Kingdom: On coronary artery bypass grafting. II. Commentary by chairman of conference. *Br. Med. J.* 291:716–18

43. Johnsson, M. 1988. Evaluation of the consensus conference program in Sweden. Its impact on physicians. *Int. J. Technol. Assess. Health Care* 4:89–94

44. Joint Natl. Comm. Detection, Evaluation, Treatment of High Blood Pressure. 1977. Report of the JNC on Detection, Evaluation, and Treatment of High Blood Pressure. *J. Am. Med. Assoc.* 237:255–61

45. Kahan, J. P., Kanouse, D. E., Winkler, J. D. 1988. Stylistic variations in Natl. Inst. Health consensus statements, 1979–1983. *Int. J. Technol. Assess. Health Care* 4:289–304

46. Kanouse, D. E., Brook, R. H., Winkler, J. D., Kosecoff, J., Berry, S. H., et al. 1989. *Changing Medical Practice Through Technology Assessment. An Evaluation of the NIH Consensus Development Program.* Ann Arbor, Mich: Health Adm. Press

47. Kanouse, D. E., Jacoby, I. 1988. When does information change practitioners' behavior? *Int. J. Technol. Assess. Health Care* 4:27–33

48. Klazinga, N. S., Casparie, A. F., van Everdingen, J. J. 1987. Contribution of medical decision-making to consensus development conferences. *Health Policy* 8:339–46

49. Kolata, G. 1985. Heart panel's conclusions questioned. *Science* 227:40–41

49a. Kosecoff, J., Kanouse, D. E., Rogers, W. H., McCloskey, L., Winslow, C., Brook, R. H. 1987. Effects of the

64   LOMAS

National Institutes of Health Consensus Development Program on physician practice. *J. Am. Med. Assoc.* 258:2708–13

50. Lane, D. A. 1988. Making recommendations on preventive practices: Methodological issues. *Am. J. Prev. Med.* 4(Suppl.):68–72
51. Logan, A. G. 1984. Report of the Canadian Hypertension Society's consensus conference on the management of mild hypertension. *Can. Med. Assoc. J.* 131:1053–56
52. Lomas, J. 1986. The consensus process and evidence dissemination. *Can. Med. Assoc. J.* 134:1340–41
53. Lomas, J. 1989. *The role of a consensus statement in changing physicians' awareness, attitudes, knowledge, and behaviour.* Presented at Ann. Meet. Int. Soc. Technol. Assess. Health Care, 5th, London
54. Lomas, J., Anderson, G. M., Enkin, M., Vayda, E., Roberts, R., et al. 1988. The role of evidence in the consensus process. Results from a Canadian consensus exercise. *J. Am. Med. Assoc.* 259:3001–5
55. Lomas, J., Anderson, G. M., Pierre, K. D., Vayda, E., Enkin, M. W., et al. 1989. Do practice guidelines guide practice? The effect of a consensus statement on the practice of physicians. *N. Engl. J. Med.* 321:1306–11
56. Lomas, J., Haynes, R. B. 1988. A taxonomy and critical review of tested strategies for the application of clinical practice recommendations; from "official" to "individual" clinical policy. *Am. J. Prev. Med.* 4(Suppl.):77–94
57. Lord, C., Ross, L., Lepper, M. 1979. Biased assimilation and attitude polarization: The effect of prior theories on subsequently considered evidence. *J. Pers. Soc. Psychol.* 37:2098–109
58. Lurie, N., Manning, W. G., Peterson, C., Goldberg, G. A., Phelps, C. A., et al. 1987. Preventive care: Do we practice what we preach? *Am. J. Public Health* 77:801–4
59. Markle, G. E., Chubin, D. E. 1987. Consensus development in biomedicine: The liver transplant controversy. *Milbank Mem. Fund Q.* 65:1–24
60. Marmot, M. G. 1986. Epidemiology and the art of the soluble. *Lancet* 1:897–900
61. May, W. E. 1985. Consensus or coercion. *J. Am. Med. Assoc.* 254:1077
62. McPhee, S. J., Richard, R. J., Solkowitz, S. N. 1986. Performance of cancer screening in a university general internal medicine practice: Comparison with the American Cancer Society guidelines. *J. Gen. Intern. Med.* 1:275–81
63. Merrick, N. J., Fink, A., Park, R. E. 1987. Derivation of clinical indications for carotid endarterectomy by an expert panel. *Am. J. Public Health* 77:187–90
64. Moore, C. 1986. *Group Decision-Making Techniques.* Beverly Hills, Calif: Sage
65. Mullan, F., Jacoby, I. 1985. The town meeting for technology: The maturation of consensus conferences. *J. Am. Med. Assoc.* 254:1068–72
66. Natl. Heart Lung Blood Inst., 1982. Management of patient compliance in the treatment of hypertension. Report of a Working Group. *Hypertension* 4:415–23
67. Naylor, C. D., Basinski, A., Baigre, R. S., Goldman, B. S., Lomas, J. 1990. Placing patients in the queue for coronary revascularization: Evidence for practice variations from an expert panel process. *Am. J. Public Health.* In press
68. Oliver, M. F. 1985. Consensus or nonsensus conferences on coronary heart disease. *Lancet* 1:1087–89
69. Off. Med. Appl. Res. n.d. *Participants Guide to Consensus Development Conferences.* Bethesda, Md: Natl. Inst. Health
70. Off. Med. Appl. Res. 1983. *Guidelines for the Selection and Management of Consensus Development Conferences.* Bethesda, Md: Natl. Inst. Health
71. Panel Natl. Consensus Conf. Aspects Cesarean Birth. 1986. Indications for cesarean section: Final statement of the panel of the Natl. Consensus Conf. Aspects Cesarean Birth. *Can. Med. Assoc. J.* 1348–52
72. Park, R. E., Fink, A., Brook, R. H., Chassin, M. R., Kahn, K. L., et al. 1986. Physician ratings of appropriate indications for six medical and surgical procedures. *Am. J. Public Health* 76:766–72
73. Pauker, S. 1986. Decision analysis as a synthetic tool for achieving consensus in technology assessment. *Int. J. Technol. Assess. Health Care* 2:83–91
74. Perry, S. 1987. The NIH consensus development program: A decade later. *N. Engl. J. Med.* 317:485–88
75. Physician Paym. Rev. Comm. 1989. *Annu. Rep. Congress*, pp. 219–30. Washington, DC: Physician Paym. Rev. Comm.
76. Rahimtoola, S. H. 1981. A consensus on coronary bypass surgery. *Ann. Intern. Med.* 94:272–73
77. Retchin, S. M., Fletcher, R. H., Buescher, P. C. 1985. The application of

official policy: Prophylaxis recommendations for patients with mitral valve prolapse. *Med. Care* 23:1156–62
78. Richmond, J. B. 1978. Statement before the subcommittee on domestic and international scientific planning, analysis, and cooperation. *Congr. Rec.* Oct. 6
79. Rogers, E. M., Larsen, J. K., Lowe, C. U. 1982. The consensus development process for medical technologies: A cross-cultural comparison of Sweden and the United States. *J. Am. Med. Assoc.* 248:1880–82
80. Romm, F. J., Fletcher, S. W., Hulka, B. S. 1981. The periodic health examination: comparison of recommendations and internists' performance. *South. Med. J.* 74:265–70
81. Roper, W., Winkenwerder, W., Hackbarth, G., Krakauer, H. 1988. Effectiveness in health care: An initiative to evaluate and improve medical practice. *N. Engl. J. Med.* 319:1197–1202
82. Sackett, D. L. 1986. Rules of evidence and clinical recommendations on the use of antithrombotic agents. *Chest* 89 (Suppl.):2S–3S
83. Sacks, H. S., Berrier, J., Reitman, D. 1987. Meta-analysis of randomized clinical trials. *N. Engl. J. Med.* 316:450–55
84. Schroeder, S. A. 1987. Strategies for reducing medical costs by changing physicians' behavior: Efficacy and impact on quality of care. *Int. J. Technol. Asses. Health Care* 3:39–50
85. Siu, A., Sonnenberg, F., Manning, W. H. 1986. Inappropriate use of hospitals in a randomized trial of health insurance plans. *N. Engl. J. Med.* 315:1259–66
86. Stocking, B. 1985. First consensus development conference in the United Kingdom: On coronary artery bypass grafting. I Views of audience, panel and speakers. *Br. Med. J.* 291:713–16
87. Task Force Pres. Advis. Group Anticipated Adv. Sci. Technol. 1976. The science court experiment: an interim report. *Science* 193:653–56
88. van Everdingen, J. J., Klazinga, N. S., Casparie, A. F. 1988. Blood transfusion policy in Dutch hospitals. *Int. J. Health Care Qual. Assur.* 1:16–19
89. van Everdingen, J. J., Rampen, F. H., Ruiter, D. J., Casparie, A. F. 1989.

Evalutie consensus melanoom van de hui op grond van pathologisch-anatomische verslagen. *Ned. Tijdschr. Geneeskd.* 133:2285–88
90. Vang, J. 1986. The consensus development conference and the European experience. *Int. J. Technol. Assess. Health Care* 2:65–76
91. White, L. J., Ball, J. R. 1985. The Clinical Efficacy Assessment Project of the American College of Physicians. *Int. J. Technol. Assess. Health Care* 1:169–74
92. Williams, A. H. 1985. Economics of coronary artery bypass grafting. *Br. Med. J.* 291:326–29
93. Williamson, J. W., German, P. S., Weiss, R., Skinner, E. A., Bowes, F. 1989. Health science information management in continuing education of physicians: A survey of US primary care practitioners and their opinion leaders. *Ann. Intern. Med.* 110:151–60
94. Winkler, J. D., Kanouse, D. E., Brodsley, L., Brook, R. H. 1986. Popular press coverage of eight Natl. Inst. Health consensus development topics. *J. Am. Med. Assoc.* 255:1323–27
95. Winkler, J. D., Kanouse, D. E., Berry, S. H., Brook, R. H. 1989. Physicians' conformity to consensus recommendations. In *Changing Medical Practice Through Technology Assessment,* ed. D. E. Kanouse, pp. 102–26. Ann Arbor, Mich: Health Adm. Press
96. Winkler, J. D., Lohr, K., Brook, R. H. 1985. Persuasive communication and medical technology assessment. *Arch. Intern. Med.* 145:314–17
97. Woo, B., Woo, B., Cook, E. F., Weisberg, M., Goldman, L. 1985. Screening procedures in the asymptomatic adult: Comparison of physicians' recommendations, patients' desires, published guidelines, and actual practice. *J. Am. Med. Assoc.* 254:1480–84
98. Wortman, P. M., Vinokur, A., Sechrest, L. 1982. *Evalution of NIH Consensus Development Program, Phase I: Final Report.* Ann Arbor, Mich: Inst. Soc. Res., Univ. Mich.
99. Wortman, P. M., Vinokur, A., Sechrest, L. 1988. Do consensus conferences work? A process evaluation of the NIH consensus development program. *J. Health Polit. Policy Law* 13:469–98

Annu. Rev. Publ. Health. 1991. 12:67–84

LONG-TERM CARE FINANCING: PROBLEMS AND PROGRESS[1]

Joshua M. Wiener and Raymond J. Hanley

Economic Studies Program, The Brookings Institution, Washington, DC 20036

KEY WORDS: private insurance, public insurance, elderly, disability, Medicaid

INTRODUCTION

There is good news and bad news about long-term care financing. The bad news is that the United States does not have, either in the private or the public sectors, satisfactory ways of helping people anticipate and pay for nursing home and home care. As the cost of a year in a nursing home exceeds $29,000, long-term care is the main cause of catastrophic health care expense for the elderly (21, 22).

The disabled elderly and their families find, often to their surprise, that neither private insurance nor Medicare covers the costs of long-term care to any significant extent. The disabled elderly must rely on their own resources or, when these have been exhausted, turn to welfare in the form of Medicaid. The aging of the baby boom generation, combined with rapidly falling mortality rates for the elderly, will lead to sharply increased demand for long-term care that will require substantially greater public and private spending far into the next century.

The good news is that long-term care financing, which has traditionally been a backwater issue, has moved up on the national political agenda. It is now widely recognized as one of the country's most pressing social policy issues. In 1988, almost all of the major health care players in Congress, including Senators Mitchell, Kennedy, and Durenberger and Representatives Stark, Waxman, and Gradison, introduced long-term care financing bills. In

---

[1]These opinions are those of the authors and should not be attributed to other staff members, officers, or Trustees of the Brookings Institution.

0163-7525/91/0501-0067$02.00

addition, long-term care financing is partly the subject of two Congressionally mandated commissions—the US Bipartisan Commission on Comprehensive Health Care (also known as the Pepper Commission) and the Advisory Council on Social Security. It is also a major component of the health policy review ordered by President Bush in his 1990 State of the Union address.

The fundamental policy question is whether we can come up with a financing system that works better than just multiplying the current unsatisfactory system by three or four. There is good news here, as well. More than ever before, a lot of thought and energy is going into the development of long-term care financing system reform.

BACKGROUND

Total nursing home and home care expenditures for the elderly were an estimated $42 billion in 1988 (23). Most spending goes toward nursing home care, which accounts for 79% of the total.

The striking fact about current long-term care financing is that only a trivial portion of the bill is paid by any form of insurance. Only 3% of the elderly have any private long-term care insurance (28); about 1% of total nursing home expenditures are paid by private insurance (8). Medicare covers short stays in skilled nursing facilities, but Medicare spending amounts to less than 3% of nursing home expenditures (8). Somewhat expanded nursing home benefits under Medicare were eliminated with repeal of the Medicare Catastrophic Coverage Act of 1988.

The disabled elderly who use long-term care pay for it out of their own or their family's income and assets—or they turn to welfare. Out-of-pocket spending accounts for 55%, and Medicaid accounts for about 43% of all spending for elderly nursing home care (23). Medicaid is the dominant source of public funding; it accounts for nearly 80% of government spending for nursing home and home care for the elderly.

The cost of an extended stay in a nursing home exceeds the financial resources of many elderly. Thus, it is not surprising that 41% of elderly nursing home discharges (26) and 49% of elderly nursing home residents rely on Medicaid as their primary source of payment (18).

In 1990, individuals generally do not qualify for Medicaid if they have liquid assets of more than $2000, excluding the value of their home. To qualify, patients must also contribute all of their income to help pay for care, after they deduct funds for a small personal needs allowance of about $30 per month, uncovered medical expenses, and maintenance of a community spouse (4). Provisions in the unrepealed sections of the Medicare Catastrophic Coverage Act of 1988 substantially liberalized the requirements for married couples, an important but small group of nursing home users. Medicaid will only help pay the bills for those nursing home patients who meet the assets test and whose medical expenses exceed their ability to pay from current income. The process by which patients deplete their income and assets to the Medicaid financial eligibility level is known as "spending down."

Over the next several decades, the bill for long-term care is certain to rise rapidly. The Brookings-ICF Long-Term Care Financing Model provides detailed projections of the number of disabled elderly to the year 2020. The model includes their income, resources, and likely use of long-term care. It assumes that mortality rates continue to decline, incomes and inflation continue to grow at moderate levels, and current long-term care financing policies do not change (23). Four results of these projections are notable.

First, the older population will grow rapidly, and the number of very elderly will rise even faster. Because more of the population over age 65 will be over 75, more of the elderly will also be disabled. The increase in disabled elderly will mean more users of long-term care, especially nursing home care. The number of persons over 65 is projected to increase 61% between 1988 and 2018; however, the nursing home population will increase 76%. Nursing home residents will also be older—51% will be over 85 in 2018, compared with 42% in 1988.

Second, older persons will be significantly better off financially by 2018. Real incomes of persons aged 65 and over will more than double over the three decades because of more and higher pensions, increases in Social Security benefits, and income from assets.

Third, spending for long-term care will increase rapidly, especially for nursing homes (see Table 1). If nursing home costs rise 5.8% a year (compared with a 4% annual increase assumed for the general price level), nursing home spending for the elderly will triple. It will rise from $33 billion in 1988 to $98 billion (in constant 1987 dollars) by 2018.

Finally, the proportion of nursing home expenditures accounted for by Medicaid will not decline, nor will the proportion of nursing home patients dependent on Medicaid. This last result is surprising. If the overall economic well-being of the elderly is expected to improve substantially over the period, why should they not become less dependent on a program intended for the poor? The answer is that long-term care costs are projected to rise as least as fast as the incomes of the very elderly, the group most likely to use long-term care. Thus, those with the greatest risk of needing care will be no better off in terms of their ability to pay for it than the same group is today.

GOALS FOR FINANCING REFORM

The most important goal for improving long-term care financing is to treat long-term care as a normal risk of growing old. The costs of long-term care should not come as an unpleasant surprise that causes severe financial distress

Table 1 Thirty-year projection: Long-term care spending for the elderly 1986–90 to 2016–20 in billions of 1987 dollars[a]

Payment source	1986–90	2016–20	Percent increase, 1986–90 to 2016–20
	Nursing home services		
Medicaid	14.1	46.2	227
Medicare	0.6	1.6	168
Out-of-pocket	18.3	50.3	176
Total	33.0	98.1	197
	Home care services		
Medicaid	1.2	2.4	95
Medicare	3.1	7.7	149
Other payers[b]	2.7	7.2	170
Out-of-pocket payments	1.6	4.6	182
Total	8.6	21.9	154

SOURCE: Brookings-ICF Long-Term Care Financing Model. Figures are rounded.
[a] Average annual expenditures. Nursing home and home care inflation is assumed to be 5.8 percent a year. General inflation is assumed to be 4% a year; long-term care inflation in excess of general inflation is assumed to be 1.8% a year.
[b] Other payers include state and local expenditures, social services block grant, Older Americans Act and Veterans Administration home care funds, charity, and out-of-pocket expenditures, by persons other than the service recipient.

to individuals and families. Right now, the pain and anxiety inherent in becoming disabled or caring for a disabled relative are compounded by worries over how to pay for care. One of the great fears of the elderly is that they will be a burden on their children. It should come as no surprise that Americans highly value their independence.

The desire to protect the elderly against the financial burden of long-term care embodies two distinct aims. One goal is to protect the elderly from depleting their life savings simply because they end up in a nursing home or need extensive home care. This goal is most important to middle- and upper-class individuals who have significant assets and it is at the heart of the concern about Medicaid spend-down.

Although highly rated by many elderly, asset protection is probably the most controversial of long-term care financing goals. While acknowledging problems with the current situation, some groups question whether protecting financial estates that will be passed on to adult children is an appropriate public policy goal: What are savings for, if not to help pay for needed care at the end of life? At the very least, this position argues for a sharply progressive financing structure, so that the expenditures associated with asset protection will be paid by the upper class individuals who are most likely to benefit.

A separate but related concern is to prevent elderly persons who have been financially independent all of their lives from depending on welfare, with its indignities and stigma. About 35% of all nursing home discharges are Medicaid at admission, an unknown but probably higher proportion of whom were not Medicaid eligible in the community (26).

Reform of the financing system should also create a more balanced delivery system by expanding home care. The rationale for such reform should be addressing unmet needs in the community, supplying the type of care the elderly overwhelmingly want, and providing respite to family caregivers. Although one wishes it were otherwise, the preponderance of research argues that cost savings do not result from expanded home care (14, 23, 29). Expanded home care generally raises, rather than lowers, expenditures because large increases in such care more than offset small decreases in nursing home care.

The financing system should also improve quality of care and the flexibility and efficiency of the delivery system. The system should encourage experimentation with new ways of organizing care designed to increase patient satisfaction and avoid nursing home placement.

At the same time, reforms should limit the rise in long-term care expenditures and moderate the inflationary pressures on the long-term care industry. As usual, the objective of ensuring more and better care conflicts with the objective of minimizing public and private costs. Policymakers must find the appropriate balance (12).

ROLES OF THE PUBLIC AND PRIVATE SECTORS

What should be the roles of the public and private sectors in financing long-term care? Some groups believe that the primary responsibility for care of the elderly should fall on individuals and their families; the government should act only as a payer of last resort for those who are unable to provide for themselves. The opposite view is that the government should provide comprehensive long-term care for all elderly persons, with little cost sharing and regardless of financial need. In this view, there is little or no role for the private sector. Between these polar views, many combinations of public and private responsibility are possible.

The choice of emphasis between public and private programs depends not just on differences in political ideology, but also on differences in which private initiatives are feasible and affordable and whom they would benefit. For example, if it were demonstrably possible to market private sector financing mechanisms that would protect a large majority of the elderly from hardship and reduce dependence on Medicaid, then many people would see little need for new kinds of government intervention. Conversely, if private initiatives were not to prove so widespread or to play a major role in paying for nursing home and home care, then the case for an expanded public role would be stronger.

PRIVATE LONG-TERM CARE INSURANCE

There are many possible private sector financing mechanisms, including tax-favored long-term care savings accounts, continuing care retirement communities, home equity, and long-term care benefits to health maintenance organizations. However, by far the most widespread of all private sector options is long-term care insurance. Private long-term care insurance is a growing and rapidly changing market. A survey conducted by the Health Insurance Association of America (HIAA) found that the number of companies selling policies increased from 75 in 1987 to 118 in 1989 (Highlights of HIAA Long-Term Care Insurance Survey, March 1990, unpublished). As of December 1989, there were about 1 million policies in force.

Demand and Supply Barriers

The availability of private long-term care insurance is a recent phenomenon, available to any significant extent only in the last four years. Development has been slow because of barriers on both the demand and the supply side.

On the demand side, there have been three major barriers. Historically, the elderly were disproportionately poor and unable to afford substantial premium payments. This barrier is much less true now, as the income of the elderly has increased substantially over the last 20 years. Although the elderly still have the highest poverty and near-poverty rates of any adult group, most current evidence suggests that the elderly as a whole are roughly as well off as the rest of the population (7, 13). Most estimates of the future income and assets of the elderly project substantial further improvements over time (32).

Despite improvements in income, private long-term care insurance remains expensive for most elderly. According to HIAA, the average annual premium for the 15 top-selling individual long-term care insurance products with some inflation protection is $1395 per person if purchased at age 65; it climbs rapidly to $4199 per person at age 79 (Highlights of HIAA Long-Term Care Insurance Survey, March 1990, unpublished). Thus, married couples must pay annual premiums of $2800–$8400, a considerable amount of money by any measure.

The second barrier is most individuals are unaware of or denied their risk of needing long-term care services. Most research suggests that persons who live to age 65 face a four out of ten chance of spending some time in a nursing home before they die and a one in five chance of spending more than a year (6, 17). People seem willing to accept the possibility that they will someday get sick and will need to visit a doctor or be admitted to a hospital, but few people will admit that they face a significant lifetime risk of becoming disabled and using expensive nursing home or home care.

Finally, there has been extensive misinformation. Although many people think that Medicare or their Medigap policies cover long-term care (9, 31), these programs do not cover such costs. The debate over the Medicare Catastrophic Coverage Act of 1988 largely exploded the myth of Medicare long-term care coverage for the Congress, the media, and the general public.

On the supply side, there have also been several barriers. Insurers have worried about whether long-term care was, in fact, an insurable risk. They worry about "moral hazard"—the increased use of services that results when individuals have insurance. As most long-term care is currently provided by family members at no formal cost, the possible increase in use is large. Because only about 25% of the disabled elderly in the community receive paid home care (Hanley and Wiener, unpublished), there is a substantial possibility of increased use of services by the many individuals who would "medically" qualify.

In addition, insurers worry about adverse selection—the possibility that people who "know" they will use long-term care services will disproportionately buy the insurance, which will drive up use beyond expectations. This creates a vicious circle: Premiums have to be raised, which causes low risk people to drop their policies, which in turn forces additional increases in premiums.

Finally, insurers have been concerned about the timing of premium payments and the ultimate use of benefits. Long-term care is needed principally by the very elderly, especially those age 85 and over. Thus, there is likely to be a very long time between initial purchase of the insurance policy and its eventual use. For example, a policy bought at age 65 might not be used for 20 years; a policy bought at age 45 might not be used for 40 years. Unforeseen changes in disability or mortality rates, utilization patterns, inflation in nursing home and home care costs, or the rate of return on financial reserves can dramatically change a profitable policy into a highly unprofitable one.

Despite these supply and demand barriers, insurers are moving into the marketplace. Although policies are improving, most of them still have major restrictions. Most insurers are still extremely cautious about whom they sell policies to. It is not uncommon for insurers to reject 10–30% of applications. In addition, they are not marketing products as aggressively as they might. Insurers still do not know if this will be a profitable line of business.

Projections of the Role of Private Insurance

Although no one knows for sure what the future will be like, simulations that use the Brookings-ICF Long-Term Care Financing Model provide an order of magnitude estimate of what the potential influence of private insurance might be over the next 30 years (see Figure 1 for detailed assumptions of the simulations and Table 2 for results). The simulations assume that mortality rates continue to decline, disability rates remain constant, nursing home and

Figure 1 Summary of private long-term care insurance simulation assumptions.

Assumptions	Big benefit	Low benefit	New policy 5%	New policy 3%	Young insurance
Nursing home payment per day	$50	$50, $40, $30	$50	$50	$50
Indexed benefit	$2.50 for 10 years	$2.50, $2.00, $1.50 for 10 years	$2.50 until age 85	$2.50 until age 85	Fully indexed at 5.8%
Deductible	100 days	100 days	100 days	100 days	90 days
Length of coverage	6 years	6 years	4 years	4 years	1 year to unlimited
Prior hospitalization required	Yes	Yes	No	No	No
Any home care benefits	Yes	Yes	Yes	Yes	No
Premiums					
50 year-old	N/A	N/A	$236	$236	See Table 1
60 year-old	N/A	N/A	$413	$413	See Table 1
65 year-old	$584	$584–$350	$583	$583	See Table 1
80 year-old	$1,642	$1,642–$985	$1,676	$1,676	See Table 1
Indexed after purchase	No	No	No	No	Yes
Purchase assumptions					
Can disabled buy	No	No	No	No	No
Premiums as % Income/assets					
Age < 55	N/A	N/A	< 1%/NA	< 1%/NA	< 1%/NA
Age 55–64	N/A	N/A	< 3%/NA	< 1%/NA	< 1%/NA
Age 65+	< 5%/$10,000	< 5%/$10,000	< 5%/$10,000	< 3%/$10,000	< 3%/$10,000
Does one person buy if couple cannot afford 2 policies	No	No	Yes	Yes	No

Table 2   Key simulation results for private insurance, 2018

Option	Percent of elderly participating	Percent of total nursing home expenditures paid by insurance*	Percent change from base case Medicaid nursing home expenditures*
Big benefit	25	7	− 5
Low benefit	45	12	− 1
New policy 5%	54	17	−15
New policy 3%	33	10	− 6
Young insurance	63	17	−12

Source: Brookings-ICF Long-Term Care Financing Model.

*For New policy 5% and New policy 3%, the simulations include spousal impoverishment and Medicare SNF changes mandated by Medicare Catastrophic Coverage Act of 1988. Big benefit, Low benefit and Young insurance do not include these changes.

home care use rates remain constant, incomes and general inflation continue to grow at moderate levels, and nursing home and home care inflation are somewhat higher than general inflation. In general, these assumptions reflect those used by the Social Security Administration in their widely-used, mid-range Alternative II-B projections (24).

We used optimistic assumptions about the willingness of people to pay for insurance and the willingness of insurers to offer it to project the potential market for private insurance initiatives for the next three decades. The purpose was to determine the most that can reasonably be expected from the private sector with respect to participation, proportion of long-term care expenses financed, and reduction of Medicaid use.

Some of the assumptions could be criticized as exaggerating the affordability and effectiveness of private insurance in meeting the need for long-term care. For example, in three simulations, 100% of persons who can buy policies for 5% of their income (and have $10,000 in nonhousing assets) are assumed to buy insurance at age 65 or 67, even though the purchase would mean a substantial increase in out-of-pocket costs for health care for most elderly.

The projections indicated substantial potential for growth of private insurance for long-term care. A potential multibillion dollar market is almost entirely untapped. Persons who purchase these products will have better financial protection than they have now.

Even under our optimistic assumptions about who would participate, private sector financing cannot be relied on to do the whole job. Private sector approaches are unlikely to be affordable by a substantial majority of elderly persons, to finance more than a modest proportion of total nursing home and home care expenditures, or to have more than a modest impact on Medicaid expenditures. For example, by 2018, private long-term care insurance sold to the elderly might be purchased by 25–54% of the elderly, might account for 7–17% of total nursing home expenditures, and might reduce Medicaid expenditures by 1–16% compared with what would have been spent without private insurance. Private insurance that is initially sold to persons under age 65 would be more affordable, but would still account for only about 17% of nursing home expenditures in 2018.

Private sector options have a relatively modest impact for two reasons. First, they are too expensive for most elderly, especially those individuals who would otherwise end up on Medicaid (33). Because total long-term care expenditures per capita age 65 and over exceed $1300 a year, this fact is hardly surprising. Total (public and private) long-term care costs roughly equal Medicare physician and other anticipated expenditures and exceed three fourths of Medicare hospital expenditures. Thus, costs never become trivial, even when they are spread over the whole elderly population.

Second, although private long-term care insurance policies are rapidly evolving and improving, policies now available are limited in the amount of financial protection that they offer. For example, policies often have preexisting condition exclusions and age restrictions on who may purchase policies and they cover relatively little home care (28, 30). Reimbursement levels usually do not increase with inflation, or if they do, benefits do not increase sufficiently to provide full protection. This can be a serious problem because a payment level that is adequate today will not be adequate in the future. An indemnity policy with a $50 per day nursing home benefit purchased at age 65, when it's relatively affordable, will need to pay over $150 per day at age 85 to have comparable purchasing power.

There is no inherent reason why insurers could not eliminate these restrictions and provide better financial protection. The problem is that improved coverage and affordability are tradeoffs within the elderly population. That is, coverage improvements are likely to make products more expensive, thus affordability is reduced. For example, if the indemnity level was fully indexed to inflation, premiums for nonindexed policies for the elderly would probably increase by about 30–40%.

Group Insurance

One potential way out of this tradeoff is through group insurance geared to the nonelderly, working population (11). Unlike most acute health care insurance, 97% of long-term care insurance is sold on an individual, rather than group, basis (28). Because administrative and marketing costs are much lower for group products, a purchaser can obtain more benefits for the dollar. In addition, because group policies are generally sold to the nonelderly, there is more time for reserves to build up. Thus premiums are lowered, and affordability is improved. Selling policies to a low-disability group of nonelderly also reduces adverse selection. Many large employers already offer acute care retiree health benefits (3).

The employer-based group long-term care market is new and untested. According to HIAA, only 11 of the 109 insurance companies that sold products in 1989 offered an employer-sponsored group plan (28). As of 1990, only about 51,000 employer-sponsored policies have been sold, roughly half to retirees, half to active employees (Highlights of HIAA Long-Term Care Insurance Survey, March 1990, unpublished). In fact, these policies are better characterized as individual policies sold in a group setting than as "real" group policies (10). Although it is a promising development that should be encouraged, employer-based insurance is unlikely to have any influence on nursing home and home care financing for years to come.

The extremely low market penetration of employer-sponsored group plans reflects several factors. For insurers, the very long-time horizon between initial purchase and use of nursing home and home care, which is associated with selling to the nonelderly, involves even more uncertainty and risk than selling to the elderly. The uncertainties, which were already large for the elderly oriented market, are compounded greatly.

Another barrier to the growth of the employer-sponsored long-term care insurance has been low consumer demand. Lack of awareness of the need for this insurance has been a recurrent theme in market research. As a result, few employees and unions have bargained for long-term care insurance. In those handful of companies that have offered active employees insurance, only a small percentage of employees have purchased policies (10).

Finally, although employers' interest in offering long-term care insurance is growing, their interest in helping to pay for the insurance is not (10). In virtually all sales of employer-sponsored long-term care insurance, the employee pays all of the costs. Employers see long-term care benefits as a financial risk that is sure to grow as the baby boom generation ages. Moreover, employers already face an unfunded liability for retiree health benefits that is commonly estimated to be $200–$300 billion (5). Thus, employers are not looking for another retiree benefit to which they must contribute.

OPTIONS FOR THE PUBLIC SECTOR

Although it is desirable for the private sector to play a much greater role in financing long-term care, our projections indicate that it is not reasonable to count on private initiatives to play more than a modest role. The question then becomes: Should the nation stick with a means-tested public welfare program as its major program for financing long-term care or should it enact a new program of social insurance?

Medicaid

The principal argument for staying with a means-tested approach is that Medicaid, despite its many deficiencies, does meet the most urgent needs of the low-income, disabled, elderly population at minimal cost to the taxpayer. For example, the entitlement character of Medicaid means that expenditures tend to rise with need and are not arbitrarily limited by the appropriation process. Although Medicaid is targeted to the poor, it also provides a safety net for the middle class. The spend-down requirements mean that Medicaid only finances the care that the income and the assets of the elderly cannot, thus public expenditures are kept down. The institutional bias ensures that persons who receive publicly financed care are predominantly the severely disabled. Finally, home care services, although not as widespread as many would like, are moderately available to program participants.

Making the Medicaid means test less onerous, reimbursement rates more adequate, and expanded home care more available would make life better for the disabled elderly, but still retain the fundamental welfare character of the program. Although incremental improvements in Medicaid are attractive, public charity always carries a stigma. Efforts to reduce taxpayer costs are likely to perpetuate a two-class system, with inferior care and status for Medicaid patients. Moreover, it is an odd welfare program whose eligibility requirements are met by a majority of the persons who use the services. In other US welfare programs, such as Aid to Families with Dependent Children and the Supplemental Security Income program, only a small minority of the population is expected to be financially eligible.

Public Insurance

The other broad approach is social insurance coverage of long-term care, most likely through expansion of the Medicare program. Under this approach, everyone would pay into the social insurance program and earn the right to benefits without having to prove impoverishment (1).

RATIONALE   There are several advantages to the social insurance approach. First, as with Social Security and Medicare, this approach would guarantee near-universal coverage. Private insurance excludes both those who cannot afford it and the disabled who cannot meet the tests of medical underwriting. Second, the costs can be spread over the largest possible base, which reduces the burden on any one individual.

Third, public insurance also offers some advantages for the way long-term care services are delivered and paid for. Although it will not completely eliminate the two-class system, public insurance will greatly reduce the access and quality gaps between private- and public-paying patients that exist under our current Medicaid-dominated public system. Moreover, public insurance can create a more balanced delivery system by expanding home care.

Finally, public insurance can be financed so that upper income people pay more than lower income people. For example, under Part A of the Medicare program, the $50,000-a-year worker pays five times in taxes what the $10,000-a-year worker pays for exactly the same set of benefits. In contrast, private insurance, with its flat premiums, is the most regressive way to finance benefits.

There are, however, major drawbacks to the social insurance approach. The most important ones are the costs and, by implication, the taxes necessary to pay for the program, both of which are certain to be substantial. The combination of an intractable budget deficit combined with a "read my lips" resistance to new taxes makes this a formidable barrier. The other potential problem is that public insurance may not provide the consumer with the choices inherent in having many private insurers competing to sell policies.

SPECIFIC PROPOSALS   Several proposals have been introduced into Congress to expand Medicare to include public long-term care insurance. One option proposed by Senator Mitchell would cover home care with a modest deductible and coinsurance, but only provide public nursing home insurance for those with lengths of stay longer than two years. The assumption is that insurers will offer and the elderly will buy insurance to cover the two-year deductible period. With this approach, the government would pay the costs of truly catastrophic care, a role that many groups feel is appropriate. Relatedly, recent analyses suggest that Medicaid spend-down is largely a problem of long-stay patients. This approach is, however, a very high risk strategy. If the supply or demand for private insurance is not what is assumed, then the program fails because nursing home residents will face $50,000–$60,000 in out-of-pocket costs.

A second option, proposed by Senator Kennedy and former Social Security Commissioner Bob Ball, would cover comprehensive home care but only six months of nursing home care. The Pepper Commission has proposed a similar approach, with the exception that just three months of nursing home care are covered. The rationale is that, in a time of limited resources, we should concentrate incremental public expenditures on patients who have some chance of going home from the nursing home or staying in the community. It is important to note that the longer-staying patients targeted by the Mitchell approach are usually discharged dead, whereas a substantial proportion of short-stay patients are discharged alive to the community. Because about one half of nursing home patients have lengths of stay of less than six months, the Kennedy plan completely covers a substantial percentage of nursing home patients (27). Furthermore, although all patients are covered, the total number of days paid for is relatively low. Thus, the plan is by far the least expensive. Short nursing home stays certainly do not provide total protection against the huge out-of-pocket expenditures that are associated with very long stays. However, short stays do mean out-of-pocket costs that would universally be regarded as catastrophic if they occurred as a result of acute care.

A third strategy, comprehensive coverage, has been introduced in two forms by Representatives Waxman and Stark. Both bills cover comprehensive nursing home and home care after a relatively short deductible and with moderate coinsurance levels. This approach provides the advantage of establishing a single payer, and thus enables the government to control payment rates and service delivery methods. The drawbacks, however, are formidable. The costs of a comprehensive program would be by far the highest of all the public approaches, and it is quite possible that a rigid, bureaucratic system will develop for its administration.

Although the differences among the proposed bills are noteworthy, there are some remarkable similarities. First, eligibility under all of the plans would be based on limitations of activities of daily living, thus the target population, rather than the range of services available, would be narrowed. Second, all proposals cover both nursing home and home care, and home care quite broadly. Third, all proposals use case management to control utilization, develop care plans, and monitor care. Fourth, all proposals attempt to be progressively financed by raising the cap on Medicare payroll tax or increasing estate tax and they call for the elderly to pay premiums. Finally, all of these approaches would be expensive. For the elderly alone, the costs are at least $25–50 billion a year.

PROGRAM DESIGN AND COST CONTAINMENT

Regardless of the final balance of public and private insurance, there are many issues of program design and cost control that need to be addressed. On the private side, the ability to control nursing home and home care expenditures is one of the factors that will make policies either profitable or unprofitable. On the public side, policymakers are concerned not only about the absolute level of expenditures, but the uncertainty that surrounds the estimates. It is part of the folklore of Washington health politics that the costs of Medicare and Medicaid turned out to be far higher than initially estimated.

In controlling expenditures, programs can try to limit the population eligible for services, the use of services, the overall cost per recipient, or the payment rate. Combinations are both possible and likely. In terms of limiting the population eligible for services, it is striking that all of the public proposals and an increasing number of private insurance policies use a number of limitations in the activities of daily living (ADL), e.g. two or more problems in eating, bathing, dressing, transferring, and toileting, or serious cognitive impairment as a screen for eligibility for benefits (25, 28). By counting ADL limitations, the eligible population can be expanded or contracted, depending on how much money is available. This approach is replacing more mechanistic screens, like prior hospital or nursing home use or need for skilled services.

The effect of insurance on use of long-term care services is not known, but many believe it will be substantial. Most disabled elderly who might qualify for paid long-term care services do not currently receive any. The principal effect of insurance or other such financing mechanisms is to reduce the net cost of a service. People tend to buy more of a service when it costs less out-of-pocket. Thus, with any insurance, admissions to nursing homes and use of home care may rise. The reluctance of the elderly to enter nursing homes, however, reduces the likelihood of very large increases in nursing home use (23). But, the inherent desirability of some home care services, such as homemaker services, means that their use is likely to increase substantially if covered by insurance. In designing long-term care programs, both private insurance and the government must take moral hazard into account.

Aggregate expenditures can also be limited by shifting the risk from the insured or government to the providers. In this strategy, fixed payments per enrollee are made to providers who are then responsible for supplying the contracted set of services within the budget constraint. Social health maintenance organizations and continuing care retirement communities are examples of this approach. Providers who can keep expenditures under budget make money; those providers that cannot are unprofitable. As with all prepaid, capitated arrangements, the greatest risk is that providers have an incentive to provide fewer services than would be desirable.

Another strategy for controlling expenditures is to limit payment rates to nursing homes and home care providers. Private insurance policies typically do so by paying on a flat indemnity basis that does not increase at all or at least is not commensurate with expected nursing home and home care inflation (28). Medicaid nursing home reimbursements have traditionally been quite low, which raises questions about their influence on quality of care and access to services for low-income patients. Medicare rates have historically been between Medicaid and private pay rates, but Congress and the President have not hesitated to trim payment rates for hospitals and physicians over the last eight years.

A major question, which overhangs all of these financing proposals, is whether the delivery system will be able to expand enough to meet demand implied by the growing number of frail elderly and changes in the financing system (2). Even without changes in financing, nursing home utilization may double over the next 30 years. Shortages in the labor supply are already evident in some parts of the country (15).

CONCLUSION

The political debacle of the repeal of the Medicare Catastrophic Coverage Act of 1988, with its strong overtones of generational conflict, has definitely cooled the ardor of Congress to tackle this problem. Indeed, for the short run, the prospects for expanded public funding for long-term care are less now than they were just one year ago, although much greater than they were five years ago.

Over the long run, neither the President nor Congress will be able to avoid addressing the issue of long-term care financing. During the 1990s, the size of the population age 75 and over will increase by 25%. Even more importantly, virtually all of the parents of the baby boom generation will have to face long-term care, not as an abstract concept, but as a real life, intensely personal issue. As a result, they are likely to put intense pressure on their elected representatives to "do something" to help them pay for nursing home and home care.

As long-term care rises on the political agenda, discussions of generational equity will become more pronounced. There are, in fact, strong public policy and moral reasons to address the problem of health care for the uninsured before additional public funds are spent on the elderly. It is a major problem that 37 million persons have no health insurance whatsoever. The difficulty is that public opinion surveys consistently show that people are willing to pay additional taxes for a public long-term care program, but not for health care for the uninsured (9, 16). In a national survey of voters sponsored by the American Association of Retired Persons and the Villers Foundation, 68% of respondents were willing to pay an additional $120–$720 in taxes, depending on their income, for a long-term care program (20). Yet in another national survey, only 25% of persons with incomes over $20,000 were willing to pay as little as $51 a year to address the problems of the uninsured (19). As a society, we may never solve the problem of health care for the uninsured and, thus, never gain the legitimacy to address the issue of long-term care. Politically, it is critical that these two issues be joined together.

Finally, as a political issue, long-term care faces a paradox. On the one hand, the major factor that is forcing long-term care onto the political agenda is that every day for the next 70 years there will be more and more disabled elderly. On the other hand, the costs associated with caring for this growing disabled population is the major factor that causes policymakers to hesitate to address this issue.

Major new initiatives are needed both in the private sector and in the public sector to improve financing of long-term care. Americans need to recognize that long-term care is a normal risk of growing old; it requires anticipation and planning. A large and virtually untapped market awaits private insurance. Continued development of that market by the private sector, with encouragement from the government, could make long-term care much more affordable for a substantial fraction of the population. However, even with maximum likely development of private options, public spending for long-term care will continue to increase rapidly for the foreseeable future. As a result, improvement of public programs will remain a crucial component of any reform effort.

Although long-term care financing has traditionally been viewed as an insolvable problem, it is actually one of the more tractable social issues facing the United States. Unlike crime, poverty, racism, and teenage pregnancy, this issue has a range of known and feasible solutions. The question is whether we as a society have enough political will and ingenuity to choose among them to put an improved system in place.

Literature Cited

1. Aaron, H. J., Bosworth, B. P., Burtless, G. 1989. *Can America Afford To Grow?*, p. 6. Washington, DC: Brookings Inst. 144 pp.
2. Brannon, D., Smyer, M. A. 1990. Who will provide long-term care in the future? *Generations* 14:64–67
3. Bureau Labor Stat. 1989. Employee benefits in medium and large firms in 1988. Washington, DC: US GPO. Bull. 2336
4. Carpenter, L. 1988. Medicaid eligibility for persons in nursing homes. *Health Care Financ. Rev.* 10:67–78
5. Chollet, D. J., Friedland, R. B. 1988. Employer-paid retiree health insurance: History and prospects for growth. In *The Sourcebook on Post Retirement Health Care Benefits*, ed. R. D. Paul, D. M. Disney, pp. 17–29. Greenvale, NY: Panel
6. Cohen, M., Tell, E., Wallack, S. 1986. The lifetime risks and costs of nursing home use among the elderly. *Med. Care* 24:1161–72
7. Danzinger, S., van der Gaag, J., Smolensky, E., Taussig, M. K. 1984. Implications of the relative economic status of the elderly for transfer policy. In *Retirement and Economic Behavior*, ed. H. J. Aaron, G. Burtless, pp. 135–71. Washington, DC: Brookings Inst.
8. Div. Natl. Cost Estimates, Off. Actuary, Health Care Financ. Adm. 1987. Natl.

health expenditures, 1986–2000. *Health Care Financ. Rev.* 8:1–135
9. Employee Benefit Res. Inst. 1989. *Public Attitudes on Long-Term Care: Full Report*, pp. 21–22. Washington, DC:Empl. Benefit Res. Inst.
10. Friedland, R. 1989. *Facing the Costs of Long-Term Care*. Washington, DC: Empl. Benefit Res. Inst. 365 pp.
11. Friedland, R. 1989. Issues concerning the financing and delivery of long-term care. *Empl. Benefit Res. Inst. Issue Brief*, No. 86
12. Holahan, J. F., Cohen, J. W. 1986. *Medicaid: The Trade-off Between Cost Containment and Access to Care*, pp. 75–95. Washington, DC: Urban Inst.
13. Hurd, M. J., Shoven, J. B. 1982. Real income and wealth of the elderly. *Am. Econ. Rev.* 72:314–18
14. Kemper, P., Applebaum, R., Harrigan, M. 1987. Community care demonstrations: What have we learned? *Health Care Financ. Rev.* 8:87–100
15. Lewin/ICF. 1988. *The Home Care Labor Market in New York State: An Analysis of Issues and Projections Through 2000*, pp. 1–3. Washington, DC: Lewin/ICF
16. Meiners, M. 1989. *Public Attitudes on Long-Term Care*. College Park, MD: Univ. Maryland Cent. Aging
17. Murtaugh, C., Kemper, P., Spillman, B. 1989. *The Risk of Nursing Home Use*

in Later Life. Rockville, Md: Agency Health Care Policy Res.
18. Natl. Cent. Health Stat., by Hing, E., Sekscenski, E., Strachan, G. 1989. *The National Nursing Home Survey: 1985 Summary for the United States*, 13:97. DHHS Publ. No. (PHS)89-1758. Public Health Service. Washington, DC:US GPO
19. Pokorny, G. 1988. Report card on health. *Health Manage. Q.* 10:3–9
20. R. L. Associates. 1987. *The American Public Views on Long-Term Care*. Prepared for the Am. Assoc. Retired Persons and Villers Found., Princeton, NJ
21. Rice, T. 1989. The use, cost and economic burden of nursing home care in 1985. *Med. Care* 27:1133–47
22. Rice, T., Gabel, J. 1986. Protecting the elderly against high health care costs. *Health Aff.* 5:5–21
23. Rivlin, A., Wiener, J., with Hanley, R., Spence, D. 1988. *Caring for the Disabled Elderly: Who Will Pay?* Washington, DC: Brookings Inst.
24. Social Security Admin. 1989. *Annual Report of Federal Old-Age and Survivors Insurance and Disability Insurance Trust Funds*. Washington, DC: Soc. Secur. Admin.
25. Spence, D., Hanley, R. J. 1990. Public insurance options for financing long-term care. *Generations* 14:28–31
26. Spence, D., Wiener, J. 1990. Estimat-

ing the extent of Medicaid spend-down in nursing homes. *J. Health Polit. Policy Law*. In press
27. Spence, D., Wiener, J. 1990. Nursing home length of stay patterns: Results from the 1985 National Nursing Home Survey. *Gerontologist* 30:16–20
28. Van Gelder, S., Johnson, D. 1989. *Long-Term Care Insurance: Market Trends*. Washington, DC:Health Insur. Assoc. Am.
29. Weissert, W., Cready, C., Pawelak, J. 1988. The past and future of home and community based long-term care. *Milbank Q.* 66:309–88
30. Wilson, C. E., Weissert, W. G. 1989. Private long-term care insurance: After coverage restrictions, is there anything left? *Inquiry* 26:493–507
31. Yankelovich Group. 1990. *Long-Term Care in America: Public Attitudes and Possible Solutions (Executive Summary)*. Prepared for Am. Assoc. Retired Persons, Washington, DC
32. Zedlewski, S. 1984. The private pension system to the year 2000. In *Retirement and Economic Behavior*, ed. H. J. Aaron, G. Burtless, 11:315–41. Washington, DC:Brookings Inst. 352 pp.
33. Zedlewski, S., Barnes, R. O., Burt, M. K., McBride, T. D., Meyer, J. A. 1989. *The Needs of the Elderly in the 21st Century*. Washington, DC:Urban Inst.

Annu. Rev. Publ. Health. 1991. 12:85–109

LYME DISEASE: A MULTIFOCAL WORLDWIDE EPIDEMIC

Leonard H. Sigal[1] and Anita S. Curran[2]

Departments of Medicine and Molecular Genetics and Microbiology and Lyme Disease Center[1] and Department of Clinical, Environmental, and Community Medicine[2], University of Medicine and Dentistry of New Jersey—Robert Wood Johnson Medical School, New Brunswick, New Jersey 08903

KEY WORDS: *Borrelia burgdorferi,* Ixodes ticks

INTRODUCTION

Lyme disease (LD) is a multisystem, inflammatory disease that is caused by the spirochete, *Borrelia burgdorferi,* and spread by Ixodes ticks. Since the isolation of the organism, we have clearly seen that many lessons learned from syphilis are applicable to Lyme disease. Syphilis, which is caused by *Treponema pallidum* (another spirochete), is also a multisystem disease that often is quite delayed after the initial infection. In the last few years, a better understanding of LD has helped us understand syphilis, as well.

In 1975, Steere, Malawista, and colleagues at Yale University described Lyme arthritis, an oubreak of "juvenile rheumatoid arthritis" in three small towns on the east bank of the Connecticut River (142). Over the next few years, we began to appreciate the multisystem nature of this newly described ailment, and the name "Lyme disease" came into usage. By 1990, researchers identified Lyme disease as an epidemic disease in the Northeast (from Massachusetts through Pennsylvania, with cases described as far south as the Carolinas and Georgia); the northern Midwest (primarily Minnesota and Wisconsin, as well as Michigan), and in northern California and Oregon. In the United States, 90% of the cases reported are from these three regions, and the total number has steadily increased each year. In retrospect, however, the story of *B. burgdorferi* infection began in Europe, more than a century ago.

85

0163-7525/91/0501-0085$02.00

In 1883, Buchwald reported an atrophic skin lesion, which, in 1902, Herxheimer and Hartmann named acrodermatitis chronica atrophicans (ACA). In 1946, Hauser reported that some patients recalled a tick bite, often at the site of the skin lesion. Occasionally, the ACA lesion had been preceded by another lesion, known as erythema chronicum migrans (ECM), also at the site of the bite.

Afzelius had described ECM previously in 1909, and in 1914 Lipschutz gave the lesion its descriptive name. In 1922, Garin and Bujadoux noted a connection between meningitis and preceding tick bite, and in 1941 Bannwarth reported tick-borne meningopolyneuritis, the syndrome that bears his name. In 1930, Hellerstrom reported that in certain patients, lymphocytic meningitis was preceded by ECM. Lenhoff described spirochetal forms in biopsies from ECM lesions in 1948, and in 1951 Hellerstrom found that ECM resolves after standard spirocheticidal therapy (including bismuth, neoarsphenamine, and penicillin). In 1955, Binder reported that ECM could be transferred by skin graft.

Scrimenti reported the first case of ECM in the Americas, which occurred in Wisconsin in 1970. Five years later, the outbreak of juvenile rheumatoid arthritis in Connecticut was also linked to proceding ECM and tick bite. Over the next few years, Lyme arthritis, became known as Lyme disease, in part because of the association with cardiac disease, but also because approximately 10% of the patients had a neurologic syndrome essentially identical to Bannwarth's syndrome. The multisystem, inflammatory nature of Lyme disease was established.

After *B. burgdorferi* was identified as the etiologic agent of LD in the United States, studies in Europe established that the same organism was the cause of ECM and ACA in Germany, Austria, and Scandinavia. Indirect immunofluorescence (IFA), enzyme-linked immunosorbent assay (ELISA), and Immunoblot for serologic testing and T-cell proliferative responses for cellular testing are now used to confirm the diagnosis of LD. Comparison of levels of specific immune reactivity between sites of inflammation and the peripheral blood help to identify locations of *B. burgdorferi*-induced inflammation. Newer techniques, like polymerase chain reaction, in situ hybridization, and immunologic antigen identification help locate organism-derived compounds at these sites.

Lyme disease is now known to have a worldwide distribution, with cases described in Africa, Asia, and Australia. The primary vector in each area has been identified as an Ixodes tick: *I. dammini* in the Northeast and Midwest, *I. scapularis* in the Southeast, and *I. pacificus* in California.

Thus, between 1883 and 1990, at least three discrete skin lesions and a multisystem, inflammatory disease have been ascribed to infection with *B. burgdorferi*. Sufficient new information has been generated to hold three international convocations and fill three volumes (12, 131, 141); the fourth such meeting was held in June 1990, in Stockholm.

CLINICAL DESCRIPTION AND CONTROVERSIES

Lyme disease is an infectious disease, capable of causing damage to a number of organ systems (18, 31). The clinical syndrome has been divided into three relatively arbitrary stages to describe the many manifestations. Stage One usually occurs within a month of inoculation with *B. burgdorferi*, the causative agent (13, 59, 137). It includes ECM, which is the skin rash that is a marker for LD, and associated symptoms. Stage Two manifestations include cardiac and neurologic disease and usually occur two to three months after the initial infection; there may be no preceding evidence of illness suggestive of Stage One LD. Stage Three includes arthritis and chronic neurologic manifestations, which have recently been described; Stage Three may occur years after ECM, or in the absence of any preceding history suggestive of earlier LD.

Stage One occurs between one day and one month after tick bite (median seven days). It consists of ECM and associated symptoms: fever, fatigue, malaise, headache, stiff neck, arthralgia, and myalgia. About 50–70% of patients will experience ECM; of these, 50% will have more than one skin lesion. Regional (and occasionally systemic) lymphadenopathy may occur. Patients may experience pain on neck flexion, conjunctivitis, erythematous throat, or temporomandibular joint pain. A few patients have hepatosplenomegaly and/or right upper quadrant tenderness (133). Only about 30% of patients will recall a tick bite (142), although animal studies suggest that the tick must remain attached for a day or longer to transmit the disease (97).

Nonspecific laboratory studies, such as erythrocyte sedimentation rate, complete blood count, and liver function tests, are not clinically helpful, even when abnormal (133). In the first weeks of the disease, specific serologic tests may be negative (30, 103, 138). Researchers have cultured *B. burgdorferi* from biopsy specimens taken at the expanding red border of the ECM lesion (138).

Two to three months following the onset of ECM, about 10–15% of untreated patients with Stage One LD will experience neurologic disease. Meningoencephalitis, meningitis, cranial nerve palsies, and peripheral neuropathies may occur (91, 95, 100). These conditions are often accompanied by extreme fatigue, malaise, headache, and photophobia; fever is usually absent. Mild encephalopathy, including difficulty with concentration and memory and emotional lability, may occur. These neurologic findings match those described in Europe in the early part of this century. They are now known as Bannwarth's syndrome (9) or tick-borne meningopolyneuritis (53).

A lymphocytic pleocytosis is found in cerebrospinal fluid with elevated protein, but normal glucose levels (91, 100). *Borrelia burgdorferi* has been grown from the cerebrospinal fluid of patients with Lyme meningitis (138).

Pachner & Steere (91) have found neuropathic changes on nerve conduction testing; Halperin et al (46) documented axonopathy in one third of patients with peripheral neuropathy. Peripheral nerve biopsies have shown heavy epineural vessel infiltration with mononuclear cells (23, 39, 46, 62, 153). Vasculitis, but no organisms, was seen in one patient (23); luminal obliteration of perineural vessels without vasculitis was found in another (39). Researchers have not seen immune complexes, immunoglobulin, and complement in biopsy specimens (23, 46).

Stiernstedt et al (148) proposed vascular disease induced by *Borrelia burgdorferi* as a possible pathogenetic mechanism for cerebrovascular disease. Midgard & Hofstad (83) have seen vasculitis on angiographic study of a patient with LD central nervous system disease.

Most patients with encephalitic symptoms have abnormalities on electroencephalography (91). Halperin et al (46) have documented reversible neuropsychiatric testing abnormalities; they found small plaques in some patients on magnetic resonance imaging (MRI); the plaques occasionally resolved after antibiotic therapy. An insufficient number of normal individuals have had MRI to know if these plaques represent *B. burgdorferi*-induced cerebral damage or if normal individuals may have such plaques.

Cardiac disease occurs in 8–10% of previously untreated patients two to three months after ECM, occasionally in association with Stage Two neurologic disease. Steere et al (134) have reported atrioventricular conduction defects, mild congestive heart failure, and ST and T wave changes compatible with myopericarditis. Researchers have described reversible (50, 55, 101) and rarely fatal (77) myocarditis. Multifocal damage has been documented in electrophysiologic studies of individual cases (101, 134). Duray (39) described focal myonecrosis and a sparse interstitial infiltrate of polymorphonuclear cells and lymphocytes in one report of myocardial biopsies; in another report, Reznick et al found *B. burgdorferi,* myonecrosis, and perivascular mononuclear cell infiltration. The finding of an organism within the myocardium (77) suggests that direct invasion occurs in Lyme myocarditis.

Arthritis is the classic feature of Stage Three LD (136). Steere et al summarized their experience with 55 LD patients who did not receive antibiotic therapy (144). A prospective study of these patients revealed that 44 experienced articular problems over a six-year period. Of this group, ten patients experienced arthralgias with or following ECM, occurring one day to eight weeks (mean, two weeks) after the onset of the lesion. Twenty-eight patients had polyarthritis, often migratory, four days to two years after the onset of ECM (mean, six months); half of this group had experienced preceding migratory arthralgias. Finally, chronic Lyme arthritis developed in six patients, usually affecting a single joint, with onset four months to four years after ECM (mean, 12 months); Five of these patients had experienced either arthralgia or intermittent arthritis before chronic synovitis developed. The migratory polyarthritis group is reminiscent of the original cohort of patients described by Steere et al in their initial report of Lyme arthritis (142).

The synovium in Lyme arthritis is hypertrophic and hyperplastic, with focal necrosis, vascular proliferation, and inflammatory cell infiltration. Mononuclear cell aggregates and lymphoid follicles, which resemble rheumatoid synovium, may be present (136), although there are histological differences between rheumatoid and Lyme synovitis (39). As in syphilis, endarteritis obliterans may be seen, with capillary arborization, dilatation, and congestion (60). *B. burgdorferi* has been seen rarely, in or near synovial vessels (60) or in synovial fluid (126), and it has been grown from synovial fluid (105).

Tertiary neuroborreliosis, a term that purposely draws upon the clinical analogy with tertiary neurosyphilis, includes chronic encephalomyelopathy and neuropathy (1, 90, 92). Like tertiary neurosyphilis, Stage Three neurologic LD may occur insidiously months to years after the onset of infection, even in the absence of clinically apparent preceding infection. Thus, subclinical infection may occur for long periods before the emergence of overt neurologic damage. This development raises serious concerns over the finding of asymptomatic seropositivity in a significant percentage of persons in areas endemic for LD.

One of the major controversies regarding LD is the question of which clinical conditions can be ascribed to *B. burgdorferi* infection. On the basis of seroepidemiologic and biopsy evidence, it has been suggested that many cutaneous lesions, including morphea, lichen sclerosis et atrophicans, eosinophilic fascitis, and certain other cutaneous fibrotic disorders, are due to *B. burgdorferi* (118). However, these claims are by no means definitive. Subclinical or asymptomatic infection may be prevalent in endemic areas (30, 145), so that seropositivity may represent no more than a coincidence (117).

An area of great interest is defining the true extent of neurologic manifestations of LD. Claims that amyotrophic lateral sclerosis (76), multiple sclerosis (29), and Alzheimer's disease (94) are due to infection with *B. burgdorferi* have been laid to rest. Many individual cases of neurologic damage have been attributed to *B. burgdorferi* infection merely because the patient has a positive serologic test, a circumstance that does not guarantee causality.

Another area of major concern is *B. burgdorferi* infection that occurs during pregnancy. Shortly after the LD epidemic in the Northeast was appreciated, reports of adverse outcomes of pregnancy began to appear. In a review of 19 pregnancies between 1976 and 1984 that were complicated by LD, Markowitz et al (78) noted 14 normal births and 5 adverse outcomes. Complications included rash, syndactyly, congenital heart anomalies, cortical blindness, prematurity, and intrauterine death. Toxemia of pregnancy has been attributed to pregnancy-related *B. burgdorferi* infection (69). Claims have been made that *B. burgdorferi* may cause fetal anomalies and fetal demise (70, 104, 155). A few large studies have been organized to evaluate the true risk of such infection. A prospective study found no evidence that asymptomatic seropositivity had any effect on pregnancy outcome (38), and a study in New York found no association between anti-*B. burgdorferi* antibody in cord blood and congenital malformations in the babies (157). A Swiss study found no reason to screen for LD during pregnancy (86), whereas a small Italian study found that LD during pregnancy might predispose to stillbirth (24). Thus, the theory that *B. burgdorferi* infection causes adverse pregnancy outcomes has not been proven. The ongoing study of Dlesk et al (38) hopefully will gain enough entrants to answer this question definitively.

There also is no evidence that LD can be passed by sexual or other intimate contact. There is evidence, however, that *B. burgdorferi* can survive in blood (10) and various blood products (11) for as long as 6–8 weeks (L. H. Sigal, unpublished observations). Whether LD can be spread by transfusion is unclear (8).

DIAGNOSIS AND DIAGNOSTIC TESTING

In early studies of LD, the presence of ECM was required to assure that diagnosis, as ECM was the only pathognomonic feature of the disease (133). Because LD has been described in more geographic areas and has been implicated in more clinical situations, a case definition became necessary. In 1982 and 1983, the Centers for Disease Control stated that ECM in an endemic area, or ECM and two or more organ systems affected in a nonendemic area, would be accepted as a case of LD. Since 1984, this has been changed: ECM or laboratory confirmation of infection (serologic positivity or isolation of *B. burgdorferi* from the site of disease) and one or more organ systems affected in an endemic area; ECM and two or greater organ systems affected in a nonendemic area; or ECM plus laboratory confirmation of infection (26). In New York State, a case is defined as a history of ECM or symptoms compatible with late disease, plus serologic evidence of preceding infection with *B. burgdorferi,* plus a history of exposure in an area (county) known to be endemic (89).

As has been well documented recently, serologic testing for LD is not well standardized, and interlaboratory variation makes interpretation difficult (52, 68, 115). An excellent summary of the issues involved in serologic tests and their interpretation appeared as part of the Third Symposium on LD (71). Cross-reactivity in serological tests for LD and other spirochetal infections can occasionally pose a problem (75). Additionally, infection with *B. burgdorferi* can cause serologic false-positivity for other organisms, perhaps because the organism nonspecificity stimulates immunoglobulin production, which is known as polyclonal B cell activation (122). Different techniques (including IFA, ELISA, and Western immunoblotting) and modification of these techniques are available. A recent antibody-capture enzyme immunosorbent assay shows promise as a more sensitive test for specific antibodies (15). Different preparations of the organism have been tried, with mixed results (49, 74). Antibodies bound in immune complexes have also been identified, which suggests another means of early serologic confirmation of the diagnosis (112).

One effective use of both serologic and cellular testing is to determine levels of specific immune reactivity at closed space sites of inflammation. In arthritis (123) and meningitis (93) caused by *B. burgdorferi,* there is evidence that antigen-sensitive cells are concentrated at the site of inflammation, and specific antibodies have been found concentrated within the cerebrospinal fluid of patients with Lyme neurologic disease (120, 147).

Recent editorials caution on the overuse of LD serologic testing (82) and repeat the need for a national program of standardization of these tests (51, 72). Many kits for rapid determination of serologic reactivity in doctor's offices are now available and more are soon to be marketed, which may further muddy the waters. One suggestion for practitioners in endemic areas is to use an academically oriented laboratory for diagnostic serologic tests.

As noted above, measurable levels of IgM and IgG immunoglobulin may not be present for up to eight weeks after the tick bite (116), so the timing of the test is crucial in its interpretation (71). Early, even incomplete, antibiotic therapy may blunt or abrogate the humoral immune response to the organism, which would render the patient inappropriately seronegative (116). Lyme disease, however, remains a clinical diagnosis. Without a set of well-substantiated criteria for the diagnosis of LD (like the Jones criteria for rheumatic fever), there is no substitute for a careful history and physical done by a well-prepared health care provider that is confirmed, as needed, by serologic evidence of preceding infection.

NEW DIAGNOSTIC TESTING: NEW ANTIGEN PREPARATIONS, ANTIGEN TESTING, POLYMERASE CHAIN REACTION

Newer diagnostic tests for LD have been developed and many show great promise. As noted above, some of the serologic negativity in patients may be because of binding of the specific antibodies in immune complexes; these antibodies are then unable to bind in the assay being used. Isolation of these immune complexes may be helpful in such cases (113).

Modification of the assays being used also may be helpful. The antibody capture technique may be able to decrease nonspecific binding, and thus is more sensitive and as specific as assays currently being used (15). Nonspecific binding by the test sera may be decreased by absorption of the sera with other microorganisms to remove these antibodies; this has been tried, with mixed results (30, 44).

Berger et al (16) used the organism cultured from an individual; however, this procedure did not increase the efficacy of serologic testing. Nevertheless, differential responsiveness to individual components of *B. burgdorferi* suggests that fractions of the organism may offer a better antigenic preparation for use in ELISA (45, 48, 49, 74).

Infected *Peromyscus leucopus* (white-footed field mice) shed large numbers of viable *B. burgdorferi* in their urine (22, 113), which suggests that the isolation of organism-derived proteins in the urine might lend itself to diagnosing LD (54). Although enough information is not yet available to assess this technique, detection of antigen does not differentiate between live and dead organisms (see below, Pathogenesis).

B. burgdorferi-derived nucleic acids can be identified in tissue (114), which allows a sensitive method for implicating the organism in local inflammation. An individual copy of a gene from a microorganism can be copied rapidly and accurately in vitro until 1 million copies are present in the test tube, by using a new technology called polymerase chain reaction. Thus, a fluid or tissue specimen with one copy of a gene can be probed and this genetic evidence of infection can be detected. This technique has been used in LD (102; M. A. Liebling, unpublished observations) to identify *B. burgdorferi*-derived genetic materials in the blood and cerebrospinal fluid of patients with LD. Although this technique is potentially very sensitive, it is prone to false-positive testing because of contamination. It also suffers from the same problem as noted above for antigen detection; after effective therapy, genetic materials may persist, so that this test does not help the physician determine if further therapy is indicated.

PATHOGENESIS

B. burgdorferi can elicit many immunologic responses and changes in the host (119). Therefore, the means by which this pathogen may cause tissue damage may be quite complicated. The organism clearly is present at many of the sites of inflammation. Complement fixation by the organism and local polymorphonuclear cell activation may cause local damage. Production of in situ immune complexes may act as a focus of persisting inflammation or producing vasculitis. *B. burgdorferi* can elicit the production of immunologically active compounds from monocyte/macrophages, including interleukin-1 and tumor necrosis factor (cachectin), which may affect immune cells locally and alter the function of fibroblasts and endothelial cells at the site of inflammation. Thus, the presence of live organism certainly plays a role in the pathogenesis of LD.

The persistence of dead organism may act as a focus of local or systemic inflammation; long after antibiotics have killed *B. burgdorferi*, there may be persistent inflammation, as immune mechanisms continue to react with the effete organism. All the mechanisms noted above could continue for months until the host's macrophages can eliminate the residue. This mechanism may explain the delayed response to antibiotics and the peristence of nonspecific symptomatology long after the end of (ultimately) curative antibiotic therapy.

Occasionally, a molecule found in a microorganism resembles a component of the potential host. In this circumstance, known as molecular mimicry, the immune response against the microorganism might identify and attack the host component and lead to host damage. There is evidence that a *B. burgdorferi* molecule, the flagellin, resembles a specific human axonal protein (125). Immunologic reactivity with flagellin might then cause tissue damage. Thus, another possible immunopathogenetic mechanism must be considered in LD. However, any suggestion that immunomodulatory therapy might be an effective treatment of LD is premature at this time.

VACCINE DESIGN

No human vaccine for LD is currently available. Passive immunization of hamsters with serum from rabbits previously inoculated with *B. burgdorferi* led to protection from subsequent inoculation of the hamsters with the organism; normal rabbit serum was ineffective (56). Passive immunization with allogeneic anti-*B. burgdorferi* serum prevented the development of Lyme arthritis in the LSH strain of hamster (106). Active immunization with dead *B. burgdorferi* also protected hamsters (57). An animal vaccine for LD is under development, and a human vaccine is being planned. The fact that the immunopathogenesis of LD may, in part, include autoimmunity predicated upon molecular mimicry (125) suggests that the safety and efficacy of whole organism vaccines may be problematic.

THERAPY AND PROGNOSIS

Antibiotic therapy in Stage One disease usually results in resolution of disease and prevents progression to later stages. Oral therapy is recommended for early disease. There is no evidence that intravenous drugs are necessary, even for severe Stage I disease. The only comparative study of antibiotic therapy in early disease suggested that either penicillin or tetracycline was more effective than erythromycin (1000 mg in 4 divided dosages for 10 days) in preventing progression to later disease; 20 days of tetracycline was no better than 10 days of treatment (139). There are many proposed antibiotic regimens for early disease, and there is no evidence that one drug is superior to another. Tetracycline, amoxicillin, ampicillin, and penicillin have been used with good success, at 4 divided dosages of 1000–2000 mg per day. Doxycycline at 100 mg 2–3 times a day is also effective. There is no evidence that the addition of probenecid to therapy with the penicillins adds any efficacy. Other agents, including cefuroxime axetil, cefixime, and minocycline have also been used. Initial studies of azithromycin, a new macrolide antibiotic with greater anti-*B. burgdorferi* activity than erythromycin, are encouraging. The optimum duration of therapy has not been determined, although current practice is generally to continue treatment for 3–4 weeks.

Within a few hours to days of the onset of therapy, approximately 15% of patients may experience a remarkable worsening of signs and symptoms of disease (139), which is often accompanied by fever, chills, malaise, headache, and myalgia. These patients may experience a rise in the peripheral blood white cell count and, occasionally, increases in liver function tests. All of these abnormalities are relatively mild and usually resolve within a day or so. This phenomenon, first described in syphilis, is known as the Jarisch-Herxheimer reaction. Such reactions are also found early in the therapy of other Borrelial infections and of Brucellosis, where the reaction may be life threatening.

If untreated, ECM will spontaneously resolve in a median of 28 days, although it may persist for as long as 14 months. Progression to later disease is most frequent in patients with more serious early manifestations (144), but progression may follow mild or inapparent Stage One LD (99).

Oral or parental antibiotics are effective in treatment of Stage Two LD. The suggested route, dosage, and duration of therapy varies with the type of manifestations (77, 91, 139, 143, 146).

The arthritis of LD is generally treated with intravenous antibiotics, including penicillin (20 million units per day in 6 divided dosages), cefotaxime (3 grams twice a day), and ceftriaxone (1 gram twice a day). Chloramphenicol, at dosage appropriate to body mass, is also effective. Steere et al (137) reported that Lyme arthritis was successfully treated with intravenous penicillin in 55% of patients. *B. burgdorferi* is sensitive to ceftriaxone (58), and this agent has been used successfully (33). One study suggests that subsequent treatment with ceftriaxone is effective in patients who have failed to respond to penicillin (34). There is preliminary evidence to suggest that prolonged oral therapy (one month) may be effective in treatment of late disease (67), but these studies must be confirmed.

The most appropriate therapy for Stage Three neurologic disease is probably intravenous antibiotics, as used for other late manifestations of LD, although there is not enough clinical experience to know if late neurologic damage is totally reversible. There are anecdotes that claim slow, but impressive, resolution.

Based on the premise that *B. burgdorferi* is a slowly growing organism, some groups have suggested that therapy for late LD should include intravenous courses for six weeks or longer and prolonged oral "maintenance" therapy for up to 18–24 months. It is not evident that these regimens are any more effective than the more traditional approaches noted above; however, it is certainly believable that the longer regimens are associated with more side effects and more expense to the patient or the third-party payer.

One argument made in favor of more prolonged therapy is the persistence of symptoms and the occasional apparent "progression" to later manifestations, often in the presence of persistent elevated levels of anti-*B. burgdorferi* antibody. The general experience has been that it may take as long as six months for some patients with arthritis to fully resolve after antibiotic therapy (137), and continuous achiness and nonspecific symptoms may occur after therapy of other late manifestations of LD. This problem may be because of the persistence of *B. burgdorferi*-derived antigens at the site of disease, which is a focus for prolonged inflammation, as described above. Our experience suggests that symptoms will develop in some patients after LD, including fibromyalgia, which are not due to ongoing infection and are not amenable to further antibiotic therapy (121). Many patients referred to the Lyme Disease Center at Robert Wood Johnson Medical School have been subjected to many courses of oral and intravenous therapy for complaints clearly not due to *B. burgdorferi* infection, but which have been mistakenly attributed to LD (121). Not every complaint in a patient who has had LD (or, for that matter, in an individual with serum antibodies to *B. burgdorferi*) is necessarily because of *B. burgdorferi* infection.

One indisputable fact is that the earlier a patient is treated, the less likely that person is to experience later manifestations. The overwhelming majority of patients with treated Stage I LD will be cured. Fatalities due to *B. burgdorferi* infection are very rare. The only LD fatalities reported in the American literature were because of carditis [although in one, coexisting babesiosis complicated the clinical picture (77)], and possibly because of adult respiratory distress syndrome related to LD (61). There is also a brief French report of a case of Lyme meningoradiculitis, which was complicated by encephalitis and phrenic paralysis (81). Permanent heart block due to LD was reported from the Netherlands (35). Lyme meningitis resolves with antibiotic therapy (65).

Lyme arthritis has proven somewhat less responsive to antibiotic therapy. In the initial report, 55% of patients treated with intravenous penicillin resolved; later studies suggest a better response rate to therapy with third generation cephalosporins. Nonetheless, some patients have required other forms of treatment, including hydroxychloroquine (as a remittive agent) and synovectomy (132).

A controversial issue in the therapy of LD is the status of asymptomatic persons who happen to test positive for antibodies to *B. burgdorferi*. We do not know how many, if any, of these individuals will ever experience tissue damage because of this infection. The policy at the Lyme Disease Center at Robert Wood Johnson Medical School is that if a true seropositive result is obtained on an individual without any preceding history of LD, oral therapy for one month, as for Stage One disease, is given.

EPIDEMIOLOGY OF THE DISEASE, TICK (AND OTHER POSSIBLE) VECTORS, AND HOSTS

As mentioned above, LD was first described as Lyme arthritis. In these early studies, LD patients occasionally recalled a preceding tick bite (142). Subsequent field studies documented that there were far fewer cases of LD on the west bank of the River, in parallel with the smaller number of deer, mice, and ticks (154). When cases were described elsewhere in the US, the distribution of LD was found to match that of Ixodes ticks (140).

Lyme disease has occurred as focal epidemics in three areas of the United States; 90% of cases are found in the Northeast, the northern Midwest, and the Pacific Northwest. Newly developing foci were documented in New Jersey (17, 111), Westchester County, NY (158), Suffolk County, NY (14), Ipswich, Mass. (65), and greater Philadelphia (4a). In each area, there has been a rapid increase in the number of cases. In the "home" of LD, there has been a three- to eight-fold increase near the mouth of the Connecticut River, and a spread of LD into inland and southern Connecticut. The highest incidence, however, is still on the east bank of the river (25).

New York State now has the dubious distinction of having the largest number of LD cases, and Rhode Island has the highest state-wide incidence (73, 84, 152). However, state figures obscure the focal nature of the disease; incidence figures in a given small area may approach 1 in 1000 residents (152). In Mount Kisco, NY, the prevalence rate in 1987 was 5 per 1000 residents (A. Curran, Westchester County Department of Health surveillance data). Approximately 4% of the residents of Lyme, Conn. have had LD (25); in smaller communities, 16% of the summer residents of Great Island, Mass. (145), and 7.5% of the summer residents of Shelter Island, NY (47), have had LD.

Nationwide, the 1988 figures represent a ninefold increase in cases compared with 1982, and a twofold increase compared with 1987 (84). In 1987–1988, 11 states reported their first cases of LD (84). Preliminary 1989 figures suggest further increases, especially in the central Midwest (84) and in the South Atlantic states. Georgia, for example, had a twelvefold increase between 1988 and 1989. The geographic distribution of *I. dammini* and *B. burgdorferi* extends into northern and inland areas not yet endemic for LD, which suggests that there may be new areas of disease in the future (7).

The increased number of cases of reported LD is probably due to many factors, including increased awareness on the part of both physicians and patients, more aggressive case finding, and the rapid development of new foci of disease (17). However, the absolute increase in cases, which is attributable to increased exposure to the vector, is probably from increased recreational, occupational, and residential exposure (17).

Lyme disease is spread by different species of Ixodes ticks, in different areas of the world. In the Northeast and northern Midwest, *Ixodes dammini*, the deer tick, is the primary vector of LD; in the West, it is *I. pacificus*, the black-legged tick (19). On the other continents other Ixodes ticks have been implicated: *I ricinus* in Europe; *I. persulcatus* in the transUral Soviet Union, China, and Japan; and possibly *I. hyocyclus* in Australia (118).

The life cycle of *I. dammini* includes dependence on hosts for each of its three stages of development. Eggs are laid in the early spring. Larvae, which emerge about one month later, seek and acquire a blood meal, usually from a white-footed field mouse. Once this is accomplished, usually between July and September, the larvae undergo a prolonged metamorphosis and emerge as nymphs in the earlier spring of the following year. The nymphs, too, single-mindedly seek a single blood meal, again usually provided by a mouse, from May through July. Having sated themselves, the nymphs molt. Adult male and female *I. dammini* emerge in the fall and obtain their blood meal, during the late fall and early winter, their preferred host being the white-tailed deer. Once engorged, the female drops to the ground and lays her eggs, and the two-year cycle starts again (20, 129).

In the Northeast and Midwest, *Peromyscus leucopus*, the white-footed field mouse, is the usual host for the larva and nymph *I. dammini*, and *Odocoileus virginianus*, the white-tailed deer, is the usual host for the adult stage. In general, *I. dammini* larvae do not carry *B. burgdorferi* (20), but acquire the organism with their first blood meal, typically from the field mouse. In *I. ricinus*, the sheep tick and principal vector in Europe, there is evidence to suggest transovarial passage of the organism (130). *P. leucopus* is a competent reservoir for *B. burgdorferi:* It is densely infested with the vector, *I. dammini;* it is the predominant host for the vector; and it has a persistent spirochetemia, which efficiently infects the vector (66, 79). The timing of the life cycle of *I. dammini* is crucial to the amplification of LD, because it is the infected nymph that then infects mice with *B. burgdorferi* before the initial blood meal of the larva. One generation of infected *I. dammini* thus is capable of passing *B. burgdorferi* on to the next. Deer are the primary hosts of adult *I. dammini* (159), insuring that the eggs can be laid, but *O. virginianus* does not act as a reservoir of *B. burgdorferi* infection (149). The crucial nature of the deer-tick interaction is clear: If, as was done on Great Island, the deer population is eliminated, the number of larval ticks and the number of new cases of LD are substantially diminished (159).

Other animals may be infected with *B. burgdorferi*, including many different mammals (3, 4, 21, 98) and birds (5, 156). Although humans can spread louse-borne Borrelial infections by distributing the lice, birds with infected ticks may distribute LD to new areas (5, 156). Once an infected tick gains a blood meal from a local mammalian potential reservoir, a new focus of LD may be established. The new outbreaks of LD in the South Atlantic states may, in part, be due to such avian distribution along migratory paths. Other deer may act as hosts to infected ticks; in California, black-tailed deer and the exotic species fallow and axis deer were found to carry *B. burgdorferi* (63).

Jack rabbits in Texas are seropositive for *B. burgdorferi*, which suggests intense exposure to the organism (21). The cotton-tailed rabbit, *Sylvilagus floridans*, found throughout the Western hemisphere, is usually infested with *I. dentatus* in the Eastern US; 50% of the *I. dentatus* isolated in one study carried *B. burgdorferi* (150). *I. spinalpis* infests rabbits in the Western US (150). Although *I. dentatus* rarely bites humans (3), *I. dammini, I pacificus*, and *I. scapularis* can feed on either humans or rabbits; thus, rabbits may represent a hidden enzootic cycle (151) and may introduce heterogeneous *B. burgdorferi* into the process (6).

In some areas of New York 100% of *I. dammini* ticks carry the organism (18), and in endemic areas 40% infection rates are common (73). In contrast, rate of infection of *I. scapularis* is usually 1% or less (73). *I. pacificus* infection rates may be as high as 10% (64), but are usually about 1–2% (18). The competence of the reservoirs in the various locations of endemic LD have a profound influence on the different tick infection rates, which in turn affect human infection rates. Thus, *P. leucopus*, which is a competent reservoir, helps amplify infection with *B. burgdorferi* in the Northeast and Midwest. However, the main hosts for nymphal *I. scapularis* and *I. pacificus* are skinks and other small lizards (127). The skink is not a competent reservoir for *B. burgdorferi*, so infection with the organism is not amplified in the South and the West.

Other ticks may also be involved in the transmission of LD. In New Jersey, another Ixodid tick, *Amblyomma americanum*, the Lone Star tick, may carry *B. burgdorferi* (107). *A. americanum* may be a secondary vector for LD (108). Occasionally other ticks, including Dermacenter (64), another Ixodid tick, and Ornithodoros (18), an Argasid tick, may carry *B. burgdorferi*. However, there is no evidence that these species serve as major vectors of LD. Individual reports suggest that other hematophagous insects, including fleas, mosquitoes, flies, stable flies, and flying insects may spread LD (5, 14, 98), perhaps by passive transfer, but the primary vector remains the Ixodid tick.

WHY NOW, WHY HERE?

I. dammini was first identified on Naushon Island, off the coast of Massachusetts, in the early 1920s. Since the 1970s, it has been collected from an increasingly large area of the US. In 1904, examples were identified in Ontario Province. This species was probably the same tick that visiting naturalists described as abundant in central New York in 1749, but virtually gone from the same area by the mid 1800s (31).

The recent expansion of LD and the domain of *I. dammini* parallel the change in abundance of deer. Before the 1600s, Native Americans engaged in a deliberate policy of forest burning to provide themselves with farmland. By the mid-1600s, virtually all large animals in southern New England and the mid-Atlantic region had been destroyed, the result of hunting for food and bartering with the colonists. After the settlers had displaced the original occupants of the region, agriculture kept the area deforested into the 1900s. Attempts to eradicate Texas cattle fever early in the twentieth century included a nationwide attempt to eradicate deer. Thus, when our first (and only) environmentalist President, Theodore Roosevelt, wished to go big game hunting, there were no deer to hunt on the continental US. He, and others, had to go to Africa or across a narrower body of water to the Elizabeth Islands, especially Naushon, where deer had long survived.

As agriculture failed in the East, and the nation was fed by the farmers of the Midwest and West, Eastern forests were gradually reestablished in the 1800s, and undergrowth, shrubbery and brush thrived again. With the earlier destruction of the forest, there had been destruction of the undergrowth, the preferred environment for field mice. Thus, a return of forest land increased the habitat for the mice.

Deer populations were reestablished in the East in the 1930s (for example, deer were taken from the upper peninsula of Michigan and imported to Nantucket Island). By the 1950s, deer were commonplace. [A parallel story of diminished and then increasing deer populations can be told in Europe during and after World War II. Deer population is a less crucial determinant of *I. ricinus* levels; unlike *I. dammini* adult *I. ricinus* have many potential hosts (31, 80).] We do not know if the imported deer carried with them *I. dammini* or whether the deer were infested by the small number of ticks that had survived on Naushon, Gardiner, and Shelter Islands and in Ontario. We do know, however, that with the increased number of deer has come an increased number of *I. dammini* and focal epidemics of LD (80, 128).

PUBLIC HEALTH CONCERNS AND PREVENTION STRATEGIES

Lyme disease has become a major public health problem in endemic areas, and these areas have expanded in recent years. As noted above, the increased number of cases of LD is attributable to greater exposure to a larger number of infected ticks. Humans are accidental hosts for *B. burgdorferi;* this disease is a zoonosis, which affects the animals noted above. Humans are only recently involved.

Forestry workers in endemic areas are at increased risk for seropositivity (37, 85), as are farmers (36), but an outdoor occupation is not required. Parks in suburban New York are an area of increased risk for LD (43), and even a private yard may not be safe. In areas of high incidence in Westchester, there is an average of one tick per square meter of lawn (41). A survey of patients with LD identified that 68.6% acquired the disease in their yard; 11.4% in school or camp; and 8.6%, in parks (42).

Recent work has suggested that dogs in areas with LD may also be afflicted. Serologic surveys of dogs may identify new foci of human LD; dogs may be used as sentinels of new areas of infection (40). Having pets, either dogs (2, 64, 88) or cats (32, 64, 135), or farm animals (135) may increase a person's risk of contracting LD, although this has been disputed (27).

Prevention of the disease can be accomplished at many levels of effort (110). Individuals can decrease their risk by taking simple precautions. Once the areas that contain the most ticks are identified—brush and undergrowth, especially in areas frequented by deer, and the lawn-shrub interface where field mice live—these areas should be avoided, where practical. When spending time outside, a person should tuck trousers into socks and wear long-sleeved shirts; nymphs live in low brush and grab onto a passing leg, then crawl upward to find a dining site. Wear light-colored clothing to spot the tiny tick more easily. It may take many hours, or even days, for a tick to bite and begin its blood meal, so there is time to remove ticks before any damage can be done (87, 96). At the end of an outdoor activity, inspect yourself and others; a shower will wash off any nonattached ticks. Tick repellents are very effective and, when used as directed, safe; application to shoes and socks may be especially useful. There is evidence that pets may carry ticks into the home; animals should be inspected carefully and frequently.

Ticks should be removed with thin tweezers or forceps, and antiseptic precautions should be used. Old wives' tales suggest that kerosene, petroleum jelly, or a lit match or cigarette are effective in tick removal; these methods should be eschewed, as they may cause the tick to regurgitate into the wound and cause infection.

Even if an engorged tick is found, Costello et al (28) estimate that in an endemic area only 10% of tick bites actually transmit the disease, which suggests that prophylactic antibiotic therapy of all tick bites is not necessary. In one study, the risk of adverse reactions from the antibiotic therapy was as great as the risk of seroconversion if no prophylaxis was given. When this experience is extrapolated to repeated prophylaxis of large numbers of residents in endemic areas, the cost and potential morbidity of therapy is tremendous. In addition, prophylactic therapy may give a false sense of security and lead individuals to abandon preventive techniques. We suggest that if no skin rash develops and no signs or symptoms of LD develop, a bitten individual should return for blood testing six to eight weeks after the bite. If seropositive, the patient can then be treated with an oral regimen. Some researchers suggest that a blood test at the time of the bite is indicated. True seropositivity would suggest prior exposure to *B. burgdorferi,* and, if treatment of asymptomatic seropositivity is considered advisable, therapy could be started at that time.

If a person lives in an area known to support a deer population, ticks carrying the organism may be on the lawn. Thus, local prevention may be indicated. One commercially available product consists of cardboard tubes that contain cotton soaked in an acaricide; mice take the cotton and use it for their nests. Any ticks present will be killed by the acaricide. This product does provide some protection, but unless all the other homeowners in the area use it, a mouse from the next yard can come onto the protected property and deposit ticks. Also, deer may deposit ticks on the lawn, and these ticks may not interact with mice or the treated nest. Finally, if use of this product leads the individual to become lax in personal preventive measures, a disservice has been done.

The use of granular acaricide may temporarily decrease the tick population locally. Ongoing studies suggest that this may be an effective means of decreasing the risk of LD, although the risk to children and pregnant women must be considered. Spraying yards with a variety of chemical acaricides usually does not allow acaricide to reach the primary habitat of the tick, i.e. the leaf litter on the ground and the underside of vegetation; thus, this method is not very effective (109, 127). Spraying larger areas at risk is not an appropriate and effective response to LD in endemic areas.

There is little else that can be done practically on a community-wide basis. On Great Island, removal of all deer was effective, but this cannot be done on the mainland. (This is perhaps the only issue that has ever united hunters, the gun lobby, and environmentalists). If we could eradicate all field mice, the ticks would probably search for a new host, in all likelihood the residents of the community. Controlled clear burning decreases the habitat for mice, but is also not practical in suburbia or more rural settings. Brush grows back, and deer, mice, and other animals return; birds might reintroduce *I. dammini* and *B. burgdorferi*.

PUBLIC HYSTERIA

The press and broadcast media have described LD as the scourge of the 1980s and 1990s and speak of LD as second only to AIDS as a public health problem in the US. Well-meaning physicians have stated as fact that LD is only very rarely cured, and that prolonged and repeated antibiotic regimens are necessary to suppress (but rarely cure) the ailment. The medical literature contains many reports of medical problems thought due to *B. burgdorferi* infection, claims supported by only a positive serologic test. The very tests practitioners use have been unfairly derided as being nearly useless, because of cross-reactivity, inaccuracy (especially early in the disease), and lack of standardization. The end result has been that patients in endemic areas often feel that their physicians do a poor job of diagnosing and treating LD, that the tests and therapeutic agents are profoundly flawed, and that LD should represent a cause for alarm (124).

Given their perception of LD as a mysterious, difficult to diagnose disease with an ever expanding and poorly defined clinical spectrum, it is no wonder that many patients have seized upon LD as the ultimate explanation for all of their ills. Given the perception of the poor quality for testing, the inability of physicians to diagnose the disease, and the inefficacy of therapy, it is no wonder that many patients view LD with alarm that borders on hysteria. Ill-advised physicians and lay groups have exacerbated the situation: If the tests are less than 100% accurate, how can you say that I don't have LD? If antibiotics are less than 100% effective, how can you tell me that I don't need further therapy? If I don't feel 100% improved, how can you tell me that I am cured and that I don't need more medicine?

What is the answer to these problems? Health care providers and planners must better educate physicians, patients, health officers, and veterinarians about the risks, manifestations, and treatment of LD. As increasing numbers of cases occur in a new area, local physicians are more aware of the disease and its signs and symptoms, are more adept at using the diagnostic laboratory tests available, and are more knowledgeable about therapy and prognosis.

We also must better educate the public about the kinds of personal and community-wide efforts that can be made to decrease the prevalence of LD. The time is long overdue for state and local health officials to become the major source of information of knowledge. They must take this role back from the "medical journals" available at the supermarket check-out. Educational materials have been developed by many groups, including our own at Robert Wood Johnson Medical School.

Finally, we must do a better job of exposing the charlatans. We must insist on scientific proof of assertions that have passed into the lay conventional wisdom. We must cooperate with the academic centers that perform clinical studies, so that a sufficient number of patients are included to provide answers to the many questions. We must insist that there are funds for such research, even in a time of fiscal restraint.

Lyme disease has become a major health concern in a growing number of communities. The problem is manageable, if we can convince our patients that Lyme disease is a cause for concern, not panic; vigilance, not hysteria.

Literature

1. Ackermann, R., Rehse-Kupper, B., Gollmer, E., Schmidt, R. 1988. Chronic neurologic manifestations of erythema migrans Borreliosis. *Ann. NY Acad. Sci.* 539:16–23
2. Aeschlimann, A., Chamot, E., Gigon, E., Jeannert, J.-P., Kesseler, D., Walther, C. 1986. *B. burgdorferi* in Switzerland. *Zbl. Bakt. Hyg. A* 263:450–58
3. Anderson, J. F. 1988. Mammalian and avian reservoirs for *Borrelia burgdorferi*. *Ann. NY Acad. Sci.* 539:180–91
4. Anderson, J. F. 1989. Epizootology of *Borrelia* in *Ixodes* tick vectors and reservoir hosts. *Rev. Infect. Dis.* 11(Suppl. 6):S1451–59
4a. Anderson, J. F., Duray, P. H., Magnarelli, L. A. 1990. *Borrelia burgdorferi* and *Ixodes dammini* prevalent in the greater Philadelphia area. *J. Infect. Dis.* 161:811–12
5. Anderson, J. F., Johnson, R. C., Magnarelli, L. A., Hyde, F. W. 1986. Involvement of birds in the epidemiology of the Lyme disease agent *Borrelia burgdorferi*. *Infect. Immun.* 51:394–96
6. Anderson, J. F., Magnarelli, L. A. LeFebvre, R. B., Andreadis, T. G., McAninch J. B., et al. 1989. Antigenically variable *Borrelia burgdorferi* isolated from cottontail rabbits and *Ixodes dentatus* in rural and urban areas. *Infect. Immun.* 27:13–20
7. Anderson, J. F., Magnarelli, L. A., McAninch, J. B. 1987. *Ixodes dammini* and *Borrelia burgdorferi* in Northern New England and upstate New York. *J. Parasitol.* 73:419–21

8. Aoki, S. K., Holland, P. V. 1989 Lyme disease—another transfusion risk? *Transfusion* 29:646–50
9. Bannwarth, A. 1941. Chronische Lymphocytare Meningitis, entzundliche Polyneuritis und "Rheumatismus." Ein Beitrag Zum Problem "Allergie und Nervensystem." *Arch. Psychiatr. Nervenk.* 113:284–376
10. Baranton, G., Saint-Girons, I. 1988. *Borrelia burgdorferi* survival in human blood samples. *Ann. NY Acad. Sci.* 539:444–45
11. Baron, S. J., Fister, R. D., Cable, R. G. 1989. Survival of *Borrelia burgdorferi* in blood products. *Transfusion* 29:581–83
12. Benach, J. L., Bosler, E. M., eds. 1988. Third Int. Symp. on Lyme Disease and Related Disorders. *Ann. NY Acad. Sci.* 539:1–513
13. Benach, J. L., Bosler, E. M., Hanrahan, J. P., Coleman, J. L., Habicht, G. S., et al. 1983. Spirochetes isolated from the blood of two patients with Lyme disease. *N. Engl. J. Med.* 308:740–42
14. Benach, J. L., Coleman, J. L. 1986. Clinical and geographic characteristics of Lyme disease in New York. *Zbl. Bakt. Hyg. A.* 263:477–82
15. Berardi, V. P., Weeks, K. E., Steere, A. C. 1988. Serodiagnosis of early Lyme disease: Analysis of IgM and IgG antibody responses by using an antibody-capture enzyme immunoassay. *J. Infect. Dis.* 158:754–60
16. Berger, B. W., MacDonald, A. B., Benach, J. L. 1988. Use of an autologous antigen in the serologic testing of patients with erythema migrans of Lyme disease. *J. Am. Acad. Dermatol.* 18:1243–46
17. Bowen, G. S., Griffin, M., Hayne, C., Slade, J., Schulze, T. L., Parkin, W. 1984. Clinical manifestations and descriptive epidemiology of Lyme disease in New Jersey, 1978 to 1982. *J. Am. Med. Assoc.* 251:2236–40
18. Burgdorfer, W. 1986. The enlarging spectrum of tick-borne spirochetoses: R. R. Parker Mem. Address. *Rev. Infect. Dis.* 6:932–40
19. Burgdorfer, W., Gage, K. L. 1986. Susceptibility of the black-legged tick, *Ixodes scapularis*, to the Lyme disease spirochete, *Borrelia burgdorferi*. *Zbl. Bakt. Hyg. A* 263:15–20
20. Burgdorfer, W., Hayes, S. F., Benach, J. L. 1988. Development of *Borrelia burgdorferi* in Ixodid tick vectors. *Ann. NY Acad. Sci.* 539:172–79
21. Burgess, E. C., Windberg, L. A. 1989.

Borrelia sp. infection in coyotes, black-tailed jack rabbits and desert cottontails in southern Texas. *J. Wildl. Dis.* 25:47–51
22. Callister, S. M., Agger, W. A., Schell, R. F., Brand, K. M. 1989. Efficacy of the urinary bladder for isolation of *Borrelia burgdorferi* from naturally infected, wild *Peromyscus leucopus*. *J. Clin. Microbiol.* 27:773–4
23. Camponova, F., Meier, C. 1986. Neuropathy of vasculitic origin in a case of Garin-Bujadoux-Bannwarth syndrome with positive *Borrelia* antibody response. *J. Neurol.* 233:698–726
24. Carlomagno, G., Luksa, V., Candussi, G., Rizzi, G. M., Trevisan, G. 1988. Lyme Borrelia positive serology associated with spontaneous abortion in an endemic Italian area. *Acta Eur. Fertil.* 19:279–81
25. Cartter, M. L., Mahar, P., Hadler, J. L. 1989. The epidemiology of Lyme disease in Connecticut. *Conn. Med.* 53:320–23
26. Ciesielski, C. A., Markowitz, L. E., Horsley, R., Hightower, A. W., Russell, H., Broome, C. V. 1989. Lyme disease surveillance in the United States, 1983–1986. *Rev. Infect. Dis.* 11(Suppl. 6):S1435–41
27. Cimmino, M. A., Fumarola, D. 1989. The risk of *Borrelia burgdorferi* infection is not increased in pet owners. *J. Am. Med. Assoc.* 262:2997–98
28. Costello, C. M., Steere, A. C., Pinkerton, R. E., Feder, H. M. Jr. 1989. Prospective study of tick bites in an endemic area for Lyme disease. *J. Infect. Dis.* 159:136–39
29. Coyle, P. K. 1989. *Borrelia burgdorferi* antibodies in multiple sclerosis patients. *Neurology* 39:760–61
30. Craft, J. E., Grodzicki, R. L., Steere, A. C. 1984. Antibody response in Lyme disease: Evaluation of diagnostic tests. *J. Infect. Dis.* 149:789–95
31. Cronon, W. 1983. *Changes in the Land: Indians, Colonists, and the Ecology of New England.* New York: Hill & Wang. 241 pp.
32. Curran, K. L., Fish, D. 1989. Increased risk of Lyme disease for cat owners. *N. Engl. J. Med.* 320:183
33. Dattwyler, R. J., Halperin, J. J. 1987. Failure of tetracycline therapy in early Lyme disease. *Arthritis Rheum.* 30:448–50
34. Dattwyler, R. J., Halperin, J. J., Pass, H. 1987. Ceftriaxone as effective therapy in early Lyme disease. *J. Infect. Dis.* 155:1322–25

35. deKooning, J., Hoogkaamp-Korstanje, J. A. A., van der Linde, M. R., Crijns, H. J. G. M. 1989. Demonstration of spirochetes in cardiac biopsies of patients with Lyme disease. *J. Infect. Dis.* 160:150–53

36. Dlesk, A., Bjarnason, D. F., Goldberg, J. W., Lee, M., Marx, J., et al. 1987. Lyme disease (LD) seropositivity by ELISA among farmers in an endemic area. *Arthritis Rheum.* 30(Suppl.):S49

37. Dlesk, A., Broste, S. K., Gries, D. J., Mitchell, P. D., Rowe, K. E. 1989. Lyme seroreactivity among U.S. Forest Service (USFS) workers from a "nonendemic" area for Lyme disease (LD). *Arthritis Rheum.* 32:S46

38. Dlesk, A., Broste, S. K., Harkins, P. G., McCarty, P. A., Mitchell, P. D. 1989. Lyme seropositivity (LS+) and pregnancy (PG) outcome in the absence of symptoms (Sx) of Lyme disease (LD). *Arthritis Rheum.* 32:S46

39. Duray, P. H. 1977. The surgical pathology of human Lyme disease. An enlarging picture. *Am. J. Surg. Pathol.* 11 (Suppl.1):47–60

40. Eng, T. R., Wilson, M. I., Spielman, A., Lastavica, C. C. 1988. Greater risk of *Borrelia burgdorferi* infection in dogs than in people. *J. Infect. Dis.* 158:1410–11

41. Falco, R. C., Fish, D. 1986. Prevalence of *Ixodes dammini* near the homes of Lyme disease patients in Westchester County, New York. *Am. J. Epidemiol.* 127:826–30

42. Falco, R. C., Fish, D. 1988. A survey of tick bites acquired in a Lyme disease endemic area in southern New York State. *Ann. NY Acad. Sci.* 539:456–57

43. Falco, R. C., Fish, D. 1989. Potential for exposure to tick bites in recreational parks in a Lyme disease endemic area. *Am. J. Public Health* 79:12–15

44. Fawcett, P. T., O'Brien, A. E., Doughty, R. A. 1989. An absorption procedure to increase the specificity of enzyme-linked immunosorbent assays for Lyme disease without decreasing sensitivity. *Arthritis Rheum.* 32:1041–44

45. Grodzicki, R. L., Steere, A. C. 1988. Comparison of immunoblotting and indirect immunosorbent assay using different antigen preparations for diagnosing early Lyme disease. *J. Infect. Dis.* 157:790–97

46. Halperin, J. J., Pass, H. L., Anand, A. K., Luft, B. J., Volkman, D. J., Dattwyler, R. J. 1988. Nervous system abnormalities in Lyme disease. *Ann. NY Acad. Sci.* 539:24–34

47. Hanrahan, J. P., Benach, J. L., Coleman, J. L., Bosler, E. M., Morse, D. L., et al. 1984. Incidence and cumulative frequency of endemic Lyme disease in a community. *J. Infect. Dis.* 150:489–96

48. Hansen, K., Asbrink, E. 1989. Serodiagnosis of erythema migrans and acrodermatitis chronica atrophicans by the *Borrelia burgdorferi* flagellum enzyme-linked immunosorbent assay. *J. Clin. Microbiol.* 27:545–51

49. Hansen, K., Hindersson, P., Pedersen, N. S. 1988. Measurement of antibodies to the *Borrelia burgdorferi* flagellum improves serodiagnosis in Lyme disease. *J. Clin. Microbiol.* 26:338–46

50. Hansen, K., Madsen, J. K. 1986. Myocarditis associated with tickborne *Borrelia burgdorferi* infection. *Lancet* 1:1323–24

51. Hedberg, C. W., Osterholm, M. T. 1990. Serologic tests for antibody to *Borrelia burgdorferi:* Another Pandora's box for medicine? *Arch. Intern. Med.* 150:732–33

52. Hedberg, C. W., Osterholm, M. T. MacDonald, K. L., White, K. E. 1987. An interlaboratory study of antibody to *Borrelia burgdorferi.* *J. Infect. Dis.* 155:1325–27

53. Horstrup, P., Ackermann, R. 1973. Durch zecker ubertragene Meningopolyneuritis (Garin-Bujadoux, Bannwarth). *Fortschr. Neurol. Psychiatr.* 41:583–606

54. Hyde, F. W., Johnson, R. C., White, T. J., Shelburne, C. E. 1989. Detection of antigens in urine of mice and humans infected with *Borrelia burgdorferi,* etiologic agent of Lyme disease. *J. Clin. Microbiol.* 27:58–61

55. Jacobs, J. C., Rosen, J. M., Szer, I. S. 1984. Lyme myocarditis diagnosed by gallium scan. *J. Pediatr.* 105:950–52

56. Johnson, R. C., Kodner, C., Russell, M. 1986. Passive immunization of hamsters against experimental infection with the Lyme disease spirochete. *Infect. Immun.* 53:713–14

57. Johnson, R. C., Kodner, C., Russell, M. 1986. Active immunization against experimental infection with *Borrelia burgdorferi.* *Infect. Immun.* 54:897–98

58. Johnson, R. C., Kodner, C., Russell, M. 1987. In vitro and in vivo susceptibility of Lyme disease spirochetes, *Borrelia burgdorferi* to 4 antimicrobial agents. *Antimicrob. Agents Chemother.* 31:164–67

59. Johnson, R. C., Schmid, G. P., Hyde, F. W., Steigerwalt, A. G., Brenner, D.

J. 1984. *Borrelia burgdorferi* sp. nov.:
Etiologic agent of Lyme disease. *Int. J.
Syst. Bacteriol.* 34:496–97

60. Johnston, Y. E., Duray, P. H., Steere,
A. C., Kashgarian, M., Buza, J., et al.
1985. Lyme arthritis. Spirochetes found
in synovial microangiopathic lesions.
Am. J. Pathol. 118:26–34

61. Kirsch, M., Ruben, F. L., Steere, A.
C., Duray, P. H., Norden, C. W.,
Winkelstein, A. 1988. Fatal adult respiratory distress syndrome in a patient
with Lyme disease. *J. Am. Med. Assoc.*
259:2737–39

62. Kristoferitsch, W. 1988. Neuropathies
in cases of acrodermatitis chronica
atrophicans *Ann. NY Acad. Sci.* 539:35–
45

63. Lane, R. S., Burgdorfer, W. 1986.
Potential role of native and exotic deer
and their associated ticks (Acari:*Ixodidae*) in the ecology of Lyme disease in
California, USA. *Zbl. Bakt. Hyg. A*
263:55–64

64. Lane, R. S. LaVoie, P. E. 1988. Lyme
Borreliosis in California: Acarological,
clinical, and epidemiological studies.
Ann. NY. Acad. Sci. 539:192–203

65. Lastavica, C. C., Wilson, M. L., Berardi, V. P., Spielman, A., Deblinger, R.
D. 1989. Rapid emergence of a focal
epidemic of Lyme disease in coastal
Massachusetts. *N. Engl. J. Med.* 320:
133–37

66. Levine, J. F., Wilson, M. L., Spielman,
A. 1985. Mice as reservoirs of the Lyme
disease spirochete. *Am. J. Trop. Med.
Hyg.* 34:355–60

67. Liu, N. Y., Dinerman, H., Levin, R.
E., Massarotti, E., Molloy, P. J., et al.
1989. Randomized trial of doxycycline
vs. amoxicillin-probenecid for the treatment of Lyme arthritis: Treatment of
non-responders with IV penicillin or
ceftriaxone. *Arthritis Rheum.* 32:
S46

68. Luger, S. W., Krauss, E. 1990.
Serologic tests for Lyme disease: In-
terlaboratory variability. *Arch. Intern.
Med.* 150:761–63

69. MacDonald, A. B. 1986. Human fetal
Borreliosis, toxemia of pregnancy, and
fetal death. *Zbl. Bakt. Hyg. A* 263:189–
200

70. MacDonald, A. B., Benach, J. L.,
Burgdorfer, W. 1987. *Stillbirth* follow-
ing maternal Lyme disease. *NY State J.
Med.* 87:615–16

71. Magnarelli, L. A. 1988. Serologic diagnosis of Lyme disease. *Ann. NY Acad.
Sci.* 539:154–61

72. Magnarelli, L. A. 1989. Quality of
Lyme disease tests. *J. Am. Med. Assoc.*
262:3464–65

73. Magnarelli, L. A., Anderson, J. F.,
Apperson, C. S., Fish, D., Johnson, R.
C., Chappell, W. A. 1986. Spirochetes
in ticks and antibody to *Borrelia burgdorferi* in white-tailed deer from Connecticut, New York State, and North
Carolina. *J. Wildl. Dis.* 22:178–88

74. Magnarelli, L. A., Anderson, J. F., Barbour, A. G. 1989. Enzyme-linked im-
munsorbent assays for Lyme disease:
Reactivity of subunits of *Borrelia burgdorferi*. *J. Infect. Dis.* 159:43–49

75. Magnarelli, L. A., Anderson, J. F.,
Johnson, R. C. 1987. Cross-reactivity in
serological tests for Lyme disease and
other spirochetal infections. *J. Infect.
Dis.* 156:183–88

76. Mandell, H., Steere, A. C., Reinhardt,
B. N., Yoshinari, N., Munsat, T. L., et
al. 1989. Lack of antibodies to *Borrelia
burgdorferi* in patients with amyotrophic
lateral sclerosis. *N. Engl. J. Med.*
320:255–56

77. Marcus, L. C., Steere, A. C., Duray, P.
H., Anderson, A. E., Mahoney, E. B.
1985. Fatal pancarditis in a patient with
coexistent Lyme disease and Babesiosis.
Ann. Intern. Med. 103:374–76

78. Markowitz, L. E., Steere, A. C., Benach, J. L., Slade, J. D., Broome, C. V.
1986. Lyme disease during pregnancy *J.
Am. Med. Assoc.* 255:3394–96

79. Mather, T. N., Wilson, M. L., Moore,
S. I., Ribiero, J. M. C., Spielman, A.
1989. Comparing the relative potential
of rodents as reservoirs of the Lyme
disease spirochete *(Borrelia burgdorferi)*. *Am. J. Epidemiol.* 130:143–
50

80. Matuschka, F. R., Spielman, A. 1986.
The emergence of Lyme disease in a
changing environment in North America
and Central Europe. *Exp. Appl. Acarol.*
2:337–53

81. Melet, M., Gerard, A., Voiriot, P.,
Gayet, S., May, T., et al. 1986.
Meningoradiculonevrite mortelle au
cours d'une maladie de Lyme. *Presse
Med.* 15:2075

82. Mertz, L. E., Wobig, G. H., Duffy, J.,
Katzmann, J. A., 1985. Ticks, spirochetes, and new diagnostic tests for
Lyme disease. *Mayo Clin. Proc.*
60:402–6

83. Midgard, R., Hofstad, H. 1987. Unusual manifestations of nervous system
Borrelia burgdorferi infection. *Arch.
neurol.* 44:781–83

84. Miller, G. L., Craven, R. B., Bailey, R.
E., Tsai, T. F. 1990. The epidemiology

of Lyme disease in the US, 1987–1988. *Lab. Med.* 21:285–89

85. Munchhoff, P., Wilske, B., Preac-Mursic, V., Schierz, G. 1986. Antibodies against *Borrelia burgdorferi* in Bavarian forest workers. *Zbl. Bakt. Hyg. A* 263:412–19

86. Nadal, D., Hunziker, U. A., Bucher, H. U., Hitzig, W. H., Duc, G. 1989. Infants born to mothers with antibodies against *Borrelia burgdorferi* at delivery. *Eur. J. Pediatr.* 148:426–27

87. Nakayama, Y., Spielman, A. 1989. Ingestion of Lyme disease spirochetes by ticks feeding on infected hosts. *J. Infect. Dis.* 160:166–67

88. Neubert, U., Munchhoff, P., Volker, B., Reimers, C. D., Pfluger, K. H. 1988. *Borrelia burgdorferi* infections in Bavarian forest workers: A follow-up study. *Ann. NY Acad. Sci.* 539:476–79

89. NY State Dept. Health. 1989. Lyme disease surveillance. *Epidemiol. Notes* 4 (8):1–4

90. Pachner, A. R. 1986. Spirochetal diseases of the CNS. *Neurol. Clin.* 4:207–22

91. Pachner, A. R., Steere, A. C. 1985. The triad of neurologic manifestations of Lyme disease: meningitis, cranial neuritis, and radiculoneuritis. *Neurology* 35:47–53

92. Pachner, A. R., Steere, A. C. 1986. CNS manifestations of third stage Lyme disease. *Zbl. Bakt. Hyg. A* 263:301–6

93. Pachner, A. R., Steere, A. C., Sigal, L. H., Johnson, C. J. 1985. Antigen-specific proliferation of CSF lymphocytes in Lyme disease. *Neurology* 35:1642–44

94. Pappolla, M. A., Omar, R., Saran, B., Andorn, A., Suarez, M., et al. 1989. Concurrent neuroborreliosis and Alzheimer's disease: Analysis of the evidence. *Hum. Pathol.* 20:753–57

95. Pfister, H.-W., Einhaupl, K. M., Wilske, B., Preac-Mursic, V. 1986. Bannwarth's syndrome and enlarged neurological spectrum of arthropod-borne Borreliosis. *Zbl. Bakt. Hyg. A* 263:343–47

96. Piesman, J., Donahue, J. G., Mather, T. N., Spielman, A. 1986. Transovarially acquired Lyme disease spirochete *(Borrelia burgdorferi)* in field-collected larval *Ixodes dammini* (Acari:Ixodidae). *J. Med. Entomol.* 23:219

97. Piesman, J., Mather, T. N., Sinsky, R. J., Spielman, A. 1987. Duration of tick attachment and *Borrelia burgdorferi* transmission. *J. Clin. Microbiol.* 25:557–58

98. Rawlings, J. A. 1986. Lyme disease in Texas. *Zbl. Bakt. Hyg. A* 263:483–87

99. Reik, L. Jr., Burgdorfer, W., Donaldson, J. O. 1986. Neurologic abnormalities in Lyme disease without erythema chronicum migrans. *Am. J. Med.* 81:73–78

100. Reik, L. Jr., Steere, A. C., Bartenhagen, N. H., Shope, R. E., Malawista, S. E. 1979. Neurologic abnormalities of Lyme disease. *Medicine* 58:281–94

101. Reznick, J. W., Braunstein, D. B., Walsh, R. L., Smith, C. R., Wolfson, P. M., et al. 1986. Lyme carditis electrophysiologic and histopathologic study. *Am. J. Med.* 81:923–27

102. Rosa, P. A., Schwan, T. G. 1990. A specific and desensitive assay for the Lyme disease spirochete, *Borrelia burgdorferi*, using the polymerase chain reaction. *J. Infect. Dis.* 160:1018–29

103. Russell, H., Sampson, J. S., Schmid, G. P., Wilkinson, H. W., Plikaytis, B. 1984. Enzyme-linked immunosorbent assay and indirect immuno-fluorescence assay for Lyme disease. *J. Infect. Dis.* 149:465–76

104. Schlesinger, P. A., Duray, P. H., Burke, B. A., Steere, A. C., Stillman, T. 1985. Maternal-fetal transmission of the Lyme disease spirochete, *Borrelia burgdorferi*. *Ann. Intern. Med.* 103:67–68

105. Schmidli, J., Hunziker, T., Moesli, P., Schaad, U. B. 1988. Cultivation of *Borrelia burgdorferi* from joint fluid three months after treatment of facial palsy due to Lyme Borreliosis. *J. Infect. Dis.* 158:905–6

106. Schmitz, J. L., Schell, R. F., Hejka, A. G., England, D. M. 1990. Passive immunization prevents induction of Lyme arthritis in LSH hamsters. *Infect. Immun.* 58:144–48

107. Schulze, T. L., Bowen, S. B., Bosler, E. M., Lakat, M. F., Parkin, W. E., et al. 1984. *Amblyomma americanum:* A potential vector of Lyme disease in New Jersey. *Science* 224:601–3

108. Schulze, T. L., Lakat, M. F., Parkin, W. E., Shisler, J. K., Charette, D. J., Bosler, E. M. 1986. Comparison of rates of infection by the Lyme disease spirochete in selected populations of *Ixodes dammini* and *Amblyomma americanum* (Acari: Ixodidae). *Zbl. Bakt. Hyg. A* 263:72–78

109. Schulze, T. L., Parkin, W. E., Bosler, E. M. 1988. Vector tick populations and Lyme disease: A summary of control

strategies. *Ann. NY Acad. Med.* 539: 204–11

110. Schulze, T. L., Parkin, W. E., Bosler, E. M. 1988. Vector populations and Lyme disease: Summary of control strategies. *Ann. NY Acad. Sci.* 539:204–11

111. Schulze, T. L., Shisler, J. K., Bosler, E. M., Lakat, M. F., Parkin, W. E. 1986. Evolution of a focus of Lyme disease. *Zbl. Bakt. Hyg. A* 263:65–71

112. Schutzer, S. E., Coyle, P. K., Belman, A. L., Golightly, M. G., Drulle, J. 1990. Sequestration of antibody to *Borrelia burgdorferi in immune* complexes in seronegative Lyme disease. *Lancet* 1:312–15

113. Schwan, T. G., Burgdorfer, W., Schrumpf, M. E., Karstens, R. H. 1988. The urinary bladder, a consistent source of *Borrelia burgdorferi* in experimentally infected white-footed field mice *(Peromyscus leucopus)*. *J. Clin. Microbiol.* 26:893–95

114. Schwan, T. G., Simpson, W. H. J., Schrumpf, M. E., Karstens, R. H. 1989. Identification of *Borrelia burgdorferi* and *B. hermsii* using DNA hybridization probes. *J. Clin. Microbiol.* 27:1734–38

115. Schwartz, B. S., Goldstein, M. D., Ribiero, J. M. C., Schulze, T. L., Shahied, S. I. 1989. Antibody testing in Lyme disease: A comparison of results in four laboratories. *J. Am. Med. Assoc.* 262:3431–34

116. Shrethra, M., Grodzicki, R. L., Steere, A. C. 1985. Diagnosing early Lyme disease. *Am. J. Med.* 78:235–40

117. Sigal, L. H. 1985. Response of mononuclear cells to *Borrelia burgdorferi*. *Ann. Intern. Med.* 103:808

118. Sigal, L. H. 1988. Lyme disease: A worldwide Borreliosis. *Clin. Exp. Rheumatol.* 6:411–21

119. Sigal, L. H. Lyme disease, 1988: Immunologic manifestations and possible immunopathogenetic mechanisms. *Semin. Arthritis Rheum.* 18:151–67

120. Sigal, L. H. 1990. *B. burgdorferi (BB)*-specific immune reactivity (IR) at the site of Lyme disease (LD) inflammation. *4th Int. Conf. Lyme Borreliosis,* Stockholm, Sweden

121. Sigal, L. H. 1990. Experience with the first one hundred patients referred to a Lyme Disease referral center. *Am. J. Med.* 86:577–83

122. Sigal, L. H., Steere, A. C., Dwyer, J. M. 1988. In vivo and In vitro evidence of B cell hyperactivity during Lyme disease. *J. Rheumatol.* 15:648–54

123. Sigal, L. H., Steere, A. C., Freeman, D. H., Dwyer, J. M. 1986. Proliferative

responses of mononuclear cells in Lyme disease: Concentration of *Borrelia burgdorferi*—reactive cells in joint fluid. *Arthritis Rheum.* 29:761–69

124. Sigal, L. H., Taragin, M. I. 1990. Public awareness and anxiety concerning Lyme disease (LD) in an endemic area. *4th Int. Conf. Lyme Borreliosis,* Stockholm, Sweden

125. Sigal, L. H., Tatum, A. H. 1988. Lyme disease patients' serum contains IgM antibodies to *Borrelia burgdorferi* that corss-react with neuronal antigens. *Neurology* 38:1439–42

126. Snydman, D. R., Schenkein, D. P., Berardi, V. P., Lastavica, C. C., Pariser, K. H. 1986. *Borrelia burgdorferi* in joint fluid in chronic Lyme arthritis. *Ann. Intern. Med.* 104:798–800

127. Spielman, A. 1988. Prospects for suppressing transmission of Lyme disease. *Ann. NY Acad. Sci.* 539:212–20

128. Spielman, A., Levine, J. F., Wilson, M. L. 1984. Vectorial capacity of North American *Ixodes* ticks. *Yale J. Biol. Med.* 57:507–13

129. Speilman, A., Wilson, M. L., Levine, J. F., Piesman, J. 1985. Ecology of *Ixodes dammini*-borne human Babesiosis and Lyme disease. *Annu. Rev. Entomol.* 30:439–60

130. Stanek, G., Burger, I., Hirschl, A., Wewalka, G., Radda, A. 1986. Borrelia transfer by ticks during their life cycle. *Zbl. Bakt. Hyg. A* 263:29–33

131. Stanek, G. L., Flamm, H., Barbour, A. G., Burgdorfer, W., eds. 1986. Proc. 2nd Int. Symp. Lyme disease and related disorders. *Zbl. Bakt. Hyg. A* 263:1–495

132. Steere, A. C. 1989. Lyme disease. *N. Engl. J. Med.* 321:586–96

133. Steere, A. C., Bartenhagen, N. H., Craft, J. E., Hutchinson, G. J., Newman, J. H., et al. 1983. The early clinical manifestations of Lyme disease. *Ann. Intern. Med.* 99:76–82

134. Steere, A. C., Batsford, W. P., Weinberg, M., Alexander, J., Berger, H. J., et al. 1980. Lyme carditis: Cardiac abnormalities of Lyme disease. *Ann. Intern. Med.* 93(Part 1):8–16

135. Steere, A. C., Broderick, T. F., Malawista, S. E. 1978. Erythema chronicum migrans and Lyme arthritis: Epidemiologic evidence for a tick vector. *Am. J. Epidemiol.* 108:312–21

136. Steere, A. C., Gibofsky, A., Patarroyo, M. E., Winchester, R. J., Hardin, J. A., Malawista, S. E. 1979. Chronic Lyme arthritis. Clinical and immunogenetic differentiation from rheumatoid arthritis. *Ann. Intern. Med.* 90:896–901

137. Steere, A. C., Green, J., Schoen, R. T., Taylor, E., Hutchinson, G. J., et al. 1984. Successful parenteral penicillin therapy of established Lyme arthritis. *N. Engl. J. Med.* 312:869–74

138. Steere, A. C., Grodzicki, R. L., Kornblatt, A. N., Craft, J. E., Barbour, A. G., et al. 1983. The spirochetal etiology of Lyme Disease. *N. Engl. J. Med.* 308:733–40

139. Steere, A. C., Hutchinson, G. J., Rahn, D. W., Sigal, L. H., Craft, J. E., et al. 1983. Treatment of the early manifestations of Lyme disease. *Ann. Intern. Med.* 99:22–26

140. Steere, A. C., Malawista, S. E. 1979. Cases of Lyme disease in the US: Locations correlated with distribution of *Ixodes dammini*. *Ann. Intern. Med.* 91:730–33

141. Steere, A. C., Malawista, S. E., Craft, J. E., Fischer, D. K., Garcia-Blanco, M., eds. 1984. Int. Symp. Lyme disease. *Yale J. Biol. Med.* 57:445–705

142. Steere, A. C., Malawista, S. E., Snydman, D. R., Shope, R. E., Andiman, W. A., et al. 1977. Lyme arthritis. An epidemic of oligoarticular arthritis in children and adults in three Connecticut communities. *Arthritis Rheum.* 20:7–17

143. Steere, A. C., Pachner, A. R., Malawista, S. E. 1983. Neurologic abnormalities of Lyme disease: Successful treatment with high dose intravenous penicillin. *Ann. Intern. Med.* 99:767–72

144. Steere, A. C., Schoen, R. T., Taylor, E. 1987. The clinical evolution of Lyme arthritis. *Ann. Intern. Med.* 107:725–31

145. Steere, A. C., Taylor, E., Wilson, M. L., Levine, J. F., Spielman, A. 1986. Longitudinal assessment of the clinical and epidemiologic features of Lyme disease in a defined population. *J. Infect. Dis.* 154:295–300

146. Stiernstedt, G. 1985. Tick-borne *Borrelia* infection in Sweden. *Scand. J. Infect. Dis.* Suppl. 45:1–70

147. Stiernstedt, G. T., Granstrom, M., Hederstedt, B., Skoldenberg, B. 1985. Diagnosis of spirochetal meningitis by enzyme-linked immunosorbent assay and indirect immunofluorescence assay in serum and cerebrospinal fluid. *J. Clin. Microbiol.* 21:819–25

148. Stiernstedt, G., Skoldenberg, B., Garde, A., Kolmodin, G., Jorbeck, H., et al. 1986. Clinical manifestations of *Borrelia* infections of the nervous system. *Zbl. Bakt. Hyg. A* 263:289–96

149. Telford, S. R. III, Mather, T. N., Moore, S. I., Wilson, M. L., Spielman, A. 1988. Incompetence of deer as reservoirs of the Lyme disease spirochete. *Am. J. Trop. Med. Hyg.* 39:105–9

150. Telford, S. R. III, Spielman, A. 1989. Enzootic transmission of the agent of Lyme disease in rabbits. *Am. J. Trop. Med. Hyg.* 41:482–90

151. Telford, S. R. III, Spielman, A. 1989. Competence of a rabbit-feeding *Ixodes* (Acari: Ixodidae) as a vector of the Lyme disease spirochete. *J. Med. Entomol.* 26:118–21

152. Tsai, T. F., Bailey, R. E., Moore, P. S. 1989. National surveillance of Lyme disease, 1987–1988. *Conn. Med.* 53: 324–26

153. Vallat, J. M., Hugon, J., Lubeau, M., Leboutet, M. J., Dumas, M., Desprogres-Gotteron, R. 1987. Tick-bite meningoradiculoneuritis: Clinical, electrophysiologic, and histologic findings in 10 cases. *Neurology* 37:749–53

154. Wallis, R. C., Brown, S. E., Kloter, K. O., Main, A. J. Jr. 1978. Erythema chronicum migrans and Lyme arthritis: Field study of ticks. *Am. J. Epidemiol.* 108:322–27

155. Weber, K., Bratzke, H-J., Neubert, U., Wilske, B., Duray, P. H. 1988. *Borrelia burgdorferi* in a newborn despite oral penicillin for Lyme borreliosis during pregnancy. *Pediatr. Infect. Dis.* 7:286–89

156. Weisbrod, A. R., Johnson, R. C. 1989. Lyme disease and migrating birds in the Saint Croix River Valley. *Appl. Environ. Microbiol.* 55:1921–24

157. Williams, C. L., Benach, J. L., Curran, A. S., Spierling, P., Medici, F. 1988. Lyme disease during pregnancy. A cord blood serosurvey. *Ann. NY. Acad. Sci.* 539:504–6

158. Williams, C. L., Curran, A. S., Lee, A. C., Sousa, V. O. 1985. Lyme Disease: Epidemiologic characteristics of an outbreak in Westchester County, NY. *Am. J. Public Health* 76:62–65

159. Wilson, M. L., Telford, S. R. III, Piesman, J., Spielman, A. 1988. Reduced abundance of immature Ixodes dammini (Acari:Ixodidae) following elimination of deer. *J. Med. Entomol.* 25:224–28

Annu. Rev. Publ. Health. 1991. 12:111–40

THE HEALTH EFFECTS OF LOW LEVEL EXPOSURE TO LEAD

Herbert L. Needleman

School of Medicine, University of Pittsburgh, Pittsburgh, Pennsylvania 15213

David Bellinger

Neuroepidemiology Unit, Children's Hospital and Harvard Medical School, Boston, Massachusetts 02115

KEY WORDS: lead poisoning, child development, environmental health, neurotoxicity

INTRODUCTION

Eight years ago, the problem of low level lead exposure in children was reviewed in the *Annual Review of Public Health* (65). (The term "low level" refers to exposure that is below those at which clinical signs of lead poisoning are apparent.) Since that time, knowledge about lead's health effects, biochemical toxicology, and sources and routes to people has grown exponentially. Real progress in lowering environmental levels of lead has been achieved, notably through the virtual ban on leaded gasoline. In some sectors, particularly housing, efforts to abate lead have failed completely. But, despite increased recognition of the widespread distribution of lead, islands of ignorance about its effects at low dose persist. Many modern pediatric textbooks contain discussions of the diagnosis and treatment of frank lead poisoning, but do not mention effects of lead at lesser dose.

In this review, we examine some of the newer biomedical and epidemiological information about lead at low dose and evaluate the recent studies. We then suggest some policy actions to redress the imbalance between the broad knowledge of lead's dangers and the limited steps to eliminate them.

111

0163/7525/91/0501-0111$02.00

At the time of the earlier review, the most prominent question under study was whether there were substantial health effects at doses below those that produce symptoms. That question, once a focus of considerable controversy, has been effectively settled by a substantial group of newer studies. The newer data on lead's effects have revised the threshold for effect downward. As more sensitive measurement techniques have been used, the recognized effect level has dropped steadily in response.

Once held to be solely an American problem, low dose exposure has become a worldwide issue in the past decade. Except for a few British studies, in the 1970s almost all the data came from American investigations. In the 1980s, good epidemiological and toxicological studies were reported from England (110), Scotland (30), Denmark (33), Germany (108), Italy (13), Greece (36), Australia (59), and New Zealand (28). Studies of human health effects have extended backward in time to examine the impact of intrauterine exposure on birth outcome (67) and subsequent growth and neurobehavioral development of infants (8, 23, 27, 59). Some ongoing studies have followed individuals from birth up to ten years of age, and one has followed a school age cohort for 11 years into young adulthood. Experimental investigations have employed the newest tools of modern biology, pharmacology, and psychology to study the effects of lead on receptor development, subcellular systems, and animal behavior.

SOURCES OF LEAD AND PATHWAYS TO HUMANS

Paint is the major source of high dose lead for American children today. Although the Lead Paint Poisoning Prevention Act was passed in 1971, many homes still have high amounts of lead in them. The recent Agency for Toxic Substances and Disease Registry (ATSDR) Report to Congress (1) estimates that there are 5 million tons of lead in household paint in the US. Of all houses built before 1960, 70% have leaded surfaces. More disturbing is the ATSDR estimate that 6 million homes, which house 2 million young children, are decayed and deteriorated with leaded surfaces. These houses are the critically dangerous dwelling units.

Lead is a natural constituent of soil and dust; it migrates only minimally in soil. Typical concentrations in uncontaminated soil range from 10–50 ppm. Human activity can raise these levels by a factor of 10–200. Within 25 meters of major roadways, concentrations in soil as high as 2000 ppm are found; these concentrations fall off exponentially with distance. Levels as high as 60,000 ppm have been measured in soil near smelters. In urban soils, the lead found is a mixture of powdered paint and atmospheric fallout of lead particles. The Environmental Protection Agency (EPA) is currently funding three demonstration projects to assess the efficiency of removing lead-contaminated soil in reducing the blood lead levels of inner-city children.

Dust is composed predominantly of the windblown, fine particle derivative of soil. Lead in dust may exceed that in soil because the smaller soil particles that become part of the dust mixture tend to have higher concentrations of lead. Indoor dust may have elevated lead concentrations because of weathering of paint, carry-in of soil, or fallout from airborne sources. Household dust lead level appears to be the strongest predictor of blood lead level among nonpoisoned children (6). Removing paint by sanding, scraping, or burning can raise dust lead levels into the hazardous range. The abatement of lead in homes can be dangerous. Lead abatement should only be done by trained workers in unoccupied dwellings; thorough cleanup is essential before residents may return.

Airborne lead derives from mobile and stationary sources. With the reducted amounts of lead added to gasoline, blood lead levels have declined (24, 78). Corresponding reductions in blood lead levels have been measured in children and in the umbilical cord blood of newborns (79).

Standing water contains only trace amounts of lead. The major source of lead in drinking water is household plumbing. There are three major contributors: the pipe from the street main (known as the "gooseneck"), lead pipes, and solder joints. Plumbosolvent water—water that is acidic and soft—can leach out large amounts of lead from the plumbing. This problem is especially true if the water has been standing in the pipes for an extended period of time. An estimated 16% of household water supplies have concentrations of lead over the proposed standard of 20 μg/dl (25). Despite the undisputed fact that lead is added to drinking water downstream from the source, the EPA's recommended surveillance method calls for measuring lead at the source, and then sampling a small number of households. This method is inadequate to protect consumers and can miss communities that have an unacceptable proportion of homes over the standard.

Food can be an important source of lead. Some lead is taken up by crops, particularly root vegetables, such as radishes, potatoes, and carrots. Some crops near heavily traveled roads can accumulate atmospheric lead deposited on them. The meat of foraging animals does not present a risk because lead is not concentrated in muscle. Most lead contamination of food occurs during processing. Food from soldered cans has much higher levels of lead than unprocessed food or food from seamless, aluminum cans. The lead comes from microdots of spattered solder and is leached from the seam. Although fired chinaware is generally safe, many ceramic products contain glazes or are made from clays that have leachable lead in them. Foreign tableware is not subject to the same control as US-made goods. Some bone meals sold in health food stores for calcium replenishment have dangerous amounts of lead.

Other, rarer sources that can be clinically significant are cosmetics and folk medicines. Some hair dye preparations for men contain lead acetate. The darkening pigment results from the reaction of lead acetate with sulfides in the air to produce lead sulfide. Kohl, an eye cosmetic used by Moslems, and surma, one used by Hindus, may have large concentrations of lead. These cosmetics may be applied directly to babies. Or, infants get the cosmetics on their hands by touching their mother's faces. The infants then put their hands in their mouths. The folk remedies *Azarcon* and *Greta* which are used by some Hispanic people for abdominal distress, may contain toxic amounts of lead.

EXPERIMENTAL DATA ON THE BIOLOGICAL EFFECTS OF LEAD

In this section, we limit discussion to studies that direct attention to three heretofore undescribed toxic mechanisms of lead. For a complete review of recent biochemical data on lead's effects, consult EPA's Air Lead Criteria Document (24).

Most of lead's toxicity is ascribed to its action on proteins, where it binds to sulfhydryl groups. Brown et al (15), in a provocative study, suggest another mechanism of equal importance. The investigators measured lead binding to yeast tRNA, and compared binding at pH5 and pH7.4. At pH7.4, they observed site-specific cleavage of the ribophosphate backbone. This cleavage took place between sites D17 and G18 and was catalytic, rather than stoichiometric, which may account for lead's ability to rapidly depolymerize tRNA. The authors suggest that this cleavage may be a toxic mechanism of at least as much generalized importance as sulfhydryl binding, and may have no apparent threshold.

Marcovac and Goldstein (58) demonstrated another potentially important toxic mechanism. They studied proteinkinase c, a calcium and phospholipid enzyme involved in growth, differentiation, and many other cellular functions. Of all metals tested, only lead activated phosphokinase c at picomolar concentrations. Phosphokinase c, which is a central part of the second messenger system, may be a fundamental route for lead toxicity in the central nervous system (CNS) and other organs.

The search for the biological substrate of lead-associated behavioral alterations has focused on changes in capillary permeability (69), neuronal development (2, 16), myelination (44), and catecholamine metabolism. Recent studies from Surrey pointed in a different direction: opioid receptor development and function. Winder et al (107) found that administration of low doses of lead to nursing rodent dams produced decreased development of pro-encephalin, an endogenous opioid precursor in offspring pups. This observation spawned many related studies. Using heat as the pain stimulus, Kitchen et al (41) found that the antinociceptive action of morphine was strongly diminished by low levels of lead in young rodents. They inferred that altered development of the μ opioid receptor was responsible for the observed effect. With similar blunting of the analgesic action of ketocyclazocine, Kitchen et al (41) reported a δ opioid receptor agonist. Bailey and Kitchen (3) then showed that the four putative peptide products of proencephalin were markedly depressed by small doses of lead in rodents at ten days of age.

Studies of rodent consumption of alcohol in relation to lead exposure suggest that these intriguing findings may have relevance for human behavior. Nation et al (61) have shown that naive rats find 15% solutions of alcohol aversive, but when given lead in their diet sufficient to raise their blood leads to 61 μg/dl, the rats increase their alcohol intake in both forced choice and free choice paradigms. Lead-fed rodents were also more responsive in the avoidance training period. The authors infer that lead increases emotionality, and that the rodents seek alcohol for its anxiolytic properties.

NEUROBEHAVIORAL EFFECTS ON INFANTS AND CHILDREN

Recent Studies of School Age Children

Childhood lead poisoning was first described in Brisbane, Australia, almost a century ago. The pioneering work of A. J. Turner (102) and J. Lockhart Gibson (31) established the environmental cause: paint on the porch railings of the dwellings. The first Australian lead paint legislation was enacted 20 years later. Fifty years after the Australian law, the first Lead Paint Poisoning Act was passed in the United States. In the early part of the twentieth century, lead paint poisoning was a frequent cause of death in city pediatric wards. As late as the 1940s, it was widely believed that a child who survived the acute phase of the illness was left without sequelae. In 1943, Byers reported on the follow-up of 20 children who had recovered from acute intoxication (17); of the group, 19 were behavior disordered or learning disabled. Byers asked how many cases of school failure or behavior disorder were in fact cases of missed lead poisoning. The pursuit of this question marked the beginning of the modern age of lead intoxication studies.

Growing interest in public health and inner-city populations stimulated screening studies of lead in asymptomatic children. Studies in the 1960s showed that as many as 20% of all children bore elevations of blood lead as high as two thirds that considered toxic (>60 μg/dl). Byer's conjecture that silent lead exposure may be a frequent cause of cognitive deficit in children was raised for reexamination. Some early studies of low level lead exposure showed a lead-related deficit (21, 45, 70); others did not (43, 46). Many reviews of studies from this period have been published (9, 65, 86). In this review, we focus instead on our own work, on more recent studies by other investigators, and on forward studies of exposure that begin with the fetus.

In interpreting these studies, there are often problems with small sample size, difficulties in measuring some of the variables, and "overcontrol" for confounding factors. There is no doubt of the effect of lead at high exposure levels; that matter is settled. What is not settled is at how low a concentration lead continues to produce harmful effects. Estimating the effect of a toxicant at low concentrations is difficult, precisely because the effects are likely to be subtle. The section *Issues in Drawing Inferences from Observational Studies* explores the difficulties in interpreting the literature and shows why an authors' conclusions cannot always be relied upon.

In 1979, Needleman and colleagues attempted to confront the common problems in design that challenge investigators of lead (64). The problems were inadequate markers of exposure, weak measures of outcome, insufficient attention to potential confounders, and selection bias. They studied a sample of 2335 children who were attending ordinary first and second grade in Massachusetts schools. Shed deciduous teeth were collected and analyzed for lead. The tooth, which is a long-term storage system, may reflect early exposure even after blood lead level has returned to normal. Of the 2335 children, those with dentine lead levels in the highest decile and lowest decile were identified; 270 were brought into the neurobehavioral laboratory for an intensive four-hour assessment. The children were given a panel of measures that examined psychometric intelligence, speech and language ability, attention, and classroom behavior. The researchers measured and compared 39 covariates that could affect child development between the high and low lead groups. Those covariates that differed between groups were controlled as potential confounders. Children with a history of clinical plumbism, head injury, or seizures were eliminated from the data analysis. After adjustment for confounders, the high lead group (>20 ppm, N=58) scored significantly lower than the reference group (<10 ppm, N=100) on intelligence quotient (IQ), speech and language processing, and attention (Table 1). For 2146 students, a tooth lead level and a teacher-completed questionnaire that sampled classroom behavior were obtained. The prevalence of nonadaptive classroom behavior has related in a dose-response fashion to tooth lead levels (Figure 1). Lead exposure disrupted the usual relationship between maternal and child exposure (10).

This study proved to be the springboard for a group of investigations using similar designs. Yule et al (110) studied British school children classified by blood lead. They reported significantly lower IQ, reading, and spelling scores in children with elevated blood lead levels, after control of age, social class, and gender. Another study by this group failed to observe an association between lead and IQ, achievement, or behavior in a group of middle-class children (48).

In another British investigation, Smith et al (98) examined 402 London

Table 1 Comparison of test outcomes between students with high and low lead levels: Analysis of Covariance (64)

Test	Mean Score in Low Lead Group	Mean Score in High Lead Group	P Value
Full scale IQ	106.6	102.1	0.03
Verbal IQ	103.9	99.3	0.03
Performance IQ	108.7	104.9	0.08
Seashore rhythm test			
Sum	21.6	19.4	0.002
Token test			
Sum	24.8	23.6	0.09
Sentence repetition test	12.6	11.3	0.04

[From Needleman et al (64)]

six-year olds who were classified by tooth lead level. The exposure of these children was lower than that of the children in the Needleman et al study (64). The Smith group administered an extensive battery of outcome measures. They adjusted for covariates related to tooth lead to evaluate the association between tooth lead and outcome. In some cases, this may have resulted in overcontrol. For instance, developmental delay, a possible effect of lead, was controlled in assessing IQ, reading level, and the Seashore rhythm test. The bivariate regression showed a statistically significant (P<.05) relationship between lead and IQ. With the adjustment for covariates, the effect size was diminished, although a consistent decrease in performance related to tooth lead was reported. Pocock et al (74) reanalyzed the Smith study. They used regression techniques and measured the interaction between lead and gender. For boys, the lead effect was statistically significant. Although Pocock et al interpret this as an explanatory finding, there is abundant evidence that males are more sensitive to many toxicants, including lead.

Winneke et al conducted two studies in the German cities Duisburg and Stohlburg. In the Duisburg study (108), they found a marginally significant decrease in IQ (5–7 points) across lead groups and a significant association between lead and perceptual-motor function. In the Stohlburg study (109), they found significant associations between tooth lead and perceptual motor integration, reaction time performance, and mothers' behavioral ratings.

Perino and Ernhart (70) were among the first to report an association between lead and children's intelligence. They studied black preschoolers who differed on blood lead level (high >40; low <30). Controlling for maternal IQ and gender, they reported that lead was inversely related to General Cognitive Index (GCI) of the McCarthy Scales. At follow-up in the first grade, early exposure was no longer significantly related to outcome

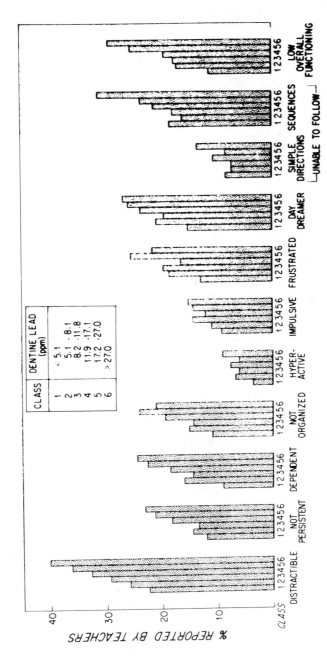

Figure 1 Teachers' ratings of 2146 students on 11-item forced-choice questionnaire. Proportion of negative comments within each dentine lead group are plotted. Teachers were blind to students' dentine lead levels, but knew each student for at least two months. (Reprinted by permission of the *New England Journal of Medicine*; see Ref. 64.)

(26). Ernhart interpreted this to mean that any effect had disappeared. But the sample size, originally 80, was reduced to 63 and then 40 because of loss-to-follow-up and missing data; the power to find an effect decreased correspondingly. Inferring no effect from studies of insufficient power is a frequent error encountered in lead studies. It and other Type II errors are discussed further in a later section of this review.

Schroeder et al (90) and Hawk et al (37) studied poor black children in North Carolina. Schroeder et al studied 104 children with blood levels between 6–59 μg/dl. Adjusting for several covariates, the authors reported that lead was significantly associated with IQ (P<.01). Five years later, with a reduced sample group, the association was weaker, but the slope of the regression of IQ on blood lead remained negative. Hawk et al (37) evaluated 80 children aged 3–7 years. The mean blood lead was 21.8 μg/dl; the highest was 26.7 μg/dl. Lead was significantly associated with IQ score after adjustment for socioeconomic status (SES), maternal IQ, and home environment.

The most recent studies have larger samples and children of higher socioeconomic status. Silva et al (97) studied 579 New Zealand children at age 11. The mean blood lead was 11.1 μg/dl. Only two children had blood leads in excess of 30 μg/dl. Significant associations were found between log blood lead and children's reading, spelling, and behavior (as reported by both parents and teachers). Although the relationship between blood lead and IQ was inverse, it did not reach the P=.05 criterion. Fergusson et al (28) studied 724 children in the Christchurch New Zealand child development project and found that high tooth lead levels were strongly related to lower reading scores, poorer spelling, lower mathematics scores, and poorer handwriting. The association between lead and IQ was inverse, but did not reach statistical significance at P=.05.

Fulton et al (30) studied 501 middle class school children in Edinburgh. They adjusted for many covariates and, using multiple regression, found a highly significant (P=.003) inverse relationship between lead and IQ. In a more recent report, lead was also related to classroom performance (101). The effects of lead in this study extended down to 10μg/dl. Hatzakis et al (36) studied 509 Greek children from Lavrion, a smelter site. Controlling for 17 covariates, they also found a highly significant inverse association between lead and IQ (P= .00007). Lead was also related to teachers' ratings of children's classroom behavior and reaction time.

Hansen et al (33) studied 162 middle class children from Aarhus, Denmark, using multivariate linear regression. They found significant associations between lead and IQ and scores on the Bender-Gestalt Test. They found no significant difference on the Seashore Rhythm Test or on the Trail-Making Test. They also found a significant increase in the risk for learning disabilities, as measured by need for remedial education in reading, speech, or math (51).

Bergomi et al (13) studied 216 children from northern Italy. Controlling for gender and SES, they evaluated the relationship between lead exposure and outcome. Outcome was measured by the Weschler Intelligence Scale for Children-Revised (WISC-R), Bender-gestalt, Trail Making, the Toulouse Pieron Test, and delayed reaction time. After adjustment for covariates, tooth lead was significantly related to WISC-R scores and performance on the Toulouse Pieron Test (a measure of attention).

Forward Studies of Lead and Infant Development

Lead crosses the placenta (89), and infant umbilical cord blood lead concentrations are correlated with maternal concentrations. In many studies, surveillance of children's exposure began during pregnancy and continued through the postnatal period. The forward nature of these investigations offers an opportunity to determine the direction of causality and to settle whether lead is a marker or a cause of cognitive deficit.

We and our colleagues identified a two-year cohort of children born at the Boston Hospital for Women (N=11, 837). We capitalized on an ongoing study of risk factors and birth outcome conducted by Linn and colleagues (50). For 5000 births, we estimated the relationship between lead and outcome at birth. Adjusting for covariates, lead was related, in dose-dependent fashion, to the rate of minor malformations (skin tags, herniae, hydrocoeles, hemangiomata). Lead was not related to birth weight or major malformations (67). In addition, infants' cord blood lead levels were associated with mothers' systolic blood pressure during labor and the prevalence of pregnancy hypertension (77).

We followed 249 of the children, from three exposure groups: low (PbB <3 μg/dl), middle (PbB= 6–7 μg/dl), and high (PbB= >10 μg/dl). We evaluated the children at 1, 6, 12, 18, 24 and 57 months of age (6), which enabled us to plot the time course of exposure and to collect environmental data at several periods. In later analyses, we evaluated the impact of exposure at each epoch on concurrent and subsequent outcome.

This cohort was unusual in comparison to most studies: The majority of children were from middle and upper middle class families, and the exposure to lead was higher in the higher classes. This latter observation was probably due to the patterns of residence; many of our more favored children lived in older homes in heavily trafficked neighborhoods. This relationship enabled us to disentangle the usually encounted collinearity between SES and lead exposure. When we adjusted for SES, the size of the lead effect became larger. When we controlled for covariates, we found that higher umbilical cord blood lead levels were associated with lower scores on the Bayley Scales

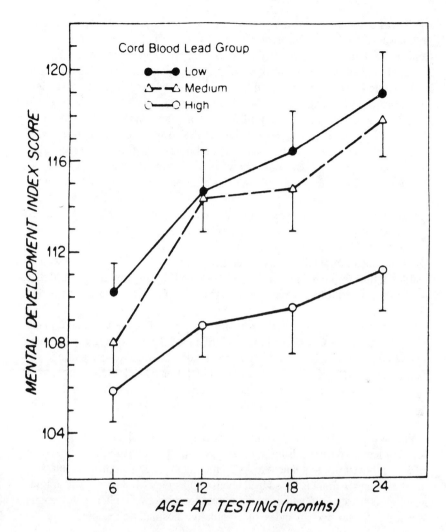

Figure 2   Mean Mental Development Index Scores at four ages in infants according to the lead level in umbilical-cord blood. (Reprinted by permission of *New England Journal of Medicine;* see Ref. 8.)

of Infant Development at all epochs between 6 and 24 months of age (Figure 2). None of the measures of postnatal exposure were associated with infants' development over this period. At 57 months of age, exposure at 24 months was significantly related to the GCI score on the McCarthy Scales, which decreased by approximately three points for each natural log unit increase in blood lead level. An increase in blood level at age 24 months from 3 to 20

μg/dl was associated with a six point decrease in GCI. The high blood lead group was bounded on the lower side by 10 μg/dl, far below the current Centers for Disease Control (CDC) screening target guideline of 25 μg/dl. Although the effect of prenatal exposure was attenuated at 57 months, it continued to be significant for children who were of lower SES, for boys, and for children whose exposure at 24 months was high (7, 12).

Dietrich et al (23) have followed forward a cohort of 300 infants born in Cincinnati. As in the Boston cohort, prenatal exposure to lead was associated with later decrements in performance on the Bayley Scales of Infant Development. At six months of age, boys showed an 8.7 point decrease in the Mental Development Index for every 10 μg/dl increase in blood lead. At 24 months, the deficits due to lead were no longer significant on the Bayley Scales. Language development at age 39 months was inversely associated with level of prenatal exposure (23). Many studies from this project have documented an association between lead at low dose and physical growth. A decrease of 114 g in birth weight for each natural log unit increase in maternal blood lead level during pregnancy was found (14), and linear growth was inhibited among infants with high exposure in both the prenatal and postnatal periods (95).

Ernhart et al (27) conducted a forward study of infants in Cleveland. This group found an association between cord blood lead levels and abnormal reflexes, and between prenatal exposure and developmental scores at age six months on the Bayley Scales and the Kent Infant Development Scale. No associations were apparent at later ages. Interpretation of this study is difficult because half the mothers in the sample were chosen because of their alcohol abuse.

Vimpani et al (104) and McMichael et al (59) reported on the relationship between lead exposure during pregnancy and postnatally in a large cohort of infants in proximity to a smelter. At 24 months of age, a significant relationship between six months blood lead levels and Bayley MDI scores was found. At 48 months, a significant association was found between GCI scores on the McCarthy Scales and an index of cumulative postnatal exposure.

FOLLOW UP STUDIES OF LOW LEVEL LEAD EXPOSURE

A few studies have been undertaken to determine whether the effects of lead exposure are lasting. Bellinger et al (11) followed 141 of the children from the Needleman et al study (64) into the fourth and fifth grades. After covariate adjustment, performance on a school administered IQ test was inversely associated with past dentine lead levels (P=.1, n=101). They also found an inverse association between teachers' rating of children's abilities and dentine lead (P=.1). High lead students had a greater need for special services.

Prevalence of grade retention was significantly related to lead level (P=.025). Direct observation of systematically sampled classroom behavior did not reveal any association with lead.

Schroeder et al (90) were able to locate 50 of their 104 original subjects after five years. Although the bivariate correlation between lead and IQ was similar, the association was not statistically significant after covariate adjustment. The reduced power to find an effect may have produced this result.

Ernhart (26) followed 63 of her original sample of 80 children five years after initial assessment. As measured by McCarthy Scales, IQ was related to contemporary blood lead level, but not past level. This study also had low statistical power.

We recently followed up 132 subjects of our 1979 sample, now young adults (mean age 18.3 years) (68). We found that high dentine lead levels in 1979 were associated with a covariate adjusted sevenfold increased risk of failure to graduate from high school, and a sixfold increased risk for reading disability, (defined as a reading score two grades below expected). Students with high levels of lead had more absenteeism in their final year of school, lower class rank, poorer vocabulary and grammatical reasoning scores, longer reaction times, poorer hand-eye coordination, and slower finger tapping. We conclude that the effects of lead are enduring and are likely to be predictors of life success (Figure 3, Figure 4).

OTHER HEALTH EFFECTS OF LEAD

Growth

Schwartz et al (92) used data on 2695 children between 6 months and 7 years of age from the National Health and Nutrition Examination Survey (NHANES) II health survey to examine the relationship between lead and several outcomes. Blood lead levels were significantly related to stature after controlling for SES and 15 nutritional variables, including hematocrit and transferrin saturation. A blood lead level increase of 26 μg/dl was associated with a 3% reduction in height. There was no apparent threshold.

In the Cincinnati prospective study, Dietrich et al (23) found that maternal blood lead levels were inversely associated with birth weight. They suggested that this association was partly responsible for the reduced development scores of infants with higher prenatal exposure. Shukla et al (95) showed that, among children with high prenatal exposure (>8 μg/dl), growth in the first year of life was inversely related to postnatal exposure. Ward et al (105) reported an inverse association between birth weight and head circumference and placental lead levels. McMichael et al studied the birth weights of infants in the Australian forward study (59) and found that the incidence of low birth weight (<2500 g) was greater in the high lead group. Blood leads tended to be

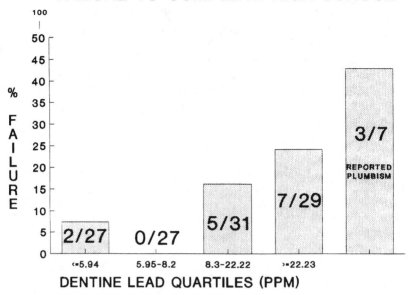

CHILDHOOD LEAD EXPOSURE AND
FAILURE TO COMPLETE HIGH SCHOOL

Figure 3   The proportion of students who failed to graduate high school classified by past exposure to lead. Asymptomatic individuals are classified by lead quartile. Seven of ten who were reported to have had clinical plumbism are also displayed. (Reprinted by permission of *The New England Journal of Medicine;* see Ref. 68.)

somewhat lower in the low birth weight group. Not all studies have reported a lead-associated decrement in birth weight, however (60, 67).

Lead's effects on growth might be an expression of its action on thyroid function. Sandstead (87) showed that lead interfered with the uptake and concentration of iodine in the thyroid gland of rats and of men poisoned by bootleg whiskey (88). Huseman (39) reported that two lead-poisoned children had impaired release of thyroid stimulating hormone after thyroid releasing hormone stimulation. Another potential mechanism is lead's inhibition of the prodution of the active form of vitamin D and the cascade of effects on calcium metabolism (54, 83).

Hearing

Robinson et al (81) found a linear increase in the 2000 Hz pure tone hearing threshold in children whose blood lead levels ranged from 6 to 47 μg/dl, with no sign of a threshold. Robinson et al (82) also studied 117 children, aged 39–66 months, from the Cincinnati study using brainstem auditory-evoked

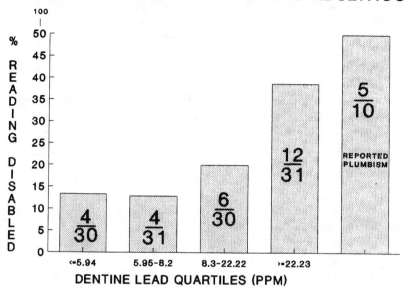

Figure 4 The proportion of reading disabled children classified by past exposure to lead. Asymptomatic children are classified by lead quartile. and ten children with a past history of clinical plumbism are displayed. The disability is defined as reading at two or more grades below expected. (Reprinted by permission of *The New England Journal of Medicine;* see Ref. 68.)

potential. They found increased latencies in the interpeak latencies III-V in relation to the prenatal blood lead level. Schwartz & Otto (93), again using data from the NHANES II study, found that lead was positively associated with hearing loss at 500, 1000, 2000, and 4000 Hz, with no evidence of a threshold.

Blood Pressure

Many recent studies have shown a positive relationship between lead exposure and blood pressure. Harlan et al (34) and Pirkle et al (72) examined data from the NHANES II study. Harlan's paper dealt with persons aged 12–74, whereas Pirkle restricted the sample to 40–59 year-olds. Both groups reported significant associations in male subjects. Schwartz (91) reported significant associations in both men and women aged 20–74 years. Pocock et al (75) examined data from the British Regional Heart Study, (N=7371 men, 40–59 years) and found significant associations between blood lead levels and both systolic and diastolic blood pressure.

ISSUES IN DRAWING INFERENCES FROM OBSERVATIONAL STUDIES

The question of whether low levels of lead are associated with deficit has provoked considerable controversy in the past. There are several reasons for this controversy: The possibility that many children have been damaged by lead, but have not been recognized, is disquieting: The effects of lead are modest in magnitude and often coexist with other risk factors that afflict the poor or minorities. And, because the financial stakes are high, vested interests have weighed in on the argument. Industry has exerted considerable energy and funds to persuade regulators and the public that lead is innocuous at lesser doses.

In making causal inferences from nonexperimental studies, the investigator must balance two opposing risks: the risk of Type I errors (accepting spurious associations as causal and the risk of Type II errors (missing true causal associations). Considerable attention has been given to avoiding Type I errors; scientific rigor is felt to be defended by focusing on this type of risk. Less attention has been given to avoiding Type II errors. Scientists must attempt to reduce the volume of spurious claims in the literature; it is time-consuming to correct false claims. But it is also important, particularly when evaluating the threats of widespread environmental pollutants, not to overlook true associations between exposures and deficits. In reviewing the literature on lead and IQ, we have encountered six flaws in design or interpretation that have systematically reduced the risk of Type I errors, but at the cost of increased risk of Type II errors:

1. OVERVALUING THE STATUS OF THE P VALUE AS A CRITERION.   Many investigators have dismissed the possibility of a causal association because the statistical significance did not reach the criterion of $P<.05$. Studies that report statistical significance of $P=.09$, or $P=.1$ are interpreted to mean that no association has been shown, or indeed, that none exists in nature (26, 98). This criterion is simply a threshold of convenience and is dependent on the sample size, as well as the effect size. R. A. Fisher (29), who is credited with introducing the criterion, was more modest in describing its use:

> It is convenient to take this point [$P=.05$] as a limit in judging whether a deviation is to be considered significant or not. Deviations exceeding twice the standard deviation are thus formally regarded as significant.

Jerome Cornfield commented (19) on this point:

> The prespecification of a significance level, e.g. .05 or .01, has no sound logical basis and remains unjustified.

2. POSTULATING PHANTOM COVARIATES.   Many factors affect child development and IQ, and careful investigators attempt to identify these factors and adjust for them in their analyses. In many, but not all cases, adjustment for confounders reduces the size of the effect of lead. Some investigators have argued from this reduced effect size: If the proper unidentified covariate had been measured or if identified covariates were measured more precisely, the effect size would drop to zero. For a variate to be a confounder, it must independently affect the outcome under examination and be associated with lead. There is a considerable, if not exhaustive, body of information on those factors that affect child development. Although the possibility of an undiscovered, lead-correlated influence on development exists, it is a tenuous reach to attribute a lead effect to residual confounding unless the variable responsible has been identified and measured.

3. BUILDING NONVERIDICAL CAUSAL MODELS.   It is an oversimplification to classify variates into three groups: independent variables, dependent variables, and covariates. A variate may have more than one position in a causal chain. It could be an effect modifier, or it could be both an outcome (dependent) variable and an independent variable. The position of a variable in a causal chain requires knowledge about the biology of the disease. In ordinary, least squares regression, attempting to control for all variates, without regard for their position in the causal nexus, risks removing variance that truly belongs to lead. For example, controlling for hyperactivity (35), developmental delay (98), or school placement (108) clearly overcontrols; such control reduces the estimate of the true effect size. The same argument applies to the hypothesis that because mothers of children with high lead and deficit tend to score lower on the IQ tests, the cause of the child's deficits is the mother's rearing competence. A mother's rearing skill might be a product of her own lead exposure as a child, a hypothesis consistent with findings in animal studies (4).

4. INADEQUATE SAMPLE SIZE AND STATISTICAL POWER.   The statistical power of a study (the probability of finding a true effect) is determined by the number of subjects, the effect size being sought, and the alpha level set by the investigator. Most studies of lead at low dose have used samples of fewer than 300 subjects. A recent review of 12 studies of lead and IQ, revealed that only four had power greater than .70 (63). One study (35) that claimed to show no lead effect had a sample size of 48 and evaluated 17 covariates. The statistical power in that study was between 0 and .30.

5. UNDERESTIMATING THE BIOLOGICAL SIGNIFICANCE OF A "SMALL" EFFECT SIZE.   In most studies, the difference between the mean IQ scores of

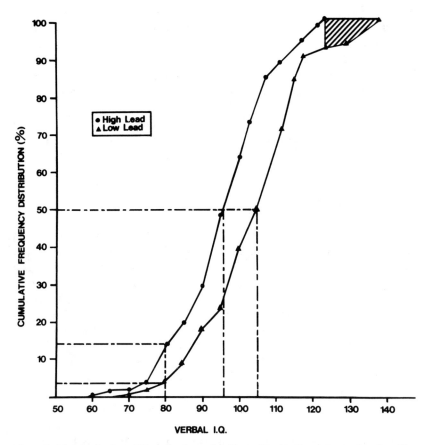

Figure 5   The distribution of IQ scores shows the effects of lead in first and second graders. The median IQ difference between groups is six points. At the low end of the scale, severe deficits occurred four times more often among children with high-lead levels. The highest score in the high-lead group was 125; among the low-lead children, 5% scored above 125. If these results are generally applicable, many children may be damaged intellectually, and others may fall short of their potential because of low-level lead exposure. (Reprinted by permission of *New England Journal of Medicine;* see Ref. 66.)

the exposed and unexposed groups studied is about 4–7 IQ points, and the partial r for lead in multiple regressions is about .14. Some researchers interpret these differences to be inconsequential. Figure 5 plots the actual cumulative frequency of IQ scores in high and low lead subjects from one of our studies (66). Although the median difference in IQ is six points, the rate of severe deficit, i.e. IQ <80, is four times greater in the high lead group (16% vs. 4%). In addition, the shift of the curve to the left that occurs among children with higher lead exposure affects the top of the distribution severely.

This shift demonstrates a previously ignored effect of major public consequence: Lead exposure may prevent about 5% of the population from achieving truly superior function. No attention has been given to lead's effects at the high end of the scale.

6. EXPECTING PROOF OF CAUSALITY.   Critics of the lead-IQ hypothesis often state that the data do not "prove" that lead caused the deficits. This assertion is true. Causality is a construct not subject to empirical proof (38, 49). The task of epidemiologists is to assemble data in a careful and rigorous fashion and then to draw the most veridical picture of nature from it. In asserting that a study has failed to prove a causal effect, the issue of possibly uncontrolled (and sometimes unidentified) covariates is often raised. But in the real world, multivariate space is infinite. There are a limitless number of factors that could influence cognition, and a finite number of subjects that can be studied. (The modal cost for a lead-IQ study is greater than $1000/subject). Thus, investigators are always dealing with unsaturated structural models, and a variety of regression lines can be drawn through the data points. In addition, both independent and outcome variables are subject to errors in measurement, and the former tends to bias the estimated coefficients, toward zero.

Epidemiologists recognize the formal and practical barriers to causal proof. They accept, instead, certain canons that permit the drawing of causal inferences (40). These canons include time precedence of the putative cause; biological plausibility; nonspuriousness, or control of appropriate confounders; and consistency.

The time precedence of exposure to developmental deficit has been demonstrated in the forward studies of lead in infants and in the elegant animal studies of Rice & Gilbert (80) and Cory-Slechta et al (20). The plausibility of the low lead-developmental deficit association is strongly supported by the resemblance of the findings at low dose to the more striking outcomes long observed in clinical plumbism. The meticulous efforts to control covariates in epidemiological investigations (and the parallel findings in experimental animal studies) satisfy the canon of nonspuriousness. Consistency is discussed in the next section.

METAANALYSIS OF THE LEAD IQ STUDIES

Individual studies of childhood lead exposure have differed in their conclusions, and review articles of the same group of studies have differed in their interpretations (9, 65, 73, 86). Narrative review articles have certain unavoidable constraints: They are subject to bias in selection of included papers. The reviewer's judgments of the papers may be biased. And, the overall conclusion may be based on simple tallies of papers that find an association and those that do not. Such an approach to research synthesis badly degrades the data.

A relatively new alternative to narrative reviews is metaanalysis, by which each study is treated as a data point in a sample of the universe of studies. Joint estimates of probability or effect size can be made with various mathematical techniques. There are three published metaanalyses of lead at low dose and IQ.

Schwartz et al (94) first summarized the data from six studies. Using Fisher's technique for aggregating probabilities, he found that the joint probability of finding the pattern of reported results by chance under the null hypothesis was .004.

Needleman & Bellinger (62) extended Schwartz's analysis to 13 studies. Using Fisher's technique, they calculated a joint probability of $3 \times 10{-}12$ for the hypothesis that lead and IQ are not associated.

Needleman & Gatsonis (63) reviewed 24 studies on lead and IQ. They excluded those studies that did not control for covariates and did not use multivariate analysis. The 12 included studies were then classified by tissue (blood or tooth) and metaanalyses conducted within groups. This study went further than its predecessors; it tested samples for homogeneity, estimated the range of effect sizes, and calculated joint probabilities on the basis of weighted and unweighted samples (weighting by subject number). To test for influential studies, probabilities were recalculated for each group after leaving out each study. The sign of the lead coefficient was negative in 11 of the 12 studies, the partial r ranged from $-.27$ to $-.003$. The joint P values for the seven blood lead studies were less than .0001 for both methods of analysis; for the tooth lead studies, the joint probabilities were .0005 and .004. The effect was robust to the removal of any study. The three metaanalyses taken together permit a strong inference that lead is causally related to IQ deficits.

INTERPRETATION OF FINDINGS

The evidence summarized above draws us to conclude that lead is a potent toxicant that acts on many organ systems. The lower limit of its "no effect" level has yet to be plumbed. Indeed, with the development of more sensitive measures of function and more rigorous experimental and quasiexperimental designs, definition of undue lead exposure has regularly been reduced. It was set at 60 μg/dl only three decades ago, and was 40 μg/dl only 15 years ago. It certainly will be lowered to acknowledge the most recent studies of effects on IQ, hearing, and growth.

There is no shortage of toxic mechanisms to explain the epidemiologic findings. Understanding of lead's toxic properties has deepened with the

Table 2 Summaries of estimated numbers of children 6 months to 5 years old in all SMSAs who are projected to exceed selected levels of blood lead, by urban status, 1984 (1)

| Characteristic | Base Population | Blood Level (μg/dl) | | |
		>15	>20	>25
In SMSAs >1,000,000	7,251,000	1,493,400	459,500	128,200
In central city	2,886,200	901,800	301,700	86,200
Not in central city	4,364,800	591,600	157,800	42,000
In SMSAs <1,000,000	3,536,400	483,000	142,400	40,300
In central city	1,504,800	301,100	93,800	27,500
Not in central city	2,031,600	181,900	48,600	12,800
In small SMSAs	3,052,600[a]	404,200	113,600	31,200
National total	13,840,000	2,380,600	715,500	200,700

[a] Total includes 6800 children who could not be stratified by income and were not included in estimates for three Pb-B levels.

application of new methods of analysis. Lead affects receptors, calcium channels, dendritic complexity, cortical connectivity during maturation, migration of cells, and the opiate system. Recent studies suggest that lead may affect RNA transcription and activate protein kinase at concentrations in the range of calcium concentrations. There is a plethora of demonstrated toxic effects; in the human host, it is reasonable that more than one phenomenon is operating at a time. Each mechanism has its own threshold and its own time constant.

In the child, the direct toxicologic expression of lead interacts with many other variables. Nutritional status and social stimulation are two of the more obvious operative factors. Iron, protein, calcium, and zinc deficiency all are associated with increased lead uptake. Lead enhances calciuria and zincuria (103). This effect provides a potential positive feedback loop, in which lead exposure results in depleted calcium and zinc stores, which in turn result in enhanced lead uptake. In those households where the parents are verbal and more inclined to stimulate the children, the toxic expression of lead at very low doses might be, to some extent, meliorated. This protective effect of highest socioeconomic status is overridden at blood lead levels greater than 10 μg/dl (5). In those homes where the possibilities for a child's enrichment are constrained, the toxic effects of lead are allowed full expression.

The newest estimates of the prevalence of elevated lead exposure are troubling (1). Table 2 displays the numbers of children exceeding 15, 20, and 25 μg/dl by area of residence. Table 3 displays the distribution of blood lead levels for children classified by race and class. There are 2.4 million children in the US with blood leads greater than 15 μg/dl (standard metropolitan statistical areas only), and there is a distinct class and race bias to the exposure patterns. An estimated 1.9 million children live in deteriorated homes with

Table 3 Projected percentages of children 0.5-5 years old estimated to exceed selected Pb-B criterion values (μg/dl) by family income, race, and urban status, who live "inside central city" of SMSAs, 1984 (1)[a]

Family Income/Race	>15 μg/dl	
	<1 M	>1 M
<$6,000		
White	25.7	36.0
Black	55.5	67.8
$6,000–14,999		
White	15.2	22.9
Black	41.1	53.6
≥$15,000		
White	7.1	11.9
Black	26.6	38.2

[a] SMSA with population <1 million (<1 M) and SMSA with population >1 Million (>1 M)

leaded surfaces. The social costs of problem of this magnitude can only be estimated. Provenzano (76) attempted to calculate the costs of acute and convalescent care and remedial education in 1980. Based on CDC prevalence data for blood leads greater than 35 μg/dl and 1979 costs for health care and remedial education, he set the annual costs at $429 million to $1 billion in 1979 dollars. The estimate requires upward revision to reflect current prevalence data, inflated health and educational costs, and lost wages.

AREAS FOR FUTURE RESEARCH

Measurement of Lead Burden

Recent research has dramatic implications for issues such as lead screening protocols an case definition. Since the early 1970s, most screening programs have relied on a hematofluorometric method to measure the concentration of erythrocyte protoporphryn in capillary blood, an index of heme synthesis derangement (71). According to the current CDC screening guidelines, a child with a blood erythrocyte protoporphyrin (EP) level greater than 35 μg/dl should be referred for follow-up evaluation of blood lead level and classified in terms of risk (18). Lead toxicity, or lead poisoning, is defined as a blood lead level greater than 25 μg/dl and a blood EP level greater than 35 μg/dl.

The utility of EP as a marker of blood lead level is greatly reduced at the lower blood lead levels that recent research indicates are toxic. The blood lead level at which EP begins to increase in response to rising blood lead levels is 16–18 μg/dl (71), although the point of inflection appears to depend on children's iron status (57). Data from the NHANES II survey indicate that among children in the general population, reliance on EP alone as the basis for screening produces many false-negatives, even at blood lead levels that exceed the current "action level." For example, in the NHANES II survey, only 47% of children with a blood lead level greater than 30 μg/dl had an EP level greater than 30 μg/dl (53). The false-negative rate is dramatically higher if the target blood lead level is shifted to 15 or 20 μg/dl.

At the time the CDC last redefined the screening guidelines, the decision was based on both biologic and practical considerations. Although the CDC acknowledged that the threshold for biologic toxicity is less than 25 μg/dl, they also recognized that the EP test has relatively poor sensitivity and specificity at blood lead levels less than 25 μg/dl. The decision to recommend reliance on the EP test was essentially a compromise. The decision balanced the deficiencies of EP concentration as a screening measure and the practical issues of analytical cost, acceptability of venous blood sampling, and laboratory proficiency required for lead analysis of micro blood samples. With a developing consensus that 25 μg/dl is unacceptable as the intervention blood lead level, the goal of screening clearly will become the identification of children with considerably lower blood lead levels. The basis for screening will have to shift either to blood lead itself or a biologic marker that is considerably more sensitive to blood lead than EP is. At this time, the former alternative appears more likely.

In Vivo Bone Lead Measurement

Efforts to identify dose-response and dose-effect relationships between lead burden and health indexes have been hampered by the shortcomings, in most circumstances, of blood lead as an index of an individual's total body lead burden. Until recently, the only way to obtain such information had been through somewhat invasive procedures, such as provocative chelation in which stored lead is mobilized and the amount excreted in urine over the subsequent 24 hours is measured. Recent progress in the development of noninvasive x-ray fluorescence-based methods for assessing bone lead stores in vivo has provided optimism that measures of total body lead burden that can be conveniently applied to the general population will be available in the near future. Currently, instruments based on K-XRF and L-XRF technology are being developed (84, 99). These instruments differ in many respects, but most significantly in the type of bone sampled (L: surface bone; K: full thickness of bone). At present, L-XRF may be especially appropriate for pediatric and K-XRF for adult populations, but ongoing research may reveal that this generalization is too simplistic. If realized, rapid, noninvasive XRF measurement of bone lead could provide the basis for screening large populations of children for lead toxicity. Before this goal will be realized, however, more work is necessary to establish the sensitivity and validity of the method at the levels commonly encountered in the general population.

Other Effects of Lead

Most studies of childhood lead exposure have focused on psychometric intelligence, i.e. reading and math achievement. Little attention has been paid to higher order behavior, such as ability to get along with peers and to accept the prevailing social mores. There is growing evidence that lead-exposed children have difficulty in attention (64); some evidence suggests that exposure is associated with aggressiveness (48). Attention deficit with hyperactivity, coupled with antisocial behavior, is a strong predictor of criminality (52, 55). Criminal behavior has been found to be higher in males, blacks, and urban dwellers. It displays itself early in life; criminals are more likely to have been hyperactive as young children and to have come from disorderly homes with poor housekeeping (106). All of these factors are associated with lead exposure. Carefully designed case control and forward studies of the association of lead exposure with antisocial behavior are clearly warranted.

The studies of Kitchen et al (42, 41) and Nation et al (61) suggest that studies of lead exposure in drug and alcohol abusers are worth pursuit. Case control studies of older individuals who are past the ages of peak exposure should benefit from new advances in the technology of in vivo lead measurement.

Almost all studies of lead toxicity have focused on young children, and more recently on fetuses in utero. Because the fetus clearly is not protected from lead, maternal exposure has become a subject of considerable interest. Hormonal changes associated with pregnancy might mobilize lead stores, which would create an endogenous source of fetal exposure, even if external exposure during pregnancy is low (56, 100). Less attention has been paid to paternal exposure and its consequences for the father and his potential offspring, despite evidence that suggests that lead is a gametotoxin. Studies of male reproductive function and fetal consequences of paternal exposure are needed.

Another ignored issue is the effect of early lead exposure on the aged. Most lead is deposited in bone, where it is relatively inert. But with aging, bone demineralizes, which possibly provides an endogenous source of ongoing exposure (96). No information on the sites of redistribution of bone lead is available. Does some of this lead get to the CNS? Is lead one factor in the disordered memory and cognition found in some older patients?

CONTROL STRATEGIES

The major sources of lead for American children are paint, dust, soil, and drinking water. What should the response of society be to this problem? To develop an informed strategy, we need to examine the forces that have impeded action in face of a large and growing body of knowledge. Activity directed at the removal of lead from the human environment has been slowed by the following factors:

1. THE BELIEF THAT THE DISEASE IS LIMITED TO POOR MINORITIES.   Related to this belief is the conviction that the disease is a product of poor mothering and unsanitary habits. The widespread tendency to assign the primary cause to human, rather than environmental, factors has relieved authorities from the obligation to act.

2. THE BELIEF THAT REDUCING THE AMOUNT OF LEAD ADDED TO GASO-LINE AND LEAD PAINT LEGISLATION HAS ALREADY SOLVED THE PROB-LEM.   The removal of lead from gasoline has resulted in a decrease in blood lead levels of about 10% per year. Although it has been impossible to purchase lead-containing paint for household use legally since 1976, half the homes in this country were built before the passage of the lead paint legislation. The ATSDR report estimates that 2 million homes in which young children live are leaded and have deteriorated surfaces.

3. THE OBDURATE OBSTRUCTIONISM OF THE LEAD INDUSTRY.   Since the 1920s the industry has worked to diminish and obscure the hazards of lead to human health and to impede legislation or regulation (32, 85). Recently mounted lawsuits, which state that knowledge of the dangers of lead paint to children were known and hidden by the industry, have added the lead industry to the list of defendants.

4. THE LACK OF MEDICAL INTEREST IN THE PROBLEM.   Lead poisoning is a low technology disease. It does not possess the drama of transplant surgery or molecular biology. Many pediatric centers have stopped screening for lead, and many house officers complete their training without having seen a case of plumbism. As a result, they do not think of the disease when constructing a differential diagnosis of developmental delay, growth failure, or behavior disorder.

To address these misplaced beliefs, we need to develop firm and repeated educational efforts for the public, regulators, educators, and pediatricians. Lead poisoning is not a disease of poor minorities alone. The ATSDR report indicates that 16% of all American children have blood lead levels in the neurotoxic range. Clearly, the poor and minorities receive a disproportionate dose of lead. For black children in poverty, the prevalence of blood lead levels greater than 15 μg/dl is 55%! Lead exists in dangerous overabundance in precisely the same areas in which there are two shameful and threatening shortages: decent housing and jobs. A rational way to manage this imbalance would be to train and then hire the unemployed in the safe deleading of houses. Lead control can be readily seen as a health program, a housing program, and an employment program. No one has spelled out the dilemma (and the hope) of lead poisoning more pointedly than the late Rene Dubos (quoted in Ref. 68a):

> The problem is so well defined, so neatly packaged, with both causes and cures known, that if we don't eliminate this social crime, our society deserves all the disasters that have been forecast for it.

Literature Cited

1. Agency Toxic Subst. Dis. Regist. 1988. *The nature and extent of lead poisoning in children in the United States: A report to Congress.* Atlanta: Dep. Health Hum. Serv.
2. Averill, D., Needleman, H. L. 1980. Neonatal lead exposure retards cortical synaptogenesis in the rat. In *Low Level Lead Exposure: The Clinical Implications of Current Research,* ed. H. L. Needleman, pp. 201–10. New York: Raven
3. Bailey, C., Kitchen, I. 1985. Ontogenesis of proenkephalin products in rat striatum and the inhibitory effects of low-level lead exposure. *Dev. Brain Res.* 22:75–79
4. Barrett, J., Livesey, P. J. 1983. Lead induced alterations in maternal behavior and offsrping development in the rat. *Neurobehav. Toxicol. Teratol.* 5:557–63
5. Bellinger, D., Leviton, A., Needleman, H. L., Rabinowitz, M. 1988. Low level lead exposure, social class and infant development. *Neurotoxicol. Teratol.* 10: 497–503
6. Bellinger, D., Leviton, A., Rabinowitz, M., Needleman, H. L., Waternaux, C. 1986. Correlates of low-level lead exposure in urban children at two years of age. *Pediatrics* 77:826–33
7. Bellinger, D., Leviton, A., Sloman, J. 1990. Antecedents and correlates of improved cognitive performance in children exposed in utero to low levels of lead. *Environ. Health Perspect.* In press
8. Bellinger, D., Leviton, A., Waternaux, C., Needleman, H. L., Rabinowitz, M. 1987. Longitudinal analyses of prenatal and postnatal lead exposure and early cognitive development. *N. Engl. J. Med.* 316:1037–43
9. Bellinger, D., Needleman, H. L. 1982. Low level lead exposure and psychological deficits in children. In *Advances in Developmental and Behavioral Pediatrics,* ed. M. L. Wolraich, D. K. Routh, 3:1–49. Greenwich, Conn: JAI
10. Bellinger, D., Needleman, H. L. 1983. Lead and the relationship between maternal and child intelligence. *J. Pediatr.* 102:523–27
11. Bellinger, D., Needleman, H. L., Bromfield, R., Mintz, M. 1984. A follow-up study of the academic attainment and classroom behavior of children with elevated dentine lead levels. *Biol. Trace Elem. Res.* 6:207–23
12. Bellinger, D., Sloman, J., Leviton, A., Rabinowitz, M., Needleman, H., Waternaux, C. 1990. Low-level lead exposure and children's cognitive function in the preschool years. *Pediatrics.* In press
13. Bergomi, M., Borella, P., Fantuzzi, G., Vivoli, G., Sturloni, N., et al. 1989. Relationship between lead exposure indicators and neuropsychological performance in children. *Dev. Med. Child. Neurol.* 31:181–90
14. Bornschein, R. L., Grote, J., Mitchell, T., Succop, P., Deitrich, K. M., et al. 1989. Effects of prenatal and postnatal lead exposure on fetal maturation and postnatal growth. In *Lead Exposure and Child Development: An International Assessment,* ed. M. Smith, L. D. Grant, A. Sors, pp. 307–19. Dordrecht/Boston/ London:Kluwer Academic
15. Brown, R. S., Hingerty, B. E., Dewan, J. C., Klug, A. 1983. Pb(II)-catalysed cleavage of the sugar-phosphate backbone of yeast tRNA(Phe)—implications for lead toxicity and self-splicing RNA. *Nature* 303:543–46
16. Bull, R. J., McCauley, P. T., Taylor,

D. H., Croften, K. M., 1983. The effects of lead on the developing central nervous system of the rat. *Neurotoxicology* 4:1–18

17. Byers, R. K., Lord, E. E. 1943. Late effects of lead poisoning on mental development. *Am. J. Dis. Child.* 66:471–83

18. Cent. Dis. Control. 1985. *Preventing lead poisoning in young children: A statement by the Centers for Disease Control,* Jan., No. 99-2230. US Dept. Health Hum. Serv., Atlanta

19. Cornfield, J. 1974. Recent methodological contributions to clinical trials. *Am. J. Epidemiol.* 104:553–58

20. Cory-Slechta, D. A., Weiss, B., Cox, C. 1985. Performance and exposure indices of rats exposed to low concentrations of lead. *Toxicol. Appl. Pharmacol.* 78:291–99

21. dela Burde, B., Choate, M. S. 1972. Does asymptomatic lead exposure in children have latent sequelae? *J. Pediatr.* 81:1088–91

22. Dietrich, K. N. 1990. Human fetal lead exposure: Intrauterine growth, maturation and postnatal neurobehavioral development. *Proc. Soc. Toxicol.,* Feb., Miami. In press

23. Dietrich, K. N., Krafft, K. M., Bornschein, R. L., Hammond, P. B., Berger, O., et al. 1987. Low-level fetal lead exposure effect on neurobehavioral development in early infancy. *Pediatrics* 80(5):721–30

24. Environ. Prot. Agency. 1986. Air quality criteria for lead. Res. Triangle Park, NC: US Environ. Prot. Agency

25. Environ. Prot. Agency. 1987. *Reducing Lead in Drinking Water: A Benefit Analysis.* Washington, DC: US Environ. Prot. Agency

26. Ernhart, C., Landa, B., Schell, N. B. 1981. Subclinical levels of lead and development deficit: A multivariate follow-up reassessment. *Pediatrics* 67: 911–19

27. Ernhart, C. B., Morrow-Tlucak, M., Wolf, A. W., Super, D., Drotar, D. 1989. Low level lead exposure in the prenatal and early preschool periods: Intelligence prior to school entry. *Neurotoxicol. Teratol.* 11:161–70

28. Fergusson, D. M., Fergusson, J. E., Horwood, L. J., Kinzett, N. G. 1988. A longitudinal study of dentine lead levels, intelligence, school performance and behavior. *J. Child. Psychol. Psychiatry* 29:793–809

29. Fisher, R. A. 1925. *Statistical Methods for Research Workers.* Edinburgh: Oliver & Boyd

30. Fulton, M., Raab, G., Thomson, G., Laxen, D., Hunter, R., Hepburn, W. 1987. Influence of blood lead on the ability and attainment of children in Edinburgh. *Lancet* 1:1221–26

31. Gibson, J. L. 1904. A plea for painted railings and painted walls of rooms as the source of lead poisoning among Queensland children. *Aust. Med. Gaz.* 23:149–53

32. Graebner, W. 1987. Hegemony through science: Information engineering and lead toxicology, 1925–1965. In *Dying for Work; Workers' Safety and Health in Twentieth-Century America,* ed. D. Rosner, G, Markowitz, pp. 140–59. Bloomington, Ind: Univ. Press

33. Hansen, O. N., Trillingsgaard, A., Beese, I., Lyngye, T., Grandjean, P. 1989. A neuropsychological study of children with elevated dentine lead level: Assessment of the effect of lead in different socio-economic groups. *Neurotoxicol. Teratol.* 11:205–13

34. Harlan, W. R., Landis, J. R., Schmouder, R. L., Goldstein, N. G., Harlan, L. C. 1985. Blood lead and blood pressure. Relationship in the adolescent and adult US population. *J. Am. Med. Assoc.* 253:530–34

35. Harvey, P. G., Hamlin, M. W., Kumar, R., Delves, H. T. 1984. Blood lead, behaviour and intelligence test performance in preschool children. *Sci. Total Environ.* 40:45–60

36. Hatzakis, A., Kokkevi, A., Katsouyanni, K., Maravelias, K., Salaminios, F. et al. 1987. Psychometric intelligence and attentional performance deficits in lead-exposed children. In *Heavy Metals in the Environment: International Conference, New Orleans,* ed. S. E. Lindberg, T. C. Hutchinson, pp. 204–9. Edinburgh:CEP consultants

37. Hawk, B. A., Schroeder, S. R., Robinson, G., Otto, D., Mushak, P., et al. 1986. Relation of lead and social factors to IQ of low-SES children. A partial replication. *Am. J. Ment. Defic.* 91:178–83

38. Hume, D. 1894. *Enquiry Concerning Human Understanding.* Oxford: Clarendon

39. Huseman, C. A., Moriarty, C. M., Angle, C. R. 1987. Childhood lead toxicity and impaired release of thyrotropin stimulating hormone. *Environ. Res.* 42:524–33

40. Kenny, D. A. 1979. *Correlation and Causality.* New York: Wiley

41. Kitchen, I., McDowell, J. 1984. Impairment of ketocyclazocine antinociception

in rats by perinatal lead exposure. *Toxicol. Lett.* 26:101–5

42. Kitchen, I., McDowell, J., Winder, C., Wilson, J. M. 1984. Low-level lead exposure alters morphine antinociception in neonatal rats. *Toxicol. Lett.* 22:119–23

43. Kotok, D. 1972. Development of children with elevated blood lead levels: A controlled study. *J. Pediatr.* 80:57–61

44. Krigman, M. R., Hogan, E. L. 1974. Effect of lead intoxication on the postnatal growth of the rat nervous system. *Environ. Health Perspect.* (May) 187–99

45. Landrigan, P. J., Whitworth, R. H., Baloh, R. W., Staehling, N. W., Barthel, W. F., Rosenblum, B. F. 1975. Neuropsychological dysfunction in children with chronic low level lead absorption. *Lancet* 1:708–12

46. Lansdown, R. G., Clayton, B. E., Graham, P. J., Delves, H. T. 1974. Blood-lead levels, behaviour, and intelligence. *Lancet* 1:1167–68

47. Lansdown, R., Yule, W., Urbanowicz, M., Hunter, J. 1986. The relationship between blood-lead concentrations, intelligence, attainment and behaviour in a school population: The second London study. *Int. Arch. Occup. Environ. Health* 57:225–35

48. Lansdown, R., Yule, W., Urbanowicz, M., Miller, I. 1983. Blood lead, intelligence, attainment and behaviour in school children: Overview of a pilot study. In *Lead versus Health*, ed. M. Rutter, R. R. Jones, pp. 267–96. New York: Wiley

49. Lave, L., Seskin, E. 1977. *Air Pollution and Human Health.* Baltimore, Md: Johns Hopkins Univ. Press

50. Linn, S., Schoenbaum, S. C., Monson, R. R., Rosner, B., Stubblefield, P. G., Ryan, K. J. 1983. Lack of association between contraceptive usage and congenital malformations in offspring. *Am. J. Obstet. Gynacol.* 147:923–28

51. Lyngbye, T., Hansen, O. N., Trillingsgaard, A., Beese, I., Grandjean, P. 1990. Learning disabilities in children: Significance of low level lead exposure and confounding factors. *Acta Pediatr. Scand.* 79:165–73

52. Magnusson, D., Stottin, H., Duner, A. 1983. Aggression and criminality in a longitudinal perspective. In *Antecedents of Aggression and Antisocial Behavior*, ed. K. T. Van Dusen, S. A. Mednick, pp. 277–302. Boston: Kluwer-Nijhoff

53. Mahaffey, K. R., Annest, J. L. 1986. Association of erythrocyte protoporphyrin with blood lead level and iron status in the second National Health and Nutrition Examination Survey, 1976–1980. *Environ. Res.* 41:327–38

54. Mahaffey, K. R., Rosen, J. F., Chesney, R. W., Peeler, J. T., Smith, C. H., DeLuca, H. F. 1982. Association between age, blood lead concentration, and serum 1,25-dihydroxycholecalciferal levels in children. *Am. J. Clin. Nutr.* 35:1327–31

55. Mannuzza, S., Kline, R. G., Konig, P. H., Giampino, T. L. 1989. Hyperactive boys almost grown up. IV: Criminality and its relationship to psychiatric status. *Arch. Gen. Psychiatry* 46:1073–79

56. Manton, W. 1985. Total contribution of airborne lead to blood lead. *Br. J. Ind. Med.* 42:168–72

57. Marcus, A. H., Schwartz, J. 1987. Dose-response curves for erythrocyte protoporphyrin vs. blood lead: Effects of iron status. *Environ. Res.* 44:221–27

58. Markovac, J., Goldstein, G. W. 1988. Picomolar concentrations of lead stimulate brain protein kinase C. *Nature* 334:71–73

59. McMichael, A. J., Baghurst, P. A., Wigg, N. R., Vimpani, G. V., Robertson, E. F., Roberts, R. J. 1988. Port Pirie Cohort Study: Environmental exposure to lead and children's abilities at the age of four years. *N. Engl. J. Med.* 319:468–75

60. Murphy, M. J., Graziano, J. H., Popovac, D., Kline, J. K., Mahmeti, A., et al. 1990. Past pregnancy outcomes among women living in the vicinity of a lead smelter in Kosovo, Yugoslavia. *Am. J. Public Health* 80:33–35

61. Nation, J. R., Baker, D. M., Taylor, B., Clark, D. E. 1986. Dietary lead increases ethanol consumption in the rat. *Behav. Neurosci.* 100:525–30

62. Needleman, H. L., Bellinger, D. C. 1989. Type II Fallacies in the study of childhood exposure to lead at low dose: A critical and quantitative review. Heavy Metals in the Environment, Edinburgh Conference, 1986. In *Lead Exposure and Child Development: An International Assessment*, ed. M. A. Smith, L. D. Grant, A. I. Sors, pp. 293–304. Dordrecht/Boston/London: Kluwer Academic

63. Needleman, H. L., Gatsonis, G. 1990. Low-level lead exposure and the IQ of children: A meta-analysis of modern studies. *J. Am. Med. Assoc.* 263:673–78

64. Needleman, H. L., Gunnoe, C., Leviton, A., Reed, R., Peresie, H., et al. 1979. Deficits in psychologic and classroom performance of children with ele-

vated dentine lead levels. *N. Engl. J. Med.* 300:689–95

65. Needleman, H. L., Landrigan, P. J. 1981. The health effects of low level exposure to lead. *Annu. Rev. Public Health* 2:277–98

66. Needleman, H. L., Leviton, A., Bellinger, D. 1982. Lead-associated intellectual deficit. *N. Engl. J. Med.* 306:367

67. Needleman, H. L., Rabinowitz, M., Leviton, A., Linn, S., Schoenbaum, S. 1984. The relationship between prenatal exposure to lead and congenital anomalies. *J. Am. Med. Assoc.* 25:2956–59

68. Needleman, H. L., Schell, A., Bellinger, D., Leviton, A., Allred, E. N. 1990. The long-term effects of exposure to low doses of lead in childhood: An 11-year follow-up report. *N. Engl. J. Med.* 322:83–88

68a. Oberle, M. W. 1969. Lead poisoning: A preventable childhood disease of the slums. *Science* 165:991–92

69. Pentschew, A., Garro, F. 1966. Lead encephalomyopathy of the suckling rat and its implications on the prophyrinopathic diseases. *Acta Neuropathol.* 6:266–78

70. Perino, J., Ernhart, C. B. 1974. The relation of subclinical lead level to cognitive and sensorimotor impairment in black preschoolers. *J. Learn. Disabil.* 7:616–20

71. Piomelli, S., Seaman, C., Zullow, D., Curran, A., Davidow, B. 1982. Threshold for lead damage to heme synthesis in urban children. *Proc. Natl. Acad. Sci., USA* 79:3335–39

72. Pirkle, J. L., Schwartz, J., Landis, J. R., Harlan, W. R. 1985. The relationship between blood lead levels and blood pressure and its cardiovascular risk implications. *Am. J. Epidemiol.* 121:246–58

73. Pocock, S. J., Ashby, D. 1985. Environmental lead and children's intelligence: A review of recent epidemiological studies. *Statistician* 34:31–44

74. Pocock, S. J., Ashby, D., Smith, M. A. 1987. Lead exposure and children's intellectual performance. *Int. J. Epidemiol.* 16:57–67

75. Pocock, S. J., Shaper, A. G., Ashby, D., Delves, T., Whitehead, T. P. 1984. Blood lead concentration, blood pressure, and renal function. *Br. Med. J.* 289:872–74

76. Provenzano, G. 1980. The social costs of excessive lead exposure during childhood. In *Low Level Lead Exposure: The Clinical Implications of Current Research*, ed. H. L. Needleman, pp. 299–315. New York: Raven

77. Rabinowitz, M., Bellinger, D., Leviton, A., Needleman, H., Schoenbaum, S. 1987. Pregnancy hypertension, blood pressure during labor and blood lead levels. *Hypertension* 10:447–51

78. Rabinowitz, M. B., Needleman, H. L. 1982. Temporal trends in the lead concentrations of umbilical cord blood. *Science* 216:1429–31

79. Rabinowitz, M. B., Needleman, H. L. 1983. Petrol lead sales and umbilical cord blood. *Lancet* 1:63

80. Rice, D. C., Gilbert, S. G. 1987. Low-level lifetime lead exposure produces behavioral toxicity (spatial discrimination reversal) in adult monkeys. *Toxicol. Appl. Pharmacol.* 91:484–90

81. Robinson, G. S., Bauman, S., Kleinbaum, S., Barton, C., Schroeder, S. R. et al. 1985. Effects of low to moderate lead exposure on brainstem auditory evoked potentials in children. In *World Health Organization Regional Office for Europe—Environmental Health Document 3*, pp. 177–82. Copenhagen: WHO

82. Robinson, G. S., Keith, R. W., Bornschein, R. L., Otto, D. A. 1987. Effects of environmental lead exposure on the developing auditory evoked potential and pure tone hearing evaluations in young children. See Ref. 36, pp. 223–25

83. Rosen, J. F., Chesney, R. W., Hamstra, A. DeLuca, H. F., Mahaffey, K. R. 1980. Reduction in dyhydroxyvitamin D in children with increased lead absorption. *N. Engl. J. Med.* 302:1128–31

84. Rosen, J. F., Markowitz, M. E., Bijur, P. E., Jenks, S. T., Wielopolski, L., et al. 1989. L-line x-ray fluorescence of cortical bone lead compared with the CaNa2EDTA test in lead-toxic children: Public health implications. *Proc. Natl. Acad. Sci. USA* 86:685–89

85. Rosner, D., Markowtiz, G. 1985. A 'gift of God'?: The public health controversy over leaded gasoline during the 1920s. *Am. J. Public Health* 75:344–52

86. Rutter, M. 1980. Raised lead levels and impaired cognitive/behavioral functioning. *Dev. Med. Child Neurol.* 22 (Suppl.):1–26

87. Sandstead, H. H. 1967. Effect of chronic lead intoxication on in vivo I131 uptake by the rat thyroid. *Proc. Soc. Exp. Biol. Med.* 124:18–20

88. Sandstead, H. H. 1973. Effects of moonshine on endocrine function. In *Trace Substances in Environmental Health*, ed. D. D. Hemphill, pp. 223–35. Columbia, Mo: Univ. Missouri Press

89. Scanlon, J. 1971. Umbilical cord blood lead concentration: Relationship to urban or suburban residency during gestation. *Am. J. Dis. Child.* 121:325–26

90. Schroeder, S. R., Hawk, B., Otto, D. A., Mushak, P., Hicks, R. E. 1985. Separating the effects of lead and social factors on IQ. *Environ. Res.* 38:144–54

91. Schwartz, J. 1988. The relationship between blood lead and blood pressure in the NHANES II survey. *Environ. Health Pers.* 78:15–22

92. Schwartz, J., Angle, C., Pitcher, H. 1986. Relationship between childhood blood lead levels and stature, *Pediatrics* 77:281–88

93. Schwartz, J., Otto, D. A. 1987. Blood lead, hearing thresholds, and neurobehavioral development in children and youth. *Arch. Environ. Health* 42:153–60

94. Schwartz, J., Pitcher, H., Levin, R., Ostro, B., Nichols, A. L. 1985. *Costs and Benefits of Reducing Lead in Gasoline: Final Regulatory Analysis.* Washington, DC:US EPA/OPA

95. Shukla, R., Bornschein, R. L., Dietrich, K. N., Buncher, C. R., Berger, O. 1989. Fetal and infant lead exposure: Effects on growth in stature. *Pediatrics* 84:604–12

96. Silbergeld, E., Schwartz, J., Mahaffey, K. 1988. Lead and osteoporosis: Mobilization of lead from bone in postmenopausal women. *Environ. Res.* 47:79–94

97. Silva, P. A., Hughes, P., Williams, S., Faed, J. 1988. Blood lead, intelligence, reading attainment, and behaviour in eleven year old children in Dunedin, New Zealand. *J. Child Psychol. Psychiatry* 29:43–52

98. Smith, M., Delves, T., Lansdown, R., Clayton, B., Graham, P. 1983. The effects of lead exposure on urban children: The Institute of Child Health, Southampton Study. *Dev. Med. Child Neurol.* 25(Suppl.):47:1–54

99. Somervaille, L. J., Chettle, D. R., Scott, M. C. 1985. In vivo measurement of lead in bone using X-Ray fluorescence. *Phys. Med. Biol.* 30:929–43

100. Thompson, G., Robertson, E., Fitzgerald, S. 1985. Lead mobilization during pregnancy. *Med. J. Aust.* 143:131

101. Thomson, G. O. B., Raab, G. M., Hepburn, W. S., Hunter, R., Fulton, M., Laxen, D. P. H. 1989. Blood lead levels and children's behaviour: Results from the Edinburgh lead study. *J. Child Psychol. Psychiatry* 30:515–28

102. Turner, A. J. 1897. Lead poisoning among Queensland children. *Aust. Med. Gaz.* 16:475–79

103. Victery, W., Miller, C. R., Zhu, S. Y., Goyer, R. A. 1987. Effect of different levels and periods of lead exposure on tissue levels and excretion of lead, zinc and calcium in the rat. *Fundam. Appl. Toxicol.* 8:506–16

104. Vimpani, G. V., Baghurst, P. A., Wigg, N. R., Robertson, E. F., McMichael, A. J., Roberts, R. R. 1989. The Port Pirie Cohort study: Cumulative lead exposure and neurodevelopmental status at age 2 years: Do HOME scores and maternal IQ reduce apparent effects of lead on Bayley Mental scores? See Ref. 62, pp. 332–44

105. Ward, N., Watson, R., Bryce-Smith, D. 1987. Placental element levels in relationship to fetal development for obstetrically "normal" births: The study of 37 elements. Evidence for effects of cadmium, lead and zinc on fetal growth, and for smoking as a source of cadmium. *Int. J. Biosocial.* 9:63–81

106. Wilson, J., Herrnstein, R. 1985. *Crime and Human Behavior.* New York: Simon & Schuster

107. Winder, C., Kitchen, I. 1984. Lead neurotoxicity: A review of the biochemical, neurochemical and drug induced behavioural evidence. *Prog. Neurobiol.* 22:59–87

108. Winneke, G., Hrdina, K. G., Brockhaus, A. 1982. I. Pilot Study. Neuropsychological studies in children with elevated tooth-lead concentrations. *Int. Arch. Occup. Environ. Health* 51:169–83

109. Winneke, G., Kramer, U., Brockhaus, A., Ewers, U., Kujanek, G., et al. 1983. Neuropsychological studies in children with elevated tooth-lead concentrations. II. Extended study. *Int. Arch. Occup. Environ. Health* 51:231–52

110. Yule, W., Lansdown, R., Millar, I. B., Urbanowicz, M. A. 1981. The relationship between blood lead concentrations, intelligence and attainment in a school population: A pilot study. *Dev. Med. Child Neurol.* 23:567–76

Annu. Rev. Publ. Health. 12:141–56

COST, CONTROVERSY, CRISIS: LOW BACK PAIN AND THE HEALTH OF THE PUBLIC[1]

Richard A. Deyo, Daniel Cherkin, Douglas Conrad, and Ernest Volinn

Departments of Medicine, Health Services, Family Medicine, and Anesthesiology, University of Washington; the Northwest Health Services Research & Development Field Program, Seattle Veterans Affairs Medical Center; and the Center for Health Studies, Group Health Cooperative of Puget Sound, Seattle, Washington 98195

KEY WORDS: backache, disability, back surgery, lumbar spine

INTRODUCTION

Low back pain is a pervasive disorder, which affects 70% to 80% of adults at some time during their lives (25, 35). Fortunately, most episodes are mild and self-limited; almost 90% are resolved within six weeks (22). Unlike cancers, heart disease, or AIDS, back pain is rarely a fatal condition. Though the differential diagnosis is broad, many (perhaps most) cases of back pain cannot be given a definite diagnosis (81). Indeed, Williams & Hadler (85) suggest that back pain is an "illness in search of a disease." Given these generally benign characteristics, the economic impact of back pain, within both the health care and the disability compensation systems, is surprising. Despite improvements in diagnostic and therapeutic strategies for back pain, use of medical services and compensation claims are rising (70). Unorthodox forms of care (e.g. reflexology, acupressure) are flourishing, new treatments appear almost daily, and there is little consensus on appropriate care. These faults

[1]Supported in part by Grant No. HS 06344 from the Agency for Health Care Policy & Research and by the Northwest Health Services Research & Development Field Program, Seattle Veterans Affairs Medical Center. The US Government has the right to retain a nonexclusive, royalty-free license in and to any copyright covering this paper.

141

point to a failure of orthodox medical care and contribute to a crisis in health care financing and worker disability. Accumulating evidence suggests that there should be a shift from passive treatments (e.g. bed rest, traction) to more active treatment, which involves the patient (e.g. exercise). Research emphasis should shift from the prevention of back pain to the prevention of back-related disability. Several public policy reforms are probably needed, because all of the parties involved (patients, health care providers, employers, third party payers) may be perpetuating and responding to perverse incentives.

COST AND IMPACT OF LOW BACK PAIN

Based on three complementary surveys by the National Center for Health Statistics (NCHS), the estimated national cost of direct personal medical care for low back pain in 1977 was $12.9 billion (approximately $17.9 billion in 1988 dollars) (59). As illustrated in Table 1, this cost far exceeds the cost of care for patients with AIDS in 1989 and exceeds future projections for AIDS, as well (33a). Table 1 includes other indicators of the cost or impact of back pain in society and in the health care system. In addition to the tabled information, the diagnosis of "herniated disc" was the fourth leading reason for Social Security Disability Insurance disability awards in 1984 (61); over 1.7 million persons reported being unable to work because of back pain (65). Back pain is the most costly ailment of working-age adults (56), although a small minority of patients account for the majority of costs (62, 76). Back symptoms are the leading cause for all visits to orthopedic surgeons and neurosurgeons, and the second leading symptom prompting all physician visits (12). "Medical back problems" comprised the second most common medical diagnosis-related group (DRG) for all hospital discharges in 1987, following only normal childbirth. Among surgical DRG's, back and neck procedures ranked only behind cesearean section and tubal ligation (31; Hospital Discharge Survey, NCHS, unpublished data).

There is little evidence that these costs are abating. Despite hopeful suggestions that surgery is being employed with increasing selectivity, the number of hospital discharges for spine surgery rose substantially in 1979–1987. Table 2 illustrates a 23% increase in laminectomy rates, a 75% increase in diskectomies (including chymopapain injection), and a 200% rise in spinal fusion rates (NCHS, unpublished data). Although these data are not age adjusted, it would be difficult to attribute such dramatic short-term changes to demographic shifts. Waddell (71) has documented a dramatic increase in disability claims because of back pain between the 1950s and the 1970s in several western nations. Webster & Snook (76) estimated a 241% increase in the total compensable cost of low back pain between 1980 and 1986. Thus, conventional preventive and therapeutic efforts are not reducing the adverse impact of back pain, and might even be contributing to it (1).

Table 1   Impacts of back pain: Comparisons with other conditions

Direct annual costs of personal medical care (33a, 59)

Back Pain	$12.9 billion (1977, in 1984 dollars, or 17.9 billion in 1988 dollars)
AIDS	$3.3 billion (1989, in 1988 dollars)
AIDS (projected)	$6.5 billion (1992, in 1988 dollars)

Annual morbidity costs: Earnings losses and productivity losses (men only) (56)

"Orthopedic Impairments of spine" plus herniated disc	$5.1 billion
Respiratory Conditions (other than asthma)	3.7 billion
Ischemic Heart Disease	2.4 billion

Symptomatic reasons for all physician visits (excludes general, prenatal, well-baby, and post-op examinations, and unspecified progress visits) (45)

Throat symptoms	16.4 million visits
Cough	16.1 million visits
Earache or infection	11.4 million visits
Back symptoms	11.3 million visits
Skin rash	10.3 million visits
Blood pressure test	9.4 million visits

Ranking of back symptoms as a reason for visit by physician specialty (1977–78) (12)

Orthopedic surgery	1
Neurosurgery	1
Occupational medicine	1
Osteopathic physicians	1
General and family practice	2
Internal Medicine	2

Reason for physician visits at which x-rays were ordered (1977) (41)

	x-ray visits
Back symptoms *plus* low back symptoms	3.2 million
General medical examination	2.8 million
Chest pain	1.8 million
Cough	1.5 million

For those cases that qualify for workers' compensation, the cost consequences of this problem are severe (32, 76). The Liberty Mutual Insurance Company, which carries about 11% of the private workers' compensation market, found their average cost per case of compensable low back pain to be $6800 in 1986, although the median was just $391. The difference between median and mean was the result of a few, high cost cases; 25% of cases accounted for 95% of costs. These investigators estimated the total compensable cost of low back pain cases in 1986 (all carriers) to be $11.1 billion (76). The efffect of compensation payments on US industry is dramatized by the following estimates: to offset a $500 work accident loss (if paid directly out of profits by the employer), a restaurant must serve 1940 three-dollar lunches; a

Table 2 Rate per 100,000 population of selected back operations in the United States. Data are from the National Hospital Discharge Survey

Procedure	1979	1981	1983	1985	1987	Percent Change, 1979–1987
Laminectomy ICD-9-CM code 3.09)	31	36	41	41	38	23%
Diskectomy (ICD-9-CM code 80.5)	59	57	81	96	103	75%
Lumbar spine fusion ICD-9-CM codes 81.06, 81.07)	5	9	10	18	15	200%

publisher must sell 25,315 newspapers at 25 cents each; and a bakery must bake 47,620 loaves of bread at 75 cents each (59).

VARIABILITY IN CARE: A LACK OF THERAPEUTIC CONSENSUS

A seemingly endless proliferation of treatments is advocated for back pain, including oral drugs, physical measures (e.g. bed rest, manipulation, physical therapy), surgical procedures, injected drugs (local, intramuscular, epidural, intradiscal), counterstimulation, and behavioral and educational approaches. Unconventional treatments, such as acupuncture, inversion gravity traction, sclerosant injections and laser stimulation of trigger points, are constantly emerging. The plethora of treatments and the uncritical use of unproven remedies suggest a poor consensus about therapy (and perhaps a lack of any treatment better than natural history plus placebo) (71). The Quebec Task Force on Spinal Disorders (63) concluded that there is "little clinical proof or epidemiologic validation to support the current methods of treating disorders of the spine."

Wide variations among hospital markets in the use of hospital care and surgery for back pain have been well documented. For example, Wennberg and colleagues (79) found approximately eightfold variations among hospital markets in the rate of both medical and surgical admissions for back pain. They compared two cities with similar demographic characteristics and medical sophistication and found that admissions for medical back problems were 3.8 times more frequent in Boston than in New Haven (78).

Although no rigorous comparisons of international rates of back surgery have been conducted, available data for the late 1970s suggest marked variation between countries (26, 36, 71). Reported rates of laminectomy for disc herniation in the United States were at least double those in six of the seven other countries for which comparison data were available. The United

Table 3 United States variations in the use of specific back operations, rates per 100,000 population. Data are from the 1986 National Hospital Discharge Survey

Procedure	Northeast	Midwest	South	West	Total US
Laminectomy (ICD-9-CM code 3.09)	26	47	35	54	40
Diskectomy (ICD-9-CM code 80.5)	60	106	123	91	99
Lumbar spine fusion (ICD-9-CM codes 81.06, 81.07)	4	14	18	35	18

States' rate was almost nine times that of the United Kingdom, but only 30% higher than that of Canada. As Wennberg and colleagues (78, 79) suggest, variability in care may reflect a poor professional consensus about appropriate care, and the use of services in high volume areas is probably excessive.

Rates for specific surgical procedures might be even more variable than aggregated data suggest. For example, Table 3 illustrates twofold regional variations in the rates of laminectomy (removing a part of the vertebra to release pressure on nerves directly or to allow removal of an intervertebral disc), but almost a ninefold difference in the rate of spine fusion (joining multiple vertebrae to reduce presumed instability) (47). Despite evidence that repeat surgical procedures are rarely indicated (72), there are documented examples of patients who have undergone as many as 20 spine operations, and back patients in many pain centers average at least two previous operations (49). Though removal of more than one disc at a single operation may almost never be necessary, some observers believe the practice is common (24).

In addition to the poor consensus about therapy, there is a poor consensus about the appropriate use of diagnostic tests and about the criteria for diagnosing (or even the existence of) certain diseases. Though spinal fusion is commonly performed for spinal "instability," there is little agreement as to what spinal instability is (23, 53). Similarly, an expert panel convened by the Institute of Medicine could not agree on the existence of myofascial trigger point syndromes (51). Like other authors, the panel also noted the ongoing controversy regarding the existence of fibrositis, or its distinctness from myofascial pain syndromes. Though muscle spasm is frequently diagnosed, specialists working in the same clinic cannot agree when it is present (73). Controversy persists about the appropriate use and sequencing of expensive diagnostic procedures, such as computed tomography, magnetic resonance imaging, and myelography (injection of contrast material around the spinal cord) (39, 77). All three of these tests may show herniated discs in 10% to 20% of normal persons who have never experienced low back pain (4, 84). Because the appearance of an anatomic change on an imaging procedure does not necessarily indicate a clinically important problem, it may be misleading to both physicians and patients. Thus, a potential cascade of ill-advised clinical interventions may result. Given these ambiguities, it is not surprising that both patients and physicians find back pain frustrating.

As if to highlight the failings of the conventional approach, an entire profession—chiropractic—has emerged, which is largely dedicated to treating back problems. Despite efforts by the American Medical Association to label chiropractic as an unscientific cult and to declare it unethical for medical doctors to associate with chiropractors, chiropractic is now recognized as a health care profession in all 50 states. In 1979, Americans made an estimated 130 million visits to 23,000 chiropractors (69). By 1987, the number of chiropractors exceeded 30,000 (2). Though chiropractic claims are made for success with other conditions, nearly half the patients who seek chiropractic care do so for back pain (50). Although chiropractors use an unsubstantiated pathogenetic concept (vertebral subluxation) and are proscribed from using many sophisticated diagnostic tests, they enjoy substantial success in the management of back pain. In a study of patients who received workers' compensation, Kane and colleagues (37) found that patients treated by chiropractors had equally good functional outcomes and greater satisfaction than those treated by medical physicians. We found that enrollees in a large Seattle health maintenance organization (HMO) who saw chiropractors for back pain reported better functional and satisfaction outcomes than enrollees seeing medical physicians (7). These cohort studies do not provide the definitive results of a randomized trial, but suggest that the traditional medical model for managing back pain is often deficient. Randomized trials (usually not involving chiropractors) have suggested that spinal manipulation may produce an immediate benefit for selected patients, but no long-term benefits (14). A very recent randomized trial in Britain, however, showed an advantage of chiropractic care over hospital outpatient care up to two years after study entry (46).

The purpose and value of nonsurgical hospitalizations are often unclear. For Washington State, 1986 data show greater hospital market area variations in medical back admissions (twelvefold) than in surgical admissions. Many such admissions have been traditionally rationalized by a "need for strict bed rest," for traction, or for other procedures, such as myelography or therapeutic injections. However, our group and others have shown in clinical trials that lengthy bed rest does not hasten the resolution of symptoms or dysfunction in most patients with back pain (17, 30). Our critical review of conservative therapy, subsequent trials, and the Quebec Task Force on Spinal Disorders concluded that there is no experimental support for the efficacy of conventional traction (14, 18, 63). Myelography and most injections can often be accomplished on an outpatient basis (9). Thus, hospital care is overused for this problem, and the variability in hospital use partly reflects ineffective care.

LACK OF SUCCESS AND CONFIDENCE IN THERAPY

The faddish proliferation of treatments for back pain suggests that there is no uniquely successful approach to this problem. The widespread public perception of failure is reflected in jokes and cartoons. Even professional confidence is limited. In our comparison of family physicians and chiropractors who treat patients in a large HMO, the family physicians felt less well trained to manage back pain (8).

A pernicious effect of conventional medical care was implied by Waddell (71), who observed that back-related disability was rare in traditional societies, such as that found in the Middle Eastern country Oman. With the introduction of western medicine to Oman, complaints of back pain and related disability rapidly increased. The implication is that modern views and practices may encourage, cause, or legitimize back-related disability in ways that were uncommon in the traditional society.

A more carefully controlled trial of conventional therapeutic approaches also suggested that some common practices are counterproductive. Fordyce and coworkers (24) found that pain-contingent recommendations for rest and medication (e.g. "rest until the pain goes away") tended to prolong symptom reports and activity limitations. Patients with acute pain who were randomly assigned to receive pain medication on a regular, rather than as needed, schedule, and whose rest and medication were prescribed for a fixed, rather than open-ended, number of days, were less disabled one year later.

White and colleagues (80) found that adding a spine fusion to removal of a herniated disc resulted in worse outcomes than a laminectomy and disc excision without fusion. The literature on surgery for back pain may be unique in the extent of its commentary on failure, and entire volumes have been written on the "failed back surgery syndrome" (44, 72, 80). Recognition of failure on this scale in abdominal or cardiac surgery might be regarded as scandalous, but it is merely an accepted aspect of care for low back disorders.

As with other clinical problems, the physician-patient communication is often lacking in therapeutic content. Many patients with back pain express a need for more and better information about their conditions, and these unmet needs may be associated with worse compliance and a desire for more evaluation (15). Part of the success of chiropractors may well lie in a more successful "bedside manner," a confident and positive approach, an easily understood conceptual model, and the immediacy and intimacy of active, hands-on therapy (7, 11, 64). In his classic book on health care in an upstate New York community, Koos quoted a patient's comment about her chiropractor (42):

> He don't hurry you none, and he lets you talk if you want to . . . he don't act as if there was a million people more important to him waiting outside, either, and he don't act as though there was nothing wrong with you, the way I could name some doctors who do . . . and

another thing, you don't feel as if this was a dollars and cents business proposition the way these high-and-mighty doctors make you feel, with their nice offices and big automobiles, and the bills they send you . . . you just feel at home in his office . . . there's another thing, too—he don't try to hide what's the matter with you from you. He comes right out and tells you—it's something no doctor will do for you . . . they all want to keep a secret from you, what you have wrong, and dress it up in big words.

PREVENTING LOW BACK PAIN AND DISABILITY

Because low back pain is primarily a condition of working-age adults, it has an enormous impact in the workplace. Furthermore, a variety of occupations have been linked epidemiologically with the occurrence of low back pain, especially those that involve prolonged sitting, lifting, twisting, driving, or exposure to vibration. Certain health care workers have particularly high risks; nursing aides have the highest rates of compensable back injuries of any occupation in several states (38). The high rates in nursing personnel may be partly related to patient lifting, but other factors also are probably involved (10, 38). Losses in productivity, compensation costs, and direct medical care costs have spurred efforts to prevent occupational low back pain.

One approach to prevention has been preemployment or preplacement screening by medical evaluation, strength testing, or low back x-rays. Unfortunately, no studies clearly demonstrate any reduction in the incidence or severity of musculoskeletal disorders as a result of these efforts (28, 60). In the case of x-ray screening, many studies have demonstrated the futility of trying to predict which workers will develop subsequent low back pain. Gibson (29) performed one of the best studies; he followed two cohorts of employees in the steel industry for a period of 12 years. One cohort of approximately 500 employees was hired before x-ray screening, and the second cohort of 500 employees was hired after the program was implemented. Over the subsequent 12 years, the overall incidence of low back pain and the proportion of lost time injuries was virtually identical in the two groups. Because the ability to predict future back problems is very limited, there is a substantial risk of erroneously labeling prospective employees as "handicapped," and such persons may be denied access to certain jobs. This issue raises legal questions; prospective employees who were denied placement could seek recourse under statutes that prevent discrimination against the handicapped (55). Thus, there is little evidence that screening approaches can reduce the prevalence of low back problems or disability costs.

A second approach to prevention is to educate workers in safe lifting techniques. Although some uncontrolled studies have suggested a reduction in back disability as a result of worker training, controlled cohort studies have failed to demonstrate any advantage (13). The National Institute for Occupational Safety and Health concluded that the value of these training programs is still open to question (66).

Another approach to prevention is related to job design. Ergonomists advocate redesigning jobs to eliminate or reduce the amount of necessary manual handling. Some studies have suggested a benefit of such job redesign programs (60), but we lack well-controlled studies. The intuitive appeal of this approach should prompt further studies, as workers with back pain could, presumably, return to work more quickly.

The high prevalence of low back pain has led some experts to conclude that prevention may be futile. They suggest redirecting the focus of research towards the prevention of high cost disability claims, rather than pain itself (62, 71). This shift in focus has called attention to a variety of social, psychological, and financial issues that may be related to high cost claims. Working environments without flexibility in task design or tempo probably will be unable to accommodate even transient problems, such as most backaches, and they will increase the likelihood of disability claims (33). In both prospective studies and national survey data, level of formal education is a stronger correlate of back-related inactivity than many clinical variables or prescribed treatment (16, 20). Income and global self-ratings of health also predict days of work absenteeism related to back problems (16, 20). In a study of industrial employees, unfavorable supervisor ratings were an important predictor of high cost disability claims (3). Several investigators have found that disability compensation or involvement in legal proceedings reduces the likelihood of symptomatic improvement with either rehabilitation or surgery (74). In a study of patients who completed a comprehensive rehabilitation program, predictors of return to work included personality traits, age, duration of back pain, and source of income (5). Thus, many determinants of work "disability" due to chronic pain are beyond the influence of medical care. These observations suggest a need for attractive and flexible workplaces and working conditions, and reforms in the disability compensation system.

Many administrative interventions appear more promising than the more conventional approaches to preventing back-related disability. For example, Wood (86) evaluated a back injury prevention program for employees in a group of geriatric hospitals in British Columbia. One intervention was a reogranization of claims procedures for employees, which centralized the process and insured immediate contact between the personnel office and both the claimant and the workers' compensation board. Regular telephone contact was maintained every ten days to assess progress of the claim, evaluate potential retraining, coordinate gradual return to work with the supervisor and the compensation board, and document communications regarding return to work. Employees who missed work because of back pain were given a strong message that they were important to the organization and that the staff was eager for their return. This intervention resulted in a lower proportion of long-term disability claims among all claims filed. There was also reversal of a trend toward increasing numbers of wage-loss accidents. The program appeared to be substantially more successful than an intensive program for teaching proper lifting techniques.

Another effective program was that of Wiesel (83). He designed a consistent algorithm for the management of employees with back problems, which required careful review of each case by an expert orthopedist and feedback to treating physicians in the community. This intervention resulted in reduced rates of back surgery, fewer days lost from work, and a decrease in both medical and compensation costs (see below). This program, which is now in place via contracts with workers' compensation agencies in seven states, covers some 6 million workers (H. Feffer, personal communication).

THE POTENTIAL FOR SAVINGS AND IMPROVED OUTCOMES

The high variability in use of services for back pain implies that some care may be unnecessary. There is a growing consensus among experts that "surgery for chronic back pain is overused and often misused, that it is seldom any more effective than nonsurgical treatment in either the short or long term and often is less effective, and that back surgery (especially repeated surgery) frequently results in serious iatrogenesis" (51).

The potential for reducing the volume of care and actually improving patient outcomes was demonstrated in the above-mentioned Wiesel study. This project was conducted at the Potomac Electric Power Company (PEP-CO) and the US Postal Service region serving the District of Columbia. When the review and feedback process was implemented, low back surgery rates fell by 88% in a single year, and work-loss days fell 51% at PEPCO. At the Postal Service, there was a 55% decrease in medical and compensation costs, and a 60% fall in work-loss days. At both sites, reported cases of low back pain decreased. An estimated savings of $225,000 accrued at the Post Office alone in a single year (83).

In an extensive review of inappropriate hospital care, Payne (52) concluded that diseases of musculoskeletal and connective tissue probably account for more inappropriate inpatient days than any other major diagnostic category. Using 1976 National Survey data, Kramer and colleagues (43) found that among common musculoskeletal conditions, including rheumatoid arthritis and osteoarthritis, low back pain resulted in the most hospitalizations and surgery. Thus, much of the inappropriate hospital care identified by Payne is probably back-related. Nonsurgical hospitalizations have fallen substantially over the past decade (66), perhaps as a result of utilization review and reimbursement restrictions. Although inappropriate hospital use may be declining, persistent and wide variations in hospitalization rates and length of stay suggest that there are still opportunities for substantial savings without reducing the quality of care (68).

Many social and economic factors influence the outcome of back pain, regardless of medical therapy. Poorly educated persons have more hospitalizations for back pain than well-educated persons, but worse outcomes (20). Local economic milieu, disability compensation, and psychological factors have powerful effects on subsequent functional disability (16, 67, 74). Such factors may account for more of the observed variance in outcomes in low back pain than do medical services (16). A wider appreciation of these influences, and better clinical investigation of them, may lead to decreases in unnecessary and invasive diagnostic evaluation and to more successful treatments.

APPROACHES TO REDUCING THE SOCIAL IMPACT OF LOW BACK PAIN

Some of the problems associated with providing effective care for low back pain have their roots in the educational experience of physicians. Primary care residents are exposed to negative attitudes about back pain patients during their orthopedic training (11) and often receive inadequate preparation to manage these patients (8). These negative attitudes, especially if they are reinforced by perceived failure to meet patients' expectations, may become deeply embedded in the physician's psyche, and subsequent educational efforts to improve patient care for low back pain might become difficult (6).

Physician training emphasizes the orthopedic surgical aspects of low back pain, but most back patients encountered by family physicians have uncomplicated, mechanical low back pain. Primary care physicians might be more effective managers of low back pain if they were given tools to approach the problem as a functional impairment, rather than as a disease. Waddell (71), who recently urged physicians to adopt a biopsychosocial perspective for back pain patients, asserts that "the physician's role as healer must be accompanied by his or her more ancient role as counselor, helping patients to cope with their problems." Primary care physicians should be aware of the excellent prognosis for acute low back pain and communicate this favorable information to their patients. Avoidance of frightening terms, such as "ruptured disc," back "injury," or "degenerative spine," would be wise. These phrases imply torn tissues or major anatomical disruptions and may encourage patients to seek legal remedies, even though we cannot demonstrate pathological changes.

Primary care physicians and surgeons should become more selective in their approach to surgery and realize that surgery is not indicated simply because "everything else has failed" (18). Clearer criteria for hospitalization and surgery are needed, particularly for conditions other than the unequivocal herniated disc. The increase in surgical rates may be related largely to operations for vague conditions that are unlikely to benefit from surgery. Some payers, such as Washington State's Department of Labor and Industries (workers' compensation), have begun to establish explicit criteria for reimbursing hospitalizations and various surgical procedures. New guidelines aside, incentives are needed for better adherence to current, widely accepted surgical criteria (34), which appear often to be expanded in practice.

Health care providers should also be aware of the growing evidence against the routine use of passive treatments, such as bed rest, traction, and transcutaneous nerve stimulation (17, 18, 21). Conversely, evidence in favor of exercise regimens is increasing, as is evidence in favor of early return to usual activities (17, 18, 21, 71). The shift from passive to active therapy represents a fundamental shift in nonsurgical treatment paradigms (71).

Enormous resources are consumed by unproven remedies that are advocated by both orthodox and unorthodox practitioners. Recent evidence challenges the efficacy of such innovations as trigger point injections (27), laser stimulation (40), colchicine drug therapy (57), and transcutaneous nerve stimulation (21). Even many traditionally accepted treatments, such as conventional lumbar traction and lengthy bed rest, are probably inefficacious and should be avoided (17, 18). Physicians, third party payers, manufacturers, and government regulatory agencies all have a role in preventing the introduction and dissemination of ineffective treatments and devices. More rigorous review of new devices, procedures, and indications for therapy is needed before their widespread use. This may often require fastidious randomized clinical trials, as are required of drug therapy by the Food and Drug Administration.

Better patient education is also necessary. In many cases, patients are unaware that low back surgery is elective and that nonsurgical management (even for herniated discs with mild neurologic deficits) will result in equivalent, long-term improvement (18, 75). Patients should understand that the natural history of almost all back problems is to improve, and that surgery itself carries some risk of neurologic injury or other serious complications. Better quantitative data and better means of conveying such information to patients would improve their own decision-making processes. Nelson (48) has advocated the use of interactive, computer-based videodisc technology to improve the process of informing patients about therapeutic options.

Managers, supervisors, and foremen should be trained in the positive acceptance of back pain, without questioning a worker's veracity and establishing adversarial situations. Because a common complaint among injured workers is that "no one cares," contact by employers or supervisors should be encouraged shortly after an episode of back pain occurs. The managerial program, described by Wood, emphasized the message that "you are a vital part of the team. Your work is important and your job is waiting for you" (86). Managers may also prolong disability by preventing workers from returning to the job until they are completely well. This strategy may be more expensive than providing modified or part-time work to accommodate the temporary predicament of back pain. An early return to the workplace maintains the work habit, prevents adversarial relationships, and avoids the impression that no one cares (60).

Labor unions also have a role in reducing low back disability. Unions may, like some managers, oppose early return to work or a return when the worker is less than "100%." The worker is thought to be entitled to time off for even a minor problem, despite medical advice that suggests that return to activity may hasten recovery. Rigid union rules, which prevent an early return to work, referrals to "friendly" physicians who prolong disability, and referrals to "friendly" lawyers who press for lump-sum settlements, rather than rehabilitation, may be detrimental to the worker (60).

Similarly, many groups advocate reform of the workers' compensation system. Potentially beneficial changes would include faster adjudication of disability and compensation claims, increased emphasis on nonsurgical intervention, and early use of physical therapy and stress management. Some countries have reduced the adversarial nature of disability claims by allowing compensation without the need to prove an injury at work, providing more rapid rehabilitation, and imposing incentives for accepting alternative employment (74).

The health services research community should be more actively involved in this expensive medical and social problem. Growing attention to outcomes research is likely to better define the indications for surgery, hospitalization, and other medical services. The quality of therapeutic research for low back problems has generally been deficient (14). Many conservative treatments, and even alternative surgical procedures, may be amenable to investigation by rigorously designed, randomized trials. Greater attention to research design will result in more definitive information and may accelerate progress in this arena.

Innovative research in the primary care approach to back pain is necessary to determine if modifications in early care can prevent subsequent high cost services and disability claims. We need better knowledge of the time course of recovery and likelihood of recurrence in primary care patients. Similarily, the proper roles of physical therapy or chiropractic care should be clarified (19). Research to improve the quality of primary care is likely to involve greater attention to the patient's psychosocial needs, better patient education, and a more confident and positive approach on the part of practitioners.

Literature Cited

1. Allen, D. B. Waddell, G. 1989. An historical perspective on low back pain and disability. *Acta Orthop. Scand.* Suppl. 234: 1–23
2. Am. Chiropr. Assoc. 1987. Chiropractic State of The Art 1987-88, Arlington, Va.
3. Bigos, S. J., Spengler, D. M., Fisher, L., Nachemson, A., Martin, N. A., Zeh, J. 1986. Back injuries in industry: a retrospective study. III. Employee-related factors. *Spine* 11:252–56
4. Boden, S. D., Davis, D. O., Dina, T. S., Patronas, N. J., Wiesel, S. W. 1990. Abnormal magnetic-resonance scans of the lumbar spine in asymptomatic subjects. *J. Bone Jt. Surg.* A-72:403–8
5. Cairns, D., Mooney, V., Crane, P. 1984. Spinal pain rehabilitation: outpatient treatment results and development of predictors for outcome. *Spine* 9:91–95
6. Cherkin, D. C., Deyo, R. A., Berg, A. O. 1990. Evaluation of a physician education intervention to improve primary care for low back pain: Part 2. Impact on patients. *Spine* In press
7. Cherkin, D. C., MacCornack, F. A. 1989. Patient evaluations of low back pain care from family physicians and chiropractors. *West. J. Med.* 150:351–55
8. Cherkin, D. C., MacCornack, F. A., Berg, A. O. 1988. Managing low back pain-a comparison of the beliefs and behaviors of family physicians and chiropractors. *West. J. Med.* 149:475-80
9. Choudhri, A. H., Rowlands, P. C., Barber, C. J., Johnson, J., Stevens, J. M. 1989. Outpatient myelography: An acceptable and cost-effective technique. *Br. J. Radiol.* 62:253–55
10. Clever, L. H., Omenn, G. S. 1988. Hazards for health care workers. *Annu. Rev. Public Health* 9:273–303
11. Coulehan, J. L. 1985. Adjustment, hands and healing. *Cult. Med. Psychiatry* 9:353–82
12. Cypress, B. K. 1983. Characteristics of physician visits for back symptoms: a national perspective. *Am. J. Public Health* 73:389–95
13. Dehlin, O., Berg, S., Anderson, G. B. J., Grimby, G. 1981. Effect of physical training in ergonomic counseling on the psychological perception of work and on the subject of assessment of low back insufficiency. *Scand. J. Rehabil. Med.* 13:1–9
14. Deyo, R. A. 1983. Conservative therapy for low back pain: distinguishing useful from useless therapy. *J. Am. Med. Assoc.* 250:1057–62
15. Deyo, R. A., Diehl, A. K. 1986. Patient satisfaction with medical care for low-back pain. *Spine* 11:28–30
16. Deyo, R. A., Diehl, A. K. 1988. Psychosocial predictors of disability in patients with low back pain. *J. Rheumatol.* 15:1557–64
17. Deyo, R. A., Diehl, A. K., Rosenthal, M. 1986. How many days of bed rest for acute low-back pain? A randomized clinical trial. *N. Engl. J. Med.* 315:1064–70
18. Deyo, R. A., Loeser, J. D., Bigos, S. J. 1990. Herniated lumbar intervertebral disc. *Ann. Intern. Med.* 112:598–603
19. Deyo, R. A., Tsui-Wu, Y. J. 1987. Descriptive epidemiology of low back pain and its related medical care in the US *Spine* 12:264–67
20. Deyo, R. A., Tsui-Wu, Y. J. 1987. Functional disability due to back pain: a population-based study indicating the importance of socioeconomic factors. *Arthritis Rheum.* 30:1247–53
21. Deyo, R. A., Walsh, N. E., Martin, D., Schoenfeld, L., Ramamurthy, S. 1990. A controlled trial of transcutaneous electrical nerve stimulation and stretching exercises for chronic low back pain. *N. ngl., J. Med.* 322:1627–34
22. Dillane, J. B., Fry, J., Kalton, G. 1966. Acute back syndrome—a study from general practice. *Br. Med. J.* 2:82–84
23. Fager, C. A. 1984. The age-old back problem: new fad, same fallacies. *Spine* 9:326–28
24. Fordyce, W. E., Brockway, J. A., Bergman, J. A., Spengler, D. 1986. Acute back pain: a control group comparison of behavioral versus traditional management methods. *J. Behav. Med.* 9:127–40
25. Frymoyer, J. W. 1988. Back pain and sciatica. *N. Engl. J. Med.* 318:291–300
26. Frymoyer, J. W. 1989. Epidemiology. In *New Perspectives on Low Back Pain,* ed. J. W. Frymoyer, S. L. Gordon, p. 21. Park Ridge, Ill: Am. Acad. Orthop. Surg.
27. Garvey, T. A., Marks, M. Z., Wiesel, S. W. 1989. A prospective, randomized, double-blind evaluation of trigger-point injection therapy for low-back pain. *Spine* 14:962–64.8
28. Gibson, E. S. 1988. The value of preplacement screening radiography of the low back. *Occup. Med: State Art Rev.* 3(1):91–108
29. Gibson, E. S., Martin, R. N., Terry, C.

W. 1980. Incidence of low back pain and preplacement x-ray screening. *J. Occup. Med.* 22:515–19

30. Gilbert, J. R., Taylor, D. W., Hildebrand, A., Evans, C. 1985. Clinical trial of common treatments for low-back pain in family practice. *Br. Med. J.* 291:791–94

31. Graves, E. J. 1987. Diagnosis-related groups using data from the National Hospital Discharge Survey: US, 1985. *NCHS Adv. Data Vital Health Stat.* No. 137. DHHS Publ. No. (PHS) 87-1250. 12 pp.

32. Haddad, G. H. 1987. Analysis of 2932 workers compensation back injury cases: the impact on the cost to the system. *Spine* 12:765–69

33. Hadler, N. M. 1988. The predicament of backache. *J. Occup. Med.* 30:449–50

33a. Hellinger, F. J. 1990. Updated forecasts of the costs of medical care for persons with AIDS. *Public Health Rep.* 105:1–12

34. Herron, L. D., Turner, J. 1985. Patient selection for lumbar laminectomy and discectomy with a revised objective rating system. *Clin. Orthop.* 199:145–52

35. Hult, L. 1954. The Munkfors investigation. *Acta Orthop. Scand.* (Suppl. 16), 35–77

36. Hurme, M., Alaranta, H., Torma, T., Einola, S. 1983. Operated lumbar disc herniation: Epidemiological aspects. *Ann. Chir. Gynaecol. Fenn.* 72:33–36

37. Kane, R. L., Olsen, D., Leymaster, C., Woolley, F. R., Fisher, F. D. 1974. Manipulating the patient—A comparison of the effectiveness of physician and chiropractor care. *Lancet* 1:1333–36

38. Kaplan, R. M., Deyo, R. A. 1987. Back pain in hospital workers. *Spine: State Art Rev.* 2(1):61–73

39. Kieffer, S. A., Cacayorin, E. D., Sherry, R. G. 1984. The radiological diagnosis of herniated lumbar intervertebral disc: a current controversy. *J. Am. Med. Assoc.* 251:1192–95

40. Klein, R. G., Eek, B. C. 1990. Low-energy laser treatment and exercise for chronic low back pain: double-blind controlled trial. *Arch. Phys. Med. Rehabil.* 71:34–37

41. Koch, H., Gagnon, R. O. 1979. Office visits involving x-rays, National Ambulatory Medical Care Survey: US, 1977. *Adv. Data Vital Health Stat.* No. 53. DHEW Publ. No. (PHS) 79-1250

42. Koos, E. L. 1954. *The Health of Regionville: What the People Thought and Did About It.* pp. 98–99. New York: Hafner

43. Kramer, J. S., Yelin, E. H., Epstein, W. V. 1983. Social and economic impacts of four musculoskeletal conditions: a study using national community-based data. *Arthritis Rheum.* 26:901–7

44. MacNab, I. 1977. Failures of spinal surgery. In *Backache*, pp. 208. Baltimore: Williams Wilkins

45. McLemore, T., DeLozier, J. 1987. 1985 Summary: National Ambulatory Care Survey. *Adv. Data Vital Health Stat.* No. 128. DHHS Publ. No. (PHS) 87-1250

46. Meade, T. W., Dyer, S., Browne, W., Townsend, J., Frank, A. O. 1990. Low back pain of mechanical origin: randomized comparison of chiropractic and hospital outpatient treatment. *Br. Med. J.* 300:1431–37

47. Nat. Cent. Health Stat. 1988. *NCHS Vital Stat. Ser.* 13, No. 95. DHHS Publ. No. (PHS) 88-1756

48. Nelson, C. 1988. Helping patients decide: from Hippocrates to videodiscs—an application for patients with low back pain. *J. Med. Syst.* 12:1–10

49. Newman, R. I., Seres, J. L., Yospe, L. P., Garlington, B. 1978. Multidisciplinary treatment of chronic pain: long term follow-up of low-back pain patients. *Pain* 4:283–92

50. Nyiendo, J., Haldeman, S 1987. A prospective study of 2000 patients attending a chiropractic college teaching clinic. *Med. Care* 25:516–27

51. Osterweis, M., Kleinman, A., Mechanic, D., eds. 1987. *Pain and Disability: Clinical, Behavioral, and Public Policy Perspectives,* p. 204. Washington, DC: Nat. Acad. Press

52. Payne, S. M. C. 1987. Identifying and managing inappropriate hospital utilization: a policy synthesis. *Health Serv. Res.* 22:709–69

53. Penning, L., Wilmink, J. T., VanWoerden, H. H. 1984. Inability to prove instability: a critical appraisal of radiological flexion extension studies in lumbar disc degeneration. *Diagn. Imaging Clin. Med.* 53:186–92

54. Deleted in proof

55. Rockey, P. H., Fantel, J., Omenn, G. S. 1979. Discriminatory aspects of pre-employment screening: low back x-ray examination in the railroad industry. *Am. J. Law. Med.* 5:197–218

56. Salkever, D. S. 1985. Morbidity cost: National estimates and economic determinants. *NCHSR Res. Summ. Ser.* DHHS Publ. No. (PHS) 86-3393. 13 pp.

57. Schnebel, B. E., Simmons, J. W. 1988. The use of oral colchicine for low-back

pain: a double-blind study. *Spine* 13:
354–57

58. Deleted in proof

59. Snook, S. H. 1988. The cost of back
pain in industry. *Occup. Med: State Art
Rev.* 3(1):1–5

60. Snook, S. H. 1988. Approaches to the
control of back pain in industry: job design, job placement, and education/
training. *Occup. Med: State of Art Rev.*
3(1):45–60

61. Social Security Bull. Annu. Stat. Suppl.
1986: Table 51, pp. 119

62. Spengler, D. M., Bigos, S. J., Martin,
N. A., Zehn, J., Fisher, L., Nachemson, A. 1986. Back injuries in industry:
a retrospective study. I. Overview and
cost analysis. *Spine* 11:141–45

63. Spitzer, W. O., LeBlanc, F. E., Dupuis,
M. 1987. Scientific approach to the
assessment and management of activity-
related spinal disorders. A monograph
for physicians: report of the Quebec
Task Force on Spinal Disorders. *Spine*
12(Suppl. 7):S1–S59

64. Thomas, K. B. 1987. General practice
consultations: Is there any point in being
positive. *Br. Med. J.* 294:1200–2

65. US Bur. Census, Curr. Popul. Rep. Ser.
P-70, No. 8. 1986. Disability, Function-
al Limitation, and Health Insurance
Coverage: 1984/85. p. 35 Washington,
DC: GPO

66. US Dep. Health Hum. Serv. 1981.
Work practices guide for manual lifting.
DHHS (NIOSH) Publ. No. 81-122

67. Volinn, E., Lai, D., McKinny, S.,
Loeser, J. D. 1988. When back pain
becomes disabling: a regional analysis.
Pain 33:33–39

68. Volinn, E., Turczyn, K. M., Loeser, J.
D. 1990. *Surgical and non-surgical hos-
pitalizations for low back pain in the US.*
Presented at Ann. Meet. Int. Assoc.
Study Pain, Adelaide, Australia

69. Von Kuster, T. Jr. 1980. *Chiropractic
Health Care, A National Study of Cost of
Education, Service Utilization, Number
of Practicing Doctors of Chiropractic,
and Other Key Policy Issues.* Un-
published document. The Found. Adv.
Chiropr. Tenets and Sci. Contract No.
HRA 231-77-0126. Prepared for the
Health Resour. Adm., Hyattsville, MD

70. Waddell, G. 1982. An approach to
backache. *Br. J. Hosp. Med.* 3:187–
219

71. Waddell, G. 1987. A new clinical model
for the treatment of low back pain. *Spine*
12:632–44

72. Waddell, G., Kummel, E. G., Lotto W.

N., Graham, J. D., Hall, H., et al.
1979. Failed lumbar disc surgery and
repeat surgery following industrial injury. *J. Bone J. Surg.* A61:201–7

73. Waddell, G., Main, C. J., Morris, E.
W., Venner, R. M., Rae, P. S., et al.
1982. Normality and reliability in the
clinical assessment of backache. *Br.
Med. J.* 284:1519–23

74. Walsh, N. E. Dumitru, D. 1988. The
influence of compensation on recovery
from low back pain. *Occup. Med: State
Art Rev.* 3(1):109–21

75. Weber, H. 1983. Lumbar disc herniation: a controlled prospective study with
ten years of observation. *Spine* 8:131–39

76. Webster, B. S., Snook, S. 1990. The
cost of compensable low back pain. *J.
Occup. Med.* 32:13–15

77. Weisz, G. M., Lamond, T. S. Kitche-
ner, P. N. 1988. Spinal imaging: will
MRI replace myelography? *Spine*
13:65–68

78. Wennberg, J. E., Freeman, J. L., Culp,
W. J. 1987. Are hospital services ra-
tioned in New Haven or overutilized in
Boston? *Lancet* 1:1185–88

79. Wennberg, J. E., McPherson, K., Ca-
per, P. 1984. Will payment based on
diagnosed-related groups control hospital costs? *N. Engl. J. Med.* 311:295–300

80. White, A. A., ed. 1986. Failed back
surgery syndrome: evaluation and treatment. *Spine: State Art Rev.* 1(1):1–175

81. White, A. A., Gordon, S. L. 1982. Syn-
opsis: workshop on idiopathic low back
pain. *Spine* 7:141–49

82. White, A. A., VonRogov, P., Zucher-
man, J., Heiden, D. 1987. Lumbar
laminectomy for herniated disc: a prospective controlled comparison with internal fixation fusion. *Spine* 12:305–7

83. Wiesel, S. W., Feffer, H. L., Roffman,
R. H. 1984. Industrial low back pain: A
prospective evaluation of a standarized
diagnostic and treatment protocol. *Spine*
9:199–203

84. Wiesel, S. W., Tsourmas, N., Feffer,
H. L., Citrin, C. M., Patronas, N. 1984.
A study of computer-assisted tomography. I. The incidence of positive CAT
scans in an asymptomatic group of
patients. *Spine* 9:549–51

85. Williams, M. E., Hadler, N. M. 1983.
The illness as the focus of geriatric
medicine. *N. Engl. J. Med.* 308:1357–
60

86. Wood, D. J. 1987. Design and evaluation of a back injury prevention program
within a geriatric hospital. *Spine* 12:77–
82

Annu. Rev. Publ. Health. 1991. 12:157–75

THE FAT KID ON THE SEESAW: AMERICAN BUSINESS AND HEALTH CARE COST CONTAINMENT, 1970–1990

Linda Bergthold

William M. Mercer, Incorporated, San Francisco, California 94111

KEY WORDS: health care politics, health policy, corporate power

INTRODUCTION

Health care politics have changed in the 1980s. In the 1960s, there was plenty of policy change, but little alteration in the balance of power among the political interest groups. In the 1990s, business alliances with the state, coalitions with other business groups, partnerships with labor, and federations with providers are readily apparent on the political landscape.

As a central part of this environment of change, American business has become the "fat kid on the seesaw" (34), which tipped the political balance of power in health care politics and policy formation. American business active-ly entered the policy arena in the 1970s and has organized itself politically in the last two decades; it intends to stay in this policy arena well into the 1990s.

If business has been so politically active, what research can we call on to explain the power and influence of this new political actor in health care? There is surprisingly little systematic research that links the role of business to the formation or implementation of health policy in the United States. The policy literature in the political sciences and political sociology has focused mainly on urban policies other than health. When studied at all, the role of business has been viewed as an intervening situational variable that is less important than economic variables, which interact with structural and cultural variables and lead to policy decisions (2, 22).

157

0163-7525/91/0501-0157$02.00

To create a study of the role of business in health care cost containment policy, several bodies of research must be drawn together: studies of business power in policy formation (1, 13, 20, 21, 27, 56, 57); studies of business and policy implementation (4, 22, 33, 54, 58); general studies of health care politics, most of which were conducted in the 1970s with little notice of any role for business (3, 25, 31, 37, 38, 53); and theoretical works on business power (12, 17–20, 35, 41–43, 49, 56). By combining these studies on power, policy, and politics, key questions emerge that link the role of business in general policy areas to its role in health care cost containment. Why does business get involved in American health policy formation? Once involved, what role does business play? What are the consequences of business involvement, both for business and the policies it promotes? And, what is the future of the business role?

The research reported in this article emerged from a series of such questions about the rise of business as an organized political interest in health care politics between 1970 and 1990.[1] What started as a solo trumpet call for business involvement in health policy by Robert Finch, Richard Nixon's Secretary of Health, Education, and Welfare in 1969, became an entire brass band by the end of the 1980s (24). The beginning year of this article is 1970, because it was the first year of the most recent cycle of corporate intervention in medical care; 1990 brings the reader into the current decade. The article focuses on the states of California and Massachusetts, which are extraordinary illustrations of the exercise of business power in health care cost containment legislation in the 1980s.

The term "business" (or "corporate"), as used in this article, describes the activities and the economic interests of big business. Most corporations involved in the formulation of policy, at either the state or federal level, are of the *Fortune* 500 variety. The organizations that express business interests are dominated, in either leadership or membership, by big business interests. Although large and important corporate interests are involved in the production and financing of medical services, I will use "business" to refer to employers as purchasers of medical care services for their employees.[2]

Business Interventions For Change

To explain how business has been involved at the local, state, and federal levels in the past two decades, I highlight three types of business interventions, with special emphasis on the business role at the state level (56):

---

[1]This research is reported in Bergthold, L. 1990. *Purchasing Power in Health: Business, the State and Health Care Politics*. New Brunswick, NJ: Rutgers Univ. Press

[2]Those businesses that provide medical care services or insure for medical care are not the focus of this article, although all providers and insurers are also purchasers for their own employees.

INSTITUTIONAL MECHANISMS   This type of intervention was organized specifically for change during this period. It includes coalitions, associations, and lobbying groups. "Organization is itself a mobilization of bias in preparation for action" (47), and business clearly intended to influence health policy. The following section briefly describes the forces that propelled business into political actitity in the 1970s through a media scan of major business journals of the 1970s and 1980s.

Business also created or promoted four specific institutional mechanisms for change in the 1970s: The Chamber of Commerce of the US and its health policy committee; the Washington Business Group on Health (WBGH); the Dunlop Group of Six, an informal national policy group consisting of the six major stakeholders in health care politics (hospitals, insurers, Blue Cross, physicians, business, and labor); and over 175 business and health coalitions around the country.

ADVISORY ROLE   Business played a key advisory role to state and federal governments, such as Reagan's first health policy advisory group and the over 30 statewide health commissions formed between 1982 and 1984. The ideology of policy change and the advisory role that business played in key national committees and commissions demonstrate another level of business participation and interaction with the state. The relationship of business and state power is complex, interactive, and central to this discussion, because the state is the central arena in which the process of politics unfolds. It makes no sense to talk about business power in policy formation without also discussing the relationship of business and the state. Successful alliances between business and the state, however, can occur only under certain conditions: a perceived policy crisis, relatively united interest groups, and a political context that encourages and allows this fusion of power. Given the fragmented nature of both national and state level American politics, it should not be surprising that this type of alliance does not occur more often.

LEGISLATIVE PARTICIPATION   Business leaders have been engaged legislatively at the state level, in such policy groups as the Roberti Coalition in California and the Health Care Coalition in Massachusetts in 1982. In both states, business was brought into the policy process by the state, and business interests and state power in alliance were able to help break the provider grip on the policy process and promote substantial policy change, particularly in the first half of the 1980s.

THE BACKGROUND OF BUSINESS PARTICIPATION

How did business get so involved in health policy in the past decade, and why is 1970 an important year with which to begin this discussion? The year

1970 marks the beginning of a decline in corporate profits, accompanied by a national involvement of both business and government in reorganizing and rationalizing health care. The passage of Medicare and Medicaid in the mid1960s had led to noticeably increased health care utilization and costs by the early 1970s, and business leaders became alarmed.

In 1970, *Fortune* magazine declared: "Our present system of medical care is not a system at all. The majority of physicians constitute an army of pushcart vendors in an age of supermarkets" (32). Both politics and economics propelled business into its widespread and active role in changing health policy and bringing the independent physicians and health care institutions into the American health care supermarket.

The intensity of business political participation increased in the 1970s, as the rising costs of employee health premiums noticeably began to affect company profits. For example, between 1970 and 1982, the nominal growth in the GNP was 208%, and US health expenditures increased 332%; however employer health benefit expenditures increased 700% (50). In 1976, the average company spent about 5% of its payroll on health benefits; in 1988, this percentage almost doubled to 9.7 (15). In 1984, the Big Three auto companies alone spent $3.5 billion for health care, which was more than each of 32 states collected in taxes and spent in that year (11). The increasing costs of health care were beginning to affect the bottom line of most major American corporations, and the amount was staggering.

Business and the Economy: 1970–1980

The American economy of the late 1960s and early 1970s was marked by the lowest level of corporate profits in the share of national income since World War II (45). "Few events discipline the corporate mind as fast as a drop in earnings": (156). Pretax rates of return for nonfinancial corporations dropped from a high of 13.7% in 1965 (the highest rate since 1948–1949) to 8.1% in 1970. Aftertax rates of return followed a similar pattern; they declined from a high of 10.3% in 1965 to 5.9% in 1970 (30). A third plunge in corporate profits occurred in the early 1980s, when, according to a study by Data Resources, the inflation-adjusted profit rate in 1982 had reached its lowest level since the early 1970s (56).

Employers continued to pay more of the total cost of health insurance for their employees, and the costs of medical care continued to increase throughout the 1970s. From 1967 to 1978, according to a study by the Chamber of Commerce, the average benefits paid by employers for health related items, including social security taxes, increased from $10.90 to $38.99 per week; all employee benefits as a portion of total payroll increased from 29.1% to 41.2% in the same period. In 1976, the average company spent 5.1% of its payroll on health benefits; by 1978, it was up to 5.8%; by 1984, it averaged 8%

nationwide; and by 1987, it had reached 9.7%. Private employers were financing nearly one of every five dollars spent on health care in America by 1984 (15, 55).

If there is a connection between economic recessions, corporate profitability, and interventions in health care, then the major corporations should have become concerned in the 1970s, with a peak of organizational and legislative activity occurring in the mid1970s and again in the early and mid1980s. That is exactly what happened.

Not every chief executive officer (CEO) of every major corporation realized the connection between medical care increases and eroding corporate profits, and even those who recognized the dilemma did not always place it high on an agenda for action (46). However, the recognition by a significant, "dominant segment" of corporate leadership is revealed by several indicators: the release of influential Committee for Economic Development's report on health care costs in 1973 and reports by the Conference Board and Business Council; the formation of various task forces and associations to deal with health care issues, such as the WBGH by the Business Roundtable in 1974; and the number of articles in the business press devoted to the health care crisis.

The Health Care Crisis and the American Press

One way of tracking a social issue and trying to decide who has the most power over its definition and solution is to scan the media for references to the problem. Not only can the frequency of articles indicate the salience of a given subject for public policy, but the type of press in which the issue is discussed can also indicate the sectors of society most concerned with the issue. As Arnold Rose has noted, "There can be little doubt that those who own and manage most of the newspapers of the United States are more pro-business than they are supportive of any other segment of the population" (44). Thus, if business is concerned about a policy issue, one can expect to find an increasing volume of articles in the business press devoted to that issue.

Starting in the 1970s, most major business magazines, as well as the *New York Times* and *The Wall Street Journal,* began to carry lead articles on the subject of health care costs. In the 1970s and 1980s, the number of articles in the business press that addressed business' role in health care cost containment steadily increased. In a 1972–1989 computerized search of articles in *Forbes* and *Business Week,* using the key words "health," "medical" or "medicine," and "cost," "control," or "containment," 336 articles were located. The largest number of articles in any two-year period appeared in 1984–1985 (see Table 1).

In a computerized search of articles in the *New York Times* between 1980

Table 1 Frequency of articles relating business to health care cost containment in *Fortune*, *Forbes*, and *Business Week*, 1972–1988[1]

Years	Number of articles appearing in any of these magazines in a two-year period
1970–1971	database not available
1972–1973[2]	7
1974–1975	17
1976–1977	24
1978–1979	43
1980–1981	25
1982–1983	52
1984–1985	82
1986–1988	70
1989	16
Total articles	336

[1]Source: Computerized database compiled by author searching issues of *Fortune*, *Forbes*, and *Business Week* between December 1971 and June 1989.
[2]The *Business Week* database does not begin until November 1972.

(the first year a computerized search was available) and the end of 1989, using "business" or "corporate" and "health care costs" as key words, 181 articles were located that linked business efforts with health care cost containment (see Table 2). The number of articles on this topic steadily increased through 1988, and although the search ends in late 1989, there is no particular decrease in interest in the topic throughout the decade.

The *New York Times'* "broad readership tends to favor general corporate coverage over specific company affairs. Quotation or citation in the *New York Times* can serve as a suitable sign of access to the media" (44). Therefore, if the issue of health care cost containment was of importance to business, and if business wanted to get that word out to the rest of the corporate and policy community, the *New York Times* would be likely to carry an increasing number of stories on the subject. By 1985, health care cost containment became so important to the business readership of the *Times* that a special column called "Business and Health" was added to its Business Section. Between 1985 and the end of 1989, 52 columns addressed purchasers' interests in health care alone.

A "health care crisis" had been announced by the business press in *Business Week's* January 1970 Special Report, "The $60 Billion Crisis Over Medical Care." The opening editorial of the *Fortune* article was an explicit volley from the business community to the medical care industry and the government. "American medicine . . . stands now on the brink of chaos. Much of US medical care . . . is inferior in quality, wastefully dispensed, and inequitably

Table 2 Frequency of articles in the *New York Times* mentioning business and health care cost containment, 1980–1989.[1]

Year	General articles	Business & health articles	Total
1980	2	—	2
1981	3	—	3
1982	8	—	8
1983	7	—	7
1984	19	—	19
1985	16	9[2]	25
1986	13	8	21
1987	11	18	29
1988	18	13	31
1989	32	4	36
Total	129	52	181

[1]Source: Computerized search of articles by author mentioning either business or corporate/corporations and health care/cost containment in the *New York Times* between 1980 and 1989.
[2]A special column entitled "Business and Health" was instituted by the *New York Times* in 1985.

financed." The article continued, "The time has come for radical change . . . The management of medical care has become too important to leave to doctors, who are, after all, not managers to begin with" (32).

The solutions that business proposed in the early 1970s were diverse. *Business Week* editors proposed a national health insurance plan and/or more efficient group practices, such as the Kaiser Permanente Health Maintenance Organization. The article quoted several academic economists who all proposed management or efficiency solutions as the way to solve the cost crisis. Of the 100 firms questioned by *Business Week,* most had an "open mind" about national health insurance (NHI), but only a few were willing to support it unequivocally. One executive said, "If what I've been reading about health are in this country today is true, then standing up against a national health plan would be like arguing against God and motherhood. My snap opinion is that a national plan would involve constantly escalating costs. But most important, a national plan would take away an item worth up to a cent an hour that you can now stack on the bargaining table" (51).

The 1970 *Business Week* article provided the first comprehensive treatment ever given national health insurance in a national business magazine. The four major bills that were proposed by the Nixon administration and Congress were reviewed, and the political advantages and disadvantages were pointed out. "Reforming the medical system is an idea whose time has come," one NHI supporter said. Well, not quite. The Nixon health care reformers saw their liaison with American business much the way the Reagan administration supporters did a decade later. There was a crisis. It needed a solution.

And, American business could provide that support. The article concluded, "Backers of a national plan see this as a good chance to get in an opening wedge" (51). Even though the right wing defeated the moderates on national health insurance in the 1970s, and the Business Roundtable and the WBGH expressed their strong reservations about it, the very real economic constraints on the profitability of American business gave liberal health policy advocates an opening in the window (or the door) of opportunity in 1970, an opening that took them more than a decade to step through.

THE ROLE OF BUSINESS IN FEDERAL HEALTH CARE COST CONTAINMENT

By the end of the 1980s, health care costs were still increasing. Business had not yet found a satisfactory mechanism by which to control these costs at either the state or national levels.

Although much attention has been paid to state level health policy change during the 1980s, much of the impetus for this change came from national legislation and policy directives. Just as the creation of Medicare and Medicaid in the 1960s had stimulated private-sector changes, federal policy initiatives in the Medicare and Medicaid programs in 1980–1982 created a window of opportunity for state health policy changes in both private and public sectors throughout the 1980s.

In 1980, some Reagan administration changes in health policy affected all levels of government. None of these dramatic ideas were particularly new, not even "new" Federalism. However, the political actors themselves were surprised by the speed with which some of these ideas were accepted and implemented into law and the degree to which the policy debate shifted from a preoccupation with regulation and national health insurance in the 1970s to the obsession with the market approach to policy change in the 1980s (9).

It is difficult to determine which role party and leadership played in accepting these policy ideas and to what degree economic, historical, and other political conditions predisposed the system to change. Certainly, the growth of medical technology, the bureaucratization and increasing corporatization of health care organizations, the rising health care costs, the economic recession and fiscal crisis, the weakening of professionals as individual entrepreneurs, and even the international debt crisis all contributed to the crisis of reform. How the system changed—to what degree and in which direction—can be most accurately explained by the way in which business leaders in the Reagan administration took advantage of the cycle of crisis and reform, which lead to further crisis, that had gripped the American health care system for almost 15 years. Instead of playing the usual pluralist game of incremental, marginal, and largely symbolic changes, the Reagan policy makers, with the support of business, went for the "big win" and what has been called the "thin end of the wedge of structural change" (14).

How important was the participation of business to the policy outcome, and did the policy solution solve the problem? The federal cutbacks in health and welfare programs acutely affected all states in 1982 and created a context in which some policy change became more likely. These federal policy changes, accompanied by increasing responsibility given to both state level policymakers and private sector business leaders, produced a minirevolution in Medicaid programs around the country in 1982–1983. All states made some changes in their Medicaid programs, and many states made some drastic changes. The federal cutbacks established a context for change, which united states on the east coast with those on the west. Massachusetts anticipated losses of up to $10 million in federal money for its Medicaid program in 1982 alone, and California faced losses of up to $40 million (16). With the new prospective payment system for Medicare, hospitals were sure to face other losses of indeterminate amounts, as they prepared to cope with caps and cutbacks in programs that provided, as in Massachusetts, up to 40% of their patient population. Business leaders recognized the magnitude of the coming cost shift to private payers, as the public sector began to take its own payer role more seriously. If caps and limits were set on public programs, where would hospitals shift their losses? To the private payers.

Just as the state level policy changes could not have occurred without the opening wedge of federal policy initiatives, neither is it likely that local business would have become as involved without the readiness of state and national business leadership to create institutional mechanisms for policy change. When the Reagan administration created its policy task forces and asked for input on the competition proposals in the early 1980s, prominent business members were always included. John Harper of Alcoa, Walter Wriston of Citibank/Citicorp of New York, and Henry Ford Jr. were informed and often participated. These individuals were not just any three business representatives, however; each had been actively involved in the influential Committee for Economic Development discussions in the early and mid1970s. They also had served on the Health Care Task Force of the prestigious National Business Roundtable.

When Reagan's second term had ended in 1988, the influence of federal health policies had temporarily slowed the growth of health care costs for some payers, but not for most. The one policy change most opposed by business and other interests—the tax cap on employer-paid premiums—had been roundly defeated, despite the enthusiastic support of conservative economists. The change from retrospective to prospective reimbursement for Medicare, an accelerated shift in federal role from regulator to prudent buyer, and increased discretionary authority at the state level promised substantial structural changes in the health care delivery system. Business support for these changes strengthened the alliance of business and the state.

BUSINESS AND THE STATE POLICY PROCESS

Once involved in the policy process[3], which role did business play at the state level and which policies has business promoted in state legislatures around the country? Business interests have helped change the cost containment policy formation process in health in several ways, including participation in setting the policy agenda. In some cases, business changed the rules of the public policy process to be consistent with private decision-making and negotiations modes; in other cases, the public, consumer interest has been made equivalent to purchaser interests, with little attention paid to the differences between these interests.

Setting the Policy Agenda

"Setting the agenda is the vital first step of policy formation, which often establishes the parameters for everything that follows. If business misses the real start of the process, it automatically reduces its effectiveness" (40). Which role did business play in the agenda formation in the early 1980s?

The policy agenda supported by business throughout the 1970s and the early 1980s was pragmatic. During the 1970s, business had supported alternative delivery systems, such as health maintenance organizations (HMOs) and the "voluntary effort" by hospitals, neither of which had affected the rising cost of health care. By the early 1980s, there was evidence that regulatory approaches, such as rate-setting for hospital charges in New Jersey and New York, could hold down health care costs. In California, business supported regulation before turning to a competitive solution in 1982 during the discussions on "MediCal Reform." In Massachusetts, business supported a regulatory all-payers solution in 1982; however, by 1988, business was promoting more competition.

The choice of policy strategies by business also depended on the relative strength of labor and the state at the location of policy decisions. In the 50 states, and particularly in those states where labor was strong, such as Michigan, Ohio, and Illinois, more regulatory strategies were selected. At the national level, where labor representation was relatively weak and management input was stronger, the market strategy of the Reagan administration was more prevalent.

---

[3]What is "policy"? Although policy and politics are closely related, and in some languages the two words are not even differentiated, I will define policy as the British social scientist Jenkins does. Policy is synonymous with decisions; patterns of decisions over time constitute policy, policy decisions are taken by political actors; policies are about both means and ends; and policies depend upon real situations and feasible projects (33).

Business and the Process of Policy Making

Business did not play a dominant role in all of the over 30 states that formed health care cost containment commissions during the 1980s. But, business participated much more frequently than labor, and thus became a permanent part of the policy process in health. Few of the statewide health advisory commissions initiated in the 1980s were formed without including representatives of key business organizations. By participating so actively and visibly at the public level, business also introduced changes in the policy process itself. Massachusetts is probably the most extreme case, as business leadership forged a legislative solution through private coalition negotiations. In 1981, the leadership of the Massachusetts Business Roundtable took a failed public commission process back to the private offices of the Roundtable in Waltham. There, in a series of closed meetings, business, the state, insurers, hospitals, and physicians created the consensus for the Chapter 372 legislation, which passed in 1982. Labor and consumers were excluded. As one participant commented, "Public policy development is different from business decision making. The Chapter 372 policy changes [the Massachusetts legislation] occurred because [Health Task Force chairman] Gifford made it a business decision making process not a public policy process" (personal interview in Boston, 1984).

In other states, business participated in a public process but often carried out a private process of lobbying and influence more compatible with private-sector decision making. In California, for example, the Roberti Coalition included all the players at the public table in 1982, but MediCal Reform was created in great secrecy and haste by legislators, their staff, and a few key interest groups.

Depending on the context and the power of business in a given state, business participation could and did lead to a change in the policy process. How is this process different from policy making processes previously controlled by the state? Although policy decisions have almost always been made in private and ratified in public, at least in the past there have been a variety of structures for participation, symbolic or otherwise, (e.g. community action program councils, Health Systems Agencies, Certificate of Need hearings). Policy alternatives and criteria for negotiation have been set, if not completely by the state, usually with strong representation, and participation was available to a wider range of stakeholders in the policy process.

In the 1980s, with business playing such a dominant role, the public process may have included labor, consumers, and minorities at the policy table if there was one. However, these groups were not invited to the back rooms and did not have the type of access to public officials that business and the providers had. In some cases, such as Massachusetts in the early 1980s, business purchaser interests were simply identified as synonymous with the public or consumer interest without challenge or discussion. Some observers doubted whether business purchasers could fairly represent all consumer interests, particularly in areas in which management concerns differed from labor or in which business leaders sided with providers rather than patients.

CONSEQUENCES OF BUSINESS PARTICIPATION

What are the consequences of business participation for health policy? In the early 1980s, the emergence of organized business interests in alliance with the state provided an opportunity for the state to tip the distributive balance away from dominant provider or producer interests and toward purchaser (state and business) interests in both Massachusetts and California. Once collectively aware of how they could benefit from political participation, business representatives in both states participated vigorously. In Massachusetts, the political and economic interests of the state and the financial interests of the commercial insurers declared a fiscal emergency and prodded the large corporate interests to get politically involved. Certainly, both states faced urgent pressure to balance their budgets. The business sectors promoted policy changes to increase public-sector productivity. To the extent that hospital and health care costs stabilized or decreased, the policy changes (along with other economic factors) successfully reduced the fiscal crisis at the state level, at least for a few years.

In both states, fiscal crisis produced the context in which policy change was possible. In neither state was the proposed policy change new. Both states had introduced similar legislation in previous years, which laid the groundwork for what was perceived as dramatic or revolutionary changes in 1982. Although business was already organized in both states, state staff and leadership brought business into the public policy debate. Once involved, business power was dominant in the Massachusetts policy process, but less so in California. Factors of political culture, fragmentation, and size of the state all contributed to the relatively less powerful role of business in California. However, the resultant policy changes from the business-state alliances in Massachusetts and California created a more powerful private sector and business presence in health policy discussions in both states for the remainder of the decade.

There have been genuine changes in the policy process in the 1980s, not just in health. At both the state and national level, varying degrees of fiscal crisis have provided the state with the opportunity to insert a thin wedge of stuctural change into a stagnant political process. Several factors have contributed to substantial policy changes in the policy process and its outcomes: the use of the budget reconciliation process as a Trojan horse filled with a variety of reform proposals; the combination of symbolic public commissions and the privatization of agenda formation; the removal of decisions from the political arena to the economic realm with the powerful sledge hammer of market ideology; and the delegation of decisions from the federal to the state level, which fragmented political opposition into 50 centers.

The role of business in the health policy process has strengthened and been strengthened by each of the above-mentioned trends. Business interests are not always served by the Trojan horse approach (e.g. passage of the 1986 COBRA extension of benefits for workers was opposed by business, and cost shifts to business from Medicare and Medicaid have continued), but the consolidation of state power usually provokes a reaction from business and can ultimately increase the exercise of private power. In combination with private negotiations, public participation by business leadership can reinforce and reproduce business power.

Decision-making by the market is not always favored by business, because the control of health care costs depends on being able to squeeze all parts of the health care cost balloon at one time. Still, business knows how to manipulate markets. When decision-making becomes stalemated in the political arena, as it has in the past, business fragments those decisions into dozens of buying and selling decisions that can benefit buyers who have some consolidated purchasing power. In Arizona, when business failed to manipulate the political process and lost its legislative initiative campaign in the early 1980s, it was forced to fall back to market solutions of HMOs and preferred provider organizations. These solutions, as business leaders pointed out, might solve cost problems for individual companies but do not contain overall costs in the system.

Decentralizing political power to the state level removes policy issues from central national attention or debate. National Health Insurance did not occur in the 1980s; Massachusetts comprehensive health insurance did. While a national commission recommended reform of physician fees in the late 1980s, Massachusetts actually passed a law that forbade physicians to bill patients for more than Medicare would reimburse. Reform and change were most dramatic at the state level in the 1980s; business leaders had considerable power and access. For multistate and multinational employers, however, a national policy solution might be preferable to policy reform in 50 different locations. The 1990s is bringing the debate back to the national level.

Points of Access in the Policy Process

There is little debate over the ability of business leaders to gain access to the policy process, but at which points of the process will business be most effective? Clarence Stone (52) has noted in his study of urban policy in Atlanta that business demands had the most impact at exactly those points at which electoral demands were weakest: That is, business had power where issues originated and where they were implemented. Business demands were least effective at the point of decision by elected officials (52). To feed policy ideas to state decision-makers in 1982, business participated in the formation of the policy agenda through the Washington, DC policy advisory groups, the WBGH's input into data disclosure legislation and physician antitrust legislation, the Massachusetts Business Roundtable's private legislative process, and the collaboration of the business membership on the Roberti Coalition and California Chamber of Commerce. Did business itself recognize its power to affect policy? Although business has extraordinary access to the policy process when it chooses to make demands, business leadership tends to deny its influence. As the *Harvard Business Review* reminds its readers, "The business community has been anything but a major player in the agenda-setting arena . . . Business and industry frequently are reactive" (40).

Staying involved in the implementation phase of policy requires a highly unified business group. Business power was exercised in 1983–1984 to maintain the gains of the MediCal Reform in California, despite efforts by the providers to overturn the contracting aspects of the legislation. To keep their coalitions together throughout the 1980s, California business leaders hired lobbyists, monitored legislation, and even introduced their own bills as challenges emerged to business gains. By the early 1990s, business was back at work; it attempted to stall state legislative plans to mandate employer-sponsored health care insurance coverage for all California workers.

The point at which decisions are made in the legislative process, however, is the weakest point of entry for business demands. Although business leaders have learned to play the legislative game in some states, they have failed rather visibly in others. In Arizona, the leaders of the business coalitions were engineers. "The [political] initiatives were drafted with the same precision that went into developing the jet airplane, and with the same kind of logic . . . This turned out to be the coalition's fundamental error: its leaders neglected political considerations when designing the initiative. For all the plan's exactness, it could not be compromised, and . . . could not fly in turbulent political air" (36). Appearing at hearings, organizing letter writing campaigns, negotiating out political settlement, and courting politicians are usually neither part of a CEO's repertoire of skills nor high on a corporate leader's agenda. Business is most effective when its leadership can mold the ideas being considered, not fight ideas already frozen into legislation.

Business Alliances for Health

One *Harvard Business Review* suggestion to business leaders who want more legislative influence is to establish network and alliances. Business learned that lesson in health policy in the 1980s. Of all potential alliances, the alliance of public and private purchasers had the most promise, but the least stability. The fragile or potential corporatism that characterized the private planning process in Massachusetts fit within a limited definition of corporatism: a strong state presence, a two-way policy process, organized constituencies, and public ratification of private decisions (12). By the late 1980s, the state role remained strong and had been strengthened in many states. However, the demands of broader consumer groups fragmented business control and melted constituencies, and the legislature more aggressively took back its responsibility for policy decisions. This limited corporatist planning has worked best in a state such as Massachusetts; the geographic area and the number of participants is small, and there is a history and acceptance of a strong state regulatory role. Even though this type of concentrated planning may not have occurred in quite the same way in other states, the activist role of the state in California and Massachusetts demands that an interpretation of the policy process include the state as a critical actor and an interest in and of itself.

The alliance of business with other interests is more common and more permanent; however, to the degree that business becomes just another interest among a medley of providers, it can lose the impact of its concentrated purchasing power. The promotion of multiparty business and health coalitions by the Robert Wood Johnson Foundation and the Dunlop Group may have diluted the effective use of business power because of the inherent instability of such coalitions (8).

An alliance of business and labor is both the most natural and the most difficult of all alliances. At the national level, where labor's political clout is strongest, alliances such as the Labor-Management Group, a national group that met actively in the 1970s, served to promote shared agendas in a powerful way. The Dunlop Group, structured to favor labor interests, was also a place where business and labor could form alliances. Although the Dunlop Group has had no demonstrated or specifiable impact on health policy thus far, the commonality of interest between the business and labor members has been noted by the other members. As Bert Seidman of the AFL-CIO has commented, "In reading over the Labor Management Group policy statements on health care in 1977 and 1987, I am surprised to see how much we agreed then, as well as now. Except for a few issues, we're together" (B. Seidman 1988, personal interview).

FUTURE OF THE BUSINESS ROLE

Business was not very active in the 1960s when Medicare was passed, but it became more central to the policy debates of the 1970s and 1980s. Few major health policies will be passed in the 1990s in which business interests are not represented and on which business does not have some influence. Business has organized a variety of both stable and fragile mechanisms for expressing its political interests. Some business and health coalitions are unlikely to survive in their present form into the 1990s; state roundtables and lobbying groups, such as the WBGH, will persist.

Although economic crisis continues to be the most powerful motivator for business political participation, other political and cultural factors both promote and impede this participation. The degree of state regulatory activity, the general level of policy innovation, and prior levels of business activism in social policy can all affect current levels of business participation. The economic turbulence of the 1970s propelled business into awareness and action in health care. Escalating costs in the late 1980s reactivated health care task forces and new strategies for cost containment on the part of large corporations, as health insurance premiums rose an average of 20% in 1987–1988 and are expected to increase annually in the double digits well into the 1990s (26, 28).

The continuing application of the economic paradigm in health care can only strengthen the political role of business, perhaps to its chagrin. The development of American health care systems is proceeding in the direction of greater efficiency, rationalization, and complexity. That trend is not likely to be reversed. Concurrently, the debate over health policy will be developed within a language in which the market and economics define the "problems" (the cost of health care more prominently that its distribution), as well as solutions (all-payer systems or competing health plans, both of which strengthen existing players and dominant ideologies) (59).

The market is viewed as a superior decision-maker by policy makers because of the difficulty of making ethical or rationing choices in the political arena. "One of the greatest virtues of the market mechanism is its ability to relieve government of a myriad of complex and difficult decisions, such as who will get artificial hearts, who will live and who will die" (29). As Sheldon Wolin asserts, the political use of economics "is to mask power by presenting what are essentially political and moral questions in the form of economic choices. As the society moves from a condition of surplus to one of scarcity, economic policies are ways of distributing sacrifices" (59).

Within the dominance of this economically constructed reality, business has emerged as the appropriate political leader, with its impeccable, ideological credentials of profit orientation and performance standards of efficiency. Business leaders, once reviled by the public, are now being asked to rescue the health care system from its irrationality and even its inequities. Republicans want to let the private sector do it all. Democrats, at least, want the private sector on the side of the state. The private sector itself, American business, has become a somewhat reluctant bride in an arranged marriage to the state. Can this marriage last?

Aside from the very problems of conducting the rescue, American business may not want to be the standard bearer of the arbiter of choices that are fundamentally political in nature. As Bob Burnett reminds us, health care cost containment is a "dirty project" (10). It is filled with time-consuming meetings, rough policy fights, dangerous public exposure, and, even at best, considerable political risks for the participants. As business continues to participate politically, even sporadically, what impact will business have on the rest of the players on the seesaw? Will increased business power lead to increased power and participation of the other interests, or will the growth and complexity in the health care system itself be reflected in a similar complexity and fragmentation of the stakeholder interests?

A final word on the substance of policy change. The last two decades are filled with examples of the pragmatism of business in its selection of health care cost containment solutions. California and Massachusetts business leaders have supported polar opposite policy solutions to similar policy problems. Fifty-state studies of business participation show business activity associated with the release and availability of data and information about health care costs, but show no pattern of business support for regulating the health system (5). Does that mean that business has had no influence on the substance of debate over health costs? Business leaders in Iowa were the primary force for financial disclosure of hospital costs and charges; in Massachusetts they were the force for regulating hospital costs. Although the patterns are not consistent, the association of business participation with substantive change is clear. Within the context of the dominant market ideology of the 1980s and 1990s, business support for alternative delivery systems, more and better data, utilization control, and occasionally rate regulation, has often been the force that tipped the balance away from the status quo. Business as the "fat kid" still sits securely on the seesaw of health care politics.

Literature Cited

1. Aiken, M., Alford,R. R. 1970. Community structure and innovation: The case of urban renewal. *Am. Sociol. Rev.* 35:650–65
2. Alford, R. R. 1969. *Bureaucracy and Participation: Political Culture in Four Wisconsin Cities.* Chicago: Rand-McNally
3. Alford, R. R. 1975. *Health Care Politics: Ideological and Interest Group Barriers to Reform.* Chicago: Univ. Chicago Press
4. Bauer, R., de Sola Pool, I., Dexter, L. 1972. *American Business and Public Policy: The Politics of Foreign Trade.* New York: Atherton. 2nd ed.
5. Bergthold, L. 1990. *Purchasing Power*

in Health: Business the State, and Health Care Politics. New Brunswick, NJ: Rutgers Univ. Press
6. Deleted in proof
7. Deleted in proof
8. Brown, L., McLaughlin, C. 1988. May the third force be with you: Community programs for affordable health care. In *Advances in Health Economics and Health Services Research,* Vol. 8, ed. R. Scheffler, L. F. Rossiter. Greenwich, Conn:JAI
9. Brown, L. D. 1982. Washington Report. *J. Health Polit. Policy Law* 6(4):822–26
10. Burnett, R. A. 1984. The CEO of Meredith Corporation, as quoted in Iglehart,

J. K., "Big Business and Health Care in the Heartland: An Interview with Robert Burnett." *Health Aff.* 3(1):40–49

11. Califano, J. 1986. *America's Health Care Revolution*, p. 31. New York: Random House

12. Cawson, A. 1986. *Corporatism and Political Theory*. New York: Basil Blackwell

13. Clark, T. 1968. Community structure, decision-making, budget expenditures and renewal in 51 American communities. *Am. Sociol. Rev.* 33:576–93

14. Cohen, S., Goldfinger, C. 1975. From permacrisis to real crisis in French social security: The limits to normal politics. In *Stress and Contradiction in Modern Capitalism*, ed. L. Lindberg, et al., p. 91. Lexington, Mass: DC Heath

15. Demkovich, L. 1980. Business as health care consumer is paying heed to the bottom line. *Natl. J.*, May 24, pp. 851–54

16. Demkovich, L. 1982. States may be gaining in the battle to curb medicaid spending growth. *Natl. J.*, Sept. 18, pp. 1584–86

17. Domhoff, G. W. 1967. *Who Rules America Now?* Englewood Cliffs, NJ: Prentice-Hall

18. Domhoff, G. W. 1970. *The Higher Circles: The Governing Class in America*. New York: Random House

19. Domhoff, G. W. 1979. *The Powers That Be: Process of Ruling Class Domination in America*. New York: Random House

20. Domhoff, G. W. 1983. *Who Rules America Now? A View for the 80's*. New York: Simon & Schuster

21. Dunlop, J. T. 1980. *Business and Public Policy* Cambridge: Harvard Univ. Press

22. Dye, R. 1966. *Politics, Economics and the Public: Policy Outcomes in the American States*. Chicago: Rand-McNally

23. Deleted in proof

24. Faltermayer, E. 1970. Better care at less cost without miracles. *Fortune*, Jan., p. 127

25. Feder, J. 1977. *Medicare: The Politics of Federal Hospital Insurance*. Lexington, Mass: Lexington Books

26. Francis, S. 1989. US industrial outlook, 1989: Health Services Washington, DC: US Dep. Commerce. *Med. Benefits* 6(3):1–2

27. Friedland, R., Palmer, D. 1984. Park Place and Main Street: Business and the urban power structure. *Annu. Rev. Sociol.* 10:393–416

28. Gabel, J., et al. 1988. The changing world of group health insurance. *Health Aff.* 7(3):64

29. Havighurst, C. 1988. The changing locus of decision making in the health care sector. *J. Health Polit. Policy Law* 13(2):723

30. Holland, D., Myers, S. 1980. Profitability and capital costs for manufacturing corporations and all nonfinancial corporations. *Am. Econ. Rev.* 70:320–25

31. Hyman, H. 1973. *The Politics of Health Care: Nine Cases Studies of Innovative Planning in New York City*. New York: Praeger

32. It's time to operate. 1970. *Fortune*, Jan., p. 79

33. Jenkins, W. I. 1978. *Policy Analysis: A Political and Organizational Perspective*, p. 15. London: Martin Robertson

34. Kirkland, R., 1981. Fat days for the chamber of commerce. *Fortune* 21:144–57

35. Kolko, G., 1967. *The Triumph of Conservatism: A Reinterpretation of American History, 1900–1916*. New York: Free Press

36. Lefton, D. 1985. Behind scenes story of coalition defeat. *Am. Med. News*, March 29, p. 9

37. Marmor, T. 1973. *The Politics of Medicare*. Chicago: Aldine

38. Marmor, T. 1983. *Political Analysis and American Medical Care*. Cambridge: Cambridge Univ. Press

39. Deleted in proof

40. Nolan, J. T. 1985. Political surfing when the issues break. *Harvard Bus. Rev.* 63(1):73

41. O'Connor, J. 1973. *The Fiscal Crisis of the State*. New York: St. Martins

42. Offe, C., Ronge, V. 1975. The theory of the capitalist state and the problem of policy formation. In *Stress and Contradiction in Modern Capitalism*, ed. L. Lindberg, et al, pp. 125–45. Lexington, Mass: DC Heath

43. Offe, C., Ronge, V. 1982. Theses on the theory of the state. In *Class, Power, and Conflict*, ed. A. Giddens, D. Held, pp. 139–47. Berkeley: Univ. Calif. Press

44. Rose, A. M. 1967. *The Power Structure, Political Process in American Society*, p. 111. London: Oxford Univ. Press

45. Salmon, J. 1978. *Corporate attempts to reorganize the american health care system*, pp. 96–126. PhD diss., Cornell Univ. Ithaca, NY

46. Sapolsky, H., Altman, D., Green, R., Moore, J. 1981. Corporate attitudes toward health care costs. *Milb. Mem. Fund Q. Health Soc.* 59(4):560–85

47. Schattschneider, E. E. 1960. *The Semisovereign People: A Realist's View*

of Democracy in America. Hinsdale, ILL:Dryden

48. Deleted in proof
49. Schmitter, P., Lehmbruch, G., eds. 1979. *Trends Towards Corporatist Intermediation.* Beverly Hills, Calif: Sage
50. Shelton, J., Ford Motor Co. 12 April 1984. Testimony before the Joint Economic Comm. of the US Congr., Washington, DC
51. Special report: The $60 billion crisis over medical care. 1970. *Business Week,* Jan. p. 56
52. Stone, C. 1976. *Economic Growth and Neighborhood Discontent.* Chapel Hill, NC: Univ. NC Press
53. Thompson, F. 1981. *Health Policy and the Bureaucracy.* Cambridge, Mass: MIT Press

54. Turk, H. 1970. Interorganized networks in urban society: Initial perspectives and comparative research. *Am. Sociol. Rev.* 35:1–19
55. US Chamber Commerce. 1985. Employee Benefits 1983. *Med. Benefits* 2(4):1–3
56. Useem, M. 1984. *The Inner Circle: Large Corporations and the Rise of Business Political Activity in the US and UK.* New York: Oxford Univ. Press
57. Walker, J. 1969. The diffusion of innovation among the American states. *Am. Polit. Sci. Rev.* 63:880–900
58. Wilson, G. K. 1985. *Business and Politics: A Comparative Introduction,* p. 30. London: Macmillan
59. Wolin, S. 1981. The new public philosophy. *Democracy,* Oct. p. 35.

Annu. Rev. Publ. Health 12:177–93

INFANT MORTALITY: THE SWEDISH EXPERIENCE

Lennart Köhler

The Nordic School of Public Health, Göteborg, Sweden

KEY WORDS: child health, health services, social security, family

INTRODUCTION

Although perinatal and infant mortality have progressively declined in most industrialized countries during the first 90 years of this century, there are still substantial differences between these countries with respect to these important health parameters. The Swedish experience, which has been well studied, provides relevant information on declines in mortality. Due to the multiple factors affecting these parameters, this article will not only show trends in these health measures in Sweden, but discuss relevant family characteristics and summarize the social support system, including health care services, which together form the "Swedish model" of the welfare state. The article concludes with a discussion of the most important factors for successful pregnancy outcomes—from the perspective of a Swedish, pediatrically oriented public health professional.

FACTS AND FIGURES

Systematic, nationwide data on Infant Mortality Rates (IMR) are available for Sweden from the mid-eighteenth century. The IMR has shown a steady downward trend since then; for many decades, it has been among the lowest in the world. In 1989, 6.5 per thousand boys and 4.9 per thousand girls died during the first year of life in Sweden. Changes in perinatal, neonatal, and infant mortality from 1915 through 1988 are displayed in Figure 1.

177

0163-7525/91/0501-0177$02.00

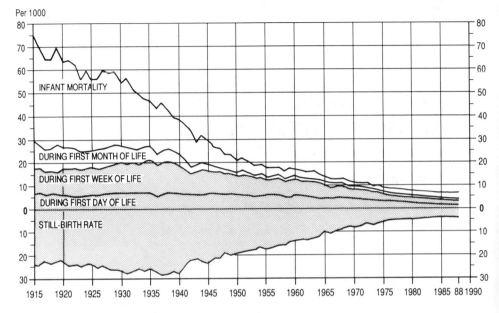

Per 1000

Figure 1   Infant and perinatal mortality in Sweden from 1915 to 1988.

The marked decrease in infant mortality is mostly due to a decrease during the latter part of the first year of life. Death in the first year of life now usually occurs shortly after birth, generally within the first week. Boys have a higher mortality than girls during the whole of infancy.

Perinatal mortality also has decreased markedly, and the number of still-borns shows approximately the same trend (the latter is part of the former.) The decrease in perinatal mortality has been steady, but not as dramatic as the decrease in postneonatal mortality (Table 1).

Causes of Infant Mortality

Traditionally, infant mortality has been used as an indicator of a society's standard of living, because mortality during the first year of life is strongly associated with the environment in which the child is conceived, born, and cared for. Improved living standards have contributed most to the decrease in infant mortality. Conditions that have influenced this favorable development have been better housing, nutrition, hygiene, and education. The environmental conditions have primarily contributed to the decrease in postneonatal mortality. The causes of death that are associated with pregnancy and delivery normally lead to the death of the child shortly after birth. These causes have relatively increased, despite their decrease in absolute terms.

The most common causes of infant mortality at present are certain perinatal

Table 1 Infant, neonatal, and perinatal mortality rates in Sweden 1989

	Boys	Girls	Both sexes
Infant mortality	6.5	4.9	5.7
Neonatal mortality	4.3	2.9	3.6
Perinatal mortality	7.0	5.9	6.5

conditions (group XV in WHO's official causes of death list) and congenital malformations (group XIV). Many deaths listed in the congenital malformations group occur in the perinatal or neonatal period. The most important cause of death after the first month of life is sudden infant death syndrome (SIDS). The incidence of SIDS in the 1970s was 0.54/1000 live births, thereafter increasing to 0.9/1000, but it is still well below the present figures from the UK and US (1.8–2.8 per 1000) (17, 24).

Changes in the age distribution of pregnant women have been given as reasons for the decrease in perinatal mortality. The maternal age-related risk for perinatal mortality is U-shaped, with the lower perinatal mortality and rate of stillbirth in women aged 20–29 years (5). As of 1990, 85% of Swedish children are now born to women aged 20–35 years. Contrary to the situation in many other countries, teenage pregnancies in Sweden have decreased markedly during the last decade, from 54.3 per thousand women 15–19 years of age in 1973 to 28.4 in 1984. A 16-year-old white girl in the US is two and a half times more likely to get pregnant than a Swedish girl of the same age (11).

Parity is also associated with perinatal mortality. The lowest infant mortality is found among second children. The firstborn and later than second-born children have a higher risk of death (22).

Meirik et al (20) estimated that changes in the age of women at childbirth in Sweden contributed 9% to the decrease in perinatal mortality from 1953 to 1975. In a 1968–1977 survey in England and Wales, the corresponding figure was 10% (4). One tenth of the reduction in perinatal mortality in Sweden during 1973–1980 has been considered attributable to a more favorable birthweight (18). In Sweden now, the incidence of low birthweight (less than 2500 g) is slightly below 4%.

Perinatal mortality is often regarded as an indicator of the quality of obstetrics and antenatal care, as well as the care of the newborn (5). Sometimes, it is also regarded as a general indicator of the standard of health services. Eksmyr (6) showed that the pregnancy outcome, in terms of perinatal mortality and incidence of cerebral palsy (CP), was the same in districts with small maternity hospitals as in districts with a more complete perinatal service. This suggests a uniformly high standard of health services in Sweden.

Anticipated risk deliveries are planned to occur in hospitals with more complete perinatal care, as well as good facilities for resuscitation of infants with asphyxia and for transports of such neonates. Similarly, an expert team from the Swedish National Board of Health and Welfare failed to find any systematic or significant differences in perinatal mortality between different types of hospitals or various levels of care (19).

As late as in the 1960s, higher infant mortality occurred among children born out of wedlock. The difficult and unprotected situation of unmarried mothers in the past has been suggested as a reason for these findings; however, now it is not possible to show any difference in mortality between children born in or out of wedlock. Other social norms and changing marriage patterns, as well as improved social welfare programs, have made these comparisons less meaningful. During the 1940s, for example, 8% of children were born out of wedlock in Sweden, compared with about 50% in 1988. Today, the fact that a child is born out of wedlock does not necessarily mean that the mother is alone or in a difficult situation, or that a stable family does not exist.

There is a well-established and overall accepted relationship between socioeconomic status of the family and infant mortality, in both developing and industrialized countries. In England and Wales, Townsend & Davidson (29) found that the risk of death at birth and during the first month of life in 1970–1972 was double in families of unskilled workers compared with professional families. A similar situation has also been documented in the US (1).

Notwithstanding the fact that infant mortality, internationally, reflects socioeconomic conditions, it is difficult to show differences in mortality between areas or groups in Sweden. The socioeconomic inequalities are no longer large enough to easily reflect such rough indicators as infant or perinatal mortality. In Sweden, however, there is little systematic reporting of such background variables as social class (3, 15).

Differences in perinatal mortality, however, have been found in certain limited studies. Comparing hospitals in the Stockholm region, Lindgren (16) found a correlation between perinatal death and the socioeconomic conditions of the hospital service areas.

In combining national data from medical birth registers for 1976–1981 with census data for 1975–1980, Zetterström & Eriksson (32) demonstrated clear differences in rates of infant and perinatal mortality and incidence of low birth weight between three socioeconomic groups (Table 2). In a more recent study, which used national birth data from 1985–1986 and census data from 1985, Cnattingius & Haglund (2) found a higher risk for fetal deaths among unskilled blue-collar workers (relative risk of 1.8) and a slightly higher risk for neonatal deaths (relative risk 1.5), but no significantly increased risk for

Table 2 Incidence of infant mortality, perinatal mortality, low birthweight, and serious malformations in Sweden in relation to socioeconomic index, 1976–1981[1]

Socioeconomic groups	Infant mortality per 1000	Perinatal mortality per 1000	Low birthweight (<2500 g) (%)	Serious malformations (%)
A	5.9	7.7	3.5	2.4
B	7.4	8.9	4.5	2.4
C	7.6	9.2	6.0	2.4
Total	7.2	8.8	4.5	2.4

A = 10% of population (high education, complete families, spacious flat or house)
B = 83% of population (middle group)
C = 7% of population (single parent, unskilled job, inferior housing)
[1]Source: Zetterström & Eriksson (32).

postneonatal deaths. Thus, infant and perinatal mortality in Sweden is still linked to socioeconomic conditions, but less obviously than in most other countries.

Child Mortality

Rates of child mortality in Sweden have been reduced in a similar manner as infant mortality. Child mortality rates began to decrease around the turn of the century and have continued to decline ever since.

In all countries mortality rates are higher in the younger age group and in boys (30). In most countries, the 10- to 14-year-olds have the lowest mortality of the whole population. Nordic children have the lowest mortality in the world in almost all age groups (Table 3).

Other Outcome Measurements

The most reliable and widely used measure of pregnancy outcome is mortality rates. However, in countries where these figures are very low, other methods of measurement are more appropriate to determine outcome, e.g. birthweight, morbidity, growth, and development. In the Nordic countries, differences in birthweight are also small, and the proportion of low birth weight children (<2500 g) is very low, ranging from 3.9% to 4.7% (23). Cerebral palsy is retrospectively closely linked to perinatal risk factors, and the prevalence is especially high in very low birthweight infants. In southwest Sweden, the epidemiological trends of CP have been followed for three decades (8). After a significantly decreasing incidence of CP in children born in 1959–1970, from 1.9 to 1.4 per thousand live births, there was a significant increase, reaching 2 per thousand in children born in 1971–1978, and 2.17 per thousand in children born in 1979–1982. Especially at risk in this increase were preterm infants, whereas full weight children showed only a marginal increase. The

Table 3 Child mortality 1986 per 1000 mean population according to age in some selected countries[1]

	0–1 year	1–4 years	5–14 years
Sweden	5.9	0.3	0.2
Finland	5.9	0.3	0.2
Norway	7.9	0.4	0.2
Denmark	8.1	0.4	0.2
Japan	5.2	0.5	0.2
Netherlands	7.8	0.5	0.2
Canada	7.9	0.5	0.2
France	8.0	0.4	0.2
W. Germany	8.5	0.4	0.2
England and Wales	9.6	0.4	0.2
USA	10.4	0.5	0.3

[1]From Maternal and Child Health Statistics of Japan 1989.

severity of motor disability and the relative frequency of mental retardation, infantile hydrocephalus, and epilepsy among preterm CP children successively increased over the same periods of time. This changing trend ran parallel with a steadily progressive decline in perinatal mortality. Thus, the increase of the perinatal survival rate seems to have brought a lowered risk of perinatal brain damage for the majority, but an increased risk for the "new," immature survivors. In this way, a considerable net gain of surviving non-CP children was achieved.

THE CHILDREN AND THEIR FAMILIES

At the end of 1988, Sweden had about 8.5 million inhabitants. Of these, 18%, or 1.5 million, were children aged 0–14 years. The average Swedish woman gives birth to 1.96 children. The low fertility figures do not automatically mean an increase in the proportion of only children. Only 13% of children aged 7–12 years had no siblings in 1985. Four- and five-child families, however, have practically disappeared.

Family Models

Of the children born in Sweden in 1988, more than 50% were born out of wedlock. As is discussed previously, this does not necessarily imply that the number of parents living alone has increased; other forms of cohabitation occur, which are not formally registered. In 1968, about 40% of the population aged 15–30 years were cohabiting in official marriages; only 0.7% were in consensual unions. In 1981, the corresponding figures were about 17% marriages and 23% consensual unions (14) (Figure 2).

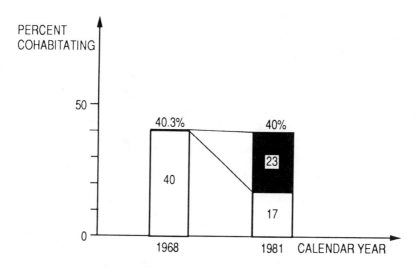

Figure 2 Percentage of population in Sweden cohabitating and mode of cohabitation. Age group, 15–30 years; calendar years, 1968 and 1981 (14).

The number of divorces has increased continuously in most industrialized countries, although in Sweden it now seems to have reached a stable level, or even begun to decrease (Figure 3). In 1988, about 18,000 marriages in Sweden ended in divorce, which involved some 20,000 children under 18 years of age. In the same year, about 40,000 marriages were entered. Altogether, some 12% of children live with only one parent, the mother in more than 90% of the cases. Approximately 5% of parents living together will break up during the child's first year of life, and within 18 years every third child has experienced a family break up (31). However, at present, 80% of children under 18 years of age live with their biological father and mother.

Abortions

The Swedish Abortion Act of 1975 allows free abortion upon request till the end of the 18th week of pregnancy. The rate of abortion has been fairly constant since the Act was introduced, around 20 per one thousand women aged 15–44 years per year. In the teenage group, however, the abortion rate has declined. In 1975, the US and Sweden had similar rates of abortion among teenagers, about 30 per one thousand women aged 15–19 years. Six years later, the Swedish rate had decreased by 30%, whereas the US rate increased by 43% (27). However, there has been a recent slight increase in

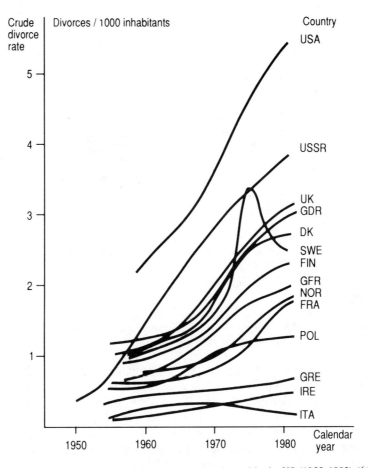

Figure 3   Crude divorce rate in selected European countries and in the US (1955–1982) (14).

Swedish abortions, which is especially disturbing in teenage girls, from 18 per thousand women under 19 years of age in 1984 to 24 per thousand in 1988 (9).

The Swedish Abortion Act strongly emphasizes preventive measures. The family planning program includes sex education (or rather living-together education) and the availability of inexpensive contraceptive advisory services. In 1983, a parliamentary committee evaluated the abortion legislation and concluded that the preventive measures had increased the use of contraceptives. Furthermore, they did not find any indications that the free abortions were used as a substitute for contraceptives. One of the reasons for the increased abortion rates might be the diminished use of contraceptive pills, mainly because of fear of complications (9).

Immigration

Immigration to Sweden during the twentieth century was fairly insignificant until World War II. However, in just a few decades, Sweden has changed from a monolingual and ethnically homogeneous society into a multilingual society with many ethnic minorities. Now, there are 150 nationalities represented: just below 5% are foreign nationals, and another 5% have become naturalized Swedish citizens. Altogether, 1 million of Sweden's population of about 8.5 million are immigrants or have at least one immigrant parent. This figure includes immigrants from other Nordic countries.

Immigration accounted for nearly 45% of the total population increase during 1944–1980; every eighth child now born in Sweden is of foreign extraction. In 1986, 48% of all foreign nationals in Sweden were from the other Nordic countries (Denmark, Finland, Iceland, Norway), 27% from other European countries, 14% from Asia, 4% from South America, 2% from Africa, and 2% from North America. Foreign nationals account for 5% of the country's work force of 4.4 million.

It is more common for immigrants to do shift work and have irregular working hours. They are also over-represented in industries that have a poor working environment. They enjoy the same housing standards as Swedes, although they often live in more crowded conditions and have a larger number of dependents. However, the difference in income between Swedes and foreign nationals is comparatively small.

In health surveys, immigrants have more physical complaints and are over-represented in hospital and outpatient care. Recent immigrants have higher perinatal mortality and more children with low birth weight than the rest of the population. However, the figures for children conceived and born in Sweden show no such differences (26, 32).

THE WELFARE STATE

Sweden is an old monarchy and it is highly industrialized and affluent. The Gross National Product (GNP) per capita in 1988 was 21,546 US $, compared with 19,558 for the United States and 14,413 for the United Kingdom. Sweden has a high standard of living, which is reasonably well-distributed among different socioeconomic groups. A high proportion of women are gainfully employed; more than 90% of 11–16-year-old children and 82% of 0–6-year-olds have working mothers. The unemployment rate is low; in March 1990, the national unemployment figure was 1.3%.

It is a pronounced welfare state, which is based on a private market economy system. However, it is balanced by a comprehensive set of public social services and a guaranteed minimum income for individuals, which is irrespective of the market value of their labor or assets ('mixed economy') and modified by a dense social security net that looks after people in illness, incapacity, and old age. However, users of the services are expected to pay a contributory charge in many cases. Typical for the Swedish model are three essential features (7): First, social policy is comprehensive in its attempt to provide welfare. The scope of public intervention is defined more broadly than in most other nations, and policy embraces an extensive range of social needs. Also, the government pursues a holistic and integrated approach to social policy, the aim of which is to ensure an unified system of social protection. The second distinct feature is the degree to which the social entitlement principle has been institutionalized. The welfare state has given citizens a basic right to a very broad range of services and benefits, which, as a whole, is intended to constitute a democratic right to a socially adequate level of living. The third feature is the solidaristic and universalist nature of social legislation. The welfare state is meant to include the entire population, rather than target its resources towards particular problem groups. Social policy is actively employed in the pursuit of a more socially just society.

More than 30% of the GNP is spent on social security, including health care, unemployment benefit, pensions, family allowances, and public assistance. Another 9% is spent on health care. For the US, the corresponding figures are 20% and 11.2% (1987).

Social Security

The modern Swedish family policy was started just before World War II. It now provides economic and social support to families with children, such as child allowances, housing assistance, parental benefit scheme, child care, and organized maternal and child health services, including a family planning program.

The annual child allowance is now SEK 6720 (US $ 1300) per child up to 16 years of age, and longer if the child is still in school. If the family has three or more children, extra allowances are paid, half the ordinary sum for the third child, and then a full sum extra for each additional child. These allowances are paid to everybody, irrespective of income, and are tax-exempted.

The parental benefit scheme includes paid parental leave for a total of 15 months in connection with childbirth and at anytime during the child's first seven years. For the mother, it could start two months before the expected delivery. Once the child is born, the parents themselves decide how to divide the remaining months between them.

During the perinatal leave, the parents are entitled to compensation at the same amounts as the sickness benefit, i.e. at 90% of their gross income for 12 months and at a reduced level for another three months. Starting in 1991, the government has promised an extension to 15 and 18 months, respectively.

Compensation from the parental insurance is taxable and qualifies for future pension in the same way as income from employment.

From 1974 to 1986, the percentage of men using the benefit rose from 3% to 23%. Furthermore, fathers are entitled to a ten-day leave of absence with parental benefit when a child is born, even if the mother is receiving parental benefit at the same time and for the same child (used by 83% of the fathers).

Parents who have to abstain from gainful employment to look after a child—their own child, adoptive child, foster child, or stepchild—who has not reached the age of 12 (16, if the child is disabled), are entitled to parental benefit in the following cases:

1. When the child is ill, or if the person who usually looks after the child falls ill.
2. When the mother is in the hospital to give birth, the father may stay at home to look after children living at home, in which case he receives parental benefit.
3. When the child is to be taken to a child health clinic, a school health clinic, a public dental care clinic, or a mental health facility, parental benefit will be paid to that parent who stays home from work to accompany the child.

Families are entitled to parental benefit for at most 90 days a year for each child. This benefit is used by mothers in 55.5% and fathers in 44.5% of cases, with an annual average of eight days. As from July 1, 1990, this benefit increased to 120 days, an important, yet inexpensive reform, as only a few parents with seriously ill children make use of it.

By law, parents have the right to stay home from work until their child is 18 months old, and then return to the same work. If the parent wants to visit the day care center or the school, parental benefits are paid for at most two days per year per child until 12 years of age.

No one can be fired because of pregnancy (or because of illness, for that matter). Parents with children under 8 years of age are entitled to reduce their work to three quarters of full time (with correspondingly reduced pay).

The total cost of the Parental Benefit Scheme is, for 1988–1989, calculated to 0.8% of the GNP.

Health Services

The health services are predominantly publicly financed and publicly provided, and hospital care takes most of the costs. More than in other industrialized countries, health services in Sweden is a task for the public sector (Figure 4). The costs of the medical services are covered by the National Health Insurance. The patient pays only a small standard charge for the outpatient service and for the drugs prescribed.

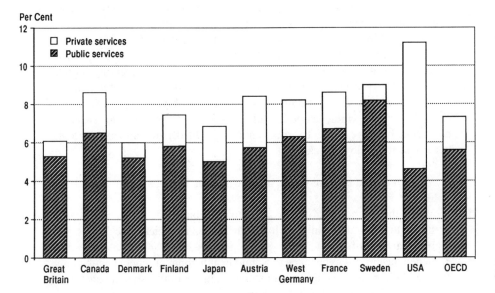

Figure 4   Expenditure on health services in percentage of GNP. 1987 (25).

Political and economic responsibilities for both individual- and population-oriented health services and for outpatient and inpatient medical care rest with the county councils. These units, with approximate populations of 60,000 to 1,500,000 (about 300,000 on average), also operate the public dental service, which provides care for everyone up to the age of 19. They also provide some adult dental care. In addition, they care for the mentally retarded. Responsibility for social welfare services and public health (environmental hygiene) rests primarily with the 284 municipalities, which have populations of 5,000–700,000.

Private health care exists on a limited scale. Only 8% of physicians work full-time in private practice. The corresponding figure for dentists, however, is more than 50%. Within the inpatient sector, there is a limited number of private medical care institutions, which are chiefly private nursing homes for long-term care.

There are 418 inhabitants per physician and 123 per nurse. Pediatricians comprise 3.3% of all physicians.

Maternal and Child Health Services

Sweden has a well-developed and broadly based system of preventive care for children and pregnant women, as a basic component in the society's health policy. These services for mothers and children enjoy a good reputation among providers and consumers, much better than other kinds of preventive care. The attendance rate is very high: during pregnancy and during the child's first year above 99%; at 4 years of age, 97%.

The overall purpose of the policy is to promote the physical, mental, and social development of pregnant women and children, which is accomplished by offering regular check-ups and screening procedures. However, the maternity health clinics and the child health clinics also function as nearby service centers for advice, education, and help for families. Thus, psychosocial support, family planning, and health education have developed into important parts of the activity. Besides the physician, nurse, and midwife, many other professionals are involved, including psychologists, dentists, dental hygienists, social workers, dieticians, physiotherapists, orthoptists, and speech therapists. All visits to the maternal and child health services and all activities offered there are free of charge.

MATERNAL HEALTH SERVICES   The recommended number of visits to the maternity health clinic is 16, 2 to the physician and 14 to the midwife, according to a plan made by the National Board of Health and Welfare. About half of the women are examined by specialists in obstetrics, and half by general practitioners. Pregnancies at risk are referred to specialists or hospitals.

Deliveries are concentrated to hospitals, with less than 1% at home, and more than 80% in special wards, where obstetricians, anesthesiologists, and pediatricians are constantly on duty. Most normal deliveries are done by nurse-midwives. After an increase in cesarian sections from 5.5% in 1973 to 12.4% in 1981, there has been a continuous decrease; the figure for 1988 was 11.2% (10). The American figure was 24.4% in 1987 (12). Only 5% of births occur in hospitals without obstetric and pediatric specialist care. With skillful and advanced intensive care, it is now possible to give extremely small low birthweight children (<900 g), a survival rate of 48% through the first year of life (28). A rooming-in system is commonly used, and practically all children are breast-fed when they leave the hospital. At four months of age, 50% are fully breast-fed; at six months, 25% (21).

For the whole country, there is a common system of records for maternal health care, deliveries, and child health care. Based on the medical birth record, statistics and evaluation of the care are published each year, which provides data on mortality, birthweight, complications, and malformations.

CHILD HEALTH SERVICES   The basis of the child health service is also frequent visits to the physician and nurse at the child health clinics. The national health supervision program recommends examinations by a physician at 2, 6, 10, and 18 months and at 4 and 5.5 years. In less than half of the health districts, the physicians at the child health clinics are pediatricians. In the remaining districts, they are general practitioners, although most of them also have additional training in pediatrics. The nurse is responsible for the continuous contact with the family, for routine weighing and measuring, for everyday support and advice, and for the parental education program. Screening programs have also been introduced for metabolic disorders, vision, hearing, speech, and general development. Vaccination and advice on nutrition and behavior are also important, as is the dental health counseling (13). Organized parental education programs are now available in 83% of the health districts. Visits to the child health services, and the educational sessions, are covered by the natural health system and included in the parental insurance scheme.

SCHOOL HEALTH SERVICES   In Sweden, a child begins school at seven years of age. School is compulsory for nine years. However, more than 90% of the children continue their education for at least an additional two or three years.

The school health services can be seen as a continuation of the child health services, but also as an occupational health service for the pupils. Health supervision by regular examinations, which is reinforced by screening programs, vaccinations, and a limited environmental supervision is the cornerstone of the services. Curative care for minor complaints is also offered. Psychologists and social workers take part in the work, together with physicians and nurses.

PARENTS' ROLE   The guiding principle of the Maternal and Child Health Programs is to create a system that covers the whole country and offers an easily accessible and attractive service to all children and pregnant women. The content of the services is based on physical surveillance, but increasingly has included mental and social aspects of health and well-being. These health surveillance programs are important in themselves, but they also reflect the society in which they are functioning. As such, they form a basic component in the society's social policy, a sign of its will and ability to care for its citizens. In the organization and execution of these programs, increasing awareness is paid to the need to involve the people in their own health promotion. Or, as it is pronounced in one of WHO's fundamental principles in the Declaration of Alma Ata: "The right and duty of the people individually and collectively to participate in the development of their health."

A good example of this changing emphasis can be seen in the Swedish health legislation for Maternal and Child Health Services, as formulated by the National Board of Health and Welfare, in 1969 and in 1979, respectively. The 1969 legislation called for the preventive services for children to be directed towards "a complete health surveillance and a handicap finding activity." In 1979, its wording was changed to "support and activate the parents in their parenthood and thereby create favorable conditions for a comprehensive development of children."

In the first formulation, the responsibility of the health supervision is still on the services. In the latter, there is a clear tendency to withdraw the professional forces and let the parents and the children themselves take over the responsibility for their health, supported and helped by the health services.

The same basic idea is found in the recent Swedish law and subsequent instructions on parental education. The goals are to increase the knowledge about children, create possibilities of contact among parents, and make parents conscious of social and economic patterns.

EVALUATION AND CONCLUSION

Social support systems, including health surveillance programs and preventive activities, are notoriously difficult to evaluate in a way that satisfies a scientific mind. Nonetheless, a history of some 50 years of practical experience from an expanding social support system and scattered evidence from evaluation studies, together with steadily decreasing childhood mortality rates, make it possible to identify the most important elements behind the extremely low infant mortality rates in Sweden. From there, we can formulate the essential points for understanding the major factors that influence the health of mothers and small children.

Characteristics of Sweden, Which Contribute to Low Infant Mortality Rates

- Sweden has a small population, which has a high per capita income and is still comparatively homogenous ethnically. The people have a high standard of living and the wealth is reasonably well-distributed. There is a high level of education, the housing is excellent, and the nutrition is good.
- The political system is based on market economy. But, it is modified by a strong public sector and a pronounced cross-party political will to support the whole population, especially the most vulnerable: pregnant women and children and sick, unemployed, handicapped, or elderly individuals.
- This welfare state has been built slowly, starting with general, compulsory schooling in the 1840s and continuing with an expanding social security system since the 1930s. It includes an extensive family policy that reaches everybody.
- The changes in fertility pattern have been noticeable during the last decades: increased maternal age at birth, fewer teenage pregnancies, decreased number of women with many children. All these factors favorably influence the perinatal mortality rate, as does the very low incidence of low birth

weight. The stigma of out-of-wedlock pregnancies has been removed, although single parents are still among the most vulnerable groups.

- There is a countrywide network of maternal and child health clinics, which are attended by practically all pregnant women and small children. They provide a wide range of preventive services, from physical check-ups to parental education. At the maternal health clinics, pregnant women at risk are identified by the midwives or physicians and referred to specialist care. Only a small minority of children are born without immediately available services of high quality from obstetricians and pediatricians.
- There is a long standing availability of sex education in all schools, not only concerned with biological and technical aspects but also with feelings, attitudes, and gender roles. There are easily accessible and inexpensive contraceptive services at the maternal health clinics, at ordinary health centers, and in school health services.

General Issues in Maternal and Child Health

- The health of a population, measured by mortality, morbidity, and growth, is more dependent on the overall socioeconomic standard and its distribution than on the health services per se.
- In countries with far reaching and extensive social support systems, the differences in mortality and morbidity between social classes are less obvious than in other countries.
- Focusing on medical intervention and on an individualistic orientation can only offer short-term and unsatisfying solutions.
- Maternal and child health services are part of the country's social policy and should act as a support for families. They should offer a wide variety of programs to promote physical, mental, and social well-being.
- To achieve success, prevention programs should be accepted as meaningful by the families and should also be easily available and accessible for all.
- The combined forces of an informed, knowledgeable public and concerned, responsive professionals are the basis of the effective health care.

Literature Cited

1. Chiles, L. 1988. *Death Before Life: The Tragedy of Infant Mortality. The Report of the National Commission to Prevent Infant Mortality.* Washington, DC: Natl. Comm. Prevent Infant Mortal.
2. Cnattingius, S., Haglund, B. 1990. Effect of socio-economic factors on late fetal and infant mortality in Sweden. *Int. Symp. Perinatal Infant Mortal.* Bethesda, Md: NIH
3. Dahlgren, G., Diderichsen, F. 1985. Sweden country paper. In *Inequalities in Health and Health Care*, ed. L. Köhler, J. Martin, pp. 167–99 Göteborg: Nordic School Public Health, NHV-Rep. 1985:5
4. Edouard, L. 1981. The dynamics of perinatal mortality. Maternal age, parity and legitimacy. *Scand. J. Soc. Med.* 9:59–61
5. Edouard, L. 1985. The epidemiology of perinatal mortality. *World Health Stat. Q.* 38:289–301
6. Eksmyr, R. 1986. *Pregnancy outcome*

in relation to paediatric care facilities at the local maternity hospital. Thesis. Karolinska Inst. Stockholm

7. Esping-Andersen, G., Korpi, W. 1987. From poor relief towards institutionalized welfare states: the development of Scandinavian social policy. In *The Scandinavian Model: Welfare States and Welfare Research,* ed. R. Eriksson. New York: Sharpe

8. Hagberg, B., Hagberg, G., Olow, I., von Wendt, L. 1989. The changing panorama of cerebral palsy in Sweden. 5: The birth year period 1979–1982. Epidemiological trends 1959–1978. *Acta Paediatr. Scand.* 78:283–90

9. Holmgren, K. 1990. Stigande aborttal i Sverige. *Nord. Med.* 105:46–48

10. Ingemarsson, I., Nielsen, T. F. 1990. Kejsarsnittsfrekvensen sjunker i Sverige. *Läkartidningen* 87:1135–37

11. Jones, E. F., Forrest, J. D., Goldman, N., Henshaw, S. K., Lincoln, R., et al. 1985. Teenage pregnancies in developed countries: determinants and policy implications. *Fam. Plann. Perspect.* 17: 53–63

12. Jones, H. S. 1989. The search for a lower cesarean rate goes on (Editorial). *J. Am. Med. Assoc.* 262:1512–13

13. Köhler, L. 1984. Early detection and screening programmes for children in Sweden. In *Progress in Child Health,* ed. A. Macfarlane, pp. 230–42. Edinburgh New York: Churchill Livingstone

14. Köhler, L., Lindström, B., Barnard, K., Itani, H. 1986. *Health Implications of Family Breakdown.* Göteborg: Nordic School Public Health, NHV-Rep. 1986: 3. 80 pp.

15. Köhler, L., Jakobsson, G. 1987. *Children's Health and Well-being in the Nordic countries.* Oxford: MacKeith, Clin. Dev. Med. No. 98, 140 pp.

16. Lindgren, L. 1979. Den perinatala dödligheten och befolkningens socioekonomiska struktur. *Socialmedicinsk Tidskrift* 56:471–79

17. McFeeley, P., Karlberg, P., Hoffman, A. 1990. SIDS as cause of death in infancy. *Int. Symp. Perinatal Infant Mortal.* Bethesda, Md: NIH

18. Meirik, O. 1983. Minskad perinatal dödlighet i Sverige 1973–80. Var har

vinsterna gjorts? *Läkartidningen* 80: 3693–96

19. Meirik, O. 1986. Expertgrupp om förlossningar vid olika sjukhustyper. *Läkartidningen* 83:3623–24

20. Meirik, O., Smedby, B., Ericson, A. 1979. Impact of changing age and parity distributions of mothers on perinatal mortality in Sweden 1953–1975. *Int. J. Epidemiol.* 8:361–64

21. Nat. Board Health Welf. 1986. *Pilot studies in breast feeding.* Stockholm: SOSFS 1986:9

22. Natl. Board Health Welf. 1990. *Medical birth registration in 1982, 1983 and 1984.* Stockholm: Natl. Board Health Welf. 33 pp.

23. NOMESKO. 1990. *Health Statistics in the Nordic Countries 1988.* Rep. 31. Copenhagen: Nord Stat Sekretariat. 108 pp.

24. Norvenius, S. G. 1987. Sudden infant death syndrome in Sweden in 1973–1977 and 1979. *Acta Paediatr. Scand.* Suppl. 333:7–120

25. OECD. 1990. *Health Care Systems in transition. The search for efficiency.* Paris: OECD, Soc. Policy Stud. No. 7

26. Smedby, B., Ericson, A. 1979. Perinatal mortality among children of immigrant mothers in Sweden. *Acta Paediatr. Scand.* Suppl. 275:41–46

27. Sundström-Feigenberg, K. 1988. Reproductive health and reproductive freedom. Maternal health care and family planning in the Swedish health system. *Women Health* 13:35–55

28. Svenningsen, N. W., Stjernqvist, K., Stavenow, S., Hellström-Westaas, L. 1989. Neonatal outcome of extremely small low birth-weight liveborn infants below 901 g in a Swedish population. *Acta Paediatr. Scand.* 78:180–88

29. Townsend, P., Davidson, N. 1982. *Inequalities in Health.* Harmondsworth: Penguin

30. United Nations. 1988. *Mortality of children under age 5. World estimates and projections 1950–2025.* New York: UN

31. *Välfärdsbulletinen 3/1989.* Stockholm: Statistiska centralbyrån

32. Zetterström, R., Eriksson, M. 1987. Hälsa och social klass. *Socialmedicinsk Tidskrift* 64:33–36

Annu. Rev. Publ. Health 1991. 12:195–207

OCCUPATIONAL HEALTH AND SAFETY REGULATION IN THE COAL MINING INDUSTRY: PUBLIC HEALTH AT THE WORKPLACE

James L. Weeks

Department of Occupational Health and Safety, United Mine Workers of America, Washington, DC 20005

KEY WORDS: coal workers' pneumoconiosis, occupational injuries, surveillance, workers' compensation

INTRODUCTION

One of the principal mechanisms for achieving occupational health and safety goals is government regulation of employers. Thus, the Occupational Safety and Health Administration (OSHA) and its sister agency, the Mine Safety and Health Administration (MSHA), both in the US Department of Labor, were established to set and enforce standards with workplace inspections and issue citations and fines for noncompliance. Administrative law agencies for both OSHA and MSHA adjudicate disputes.

The underground coal mining industry's experience with MSHA is a useful and informative case study in the efficacy of regulation: The coal mining industry is sufficiently large and hazardous, regulatory intervention is substantial, and the distinction between relatively less and more regulated time periods is well defined (before and after the 1969 Coal Mine Health and Safety Act).

Following passage of the Mine Act, the rate of fatal injuries in the coal mining industry decreased significantly (19). Exposure to respirable coal mine dust, the cause of coal workers' pneumoconiosis (CWP) and other

195

0163-7525/91/0501-0195$02.00

chronic lung diseases, also decreased (18). This historical record is consistent with the proposition that regulation works—when standards are set and conscientiously enforced, hazards can be controlled.

In addition to setting and enforcing standards, the Mine Act implemented many basic methods of public health. It provided for technical assistance, research and development, surveillance, worker training and education, and compensation for persons afflicted with CWP and other chronic occupational lung diseases commonly referred to as black lung. It provided for both risk assessment and risk management.

These developments took place in an industry with a high proportion of workers organized into one union, the United Mine Workers of America (UMWA), which has a long history of advocacy of workers' health and safety. Worker involvement in health and safety is a key ingredient in success (7, 20).

In this review, we will describe these elements as a case study of a coherent, multifaceted, and effective strategy for achieving occupational health and safety objectives. Occupational health and safety does not exist in a social or economic vacuum. Indeed, occupational disease and injury occur at the core institution in a society's welfare. This institution is the workplace, in which goods and services and wealth and income are produced. Occupational diseases and injuries do not necessarily share certain pathologies, rather they share this common social context. Thus, in this review we also will examine some measures of economic effects of regulatory intervention in the affairs of the coal mining industry. Because a comprehensive analysis of this important topic is well beyond the scope of this review, we will suggest a few indicators of economic effects.

ELEMENTS OF A PUBLIC HEALTH STRATEGY TO PREVENT OCCUPATIONAL DISEASE AND INJURY

In a high hazard occupational environment, such as an underground coal mine, many injuries result in death or permanent disability; many occupational diseases, such as chronic lung disease and hearing loss, are irreversible. Therefore, primary disease prevention is the principal public health objective. Like other public health objectives, the strategy for achievement has many elements. In the coal mining industry, these elements are regulation, technical assistance, research and development, surveillance, and compensation for persons with occupational lung diseases. Active participants include government officials, health scientists, employers, and miners themselves, both individually and collectively. This list simply represents the standard public health methods. However, their effective application to the workplace is important to document.

Regulation

The Mine Act of 1969 (with amendments in 1977) is similar to the Occupational Safety and Health Act of 1970. The Mine Act authorizes MSHA to write standards, inspect mines, and impose penalties for noncompliance. It also establishes an administrative law court to adjudicate disputes. Employers and employees (referred to as mine operators and miners) have appeal rights to federal courts of appeal. Like OSHA, MSHA can make both civil and criminal charges. There are significant differences between the two, however, with respect to standards, enforcement, and other matters.

Many mining standards are specified by statute in the Mine Act. For example, it contains many prescriptions for mining practice, including detailed requirements for roof support, ventilation, electrical equipment, fire protection, mine maps, use of explosives, hoists, emergency shelters, and communications. It sets a statutory permissible exposure limit on personal exposure to respirable coal mine dust. Because of these statutory requirements, MSHA has less flexibility for rule-making than does OSHA.

The Mining Safety and Health Administration's safety standards also tend to be more specific than performance-type standards. The additional specificity is sometimes thought to inhibit innovation and flexibility (1), but specific standards are easier to implement and to enforce. This specificity also can provide a certain reduncancy that is appropriate for a highly hazardous environment. For example, the mine face, from which coal is cut, is the most dangerous and difficult place to ventilate in a mine. Most often, it is the site from which most methane is liberated and most dust is generated. A pure performance standard, designed to prevent excessive respirable dust and methane, would set limits on their concenctrations and let the operator to find a way to comply with these limits. Current standards, however, not only set limits on concentration, they require regular monitoring by the operator, minimum quantities and velocities of air in the last cross-cut before the face and into the face area, and certain actions when limits are exceeded. (See the appendix for a description of mining methods and terminology.)

Proposed changes in ventilation regulations, however, move away from specification and towards performance standards. For example, proposed changes in ventilation regulations would allow ventilation controls to be farther than the currently required ten feet from the face, provided average exposure to respirable dust was less than the permissible exposure limit. Such a standard is significantly more difficult to enforce. Ten feet can be measured with a ten-foot pole; measurement of respirable dust requires a full shift sample that must be weighed by a laboratory away from the mine site. This procedure usually takes several days. During that time, conditions change as the mining machine advances further into the seam of coal.

In addition, MSHA has significantly greater and different enforcement powers than does OSHA. These differences largely derive from the nature of mining as an activity—it is very hazardous and constantly changing. And, because the work-site is literally carved out of the earth, many hazards are unpredictable. [The agriculture, construction, fishing, and logging industries, which also have high fatal and nonfatal injury rates, share some of these features (3).] Therefore, constant vigilance by MSHA, the mine operator, and miners is essential.

The Mining Safety and Health Administration is required to conduct frequent inspections. Under MSHA, all underground mines must be inspected quarterly, and surface mines must be inspected semiannually. Mine inspections also may be requested by workers or may be initiated by the agency for special reasons, such as modifications in ventilation or roof control plans. For the 75,000 underground and 46,000 surface miners, there were 2745 inspectors in 1989. For the 85.7 million workers under OSHA's jurisdiction, there were 2404 inspectors. Mine inspectors have the authority to shut down all or part of a mine when there is an imminent danger. However, OSHA inspectors must obtain a federal court order to close workplaces where there is an imminent danger, a far more cumbersome procedure. Unlike employers under OSHA's jurisdiction, mine operators must submit plans for mine ventilation and roof control to MSHA before operating a mine. In effect, they must obtain a permit.

Before an individual can work as a miner, the Mine Act also requires mine operators to provide the individual with 40 hours training. Miners also must receive eight hours of refresher training annually. Under OSHA, there is no such requirement.

Technical Assistance

Like OSHA, MSHA can provide technical assistance to mine operators with specific problems. This assistance can be provided either by the Technical Support Division within MSHA or by the US Bureau of Mines in the Department of the Interior. Thus, along with the stick of regulation comes the carrot of technical assistance. Because of a long tradition of research and development in mining health and safety problems, this assistance is practical and of high quality.

Research and Development

The Mine Act also authorizes research into several aspects of mine safety and health. Responsibility is delegated to the Bureau of Mines and to the National Institute for Occupational Safety and Health (NIOSH) for research into safety and health, respectively.

The Bureau of Mines conducts engineering research into several aspects of mine fires and explosions, roof and ground control, ventilation, gas control, dust measurement and control methods, and noise control. This research is typically applied and practical, rather than basic and theoretical. For example, the Bureau has published handbooks on dust control methods and catalogues of noise control technology for use by operators, foremen, and union representatives.

Research of this type complements enforcement efforts. For example, when MSHA identifies a hazard and compels an operator to eliminate it, control techniques from which the operator can choose are often well defined. If the problem has been successfully addressed by research, the question of feasibility is moot.

The National Institute for Occupational Safety and Health conducts epidemiologic, clinical, and industrial hygiene research concerned with a variety of occupational diseases and hazards among miners. This research is used to evaluate standards and controls and to identify health hazards in the industry. Under NIOSH, the largest coal mining-related project is the National Study of Coal Workers' Pneumoconiosis, which was originally intended to be a longitudinal study of CWP in a cohort of miners. Initiated in 1969 and still underway, it should prove useful for evaluating the efficacy of the respirable dust standard.

Surveillance

Surveillance is an essential part of a public health effort to prevent disease and injury. Surveillance for both disease and injury is more extensive under MSHA than OSHA. All operators are required to report quarterly on all injuries, hours worked, tons produced, and certain accidents, such as roof falls, fires, and flooding, regardless of whether injuries occurred. Thus, it is possible to compute crude, mine-specific injury rates and to identify "near-miss" incidents. Operators also must measure and report exposure to respirable dust six times each year for each mining section. In 1989, dust monitoring requirements resulted in approximately 65,000 dust samples for the 1619 underground coal mines. The MSHA inspectors also take dust measurements. These monitoring and reporting requirements make it possible to evaluate performance of the industry as a whole and to focus on those operators with the most significant problems.

Surveillance requirements under OSHA, however, are different. Employers are required to report only fatalities and injuries that result in hospitalizations for five or more persons; other injuries only are required to be recorded, but not reported. Consequently, setting priorities for inspections is difficult. This problem is significant for an agency with already scarce resources and, therefore, compelling reasons to be selective in how they are used (13).

The Mine Act also provides for surveillance of CWP. Mine operators are required to provide underground miners with a chest x-ray when first employed and at regular intervals thereafter. Chest x-ray facilities and film readers are required to be certified by NIOSH, which provides for some degree of quality control on films and their interpretation. There are two purposes to this program: to monitor progress in preventing CWP and to offer miners who have positive films the opportunity to transfer to a less dusty job. Transfer is supposed to occur at no loss of income to the miner; over time, however, the income of transferred miners is less than expected.

This medical removal program was set up earlier than OSHA's program under its lead standard and is different in one important respect. Coal workers' pneumoconiosis is irreversible, and lead poisoning is not, at least not at the blood lead concentration at which the medical removal program becomes an option under OSHA's programs. Therefore, once a miner exercises the opportunity to transfer, he or she becomes known as a person with a positive film for CWP. This knowledge could make future employment in the mining industry difficult. An employer may not wish to accomodate such a miner. And, because under the federal black lung program, payment of black lung awards must be made by the operator who last employed the miner, an employer may not wish to risk liability.

Other problems plague this program, too. For example, the chest x-ray is the only diagnostic tool used to evaluate early lung disease among miners, in spite of its imperfections and a broad legislative mandate. Especially for early diagnosis of CWP, the chest x-ray is an uncertain measure of effects. Other procedures, such as spirometry, also could be used (16). Furthermore, many aspects of the program are delegated to mine operators, which creates the common impression among miners that it is an operator's program. For these and other reasons, participation in the chest x-ray surveillance program and in the transfer program is relatively poor.

Compensation

The Mine Act also created a unique program to compensate miners with black lung, the everyday term applied to chronic occupational lung disease among coal miners. We will not analyze this controversial and expensive program (2, 15), but rather to describe its role as one element in a strategy for prevention. In this regard, its expense alone is a clear object lesson of the consequences of systematic neglect. In the 20 years of its existence, over $20 billion have been paid out in benefits to miners and their families. Current annual payments are $1.2 billion (12).

Compensation for occupational disease rarely provides incentive for prevention, but the black lung program may be an exception. Its expense is visible—it is centralized in one national program—and it is combined with the other elements of prevention described above. In contrast, compensation payments for back injuries among the nation's entire workforce, which is estimated at $16 billion annually, attracts much less attention because these payments are made by state compensation agencies.

Union Involvement

In the coal mining industry, worker and union participation occurs in two arenas: collective bargaining and regulation, which are governed by the National Labor Relations Act and the Mine Act, respectively. The most tangible product of collective bargaining is the contract between the UMWA and Bituminous Coal Operators Association (BCOA): the National Bituminous Coal Wage Agreement. The health and safety provisions were first agreed upon in 1978 and have changed little with subsequent renegotiations.

Provisions of this contract are exceptional in labor-management agreements in the US. They include recognition of a union-elected health and safety committee at each mine, creation of a joint industry-wide BCOA-UMWA committee for the purpose of training mine-site committee members and for other purposes, and recognition of the right of union staff to enter and inspect a mine. Individual workers have a right to refuse work they consider unsafe, and committee members have the right to shut down part of a mine in case of imminent danger. Both of these controversial rights are carefully circumscribed and have been subject of several arbitration decisions. Mine operators are required to notify the union before introducing new technology. Both sides also agree to comply with requirements of the Mine Act, a provision that allows some disputes to be resolved through collective bargaining in addition to whatever remedies exist under the Act.

The International Union also has a large staff, with administrative personnel at the headquarters office; most staff work in field offices. Field representatives have had the same training as OSHA inspectors, a total of 13 weeks in all aspects of mine health and safety at the Mine Safety and Health Academy. The principal responsibility of field representatives is to provide training and technical assistance for the mine committees. The Union has the highest per capita budget for health and safety of any international union in the US (21).

The other arena in which the union operates concerns regulatory affairs of MSHA. Under the Act, miners individually and collectively have many rights concerning both enforcement and standards setting. Miners have the right to request and to participate in inspections, to obtain copies of the records required by the Act, to petition for a modification of a standard, to object to petitions for modification filed by the operator, to comment on mine plans or changes in mine plans, and to participate in all aspects of rule-making. When citations are issued by MSHA against the operator, miners may contest the citation, period of abatement, or the termination of a citation, but they may not contest the size of a penalty or the failure to issue a citation. Miners also may appeal any decision made by the Mine Safety and Health Review Commission, which is an administrative law court established by the Act. Miners also are supposed to be protected from discrimination for having exercised rights under the Act.

Union miners are active participants in both mine inspections and rule-making. For example, when a MSHA inspector visits a union mine, the designated union representative—typically a member of the mine health and safety committee—usually accompanies him or her during the inspection. At nonunion mines, a designated representative of miners is the exception, rather than the rule. At union, compared with nonunion mines, special inspections are requested more often and are more thorough, and MSHA requires abatement more promptly. Although initial fines are about the same at union and nonunion mines, they are less likely to be reduced at union mines (20). Thus, the presence and participation of workers, which is provided for in occupational safety and health policy and necessary for thorough inspections and enforcement, is facilitated by union organization.

The UMWA also participates in rule-making. In recent years, MSHA has undertaken major revisions of nearly all mining regulations. These revisions include proposed changes in roof control, ventilation, electrical regulations, use of explosives, permissible exposure limits, noise, and record-keeping. Currently, MSHA is considering new regulations, which concern the use of diesel-powered equipment in underground mines and hazard communication. The UMWA has been active in all phases of this rule-making. When MSHA held public hearings on proposed changes in ventilation regulations, over 10,000 miners attended and dozens testified. The UMWA also invoked a seldom-used section of the Act by petitioning for an Advisory Committee to assist MSHA with writing rules on the use of diesel-powered equipment in underground mines.

COSTS

What is the cost of this public health intervention? One measure of cost is changes in productivity, or tons of coal produced per hour worked. This measure is independent of cost estimates based on dollars, and data are available from the same source—operator reports to MSHA—as data for computing fatality rates. Figures 1, 2, and 3 illustrate industry-wide annual fatality rates based on hours worked, annual productivity, and the ratio of these two rates, i.e. annual fatality rates based on tons produced, for underground mines for 1950 to 1989. These data suggest not only that the public health plan for mine safety described above has been effective in reducing the risk of fatalities but also that it is associated with a temporary decline in

Annual Fatality Rates (by hours) 1950-1989

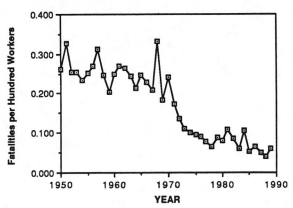

Figure 1   Fatality rates show little change for the period before passage of the Mine Act in 1969 and a sharp consistent decline for the 1970s, following passage of the Act. For the 1980s, the rate of decline is less.

productivity. These trends are not apparent when fatalities rates are based on tons produced.

At present, there are other indicators that suggest that productivity and risk of nonfatal injury are positively related. A National Research Council investigated the distinction between safe and unsafe mines. The Council concluded in part that mines with lower injury rates also had higher productivity (4). A similar conclusion was reached in a study contracted by the Bureau of

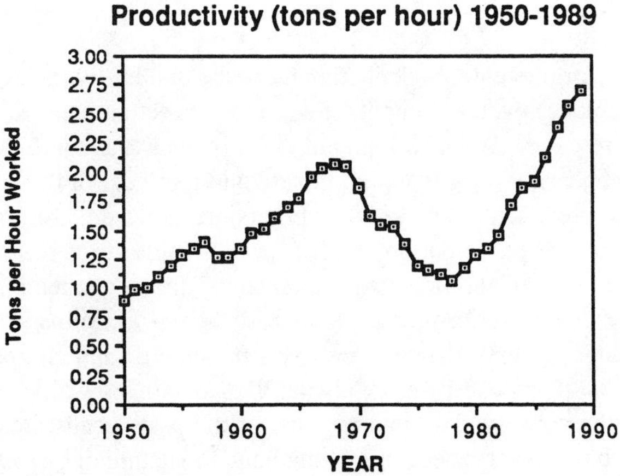

Productivity (tons per hour) 1950-1989

Figure 2   Productivity increased for the period before 1970, declined for a decade, then increased to its present, higher level.

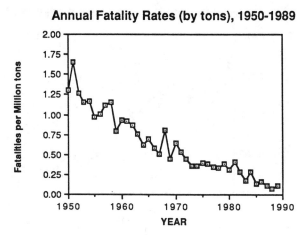

Figure 3   Fatalities based on tons produced shows a consistent decline over this time period.

Mines (6). These conclusions suggest that safety practices promoted by the Mine Act are consistent with management practices that promote increased productivity.

Trends in exposure to respirable dust differ among various mining methods. With continuous mining methods, the trend in dust exposure is consistently down while productivity is up (8, 9). With longwall methods, the industry-wide trend also shows decreasing exposure. However, increases in productivity in individual mines appear to be associated with increases in exposure to respirable dust (10, 17).

SUMMARY

The strategy for preventing occupational disease and injury in the coal mining industry employs several elements. Standards are set and enforced; technical assistance, research, and development are provided; and surveillance is conducted. Compensation for black lung is a vivid reminder of the consequences of failure to prevent disease. And, workers are represented by a union that encourages active participation in all aspects of this strategy.

There are significant problems in each of these elements. Regulatory reform threatens to weaken many standards, there is a decline in government research budgets, surveillance is not well monitored, and compensation for black lung is significantly more difficult to obtain now than in the past. Moreover, the conservative governments of the past decade are not friendly towards unions. Nevertheless, the fundamental structure of disease and injury prevention remains intact and, more importantly, it has a historical record of success.

The Mine Safety and Health Act provided for a wide array of basic public health measures to prevent occupational disease and injury in the mining industry. These measures have been effective in reducing both risk of fatal injury and exposure to respirable coal mine dust. They are also associated with temporary declines in productivity. In recent years, however, productivity has increased, while risk of fatal injury and exposure to respirable dust have declined. At individual mines, productivity and lower injury rates appear to rise and fall together, and increases in productivity with longwall mining methods appear to be associated with increases in exposure to respirable dust.

These trends are not inconsistent with similar trends following implementation of regulations by OSHA. When OSHA promulgated regulations to control exposure to vinyl chloride monomer, enforcement of the standard promoted significant efficiencies in vinyl chloride production (5). Similarly, when OSHA promulgated its standard regulating exposure to cotton dust, this effort provoked modernization in the cotton textile industry (14).

It is not inevitable that occupational health and safety regulations are associated with negative economic performance. On the contrary, in some instances, public health on the job and productivity are complementary.

ACKNOWLEDGEMENT

The author wishes to acknowledge the useful criticisms and comments of Ruth Ruttenberg.

APPENDIX: Coal Mining Technology (11)

The two most common underground mining methods in use today are continuous mining and longwall mining. Continuous mining accounts for most production and is more common, but its proportion of production is declining. Longwall mining, on the other hand, is more productive (about 2.62 tons per hours worked compared with 2.48 tons per hour for continuous mining) and more efficient (9). The most productive mines employ both methods; continuous mining machines are used to develop longwall sections. In a large mine, as many as 12 continuous mining machines and two to three longwall machines may operate at the same time in separate sections of the mine. The trend is to use more moderate-sized mines with one large longwall section and three to five continuous mining sections.

The continuous mining machine cuts coal from the face with a large rotating drum studded with picks. As it is cut from the face, coal falls and is gathered into a conveyor that transports it to the tail-end of the machine. From there, it is loaded to a shuttle car or conveyor belt.

Continuous mining was a significant advance over conventional mining, which depended on explosives to loosen coal from the face. With continuous mining, hazards of blasting were eliminated, there were fewer machines and less movement of machines, and productivity increased. However, basic mine design—room and pillar mining—was unchanged. Rooms are areas from which coal has been extracted.

Pillars, which are blocks of coal left in place to support the roof, are typically 40 ft by 40 ft. Deeper mines require larger pillars because of the increased load. Roof support also is provided by roof bolts, which anchor and stabilize rock strata above the rooms. Less commonly, roof support is provided by timbers, which may be laid horizontally to construct a crib or installed vertically as posts. Rows of pillars form entries whose purpose is to allow transportation of miners, materials, and coal; to provide escapeways in event of emergency; and to facilitate mine ventilation. Entries are usually designated as intakes or returns. These designations correspond to whether they are an intake for fresh air or a return for air contaminated with dust and methane. Several entries usually make up a mine section in which the continuous mining machine, roof bolter, shuttle cars, and other machinery operate. The mine face, from which coal is extracted, is at the end of each entry.

Many problems of productivity, safety, and health are inherent in room and pillar mining. Pillars are blocks of coal that often were left behind (because removing them posed considerable danger of roof falls) when the limits of a coal deposit were reached. Furthermore, even with pillars, bolts, and timbers, roof falls are common and are the leading cause of fatal mine injuries. And, for more than half the time of a workshift, continuous mining machines are not cutting coal; they must move from one face to another or they must wait for a shuttle car to return from the conveyor belt to receive another load.

Longwall mining solves many of these problems and is a more fundamental change in mine design. It eliminates shuttle cars and, at the longwall face, it eliminates pillars and permanent roof supports. It is more efficient at removing coal because pillars need not be left behind. It also is more productive. Machinery need not move as frequently from one place to another, and there is no need to wait for a shuttle car. In place of the 20-ft wide face from which continuous miners extract coal, the average width of a longwall face is 600 ft. Some faces extend up to 1000 ft.

Unlike a continuous mining machine, which cuts as it advances into the coal, the longwall mining machine moves from one end of the face to the other. It cuts coal to a depth of about 36 in at a time and slowly advances into the block of coal. The mine roof is temporarily supported by large hydraulic jacks and shields that advance with the mining machine, which allows the roof to fall as the machine, jacks, and shields advance into the block of coal. Dust exposure on longwall sections is a significant problem. Average dust exposure is twice that found on continuous mining sections. Thus, with increased productivity, there is improved roof support (but only on the section) and much more dust exposure.

Literature Cited

1. Ashford, N. A., Ayers, C., Stone, R. F. 1985. Using regulation to change the market for innovation. *Harv. Environ. Law Rev.* 9:419–66
2. Barth, P. S. 1987. *The Tragedy of Black Lung. Federal Compensation for Occupational Disease.* Kalamazoo, Mich: Upjohn Inst. Employ. Res. 292 pp.
3. Bell, C. A., Stout, N. A., Bender, T. R., Conroy, C. S., Crouse, W. E., Myers, J. R. 1990. Fatal Occupational Injuries in the United States, 1980 through 1985. *J. Am. Med. Assoc.* 263:3047–50
4. Comm. Undergr. Coal Mine Saf., Natl. Res. Counc. 1982. *Toward Safer Underground Coal Mines.* Washington, DC: Natl. Acad. Press
5. Dirks-Mason, S. 1979. *The Effects of the OSHA Vinyl Chloride Standard on the Vinyl Chloride Industry.* Prepared for OSHA Policy Office, 15 pp.
6. Gaertner, G. H., Newman, P. D., Perry, M. S., Fisher, G. P., Whitehead, K. 1987. *Determining The Effects of Management Practices on Coal Miners' Safety.* Res. Contract Rep. Washington, DC: US Bur. Mines. 348 pp.
7. Goldsmith, F., Kerr, L. E. 1983. Worker participation in job safety and health. *J. Public Health Policy* 4:447–66
8. Jankowski, R. A., Hake, J. 1989. Dust sources and Controls for High Production Longwall Faces. *Proc. Longwall USA Conf.* Pittsburgh, June 19–22, p. 118–32
9. Jayraman, N. I., Jankowsky, R., Stritzel, D. 1987. Improving health, safety, and productivity through the use of machine mounted scrubbers. *Proc. Ill. Min. Inst.* 23:62–75
10. Lewis, B. C. 1989. *Longwall mining: Future concerns technology must address.* Presented at Bur. Mines Conf., Pittsburgh
11. Marovelli, R. L., Karnak, J. M. 1982. *The mechanization of mining.* Sci. Am. 252(Sept):30–42
12. Nase, J. P. 1988–1989. *The surprising cost of benefits: The legislative history of the Federal Black Lung Benefits Program. J. Miner. Law Policy* 4:277–319
13. Pollack, E. S., Keimig, D. G., eds. 1987. Panel Occup. Saf. Health Stat. *Counting Injuries and Illnesses in the Workplace: Proposals for a Better System.* Washington, DC: Natl. Acad. Press
14. Ruttenberg, R. 1983. *Compliance with the OSHA Cotton Dust Rule—The Role of Productivity Improving Technology.* Final Rep. Off. Technol. Assess., US Congr.
15. Smith, B. E. 1987. *Digging Our Own Graves: Coal Miners and the Struggle over Black Lung Disease.* Philadelphia: Temple Univ. Press. 270 pp.
16. Speiler, E. 1989. *Can coal miners escape black lung? An analysis of the coal miner job transfer program and its implications for occupational medical removal protection programs. W. Va. Law Rev.* 91:775–816
17. Webster, J. B., Chiaretta, C. W., Behling, J. 1990. *Dust control in high productivity mines.* Presented at Ann. Meet. Soc. Mining Metal. Explor. Salt Lake City
18. Weeks, J. L. 1989. *Is regulation effective? A case study of underground coal mining.* Ann. NY Acad. Sci. 572:189–99
19. Weeks, J. L., Fox, M. B. 1983. *Fatality rates and regulatory policies in bituminous coal mining,* United States, 1959–1981. *Am. J. Public Health* 73:1278–80
20. Weil, D. 1987. *Government and labor at the workplace: The role of labor unions in the implementation of federal safety and health policy.* PhD dis. Harv. Univ. 390 pp.
21. Wolfe, S. M., Abrams, L. 1983. *Fourteen Union Occupational Safety and Health Programs.* Washington, DC: Public Citiz. Health Res. Group 19 pp.

Annu. Rev. Publ. Health. 1991. 12:209–34

SMOKING CONTROL AT THE WORKPLACE

Johnathan E. Fielding

Departments of Public Health and Pediatrics, University of California, Los Angeles, California 90024; Johnson & Johnson Health Management, Santa Monica, California 90404

KEY WORDS: health promotion, smoking policies, smoking cessation, worksite health promotion, smoking regulation

---

"In business corridors . . . cigarettes are no longer a symbol of strength, machismo and style, and smoky rooms, no longer synonymous with serious business. Executives who smoke these days tend to feel weak, embarrassed and ashamed. Smoking makes them feel less in control. It can shake their self-confidence" (29).

Rationale for Smoking Control Programs at the Worksite

Until recently, employers supported restrictions or bans on smoking primarily to prevent fires, protect equipment, or avoid product contamination (81). In a few instances, restrictions or bans were imposed because of demonstrated synergy between smoking and a worksite exposure to a product that increased risk of lung cancer, such as asbestos. That rationale was used by Johns-Manville Company when, in 1977, smoking was banned and smokers were no longer hired (22, 26). Based on comparable patterns of demonstrated synergy, a similar rationale could also apply to workers exposed to ionizing radiation and some occupational chemicals (68). In 1979, the National Institute for Occupational Safety and Health described the interaction of cigarette smoke with numerous occupational exposures and summarized six mechanisms by which these interactions occur (9).

In recent years, protection of employee health through reduction of expo-

209

0163-7525/91/0501-0209$02.00

sure to second-hand smoke has become a common justification for smoking restrictions. Stimulating these actions is the growing epidemiologic data base, which shows that environmental smoke exposure can have adverse health effects (30). In 1986, landmark reports by the Surgeon General and by the National Academy of Sciences independently concluded that exposure to environmental tobacco smoke (ETS) had adverse health effects on healthy adults and children (56, 81). The publication of these studies, along with the attendant publicity, has contributed to the creation of working environments that are conducive to health through a variety of policies and programs. Employers have cited their desire to create such an atmosphere as a principal reason to discourage smoking.

The Surgeon General's report concluded that, although the risks of passive smoking were considerably less than those of active smoking, the number of persons injured by involuntary smoking was much larger than the number injured by other environmental agents already under regulation to limit exposure (81). Few studies have focused exclusively on the duration and dose of exposure to sidestream smoke at the worksite. In one population study of 37,881 nonsmokers and former smokers, 63% of nonsmokers reported some daily exposure from a variety of sources, including homes and workplaces. Of this group, 35% reported more than ten hours per week of exposure, and 16% reported more than 40 hours per week (35). Other studies have documented measurable increases in work area concentrations of carbon monoxide, nitrogen dioxide, and respirable-sized particulates when these are occupied by smokers, and in urinary cotinine concentrations of nonsmokers who work with smokers (24, 54, 92).

Most of the published studies that assess possible effects of passive smoking have used spousal smoking as the primary independent variable. Although worksite exposure has sometimes been queried, few studies have provided results that permit assigning an independent risk contribution from this source.

Improved methods of determining exposure will permit much more accurate assessments of involuntary smoking dose from the worksite and other settings (51, 75). Cotinine is increasingly accepted as the short-term marker of choice because of its relatively long half-life (20 hours), lack of susceptibility to fluctuations during smoke exposure, and suitability for noninvasive ascertainment in urine and saliva (56, 81). Self-reported ETS exposure correlates well with urinary cotinine levels. For example, in one group of municipal workers, mean urinary cotinine levels were more than twice as high in both men and women nonsmokers who reported they lived with a smoker than were levels in respondents who denied exposure. Although ETS exposure in the home was the greatest contributor to increased cotinine levels in exposed nonsmokers, individuals exposed only at work had significant cotinine elevations; the reported degree of exposure agreed well with mean urinary cotinine levels (39). The recent development of small, passive nicotine monitors and the validation of questionnaires and diaries to assess cumulative ETS exposure against chemical assays will greatly improve the quality of studies that link various patterns of ETS exposure and health problems (23, 39).

To date, the strongest evidence for adverse effects of involuntary smoking is on the rate of lung cancer, with a weighted average relative-risk value of 1.34 for all studies of passive smoking and lung cancer through 1986 (95% confidence interval, 1.18 to 1.53) (56, 88). Although some studies that show positive relationship between involuntary smoking and lung cancer have reported a dose response relationship, most have important methodological limitations that preclude firm conclusions (87, 94). Estimates of relative risks translate to 2500–8400 annual lung cancer deaths in the United States attributable to ETS (56). As the studies associating ETS with lung cancer risk primarily rely on spousal exposure, the contribution of possible exposure at the worksite to the increased lung cancer rate is indeterminate.

Evidence of the effect of passive smoking on other diseases of the respiratory tract in adults is equivocal (32). However, a well-designed, 20-year study, which investigated passive smoke exposure at the workplace, found that exposed nonsmokers had significant reductions in forced midexpiratory flow (14%) and FEV1 (forced expiratory volume in one second) (6%), as compared with nonsmokers not exposed to environmental tobacco smoke in the workplace ($P < 0.005$) (93). This reduction in air flow in midexpiration is comparable with that observed in light smokers, who smoke one to ten cigarettes per day. However, other unmeasured worksite exposures may complicate the interpretation of risk of chronic obstructive lung disease for both smokers and nonsmokers.

Possible relationships between passive smoking and acquired cardiovascular diseases remain conjectural, absent definitive studies. Although several studies have shown a significant association between exposure to ETS and increased risk of cardiovascular disease, no firm conclusion of a causal relationship is yet justifiable (36, 56, 72).

The increased evidence about adverse effects of ETS adds weight and urgency to addressing employee complaints about workplace exposure. Such complaints can be a potent spur to employers' adoption of restrictive smoking policies.

In most surveys of employee smoking attitudes, 80% or more of employees support smoking restrictions at the workplace (6, 27, 66). Results of worksite or employer surveys of smoking attitudes agree with results of surveys of the American public. In 1983, for example, a nationwide survey by the Gallup Organization, sponsored by the American Lung Association, reported that, when asked whether there should be restrictions on smoking at the workplace,

75% of smokers and 87% of nonsmokers favored either designated areas or a total prohibition (2).

The recent accumulation of evidence on the adverse effects of ETS has focused attention on the risk to nonsmoking employees. Smokers, meanwhile, have been the target of employers' smoking control efforts, initiated in the hope of improving employee health and reducing health-related employer costs.

A 1985 Office of Technology Assessment study estimated smoking-related lost productivity cost $27–$61 billion yearly, of which approximately 90% was for those below age 65 (61). In the same year, the Department of Health and Human Services estimated that the total direct health care costs associated with smoking were $34 billion per year (85).

A significant portion of the health care and productivity costs attendant upon smoking is borne by employers. Several studies have reported higher morbidity, mortality, and health benefit costs for smoking employees compared with nonsmokers. For example, in a three-year study of 7863 full-time refinery and petrochemical plant workers, diseases of the circulatory system, respiratory system, and all other morbidity combined were significantly associated with current and previous cigarette smoking by both sexes. In addition, current men smokers had a motor vehicle accident rate 75% greater than nonsmokers ($P < .05$). Both men and women smokers had a frequency of nonmotor vehicle accidents more than 60% higher ($p < .05$) than nonsmokers (77). Whether the relationship between smoking and higher risk of trauma is causal has not been well explored. Control Data Corporation reported that when employees were trichotomized into risk categories based on smoking behavior, the excess claims cost of the high-risk group over the low-risk group was 118% (12). The excess smoking-related health care costs of dependents are also largely borne by employers, and these may equal or exceed the excess costs for smoking employees.

Absenteeism also tends to be more prevalent among smoking employees than among nonsmokers. In both intervention and control worksites used in conjunction with an economic evaluation of the Johnson & Johnson LIVE FOR LIFE® Program, mean sick time per year for smokers was approximately 15 hours (>40%) greater than that for nonsmokers; this pattern was persistent over a three-year period (46). In the Shell Oil Company study cited above, over a three-year period, current women smokers had 2.5 times more days of absence than nonsmokers (31.3 vs 11.7). Men smokers had 40% more days of absence than their nonsmoking coworkers (22.3 days vs 15.9) (77).

In addition, exposure to ETS by both employees and nonemployees covered by an employer-sponsored health benefit plan may lead to employer costs attributable to passive smoking. Environmental tobacco smoke exposure of the fetus due to maternal smoking has been strongly associated with a reduction in average birth weight, which in turn is consistently associated with increased neonatal and infant mortality (72). However, it is not known if exposure to ETS by nonsmoking pregnant women affects birth weight or health outcomes for the fetus and infant.

Parental smoking consistently has been shown to have an adverse effect on the incidence and/or severity of many acute respiratory illnesses, including tracheitis, bronchitis, bronchiolitis, and pneumonia. Environmental tobacco smoke exposure also increases the risk of middle-ear effusions and middle-ear infections in young children (32).

Costs of ventilation are much higher in buildings in which smoking is widely permitted. A 30% prevalence rate for smoking, with an average consumption of 30 cigarettes per day, increases the ventilation rate requirement by at least 2.5-fold (42). Smoking also is reported to increase the costs of cleaning, maintenance, and fire insurance in buildings (28).

Finally, the presence of laws or regulations that require or encourage smoking policies can lead to the adoption or extension of smoking policies at worksites. As of July 1988, 20 state jurisdictions and the District of Columbia had enacted legislation to restrict smoking in the workplace. Restrictions vary widely and, in some states, apply only to public employers. Ten states had prohibited or restricted smoking to designated areas in all enclosed or indoor areas, including private worksites. Of the 20 largest metropolitan areas in the United States, as of July 1988, nine had required that a smoking policy be in effect at private worksites. Of these nine, three required that preference be given to nonsmokers, and three prohibited retaliation against nonsmokers who insisted that the policy be enforced. Most laws pertaining to smoking at private worksites refer to public areas (hallways, stairways, elevators); areas in which large groups of people gather (auditoria, classrooms, conference and meeting rooms); and, less frequently, cafeterias and lunchrooms. In six of the 20 largest municipalities, a nonsmoking area was required. Four of the six required special ventilation, partitions, or other separation of smokers and nonsmokers (85).

As of September 1989, of the largest 397 municipalities, 297 had some type of policy to restrict smoking at the workplace. All but 13 of the 297 had policies that covered both public and private offices. However, the policies commonly leave employers considerable latitude to decide on the specifics of the policy. For example, policies of most municipalities do not permit employees to decide if an area is to be nonsmoking and do not usually provide employees who protest ETS with protection from retaliation (84).

Adoption of a formal smoking policy may reduce the likelihood of a legal action brought against the employer by nonsmoking employees concerned about exposure to ETS. However, formal smoking policies bring the potential of suit by employees or unions on the grounds that such policies constitute infringement of constitutional rights or unfair labor practices.

Reported rationales for establishing smoking policies reflect reasons for employer sponsorship of a combination of smoking control activities. In general, concern about the health effects of environmental exposure to cigarette smoke, the need to respond to employee complaints, and the increasing number of regulations that require smoking policies appear to be the primary factors that are driving smoking policies. In the 1985 National Worksite Health Promotion Survey, in response to a forced-choice question on the primary purpose of installation of a smoking policy, 39% of 372 worksites were protecting nonsmokers, 32% complying with a regulation, 12% protecting equipment, and 7% protecting high-risk employees (31).

In 1987, a survey was mailed randomly to 2132 members of the American Society for Personnel Administrators (response rate, 29%). Multiple reasons were cited for adopting a smoking policy: concern for employees' health/comfort (71%), complaints from employees (54%), state or local law (39%), order by top executive (17%), insurance cost concerns (10%), absenteeism concerns (10%), productivity concerns (8%), and other (10%) (17).

In the June 1990 Environmental Protection Agency Draft Report, ETS was classified as a Group A (known human) carcinogen, and 3800 lung cancer deaths among nonsmokers (never smokers and former smokers) a year were attributed to passive smoking. This report has validated the dangers of second-hand smoke. It recommended that organizations eliminate involuntary exposure to ETS at work wherever possible (87). This report and the related recommendations (86) could accelerate the adoption by worksites of voluntary nonsmoking policies.

Employee Smoking Behavior

Although smoking is common among employed populations, unemployed men and women are substantially more likely to be smokers. Based on data from a 1985 Current Population Survey, white employed men and women had current smoking rates of 34% and 29%, versus 45% and 36% for their unemployed counterparts. Among blacks, the same phenomenon was observed, with comparable differential smoking rates of 9% among men (50% of unemployed versus 41% of employed), but a high 18% difference among women (46% of unemployed versus 28% of employed) (89).

Large differences exist in the frequency of smoking among different groups of employees. Smoking prevalence is higher among blue-collar and service workers and among minorities. In 1985, 40% of male blue-collar workers and 40% of male service workers smoked, compared with 33% of male white-collar workers. The subgroup of professional and technical workers within the white-collar category had a prevalence rate of only 26% (83).

Analysis of data from the 1978–1980 National Health Interview Survey revealed that the types of occupations and industries with the highest smoking prevalence were fisheries (63% current smokers), tobacco (54%), general contractors (51%), water transportation (50%), trucking and warehousing (50%), coal mining (49%), and taxis and buses (47%), whereas retail was at 30%, and banking at 29%. The lowest five were education services (25%), private households (25%), security investigations (25%), credit agencies (24%), and metal mining (21%) (10).

Such broad occupational categories as managers, administrators, or secretaries do not define smoking prevalence as well as the industries in which those positions are held. For example, among managers the overall percentage of current smokers was 36%, but 57% in trucking and warehousing, 36% in wholesale trade, and 26% in restaurants. Likewise, sales clerks had an average prevalence of 30%, with a wide range from 58% in motor vehicle dealers to 27% in lumber and building trades (10).

A significantly lower percentage of women in blue-collar occupational groups were current smokers than were their male counterparts; in other occupational groups, there were no significant sex differences for smoking behavior. Overall, female smoking rates were 38% for blue-collar workers and 32% for white-collar workers.

Minority status influences smoking prevalence. Blacks in professional or technical occupations had a higher percentage of smokers than whites (38% vs 25%) (10). However, in all occupational groups, there are proportionately fewer heavy smokers among the currently smoking blacks (10).

Similar patterns are seen in at least some other industrialized countries. In Britain, a clear gradient is seen by social class, with prevalence rates increasing from 17% among male professionals to 30% of managers, 40% of skilled manual workers, and 49% of unskilled manual workers (60).

Workers exposed to occupational hazards are more likely to smoke than other workers, despite known synergistic effects of smoking and some of these exposures on specific organ systems (80). In a 1982 American Cancer Society study, men exposed to such occupational exposures as asbestos, chemicals or coal tar pitch, coal or stone dust, dyes, formaldehyde, textile fibers, or ionizing radiation were, in nine of ten categories, more likely to be current smokers than nonexposed workers. Women with these exposures, however, did not exhibit increased smoking prevalence, compared with the nonexposed, except for those with asbestos exposure (73). In summary, although overall smoking prevalence in the US has declined, a substantial minority of adults in the workforce continues to smoke.

Frequency of Worksite Smoking Control Activities

Approaches to smoking control at the worksite can be divided into legalistic mechanisms, educational activities, and economic incentives (91). Often a worksite utilizes two or all three approaches. In conjunction with issuing a more restrictive smoking policy, employers usually offer smoking cessation activities to employees. Economic incentives often are provided for participating in smoking cessation activities or in quitting smoking. To minimize smoking over time, the same employer may institute a differential on health insurance premiums and life insurance premiums based on smoking status. Some smoking control activities, particularly educational efforts, often are undertaken as part of comprehensive employer-sponsored programs.

Smoking control efforts by employers have been surveyed by many organizations. Most surveys have been of a selected, nonrandom sample of employers, often the members of a particular trade or membership organization, and often have been characterized by low response rates. In 1978, The Washington Business Group on Health surveyed its nearly 200 member companies, all part of the *Fortune* 500, and found that of respondents, 56% reported sponsoring some kind of "smoking cessation program." Most of these programs were offered only once or very occasionally, were usually left to the discretion of local management, most commonly were not conducted on company time, and were not always financially supported by the employer (90). However, a 1979 survey by the National Interagency Council on Smoking and Health, which used a random sample of 3000 businesses (response rate 29%), found that only 15% offered assistance in smoking cessation (20). This lower prevalence is in agreement with 14% rate found in a 1981 Bureau of National Affairs (BNA) survey of 313 businesses (15).

The most comprehensive survey of smoking control efforts at the workplace was the 1985 National Survey of Worksite Health Promotion Activities, which queried a random sample of worksites with 50 or more employees nationwide about nine health promotion activities, including smoking control (33). Of the 1358 worksites with completed surveys (response rate 84%), smoking control activities, including smoking policies, were found at 36%. The prevalence of smoking control, the most common of the health promotion activities surveyed, varied from 30% in the South to 44% in the West. Frequency varied directly with worksite size, from 30% in worksites with fewer than 100 employees to 58% in worksites with more than 750 employees. Among industry types, frequencies varied from 19% in other (mining, fishing, construction) to 42% in services (31).

At worksites with smoking control activities, other health promotion activities offered were health risk assessment (45%), exercise and fitness (39%), stress management (46%), and weight control (31%) (31). Table 1 displays the frequency of different types of smoking control activities at worksites with at least one such activity. These worksites reported an average of 2.5 types of smoking control activities: 0.7 activities involving employee participation and 1.8 other activities (31).

Smoking Policies

The nature of the debate over smoking policies at the worksite has changed substantially over the past decade. In the early 1980s, the question for employers was whether to implement a smoking policy. As recently as 1984, a review of corporate smoking policies stated that "Employers have . . . exhibited understandable ambivalence toward the smoking issues" (90). In that review, Walsh cited two criticisms leveled at companies that adopted such policies. One was the claim that smoking policies violated the rights of smokers and raised the specter of paternalism. The other common claim was that vigorous antismoking efforts by employers blamed the victim. A decade later, such criticisms are rarely reported. The question has turned from should a policy be considered to which restrictive policy should be adopted, what is the best process for adoption, and how far should the policy go. Total worksite bans on smoking, rare even five years ago, are increasingly common, particularly in health care institutions and in some industries, such as telecommunications.

Smoking policies have become common in work environments (48). In 1984, the Tobacco Institute sponsored a survey of the *Fortune* 1000 service and industrial companies and *Inc.* magazine's 100 fastest growing companies. Of the 40% responding, 26% reported a formal smoking policy (43). In the 1985 National Survey of Worksite Health Promotion Activities, 27% of worksites reported a formal smoking policy (31). Two BNA surveys of members of the American Society of Personnel Administrators, in 1986 and 1987, suggest accelerated growth of formal smoking policies, from 36% of respondents in 1986 to 54% in 1987 (16, 17). In the 1987 BNA Survey (the most recent available), 85% of those companies reporting smoking policies had adopted them in 1985, 1986, or 1987, which suggests a very rapid recent rise in frequency.

The largest employer in the United States, the federal government, took a leadership role in 1987 by limiting smoking to specially designated areas in the 6800 buildings controlled by the General Services Administration in which 890,000 persons work (17). Smoking is prohibited in auditoria, classrooms, conference rooms, elevators, medical care facilities, libraries, and hazardous areas. Smoking also is banned in general office spaces, except those designated for smoking and configured to protect nonsmokers from involuntary exposure to smoke.

Under orders from the Secretary of Defense, each branch of the Armed Forces has initiated action to discourage smoking. Common features include prohibition of smoking in auditoria, conference rooms, classrooms, elevators, buses, and vans. Smoking is not permitted in common work areas shared by smokers and nonsmokers unless adequate space and ventilation are available to provide nonsmokers with a healthy environment (78).

Table 1 National survey of worksite health promotion activity, 1985; percentage of smoking control activity at worksites with any smoking control activity (95% confidence interval)

	Participatory					Nonparticipatory		
	Any participatory activity	Individual counseling	Group class/ workshops	Follow-up support[b]	Special Events	Policy	Information	Self help material
Worksites with any smoking control activty	38.3 (32.9-43.7)	15.1 (11.1-19.1)	19.9 (16.3-23.5)	43.2 (34.2-52.2)	23.7 (18.9-28.5)	76.5 (71.7-81.3)	54.3 (48.7-59.9)	49.6 (44.4-54.8)
Worksite Size[a]								
<100 n=121	22.6 (12.8-32.4)	7.1 (1.3-12.9)	5.5 (0.9-10.1)	34.4 (17.6-51.2)	13.3 (5.7-20.9)	85.6 (77.4-91.8)	40.4 (30.4-50.4)	36.9 (27.1-46.7)
100-249 n=207	39.5 (32.2-46.9)	14.0 (8.2-19.8)	22.1 (15.7-28.5)	40.3 (23.3-57.3)	26.0 (19.2-32.8)	76.2 (68.8-83.6)	58.9 (50.9-66.9)	51.7 (42.7-60.7)
250-749 n=113	46.1 (35.5-56.7)	19.2 (11.0-27.4)	29.3 (20.1-38.5)	41.6 (24.0-59.2)	26.9 (17.5-36.3)	63.8 (54.0-73.6)	62.0 (51.6-72.4)	59.4 (48.8-70.0)
750+ n=70	85.9 (75.1-96.7)	44.2 (29.4-59.0)	57.8 (43.4-72.2)	54.1 (38.7-69.5)	53.5 (38.7-68.3)	62.3 (48.3-76.3)	84.9 (73.9-95.9)	80.5 (68.5-92.5)
Region[a]								
Northeast n=122	38.6 (30.0-47.2)	11.4 (6.6-16.2)	17.8 (10.4-25.2)	45.2 (27.2-63.2)	23.2 (13.4-33.0)	73.6 (63.6-83.6)	50.3 (38.7-61.9)	49.1 (38.1-60.1)
North Central n=139	43.1 (35.7-50.5)	19.2 (8.6-29.8)	21.4 (14.4-28.4)	46.4 (33.0-59.8)	20.1 (13.9-26.3)	81.5 (75.3-87.7)	58.3 (48.1-68.5)	52.2 (42.6-61.8)
South n=152	33.6 (24.0-43.2)	14.8 (9.6-20.0)	19.7 (14.1-25.3)	52.7 (37.7-67.7)	23.6 (16.0-31.2)	75.3 (66.5-84.1)	60.7 (50.5-70.9)	54.8 (44.6-65.0)
West n=98	38.3 (22.5-54.1)	14.6 (6.0-23.2)	20.8 (9.4-32.2)	27.8 (9.3-45.8)	28.3 (14.9-41.7)	75.5 (64.7-86.3)	46.1 (32.2-59.9)	40.9 (30.1-51.7)

Industry type[a]									
Manufacturing (MAN) n=154	25.7 (19.1-32.3)	11.4 (6.2-16.6)	16.4 (10.8-22.0)	45.2 (27.2-63.2)	14.5 (9.5-19.5)		78.7 (72.5-84.9)	46.8 (38.0-55.6)	48.2 (3.4-57.0)
Wholesale/Retail (WR) n=60	31.2 (14.4-48.0)	11.5 (0-23.9)	8.8 (0-17.8)	26.0 (1.8-50.2)	20.4 (6.6-34.2)		74.6 (60.8-88.4)	39.1 (23.3-54.9)	41.7 (27.7-55.7)
Utility/transportation/communication (UTC) n=15	61.8 (29.6-94.0)	44.7 (16.1-73.3)	50.5 (20.5-80.5)	27.9 (0.7-55.1)	22.7 (1.1-44.3)		65.8 (40.0-91.6)	67.2 (34.0-100)	55.9 (24.7-87.1)
Financial/real estate/insurance (FRI) n=36	66.6 (52.2-81.0)	17.6 (0-36.6)	42.6 (19.4-65.8)	57.4 (27.6-87.2)	51.7 (35.7-67.7)		56.8 (39.4-74.2)	87.6 (76.8-98.4)	72.4 (55.8-89.0)
Services (SER) n=226	44.6 (35.8-53.4)	16.3 (10.7-21.9)	21.7 (16.1-27.3)	43.1 (29.3-56.9)	28.5 (20.7-36.3)		81.8 (75.4-88.2)	58.5 (49.9-67.1)	48.9 (40.5-57.3)
Other (OTH) n=20	32.3 (11.1-51.5)	21.8 (4.4-39.2)	18.8 (4.8-32.8)	63.3 (32.1-94.5)	9.5 (0-20.7)		42.8 (16.0-69.6)	64.6 (38.2-91.0)	62.2 (34.2-90.2)

[a] percent of worksites with smoking control activity by level of stratifying variable.
[b] percent of worksites with either individual counseling or group/workshop activity.

Source: Fielding, 1990, Prev. Med. In press.

Another perspective on the extent of smoking policies comes from the 1986 Adult Use of Tobacco Survey, a national probability sample of over 13,000 adults. Of employed adults, 45% reported some restrictions on smoking at their workplace, including 3% who reported that smoking was banned (21, 83).

Restrictiveness of Smoking Policies

Smoking policies range from limited restrictions to a total smoking ban at the worksite. A gradient of restrictiveness might include the following progression:

1. Nonsmoking sections in cafeteria and auditoria.
2. Nonsmoking in conference rooms and bathrooms.
3. Nonsmoking in shared work areas.
4. No smoking in front of customers.
5. Smoking only in private offices.
6. Separation of work areas for smokers and nonsmokers.
7. Smoking only allowed in limited designated areas.
8. No smoking indoors.
9. No smoking on employer premises.
10. No smoking in company vehicles.
11. No smoking at any company function.

In general, employers initially developed policies to accomodate the competing interests of the smokers and nonsmokers. Most policies prohibit smoking in common areas, such as hallways, rest rooms, conference rooms, visitor areas, and auditoria (18, 38); however, there is considerable momentum to increase the stringency of smoking policies, and virtually all reported policy changes are in this direction. For example, between the 1986 and 1987 BNA surveys, the percentage of respondent firms that banned smoking in all open work areas increased from 41% to 51%. During this same period, the percentage of companies with policies that totally banned smoking in cafeterias and eating areas increased from 14% to 27%, in private offices from 21% to 33%, in conference and meeting rooms from 63% to 73%, and in customer/visitor areas from 14% to 27% (16, 17) (Figure 1). Prohibiting smoking in more areas and giving primacy to nonsmokers in determining when and where smoking will be permitted reflect an important shift to nonsmoking as normative behavior (83). What started out as smoking policies are now better characterized as nonsmoking policies.

Complete smoking bans are becoming more common. In the 1986 BNA survey, 6% of respondent firms with policies banned smoking in all company buildings; the comparable percentage in the 1987 survey was 12%. In a 1989

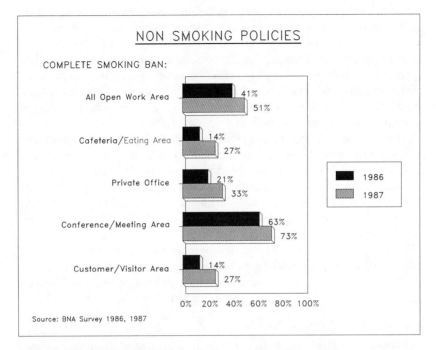

Figure 1 Non-smoking policies

survey of a random sample of manufacturing companies in King County, Washington, 36% of respondents, or 53% of companies with policies, banned smoking completely (48).

In the 1987 BNA survey, 12% of all responding companies reported giving preference in hiring to nonsmoking job applicants, with only 1% hiring nonsmokers exclusively. For one third of those giving preference to nonsmokers, the policy is companywide; in the other two thirds, the individual supervisor is allowed to give preference to nonsmokers (17).

Implementation of Smoking Policies

Many guides are available to help employers implement smoking policies (3, 16, 28, 59). In general, companies that introduce a smoking policy, or make one more restrictive, work to minimize adverse employee reaction. Techniques that are commonly utilized by nonunion employers, with some modifications in unionized environments to facilitate smooth implementation and minimize negativity, include developing an economic justification by comparing the claims and absenteeism experience of smokers and nonsmokers; surveying employees about their smoking habits and attitudes and supporting alternative potential smoking policies; obtaining committed top management support; involving employee groups in the decision-making process, particularly with respect to implementation issues; announcing and widely publicizing the policy change at least several months before its effective date; and offering, often with financial support, smoking cessation activities of various types, on or off site, during the period between policy announcement and implementation and periodically thereafter. If the policy to be implemented is prohibition of smoking, there may be intermediate stages when smoking is permitted in designated areas.

Most of the information available on the development of support, implementation, and effects of smoking policies is from large companies. In smaller firms, where the majority of employees work, the process may not be the same. In public sector organizations, there appears to be a greater likelihood that the policy will be established by law or regulation and/or that the agency administrator will determine the policy, as the Secretary of Defense did for all US military personnel.

In response to prepolicy survey questions, the vast majority of employees at most worksites support restrictions on smoking and report that their coworkers also support such restrictions. The notion of limiting areas for smoking generally receives a higher approval rating than banning smoking (83).

Effects of Smoking Policies

Approval for a restrictive policy, including a ban, generally increases after implementation, among both smokers and nonsmokers, although nonsmokers generally have higher approval ratings both before and after (4, 6, 66, 71). In one study, among smokers and recent ex-smokers, the strongest support for nonsmoking was from those who were most interested in quitting, had the greatest concerns about the health effects of smoking, worked primarily with nonsmokers, were asked by coworkers not to smoke, and reported support from their coworkers in their efforts to quit (71). Although most companies that have greatly restricted or banned smoking at the workplace have experienced some objections and informal complaints by employees, such reactions tend to be short-lived and limited to a small percentage of smokers (13). Once a smoking policy is in place, contrary to forecast or expressed employee intentions, it is rare for any smoker to leave his/her job because of smoking restrictions.

Reports of measured reduction in exposure to ETS following smoking policy implementation are lacking. Subjective reports support a diminution of ETS; however, unless it is a totally smoke-free worksite, workers will still be exposed to some ETS (83). As smoking policies tend to reduce the proportion of employees bothered by coworkers' smoke, nonsmokers are presumably less likely to complain about smoke and odor to a smoking coworker. In one study, implementation of a restrictive smoking policy led to a drop in the percentage of survey respondents bothered daily by coworkers' smoking from 22% to 4% (38). Ironically, however, if smokers must smoke in situations where they are unlikely to bother nonsmokers, they may experience less pressure to quit from their nonsmoking colleagues, thereby reducing, rather than increasing, their motivation to quit. In one report, the cessation rate among smokers whose coworkers never requested them not to smoke (after controlling for sex, education, age, coworker nonsmoking, and treatment group) was 4%, compared with 27% among those whose coworkers frequently asked that they not smoke (70).

It is unclear whether adoption of restrictive smoking policies will lead to reductions in the overall frequency of smoking or average number of cigarettes smoked per individual in employed populations. Although some employees feel motivated to quit in advance of implementation of a policy, which results in a spurt of participation in cessation programs, reductions in smoking prevalence over time have been difficult to demonstrate.

Some reports suggest that the percentage of smokers who quit after installation of a smoking ban is very small (8, 67). For example, changes in responses to three cross-sectional surveys of a worksite population, in which a restrictive smoking policy was adopted, revealed no significant changes in smoking prevalence, the proportion of smokers attempting to quit, or the total daily consumption of cigarettes. However, the daily consumption of cigarettes at work declined significantly. Before the policy became effective, 17% of workers reported smoking 15 cigarettes per day at work. Six months after implementation, the comparable percentage had decreased to 5% (38). These response patterns and other data suggest that, although smokers can adapt their smoking patterns to the policies by smoking less during the workday, compensatory increases in smoking frequently occur during nonworking hours (19, 47, 55, 81). In interpreting data on changes in smoking prevalence associated with smoking policy implementation, caution is warranted because most studies have methodological limitations, including limited power to detect reasonably expected changes in cessation rates. In addition, most are from a single industry (health care), which limits external validity.

Little is known about the time response curve for effects of smoking policies on smoking behavior. As they constitute an indirect intervention, they may not lead to rapid cessation, as clinical cessation programs are designed to achieve (37). Restrictive policies may also have effects other than cessation, such as abstinence. In one worksite study, the strongest predictors of abstinence were light smoking, more perceived social support, and less perceived stress (25). In the same study, the strongest predictors of initial quitting were less difficulty quitting, longer periods of prior abstention, and a higher desire to quit. These different predictors support a multistage model of quitting in which restrictive policies are likely to have a greater effect on those who have already quit than they do on motivating others to attempt quitting.

The military is a well defined, though atypical, working population in which a series of measures have been implemented to discourage tobacco use. Survey results show that from 1985 to 1987, smoking prevalence in the Army declined from 52% to 44%, in the Navy from 49% to 45%, and in the Air Force from 39% to 37% (78, 79). Multiple efforts to support cessation and abstinence preclude assessment of the independent effect of policies, but the strong overall trend suggests that the antismoking campaign, of which restrictive policies are an essential component, is effective. As the levels of smoking in the military are much higher than US averages, and the military workforce is very large, programs in the Armed Forces have the potential to effect a major reduction in the burden of smoking in this country.

A worksite where smoking policies affect not only current smokers, but the next generation, is the school. In 16 states, the sale, use, or possession of tobacco products is banned for minors. As of 1988, 32 states restricted or banned smoking in schools: Student smoking was banned in schools in 15 of these states and limited to designated areas in 17 other states (76).

Only one state, however, had banned smoking by teachers. A 1986 survey of smoking policies by the National School Boards Association of a stratified random sample of 2000 school districts nationwide found that 87% of respondents reported written policies or regulations on smoking in schools (57, 58, 83). Nearly one half the districts had a comprehensive policy banning student smoking in school buildings, on school grounds, and at school-sponsored functions. Although 91% of respondents prohibited student smoking in schools, only 10% had equivalent restrictions for teachers. Over four of five school districts provided designated smoking areas in school buildings for faculty and staff. Thirty-seven percent of schools indicated that they had revised their policies over a five-year period; of these schools, 80% initiated stricter policies vis-a-vis students, and 56% strengthened restrictions for faculty and staff (57, 83).

Unions and Smoking Policies

Union leaders have opposed unilateral management action to adopt smoking policies, but generally have not opposed the principle of restricting smoking at the worksite. In 1986, the AFL-CIO Executive Council declared its opposition to both legislated and employer-mandated smoking restrictions and adopted the position that workplace smoking disputes should be "worked out voluntarily in individual workplaces between labor and management in a manner that protects the interest and rights of all workers" (1). Local union leaders often are uncomfortable with the smoking issue, as it pits the interests of smoking members against those of their nonsmoking colleagues (16).

Unions tend to react to management initiatives regarding smoking restrictions, rather than take proactive positions. A common union concern is that attention to ETS exposure at the worksite will obscure more hazardous occupational exposures that receive inadequate attention. Unions also fear that employer emphasis on smoking as the major cause of preventable morbidity and mortality among workers will lead to reduced worker compensation awards from toxic exposures, which cause diseases that also may be caused by smoking (17). However, union members found smoking control policies more acceptable in the context of a strong company health and safety program (14).

Smoking Cessation Activities

Many worksites offer the same types of smoking cessation programs originally developed and offered in clinical settings. Most of these worksites utilize standard behavioral approaches, sometimes accompanied by a prescription for nicotine gum. Voluntary health organizations (e.g. affiliates of the American Cancer Society and the American Lung Association), for-profit smoking cessation organizations (e.g. Smoke Enders), some university-based research groups, health care organizations, and providers of broad-based worksite health promotion programs (e.g. Johnson & Johnson) are diverse sources for specific smoking control programs. In addition, some worksites develop their own programs; they use purchased materials or develop them de novo. As indicated in Table 1, of worksites with any smoking control activity, about 50% provided self-help materials, about 20% offered group classes/workshops, and 15% provided individual counseling (31). Counseling by physicians as an intervention generally has a low long-term quit rate and is limited to those companies with an occupational health department (40).

In general, the published studies support the hypothesis that more intensive programs, with multiple sessions and multiple components, have higher quit rates than shorter term, less intensive interventions (82). Results of clinically based versus worksite-based programs should be generalized only with an abundance of caution. Compared with clinical settings, worksite group cessation programs generally achieve lower short-term quite rates, but higher long-term quit rates (85). A recent metaanalysis of 20 worksite cessation programs, chosen for their scientific rigor, realized a 12-month initial quit rate of 13% (34). The addition of nicotine gum appears to enhance short-term cessation rates in worksite settings, but does not have a reproducible significant effect on long-term cessation (52, 82). In a British worksite study, nicotine gum, combined with individual counseling, achieved an initial quit rate of 16%, which was sustained for at least 12 months (74).

Interpretation of most published studies of worksite single component smoking cessation programs is limited by design or methodological problems.

The most common problem is lack of biochemical validation of cessation and abstinence. Other problems include failure to define the characteristics of the population offered participation in the study, failure to include dropouts in the calculation of quit rates, or use of very small samples.

Often the degree to which the environment supports smoking cessation and other health promotion objectives is not clear. Issues infrequently addressed in published reports include the existence of a formal health promotion program and its nature, intensity, and duration; the existence of a formal smoking policy and its time of adoption and enforcement; the presence and timing of other smoking control activities; and the presence of local regulations that restrict smoking and whether they apply to the worksite offering the program. Although other worksite characteristics, such as demographic factors, organization of work, and management style, might affect the success of smoking control efforts, the impact of these characteristics has not been studied in published reports.

Factors that influence participation in worksite group and individual cessation activities are not well understood (40). Even with the incentive of an impending restrictive smoking policy or ban, participation rates in formal programs vary widely. In the Group Health Cooperative Study (67) and a study of an insurance company (64) only 2% and 4%, respectively, of eligible smokers enrolled in smoking cessation classes, whereas over 25% of smoking employees at Pacific Northwest Bell participated in a company-sponsored smoking cessation program before a ban was implemented (53, 91). At Johns-Manville, 15% of smokers participated in the employer-sponsored smoking cessation classes at the time a smoking ban was established (40).

Organized smoking cessation efforts, such as classes, individual counseling, and provision of self-help materials, lend themselves to studies of relative efficacy and of relative cost-effectiveness. Cessation for a defined time period is the common outcome measure.

A careful study at a US Department of Energy installation in Washington State randomly assigned smokers (based on preference for self-help or group-help) to three cessation programs: a didactic, three-week program that utilized behavior skills training, aversive stimuli, imagery, and stress management; an eight-week interactive relapse prevention program; or a minimal treatment program that provided the American Cancer Society's "Quitters Guide" seven-day plan to stop smoking. Twelve months after the program ended, self-reported cessation rates for group- and self-help preference cohorts were, respectively, 26% and 16% for the three-week group program, 25% and 20% for the relapse prevention program, and 24% and 16.5% for the minimal treatment program (62). Although the minimal treatment group results appear impressive, less than 50% of participants in that group submitted saliva for cotinine validation at 12 months. Group preference smokers had higher quit rates than self-help preference smokers. All of these cessation rates exceed the average 5% estimated annual spontaneous quit rate. A high 11% of the total smoking population participated in these smoking cessation programs.

A study in a worksite population, which examined the relative efficacy and cost-effectiveness of a stop smoking clinic and self-help kit, both offered by the American Lung Association, found that the clinic client abstinence rate was 15%, versus 11% for the self-help group. These rates were based on self-report data covering an 18-month follow-up period. Although cost per participant was twice as high for the clinic method, the cost per successful quitter was similar, about $150 (5).

Assessments of worksite smoking control efforts on frequency and level of smoking in the entire worksite population (rather than for those employees who volunteer to participate in a formal program) have been carried out in two contexts: comprehensive health promotion programs directed at many health behaviors, including smoking, and specific smoking control programs, including policies that restrict smoking. The best-studied worksite health promotion program targeted at the entire worksite population is LIVE FOR LIFE®. Using a quasi-experimental design, four companies offered this comprehensive worksite health promotion program, while three comparison companies offered only annual health screens. Based on both self-report and serum thiocyanate validation at two years after baseline measurements, 23% of LIVE FOR LIFE® smokers were not smoking versus 17% of the smokers at the health screen only companies (69). Mean abstinence duration for the LIVE FOR LIFE® group was 14.8 months versus 12.3 for the health screen only group. Of smokers at high risk for coronary heart disease, 32% quit versus 13% at the health screen only companies. The high rate of cessation at the health screen only companies suggests that the screening, a one-hour assessment and risk reduction counseling session by a specially trained nurse, can have substantial independent impact. In programs directed against many health risks, it is not possible to assess the independent contribution of a particular program component. In the LIVE FOR LIFE® evaluation, only 21% of the baseline smokers in the intervention companies participated in formal smoking-cessation clinics (69). Participants had a 32% quit rate, compared with 20% for nonparticipants. These results support the possibility of synergistic effects of program components directed at different risks on smoking behavior.

Incentives and Competition

In contrast to clinically based programs, the worksite setting offers the opportunity to incorporate two unique elements, incentives and competition. Incentives may be monetary or nonmonetary. A ban on smoking at the workplace may provide an incentive for smokers to quit, as may a less strict smoking policy that nonetheless sends a clear message that primacy is accorded the rights of nonsmokers. Creating, intentionally or not, the impression that smokers are less likely to be promoted or banning smoking (including pipes and cigars) among top executives, can promote normative beliefs that smoking is not a desirable employee behavior and can affect motivation to quit or to stay quit.

Monetary incentives are a tool with which all private employers are comfortable, as a company's success is based on the ability to succeed in competitive markets in response to economic incentives. Many employers thus provide monetary incentives for smoking cessation and maintenance of a nonsmoking state. The most common incentive is reduction in the cost of participation in a cessation program to the employee by employer payment of part or all of the program cost. In the 1987 BNA program survey, 20% sponsored quit-smoking programs on work time, and 14% reimbursed workers for participation in outside quit-smoking programs (17).

Some employers provide contingency payments for smoking cessation, by giving a bonus to an employee who quits for a defined period of time. A commonly cited example is Bonne Bell Company, which offers its employees the opportunity to accept $250 from the company to quit smoking; however, the employees must pledge to pay the company $500 if they do not quit or resume the habit at any time (18). In some cases, employees are asked to contribute a portion or all of the cost of the smoking cessation activity or to deposit into a separate account an amount deemed "personally relevant" to the individual. The amount is paid back to the employee, sometimes with an employer supplement, if he/she quits for some period of time, usually measured in months and almost never greater than one year (45).

Smoking cessation competitions, combined with incentives, are increasingly utilized at worksites. Compared with other smoking cessation programs, they tend to have a much higher participation rate; in one study, as many as 80% of smokers in small-and medium-size worksites participated (44). Competitions may be between different employers, between different groups of the same employer at one or more worksites, or between employee-defined groups constituted specifically for the cessation competition.

Monetary incentives may be offered for participation in these competitions, as well as for short- and long-term results. For example, in one competition participants could earn $10 for attending each of six group smoking cessation meetings during a three-week period. Thereafter, they could earn $1 for each day of abstinence over the next 180 days and an extra $30 for every 30 continuous days of abstinence. Participants abstinent for at least 60 days during this period were eligible for a lottery, in which the company contributed $50 for each person quitting. Employees developed three-person teams, which worked together to quit and remain abstinent, and competed for a cash prize of $300 awarded to the team with the largest number of days abstinent. Finally, participants could select a coworker as a buddy to help them stop, and the buddy would select an item from a list of gifts at the end of the program (44). Although this array of incentives is more complicated than most, it suggests the different ways financial incentives may be used to achieve initial cessation, reduce recidivism, and, when recidivism occurs, support attempts to quit again.

Another use of incentives is to provide premiums for persons who participate in smoking control programs. For example, LIVE FOR LIFE® provides LIVE FOR LIFE® dollars, redeemable for a variety of athletic clothing and other health-oriented products (a wok, tennis balls, etc.) for participating in the smoking cessation program, regardless of outcome (11).

Overall, the use of incentives appears to increase both initial and longer term (one year) cessation rates. For seven studies reporting incentives and/or competition, the average 12-month cessation rate was 26% (49, 50, 69). The study that employed the above-mentioned complicated incentive scheme had a six-month cessation rate of 42%, compared with 13% for the control group (44). In general, reported results support the conclusion that competition strategies can increase participation rates and that incentives alone or coupled with competitive approaches tend to increase one-year abstinence levels. Most significantly, these combined approaches are associated with a higher percentage of the total smoking employee population quitting than behavioral approaches alone, which potentially reduces greatly the population-attributable risks due to smoking. How the institution of restrictive smoking policies interacts with smoking cessation programs that employ competition and economic incentives is not known, but some synergistic effects might reasonably be expected.

A continuing incentive for not smoking is differential premiums for employer-sponsored group health or life insurance benefits for smokers and nonsmokers. Because smoking behavior is associated with shorter life expectancy and with higher health benefit cost experience, smoking employees arguably should pay a commensurately higher amount for this coverage. For life insurance, age- and sex-specific average premium differentials between smokers and nonsmokers have been developed through extensive actuarial experience, supplemented by the results of epidemiological studies on differential life expectancy. However, employers may or may not set differential premiums to accurately reflect risk differences, sometimes considering the perceived fairness of premium differences and other factors in setting them. Although fewer published studies cover differential health insurance experience, there is little question that smokers have higher utilization and related health benefit costs. Based on data from the 1979 Health Interview Survey, smokers have 12% more physician visits and 22% more hospital days than nonsmokers (65). Of 124 health insurance companies that responded to an industry survey in 1985, about one third reported offering discounts to groups, usually 6%–10%, on health insurance to nonsmokers (41). At least two states, Kansas and Colorado, have instituted discounts for their nonsmoking state workers of $10 and $6 per month, respectively, available upon a signed request from an employee that indicates he/she is a nonsmoker. In Kansas, the penalty for falsification is payment of a full year of the differential, plus possible adverse impacts on employee performance evaluations. Kansas state employees, as other insured groups, appear to respond accurately to questions of smoking status. In that state, the 21% of employees who did not apply for the discount conforms to the estimate of 20% prevalence of smokers in the workforce (63). Large businesses that are self-insured, such as Johnson & Johnson and Southern California Edison, Inc., may provide discounts for life and health insurance based on health status and/or health behaviors, of which nonsmoking is just one part.

Conclusion

During the 1980s, a profound change occurred in the response of employers to smoking among employees. Increasing epidemiological data on the adverse effects of ETS have been coupled with repeated demonstrations that smokers cost employers more, both directly and indirectly, than nonsmokers. Weight of scientific evidence, combined with increasingly prevalent legal restrictions on smoking in private and public workplaces, has led employers to take more aggressive approaches to discourage smoking and encourage employees who quit to remain abstinent.

Traditional smoking cessation classes, self-help materials, and one-on-one counseling, which together reached a small percentage of smokers, have been complemented by increasingly restrictive smoking policies that discourage worksite smoking and sometimes ban smoking on employer premises and in employer-owned vehicles. Restrictive smoking policies, coupled with other smoking control activities, have widespread employee support, including that of a significant percentage of smokers. Various activities have been associated with declines in the percentage of smokers in the population, but the independent effects of restrictive smoking policies on smoking prevalence have not yet been elucidated.

The most important trend among management and workers in private and public workplaces is the shift from acceptance of smoking and the primacy of the rights of the smoker to discouragement of smoking. Intensive efforts to discourage tobacco use and to establish nonsmoking as normative behavior at the worksite have become commonplace. Should present trends continue, smoking prohibition in the worksite could be common within the next decade.

Literature Cited

1. AFL-CIO Statement on Smoking Policies. February 19, 1986. American Federation of Labor-Congress of Industrial Organizations Executive Council
2. Am. Lung Assoc. 1983. *Survey of Attitudes Towards Smoking*. New York: Lung Assoc.
3. Am. Lung Assoc. 1985. *Creating Your Company Policy*. San Diego: Am. Lung Assoc.
4. Andrews, J. L., Jr. 1983. Reducing smoking in the hospital: An effective model program. *Chest* 84:206–9
5. Bertera, R. L., Oehl, L. K., Telepchak, J. M. 1990. Self-help versus group approaches to smoking cessation in the workplace: Eighteen-month follow-up and cost analysis. *Am. J. Health Promot.* 4:187–92
6. Biener, L., Abrams, D. B., Emmons, K., Follick, M. J. 1989. Evaluating worksite smoking policies. Methodologic issues. *NY State J. Med.* 89:5–10
7. Deleted in proof
8. Biener, L., Abrams, D. B., Follick, M. J., Dean, L. 1989. A comparative evaluation of a restrictive smoking policy in a general hospital. *Am. J. Public Health* 79:192–95
9. Blackwell, M. J., French, J. G., Stein, H. P. 1979. Adverse health effects of smoking and the occupational environment. NIOSH Current Intelligence Bulletin No. 31. *Am. Ind. Hyg. Assoc. J.* 40:A38–A47
10. Brackbill, R., Frazier, T., Shilling, S. 1988. Smoking characteristics of US workers, 1978–1980. *Am. J. Ind. Med.* 13:5–41
11. Breslow, L., Fielding, J., Herrmann, A. A., Wilbur, C. S. 1990. Worksite health promotion: Its evolution and the Johnson & Johnson experience. *Prev. Med.* 19:13–21
12. Brink, S. D. 1987. *Health Risks and Behavior: the Impact on Medical Costs*. Milwaukee: Milliman & Robertson
13. Broffman, P. 1989. Ranier Bancorporation's policy on smoking. *NY State J. Med.* 89:48–49
14. Brown, E. R., McCarthy, W. J., Marcus, A., Baker, D., Froines, J. R., et al. 1988. Workplace smoking policies: Attitudes of union members in a high-risk industry. *J. Occup. Med.* 30:312–20
15. Bur. Natl. Aff. 1981. Services for employees, in *Personnel Policies Forum Survey 133*. Washington, DC: Bur. Natl. Aff.
16. Bur. Natl. Aff. 1986. *Where There's Smoke: Problems and Policies Concerning Smoking in the Workplace*. Washington DC: Bur. Natl. Aff.
17. Bur. Natl. Aff. 1987. *Where There's Smoke*. A BNA special report. Washington, DC: Bur. Natl. Aff., 2nd ed.
18. Bur. Natl. Aff. 1989. *Workplace Smoking: Corporate Practices & Developments*. Washington, DC: Bur. Natl. Aff.
19. Carey, K. B., Abrams, D. B. 1988. Properties of saliva cotinine in light smokers. *Am. J. Public Health* 78:842–43
20. Cenci, L. 1980. *Smoking and the Workplace: A Paper on the National Interagency Council on Smoking and Health Business Survey of Smoking Programs and Health Education by Corporate Industry*. New York: NY Acad. Med.
21. Cent. Dis. Control. 1988. Passive smoking: Beliefs, attitudes, and exposures—United States, 1986. *Morbid. Mortal. Wkly. Rep.* 37:239–41
22. Clutterbuck, D. April 1981. Persuading employees to break the smoking habit. *Int. Manage.* 27–29
23. Coghlin, J., Hammond, S. K., Gann, P. H. 1989. Development of epidemiologic tools for measuring environmental tobacco smoke exposure. *Am. J. Epidemiol.* 130:696–704
24. Cummings, K. M., Markello, S. J., Mahoney, M., Bhargava, A. K., McElroy, P. D., Marshall, J. R. 1990. Measurement of current exposure to environmental tobacco smoke. *Arch. Environ. Health* 45:74–79
25. Curry, S., Thompson, B., Sexton, M., Omenn, G. S. 1989. Psychosocial predictors of outcome in a worksite smoking cessation program. *Am. J. Prev. Med.* 5:2–7
26. Danaher, B. G. 1980. Smoking cessation programs in occupational settings. *Public Health Rep.* 95:149–57
27. Eriksen, M. P. 1985. Smoking policies at Pacific Bell. *Corp. Comment.* 1:24–34
28. Eriksen, M. P. 1986. Workplace smoking control: Rationale and approaches. *Adv. Health Educ. Promot.* 1(A):65–103
29. Fanning, D. March 18, 1990. Humiliating times for a boss who smokes. *NY Times*
30. Fielding, J. E. 1985. Smoking: Health effects and control. *N. Engl. J. Med.* 313:491–98

31. Fielding, J. E. 1990. Worksite health promotion survey: Smoking control activities. *Prev. Med.* 19:402–13
32. Fielding, J. E., Phenow, K. J. 1988. Health effects of involuntary smoking. *N. Engl. J. Med.* 319:1452–60
33. Fielding, J. E., Piserchia, P. V. 1989. Frequency of worksite health promotion activities. *Am. J. Public Health* 79:16–20
34. Fisher, K. J., Glasgow, R. E., Terborg, J. R. 1990. Work site smoking cessation: A meta-analysis of long-term quit rates from controlled studies. *J. Occup. Med.* 32:429–39
35. Friedman, G. D., Petitti, D. B., Bawol, R. D. 1983. Prevalence and correlates of passive smoking. *Am. J. Public Health* 73:401–5
36. Glantz, S. A., Parmley, W. W. 1991. Passive smoking and heart disease: Epidemiology, physiology, and biochemistry. *Circulation* In press
37. Glasgow, R. E. 1989. Assessment of smoking behavior in relation to worksite smoking policies. *NY State J. Med.* 89:31–33
38. Gottlieb, N. H., Eriksen, M. P., Lovato, C. Y., Weinstein, R. P., Green, L. W. 1990. Impact of a restrictive work site smoking policy on smoking behavior, attitudes, and norms. *J. Occup. Med.* 32:16–23
39. Haley, N. J., Colosimo, S. G., Axelrad, C. M., Harris, R., Sepkovic, D. W. 1989. Biochemical validation of self-reported exposure to environmental tobacco smoke. *Environ. Res.* 49:127–35
40. Hallett, R. 1986. Smoking intervention in the workplace: Review and recommendations. *Prev. Med.* 15:213–31
41. Health Insur. Assoc. Am. 1986. Survey of health promotion insurance underwriting practices. *Res. Stat. Bull.* No. 1–86
42. Hodgson, M. J. 1989. Environmental tobacco smoke and the sick building syndrome. *Occup. Med.* 4:735–40
43. Human Resources Policy Corporation. 1984. *Smoking Policies in Large Corporations.* Los Angeles: Human Resour. Policy Corp.
44. Jason, L. A., Jayaraj, S., Blitz, C. C., Michaels, M. H., Klett, L. E. 1990. Incentives and competition in a worksite smoking cessation intervention. *Am. J. Public Health* 80:205–6
45. Jeffery, R. W., Pheley, A. M., Forster, J. L., Kramer, F. M., Snell, M. K. 1988. Payroll contracting for smoking cessation: A worksite pilot study. *Am. J. Prev. Med.* 4:83–86
46. Jones, R. C., Bly, J. L., Richardson, J. E. 1990. A study of a work site health promotion program and absenteeism. *J. Occup. Med.* 32:95–99
47. Kauffmann, F., Dockery, D. W., Speizer, F. E., Ferris, B. G. 1986. Respiratory symptoms and lung function in women with passive and active smoking. *Am. Rev. Respir. Dis.* 133(Suppl.): A157
48. Kinne, S. 1990. Prevalence and restrictiveness of smoking policies in King County (WA). *Am. J. Public Health* 80:1498–1500
49. Klesges, R. C., Cigrang, J. A. 1989. Worksite smoking cessation programs: Clinical and methodological issues. In *Progress in Behavior Modification,* ed. M. Hersen, R. M. Eisler, P. M. Miller. New York: Sage
50. Klesges, R. C., Cigrang, J., Glasgow, R. E. 1987. Worksite smoking modification programs: A state-of-art review and directions for future research. *Curr. Res. Rev.* 6:26–56
51. Leaderer, B. P. 1990. Assessing exposures to environmental tobacco smoke. *Risk Anal.* 10:19–26
52. Maheu, M. M., Gervirtz, R. N., Sallis, J. F., Schneider, N. G. 1989. Competition/cooperation in worksite smoking cessation using nicotine gum. *Prev. Med.* 18:867–76
53. Martin, M. J. 1988. Smoking control—Policy and legal methods. (Letter) *West. J. Med.* 148:199
54. Matsukura, S., Taminator, T., Kitano, N., Seino, Y., Hamada, H., et al. 1984. Effects of environmental tobacco smoke on urinary cotinine excretion in nonsmokers: Evidence for passive smoking. *N. Eng. J. Med.* 311:828–32
55. Meade, T. W., Wald, N. J. 1977. Cigarette smoking patterns during the workday. *Br. J. Prev. Soc. Med.* 31:25–29
56. Natl. Res. Counc., Comm. Passive Smoking. 1986. *Environmental Tobacco Smoke: Measuring Exposures and Assessing Health Effects.* Washington, DC: Natl. Acad. Press
57. Natl. Sch. Boards Assoc. 1986. *Study on Nonsmoking Policies in the Nation's School Districts.* Washington, DC: Natl. Sch. Boards Assoc.
58. Natl. Sch. Boards Assoc. 1987. *No Smoking: A Board Member's Guide to Nonsmoking Policies for the Schools.* Alexandria, Va: Natl. Sch. Boards Assoc.
59. Off. Dis. Prev. Health Promot. and Off. Smoking Health, Public Health Serv., US Dep. Health Hum. Serv. 1985. *No Smoking. A Decision Maker's Guide to*

Reducing Smoking at the Worksite. Washington, DC: Wash. Bus. Group Health

60. Off. Popul. Censuses Surv. (London). 1985. *OPCS Monitor,* General Household Survey, Ref. GHS 85/2, Cigarette smoking: 1972–1984

61. Off. Technol. Assess. 1985. *Smoking-Related Deaths and Financial Costs.* Washington, DC: Off. Technol. Assess., US Congress

62. Omenn, G. S., Thompson, B., Sexton, M., Hessol, N., Breitenstein, B., et al. 1988. A randomized comparison of worksite-sponsored smoking cessation programs. *Am. J. Prev. Med.* 4:261–67

63. Penner, M. 1989. Economic incentives to reduce employee smoking: A health insurance surcharge for tobacco using State of Kansas employees. *Am. J. Health Promot.* 4:5–11

64. Peterson, L. R., Helgerson, S. D., Gibbons, C. M., Calhoun, C. R., Ciacco, K. H., Pitchford, K. C. 1988. Employee smoking behavior changes and attitudes following a restrictive policy on worksite smoking in a large company. *Public Health Rep.* 103:115–20

65. Rice, D., Hodgson, T., Sinskeimer, P., Browner, W., Kopstein, A. 1985. The economic costs of the health effects of smoking. *Milb. Q.* 64:489–546

66. Rigotti, N. A., Hill Pikl, B., Cleary, P., Singer, D. E., Mulley, A. G. 1986. The impact of banning smoking on a hospital ward: Acceptance, compliance, air quality and smoking behavior. (Abstract) *Clin. Res.* 34:833A

67. Rosenstock, I. M., Stergachis, A., Heaney, C. 1986. Evaluation of smoking prohibition policy in a health maintenance organization. *Am. J. Public Health* 76:1014–15

68. Saracci, R. 1987. The interactions of tobacco smoking and other agents in cancer etiology. *Epidemiol. Rev.* 9:175–93

69. Shipley, R. H., Orleans, C. T., Wilbur, C. S., Piserchia, P. V., McFadden, D. W. 1988. Effect of the Johnson & Johnson Live for Life Program on employee smoking. *Prev. Med.* 17:25–34

70. Sorensen, G., Pechacek, T. F. 1985. Smoking cessation at the workplace. *Circulation* 72 (part II):III-345

71. Sorensen, G., Pechacek, T. F. 1989. Implementing nonsmoking policies in the private sector and assessing their effects. *NY State J. Med.* 89:11–15

72. Spitzer, W. O., Lawrence, V., Dales, R., Hill, G., Archer, M. C., et al. 1990. Links between passive smoking and disease: A best-evidence synthesis. A report of the Working Group on Passive Smoking. *Clin. Invest. Med.* 13:17–42

73. Stellman, S. D., Boffetta, P., Garfinkel, L. 1988. Smoking habits of 800,000 American men and women in relation to their occupations. *Am. J. Ind. Med.* 13:43–58

74. Sutton, S., Hallett, R. 1988. Smoking intervention in the workplace using videotapes and nicotine chewing gum. *Prev. Med.* 17:48–59

75. Tager, I. B. 1989. Health effects of involuntary smoking in the workplace. *NY State J. Med.* 89:27–31

76. Tobacco-Free America Project. 1988. *State Regulations Limiting Smoking on School Property.* Washington, DC: Legis. Clearinghouse

77. Tsai, S. P., Cowles, S. R., Ross, C. E. 1990. Smoking and morbidity frequency in a working population. *J. Occup. Med.* 32:245–49

78. US Dep. Def. 1986. *The 1985 Worldwide Survey of Alcohol and Nonmedical Drug Use Among Military Personnel.* Rep. of Res. Triangle Inst. to Off. of Assist. Secr. Def. (Health Affairs), Dep. Def., June 1986

79. US Dep. Def. 1988. *The 1988 Worldwide Survey of Substance Abuse and Health Behavior Among Military Personnel.* Rep. of Res. Triangle Inst. to Off. of Assist. Secr. Def. (Public Affairs), Dep. Def.

80. US Dep. Health Hum. Serv. 1985. *The Health Consequences of Smoking: Cancer and Chronic Lung Disease in the Workplace. A Report of the Surgeon General.* US Dep. Health Hum. Serv., Public Health Serv., Off. Smoking Health. DHHS Publ. No. (PHS) 85-50207

81. US Dep. Health Hum. Serv. 1986. *The Health Consequences of Involuntary Smoking: A Report of the Surgeon General.* US Dep. Health Hum. Serv., Public Health Serv., Cent. Dis. Control, Cent. Health Promot. Educ., Off. Smoking Health. Washington, DC: GPO

82. US Dep. Health Hum. Serv. 1987. *Smoking and Health: A National Status Report.* A Report to Congress. US Dep. Health Hum. Serv., Public Health Serv., Cent. Dis. Control, Cent. Health Promot. Educ., Off. Smoking Health. HHS/PHS/CDC Publ. No. 87-8396

83. US Dep. Health Hum. Serv. 1989. *Reducing the Health Consequences of Smoking: 25 Years of Progress.* A Report of the Surgeon General. US Dep. Health Hum. Serv., Public Health Serv., Cent. Dis. Control, Cent. Chronic Dis.

Prev. Health Promot., Off. Smoking Health. DHSS Publ. No. (CDC) 89-8411

84. US Dep. Health Hum. Serv. 1989. *Major Local Smoking Ordinances in the United States.* US Dep. Health Hum. Serv., Public Health Serv., Natl. Inst. Health, NIH Publ. No. 90-479

85. US Dep. Health Hum. Serv. 1990. *Smoking and Health. A National Status Report. A Report to Congress,* 2nd ed. US Dep. Health Human Serv., Public Health Serv., Cent. Dis. Control, Cent. Chronic Dis. Prev. Health Promot., Off. Smoking Health. DHHS Publ. No. (CDC) 87-8396 (Revised 2/90)

86. US Environ. Prot. Agency. 1990. *Environmental Tobacco Smoke: A Guide to Workplace Smoking Policies.* EPA/400/6-90/004. Indoor Air Div., Off. Atmos. Indoor Air Program, Off. Air Radiat., US Environ. Prot. Agency

87. US Environ. Prot. Agency. 1990. *Health Effects of Passive Smoking: Assessment of Lung Cancer in Adults and Respiratory Disorders in Children.* EPA/600/6-90/006A. Off. Health Environ. Assess., Off. Res. Dev. Indoor Air Div., Off. Atmos. Indoor Air Program, Off. Air Radiat., US Environ. Prot. Agency

88. Wald, N. J., Nanchahal, K., Thompson, S. G., Cuckle, H. S. 1986. Does breathing other people's tobacco smoke cause lung cancer? *Br. Med. J.* 293:1217–22

89. Waldron, I., Lye, D. 1989. Employment, unemployment, occupation, and smoking. *Am. J. Prev. Med.* 5:142–49

90. Walsh, D. C. 1984. Corporate smoking policies: A review and an analysis. *J. Occup. Med.* 26:17–22

91. Walsh, D. C., McDougall, V. 1988. Current policies regarding smoking in the workplace. *Am. J. Ind. Med.* 13:181–90

92. Weber, A., Fisher, T. 1980. Passive smoking at work. *Int. Occup. Environ. Health* 47:209–21

93. White, J. R., Froeb, H. F. 1980. Small-airways dysfunction in nonsmokers chronically exposed to tobacco smoke. *N. Engl. J. Med.* 302:720–23

94. Wu-Williams, A. H., Samet, J. M. 1990. Environmental tobacco smoke: Exposure-response relationships in epidemiologic studies. *Risk Anal.* 10:39–48

Annu. Rev. Publ. Health 1991. 12:235–55

OCCUPATIONAL AND ENVIRONMENTAL EXPOSURES TO RADON: CANCER RISKS

Olav Axelson

Department of Occupational Medicine, University Hospital, 581 85 Linköping, Sweden

KEY WORDS: indoor radon, interaction, mining, radon epidemiology, smoking

INTRODUCTION

Radon is a naturally occurring radioactive gas in our environment. This element can reach high concentrations in uranium and other mines, thereby causing lung cancer in various mining populations. Recently, it has also become clear that high levels of radon may occur in dwellings. In some places, changes in the construction and ventilation of houses may even have caused the radon levels to increase over time. This increase, which may impose a health hazard to the general population in many countries, may also partly explain the increasing lung cancer rates in this century.

Some epidemiological observations, which were made long ago, suggest that factors other than smoking influence the incidence of lung cancer; for example, many criticisms have been made about the causality of the association between smoking and lung cancer (20, 21, 81). Indoor radon might turn out to be a major factor that could account for part of the urban-rural differences in lung cancer rates (remaining after adjustment for smoking); it might also explain the influence of immigration on lung cancer incidence, as ethnic groups differ in indoor and outdoor activities, house constructions, ventilation habits, etc. Finally, radon might also explain some of the dif-

235

0163-7525/91/0501-0235$02.00

ferences in cancer incidence throughout the world, after controlling for smoking (20, 29, 30).

Fisher (39) and Higenbottam et al (47) reported another puzzling observation: the inverse relation between lung cancer and inhalation of cigarette smoke. Axelson (9) has suggested indoor radon as a factor, but there may be some other explanation (103). Remarkably bronchitis is more closely correlated with air pollution than is lung cancer (108). Assuming indoor radon plays some role for these various findings, the epidemiology of lung cancer may become better understood. Furthermore, reducing indoor radon may supplement antismoking activities in preventing lung cancer.

This review will elucidate the health hazards associated with radon, especially in the indoor environment. Radon is likely to be a major public health problem of growing importance. I start with an overview of the epidemiological findings regarding lung cancer among miners exposed to radon. Many mining populations have been studied. In contrast, little data are available on the effects of indoor radon. Isolating the effects of radon poses difficult problems, which will be mentioned briefly in interpreting the results of these studies.

RADON AND ITS DECAY PRODUCTS

Radon, or more precisely the isotope radon-222, is a noble gas that originates from the decay of uranium through radium. The further decay of radon leads to a series of radioactive isotopes of polonium, bismuth, and lead. These isotopes are referred to as short-lived radon progeny (or radon daughters) and have half-lives from less than a millisecond up to almost 27 minutes. There is another decay chain from thorium through radon-220, or thoron. Even if some thoron occurs together with radon, the elements in this series usually reach only modest concentrations and are less of a public health concern. Like radon-222 itself, the decay products polonium-218 and polonium-214 emit α-particles. Because these decay products get electrically charged when created, most of them attach to surfaces and dust particles in the air. When the air is dusty, the unattached fraction tends to decrease. This decrease is important because the unattached progeny usually is considered to be responsible for the major part of the α-irradiation to the bronchial epithelium when these isotopes are inhaled and deposited in the bronchii. The contribution of α-irradiation from the radon gas is thought to be marginal, however, as it is not deposited on the epithelium like the decay products.

Although the α-particles travel less than 100 μm into the tissue, their high energy causes an intense local ionization, which damages the tissue with a subsequent risk for cancer development. There is also β- and γ-radiation from some of the decay products of radon, but because these types of radiation have a much lower energy content than the α-radiation, the effect is marginal.

Mining and Exposure to Radon and Decay Products

Radon in mines depends on the presence of uranium in the rock; very high levels are seen in uranium mines. There are trace amounts of uranium present in many types of minerals, so a high radon emanation may occur in iron, zinc-lead, and other mines. Wet mines tend to have relatively higher radon concentrations, because water desolves radon and may carry it out of the rock into the mine, where the gas vaporizes.

An important step towards risk assessment for miners was taken in the 1950s, when the working level (WL) concept was introduced to measure the level of exposure to radon progeny (49). One WL is any combination of short-lived radon progeny in 1l of air that will ultimately release 1.3×10^5 MeV of alpha energy by decay through polonium-214. This amount of radon progeny may also be taken as equivalent to 3700 Bq/m^3 EER [Equilibrium Equivalent Radon; (55)] or 2.08×10^{-5} J/m^3. Bq (becquered) is the SI-unit for radioactive decay, which replaces the Ci units; one Bq means an activity of one decay per second. The accumulated exposure to radiation is expressed in terms of working level months (WLM). In this context, one month corresponds to 170 hours of exposure. The corresponding SI-unit is the joule-hour per cubic meter, and 1 WLM equals 3.6×10^{-3} Jh/m^3 and may also be taken as 72 Bq-years/m^3. Radon concentrations may be referred to as Bq/m^3 or pCi/l; 1 pCi/l corresponds to 37 Bq/m^3. As a rough average, especially when considering indoor situations that are dependent on ventilation to affect the build up of decay products in the air, 100 Bq/m^3 of radon usually indicates the presence of 50 Bq/m^3 EER of radon progeny, or 0.014 WL.

Occupational exposure levels have been high in the past, especially in uranium mines. The extreme exposure situation is well illustrated in one study of uranium miners, in which Lundin et al (73) reported the need for an exposure category of 3720 WLM and above. A modern miner would expect to receive less than 15 WLM. The radon progeny concentrations in many nonuranium mines also have been relatively high, often 1 WL or more. For example, the hematite mines in West Cumberland, Great Britain, used to have exposure levels of 0.15–3.2 WL (18). The cumulated annual exposure for a French miner has been reported as 2.5–4.3 WLM during the late 1950s and 1960s, but decreased to 1.6–3.2 WLM during the 1970s (101).

The hygienic conditions in many mines were improved considerably during the 1970s, when many countries introduced the 4 WLM per year as an exposure limit. For example, the average exposure levels in Swedish mines are now rarely exceeding 0.1 WL, in contrast to commonly occurring levels of 0.5 to 1 WL or more around 1970. However, in 1986, the US Mine Safety and Health Administration reported 19 of 254 operating nonuranium mines to have exposure levels at 0.3 WL or more (79). Such levels would lead to cumulated exposures close to or above the limit of 4 WLM per year.

Radon in Homes

The occurrence of indoor radon depends on both building material and ground conditions. Because the leakage of radon from the ground is a somewhat irregular phenomenon, which may vary locally within a few meters because of cracks and porosity of the ground, very high indoor concentrations can occur in one house, but not in another, even if the two are located near each other. In general, the leakage of radon from the ground is more important than its emanation from stony building materials of a house (1). Air pressure, temperature, and wind conditions, as well as various behavioral factors, influence ventilation, which plays a major role for the concentrations that may build up in a room. Central heating, as introduced in this century, is likely to have reduced the ventilation, compared with older houses with fireplaces. Thus, central heating probably increased indoor radon concentrations over the past 50 years. The more recent efforts to improve insulation and preserve energy, may have worsened the situation (32, 74, 97).

Indoor radon was first measured in Swedish dwellings in the 1950s (52), but these investigations attracted little public health interest. The levels found at that time ranged from 20 to 69 Bq/m^3 (0.54–1.86 pCi/l). Recent measurements of indoor radon in Swedish homes have revealed higher levels, i.e. 122 Bq/m^3 (3.30 pCi/l) as an average in detached houses and 85 Bq/m^3 (2.30 pCi/l) in apartments, but concentrations vary from 11–3300 Bq/m^3 [0.30–89.2 pCi/l (100)]. The differences found between the earlier and the more recently measured concentrations suggest a general increase in the levels over time.

Indoor radon with concentrations in the range of 40–100 Bq/m^3 (1.08–2.70 pCi/l) have been reported as an average from many countries, e.g. the US (80), Norway (96), Finland (22), and the Federal Republic of Germany (90). Considerably higher levels, such as 2000–3000 Bq/m^3 (about 50–80 pCi/l) may occur in many houses. These levels would indicate radon progeny concentrations corresponding to or exceeding the tolerance level in mines in most countries (about 1100 Bq/m^3 EER or 0.3 WL). The rather large variation in concentrations that have been found between houses and over time underscores the potential difficulties of assessing individual exposures for epidemiologic studies. In principle, however, these difficulties result in nondifferential (or random) misclassification of exposure, which leads to an underestimation of an effect (if present); subjects with high exposure may be thought to have low exposure, and vice versa. These aspects will be discussed further.

FROM HISTORICAL OBSERVATIONS TO RECENT REPORTS ON LUNG CANCER IN MINERS

One of the first observations of occupational cancer concerned lung cancer in miners. This observation was first reported in 1879 from Schneeberg, Germany, by Härting & Hesse (44); some decades later it also was reported from Joachimsthal, Czechoslovakia, by Arnstein (8). In the sixteenth century, however, both Paracelsus and Agricola described a high mortality from pulmonary disorders among miners, presumably predominated by lung cancer. In 1924, radioactivity was first suggested to be responsible for this disorder (72). Not until the 1950s and 1960s, however, was the etiological role of radon and its decay products more fully understood and agreed upon. Hence, as late as 1944, a researcher still argued that a genetic susceptibility of the miners could be responsible for their lung cancer (69).

Since the early 1960s, many mining populations with exposure to radon and its decay products have been studied by both cohort and case-control techniques, e.g. uranium miners in the US, Canada, Czechoslovakia, and France (24, 51, 62, 73, 77, 83, 86, 88, 89, 92, 93, 101, 105); iron and other metal miners in the US, UK, China, France, Italy, and Sweden (12, 13, 15, 19, 27, 35, 42, 57, 58, 60, 71, 84, 85, 102); and fluorspar miners in Canada (31, 75, 76). Some results of these studies are summarized in Tables 1 and 2.

It is relatively uncommon for all studies on a particular occupational exposure to be totally consistent in their findings. However, all the exposed mining populations show a consistently increased risk of lung cancer, even if the overall risk ratios in the various studies have ranged from about 1.5 to 15. In this context, malignant disorders other than lung cancer have not yet been clearly related to radon progeny exposure in mines. A few studies have shown a tendency towards an excess of stomach cancer, however (17).

Many agents other than radon and its decay products are present in the mine atmosphere and could be important for lung cancer risk among miners. The series of reports in recent years on silica dust exposure as a probable cause of lung cancer is interesting in this context (53). The occurrence of silicosis and lung cancer in various mining populations has, therefore, been evaluated in reference to exposure to silica dust and radon progeny, respectively, based on various American and Swedish mining populations (6). The data clearly demonstrated that there was no correlation between exposure to silica dust and radon progeny in many uranium mines. The data also indicated that the lung cancer risk followed from high exposure to radon progeny, rather than from silica exposure. This conclusion does not rule out the possibility of lung cancer from silica exposure, but only the possibility that this kind of exposure would have played a major role in the excess of lung cancer seen among miners with exposure to radon progeny.

Table 1 A summary of some cohort studies of lung cancer in miners with exposure to radon and radon progeny (table expanded from Ref. 79)

Type of miners, country	Exposure or concentration (means)	Person—years	Lung cancer deaths			Reference number
			Observed	Expected	SMR[1]	
Metal, USA	0.05 to 0.40 WL	23,862	47	16.1	292	102
Uranium, USA	821 WLM	62,556	185	38.4	482	73, 105
Uranium, Czechoslovakia	289 WLM	56,955	211	42.7	496	62, 83
Tin, UK	1.2 to 3.4 WL	27,631	28	13.27	211	42
Iron, Sweden	0.5 WL	10,230	28	6.79	412	58
Iron, Sweden	81.4 WLM	24,083	50	12.8	390	85
Fluorspar, Canada	Up to 2040 WLM	37,730	104	24.38	427	75
Uranium, Canada	40–90 WLM	202,795	82	56.9	144	77
Uranium, Canada	17 WLM	118,341	65	34.24	190	51
Iron, UK	0.02 to 3.2 WL	17,156	39	25.50	153	60
Uranium nonsmokers, USA	720 WLM	7861	14	1.1	1270	86
Pyrite, Italy	0.12 to 0.36 WL	29,577	47	35.6	131	15

[1] SMR = standardized mortality ratio, i.e. (observed/expected) $\times$ 100

Mur et al (78) reported a somewhat contradictory and puzzling observation regarding proportional mortality among miners in Lorraine, France. These miners supposedly had rather low exposure to radon progeny (about 0.03–0.07 WL); however, they had a clearly increased proportional mortality of lung cancer. Furthermore, the risk increased with years of underground work, and the lung cancer occurred especially among those considered to have pneumoconiosis.

Table 2 A summary of some case-control studies of lung cancer in miners with exposure to radon progeny

Type of miners, country	Exposure or concentration (means)	Number of cases to controls	Number of exposed cases	Rate ratio (max.)	Reference number
Zinc-lead, Sweden	1 WL	29/174	21	16.4	13
Iron, Sweden	0.1–2.0 WL	604/(467 ×	20	7.3	27
Iron, Sweden	0.3–1.0 WL	38/403	33	11.5	35
Uranium, USA	30–2,698 WLM	32/64	23	Infinite	88
Uranium, USA	472 WLM in cases	65/230 (nested)	all	1.5% per WLM	89
Tin, China	515 WLM in cases	107/107	7	(20.0)	84
Tin, China	373 WLM	74/74	5	(13.2) 1.7% per WLM	71 (subset of 84)

Many other agents may also contribute to miners' lung cancer risk, e.g. diesel fumes and carcinogenic trace metals in the dust and especially arsenic, when present. Asbestiform fibers have occurred in some Swedish mines, but have been considered less likely to have played any substantial role for the miners' lung cancer (34).

Miners with very low exposure to radon and decay products also have had little or no excess of lung cancer, i.e. in coal (54) and potash mining (106) and in iron mining (65). Other agents of some potential etiologic interest also are likely to have occurred in these low-risk mines, at least to some extent, but without much influence on the lung cancer morbidity. Therefore, the radioactivity, rather than other factors in the mine atmosphere, is mainly responsible for the lung cancer risk in mining populations, even if other factors contribute to the risk. The comparison of risk estimates derived from mining populations with those that may be obtained from studies of indoor radon might finally permit a more precise assessment of the lung cancer risk from radon progeny exposure for both miners and the general population.

ON THE PROBLEMS OF STUDYING EXPOSURE TO INDOOR RADON

The lack of proper exposure information always is a major problem in epidemiologic studies. Attempts to study the health affects of indoor radon exposure and lung cancer is no exception; indeed, the problem seems even greater than in many other studies. If the assessment of exposure suffers from uncertainty of a random character, an epidemiologic study would find a decrease, or even a disappearance, of an existing risk. In principle, studies of indoor radon require proper information over decades about the epithelial irradiation dose as affected by the radon progeny concentrations over time, the work load and respiration, the dustiness of the air that affects attachment of the short-lived decay products (as later discussed), etc. The individual has no sensation of radiation dose and, thus, cannot report past exposure. Therefore, no good exposure assessment is achievable, and many studies should be expected to give weak or unclear results. Some studies will not show any association. A blurring effect may also result from other factors, especially of occupational exposures that cause lung cancer, whereas smoking may be more easily accounted for.

Measurements of indoor radon might be thought of as a reasonable exposure ascertainment, but even extensive measurements in several homes in which an individual has lived would not provide a good estimate of the cumulated exposure over many decades. Nevertheless, a combination of measurements and judgments with regard to pertinent characteristics of a house might give a usable estimate of radon progeny exposure.

In a few studies, the chosen study population has been rural in order to improve the assessment precision of individual exposure. The rationale is that the persons involved in such a study, especially the women, would be likely to have spent the most time in their homes and not in other buildings. Rural populations also tend to be stable, and many individuals even are born and die in the same house.

For the above-mentioned reasons, some of the first studies were restricted to rural populations (11, 38). The exposure was considered in terms of the building materials of the house in which a person had lived just before death. Hence, the early measurements reported by Hultqvist (52) had shown a difference of indoor radon in stone and wooden houses. When it became increasingly clear during the late 1970s that indoor radon concentrations were dependent on leakage from the soil underneath the house, geological features had to be controlled. This requirement lead to attempts to allocate studies in areas with specific geological characteristics, such as the island of Öland in the Baltic Sea (38). This island has specific geological features with an alum shale strip that leaks radon along the west coast, which contributes to indoor radon. Cellulose nitrate film measurements of radon decay products also were undertaken and found to agree relatively well with the exposure estimates based on various characteristics of the houses.

Other investigators in the field have applied a similar classification of assumed exposure with regard to type of house construction and building material (94). Some specific, but still uncertain, assumptions were made in another study, as the exposure was estimated even in terms of $kBq/m^3 \times$ months (82). A more crude classification has been applied in other studies, however, which only distinguish between wood and various stony materials in the walls (28).

A study of women in the Stockholm area classified highly exposed individuals as those living either in a detached house or on the bottom floor of a multifamily house (98). Measurements were made in 10% of the houses. In addition, there also was information available regarding radon that emanated from the ground in certain sectors of the geographical area involved. In a few studies, the exposure has been entirely based on direct measurements (63, 64). For many correlation studies, some general information has been used about background radiation. Data also has been used on radon in water and geological features, for example (3, 16, 33, 37, 41, 46, 48).

CASE-CONTROL AND COHORT STUDIES ON INDOOR RADON AND LUNG CANCER

Until 1990, most of the studies on indoor radon were of the case-control type, with rather small numbers involved. The results are relatively consistent: They show some degree of an increased lung cancer risk in relation to assumed or measured levels of indoor radon progeny. The risk ratios have averaged around 2, but have been higher for some subgroups. The main results from these various early studies are summarized in Table 3.

Usually, no distinction has been made with regard to histologic types of lung cancer in these studies, but Svensson et al (98) specifically considered oat-cell and other anaplastic lung cancers in women only. Damber & Larsson (28) demonstrated an interesting predominance of squamous and small cell carcinomas among individuals who had lived in nonwooden houses. We may recall that a considerable relative excess of small cell undifferentiated lung cancers appeared especially in the early studies on uranium miners, even if the spectrum of histologic types has become less extreme with a longer follow-up (7, 50, 87).

Three recent case-control studies, two Swedish and one American (10, 91, 99), used larger numbers and better exposure measurements. The results of these new studies are largely consistent with the previous studies, which suggest a lung cancer risk from indoor radon.

Table 3   A summary of some earlier case-control studies of lung cancer and exposure to indoor radon and progeny

Number of cases to controls	Rate ratio	Confidence interval, CI %	Remarks	Reference number
37/178	1.8	CI 90:0.99–3.2	Significant trend	11
50/50	2.1		Published abstract only	64
23/202	Up to 4.3	CI 90:1.7–10.6		38
Two sets of 30/30			Significant high exposure for smoking cases	82
604/(467 × 2 + 137)	Up to 2.0	CI 95:1.0–4.1	For more than 20 years in wooden houses	28
292/584	2.2	CI 95:1.2–4.0	Women with oat-cell cancer	98
27/49	Up to 11.9		Risk of 11.9 for 10 WLM	66

In one of the Swedish studies (10), the method is similar to that which was used in the earlier investigation from the island of Öland (38). Hence, this new study focused on an area with alum shale deposits in central south Sweden. Building material and other characteristics of the houses also were accounted for in the assessment of exposure. Measurements were made in 143 of 177 case houses; economic constraints limited direct measurement to 251 of the 673 controls. As in the previous study, individuals were again required to have lived at the same (and last) address for at least 30 years.

The current levels of indoor radon progeny that correspond to the chosen exposure categories were 112 (0.030 WL), 97 (0.026 WL), and 57 Bq/m^3 EER (0.015 WL), respectively, in those houses that were measured with α-sensitive film. Alternative, dichotomized categories, which were based on wall materials only, measured values that varied from 151 Bq/m^3 EER (0.041 WL) for lightweight alum shale concrete or mixed materials to 87 Bq/m^3 EER (0.024 WL) for wood, brick, and other stony material. This other stony material apparently did not have any particularly high radioactivity.

The result of the study well reproduced the findings from the earlier studies by the same group of investigators (11, 38). Hence, the risk ratios over the exposure categories were 1.0, 1.5, and 1.8, respectively. However, by considering age, sex, smoking habits, and urban-rural distribution, nonsmokers, passive smokers, and occasional smokers in rural areas showed an increasing risk with higher category of assumed exposure. There was no such pattern, however, for the smokers, nor for the urban population irrespective of smoking habits. The same findings also appeared for the subset of cases and controls for whom there were measurements of indoor radon daughter levels. However, only cases, albeit in small numbers, but no controls appeared among the smokers in the highest exposure category based on the measurements. With regard to wall materials in the homes, the risk ratio was 2 (the 90% confidence interval, CI 90 was 1.1–3.7) for residents of houses with high, in contrast to low, radon daughter levels, when both rural and urban subjects were included.

Another Swedish study (99) was based on 210 incident female lung cancer cases and two control groups, i.e. one series involved 209 matched population controls and the other involved 191 hospital controls. Exposure to indoor radon progeny was estimated, but the estimates were checked by measurements in 10.9% of the dwellings that had been lived in for more than two years. In addition, the dwellings were classified with regard to whether ground contact was likely to have increased the level of indoor radon. Risk ratios of 1.8 and 1.7 were obtained for the medium and high categories of cumulated exposure, respectively, with the strongest effect for small cell carcinoma and the weakest for adenocarcinoma. Together, squamous and small cell carcinomas resulted in risk ratios of 2.3 and 3.1 in the respective exposure categories. Furthermore, these risks operated primarily among the smokers. Interestingly, smoking, as controlled in the study, was negatively associated with estimated radon progeny exposure, i.e. it exerted negative confounding.

Schoenberg et al (91) have reported a case-control study for women with lung cancer that had 433 cases and 402 controls. This study was a subset of a larger case-control study of women with lung cancer in New Jersey. The women included in the radon study were those who had lived for at least ten years in a New Jersey dwelling 10–30 years before a lung cancer diagnosis. Measurements of indoor radon concentrations were made for a one-year period by α-track detectors and supplemented by short-term charcoal canister measurements in the basements. The information obtained from the latter measurements was used for 171 of the 835 women involved in the study, when the α-track measurements failed.

No significant difference was obtained for the radon concentrations measured for cases and controls, but there was a statistically significant trend for an increasing risk of lung cancer with increasing radon levels. The reported risk ratios for the four exposure categories were 1.0, 1.1, 1.3, and 4.2. Considering cumulative exposure, the trend remained, although not significant. The risk ratios were 1.0, 1.2, 0.9, and 7.2 for the respective exposure categories.

In both these evaluations, only the risk ratios for the highest exposure categories had the lower 90% confidence limit at unity, all the others had 90% confidence limits that extended below unity.

Two US studies examine cohorts. Simpson & Comstock (94) followed a mixed rural-urban population of 39,636 individuals with 298 lung cancer deaths in 1963–1975. This population had lived in houses of different constructions and building materials, but no clear effect was seen. However, a somewhat higher lung cancer rate was associated with concrete in the walls and with a construction on a concrete slab, especially for those having lived in such houses for 15 years or longer. These relationships may indicate an effect of radon progeny exposure, but they are inconclusive.

Klotz et al (61) followed another, rather small, cohort of 752 persons, who had inhabited 45 houses that were contaminated by radon from radium processing waste. A risk ratio of 1.7 (CI 95: 0.8–3.2) was found for lung cancer among white males compared with local rates. No excess of lung cancer appeared in females and nonwhites. As smoking histories were not available, and the results were somewhat inconsistent for the various subpopulations considered, the study only provides a weak indication, if any, for a health risk of indoor radon.

CORRELATION STUDIES ON INDOOR RADON AND LUNG CANCER AND OTHER TUMORS

The results obtained in correlation studies represent rather weak evidence for or against an effect of a particular agent or exposure. Correlation studies have supported the association of radon with lung cancer and other cancers in some, but not all, cases (3, 16, 33, 37, 40, 41, 45, 46, 48, 67). However, these studies do not have good indicators of radon exposure, and we might expect the results to be muddled.

In some of these studies, a correlation also has been obtained for cancers other than lung cancer, e.g. pancreatic cancer and male leukemia (35), bladder and breast cancer (16), and reproductive cancer in males, as well as for all cancers taken together (46). A high mortality rate from stomach cancer has been reported from New Mexico in an area with uranium deposits (109). A recent correlation study considered the incidence in various countries of myeloid leukemia, cancer of the kidney, melanoma, and certain childhood cancers in relation to radon exposure in the homes (45).

The stronger correlation with indoor radon of cancers other than lung cancer in this study, as in other studies, is puzzling because of a lack of any clear excess of such other cancers among miners. Henshaw et al (45) suggest however, that inhaled radon, as deposited in fat cells, rather than the radon progeny as deposited in the lungs, might be responsible for the induction of myeloid leukemia (by its further decay). The filtering of radon progeny through the kidney and the accumulation of these elements on the skin might explain the other correlations seen.

EXPOSURE TO RADON PROGENY AND SMOKING

Because smoking is a major risk factor for lung cancer, there has been considerable interest to evaluate the combined effect of radon progeny exposure and smoking. Most of the studies of miners, for which adequate information on smoking has been available, have found a more than additive relationship to a more or less clearly multiplicative interaction or synergism (5, 17, 27, 107). But, a few studies have suggested a merely additive relationship (34, 85), and sometimes even less than an additive effect (13, 26). Such observations also have been obtained from sputum cytology of uranium miners (14).

The discrepancy between the various studies regarding the joint effect of smoking and exposure to radon progeny may seem disturbing, but conceptually there is not necessarily any definite inconsistency. For example, there might be an influence of smoking on the dose received by the epithelium. Hence, especially for workers in a dusty environment, smoking would increase mucous secretion. The thickness of the mucous sheath also would increase, which in turn would determine the number of α-particles able to penetrate to the basal cells of the epithelium from which cancer may develop (9). The clearance of the mucous and the deposited radon decay products also may be influenced by smoking with consequences for the ultimate radiation dose delivered to the epithelium.

In support of this view, there is a considerably increased prevalence of bronchitis among miners who smoke (59, 95). However, the criteria used for the diagnosis of this disorder may not distinguish simple mucous hypersecretion from true bronchitis. An increase in thickness of the mucous layer of only about 10 μm would decrease the dose to the epithelium by about 50% (2, 104).

With regard to cancer development, there likely is a synergism between chemicals in tobacco smoke and the actual dose of radiation that reaches the sensitive part of the epithelium. This might explain why a more or less multiplicative interaction between smoking and radon progeny exposure has been seen in most of the studies of miners (70), especially as the more modern mines are much less dusty than some of the older ones. However, the model for the combined effect also might be a function of latency time (from exposure to tumors); this lag time might be shorter in smokers than in nonsmokers. If so, a multiplicative model would fit better to the younger populations, whereas an additive model would fit the older populations better (4).

This somewhat complex view on the interaction of smoking and radon progeny exposure is supported by animal experiments. For example, Cross et al (25) reported that smoking dogs were less affected by respiratory cancer than nonsmoking dogs when both groups were exposed to uranium ore dust and radon progeny. However, experiments with rodents have indicated that radon progeny exposure followed by exposure to cigarette smoke stimulated tumor development, whereas the reverse combination did not (23). It seems, therefore, plausible that smoking may have a double role; namely, by activating the mucous secretion, smoking reduces the radon dose. Smoking is also likely to directly act in the cancer process itself. From the epidemiological point of view, such a complex type of interaction could lead to almost any overall result, i.e. from a multiplicative to an even less than additive effect, depending on individual characteristics in the reaction pattern to dust and cigarette smoke and on the particular circumstances under which this kind of combined exposure may occur.

For exposure to indoor radon progeny and smoking, a more or less multiplicative effect has been indicated (28, 38, 68, 98), but again the findings are not consistent through all studies. Hence, the effect of this combined exposure has been less, and sometimes much less, than expected in some studies (10, 91, 99), i.e. the effect of radon progeny exposure has been weaker or absent among heavier smokers. The reason for this inconsistency is unclear, and there is no biologically meaningful interpretation to suggest at present. However, the simplest, and perhaps most likely, explanation is probably just an instability of the estimates because of the relatively small numbers involved in the various smoker categories. This assumption also may have some indirect support through the variability of the effects as indicated for the various histological types of lung cancer (99). As in studies of miners (7, 50), small cell carcinomas have shown the strongest association with indoor radon exposure (28, 98), at least with the relatively more recent and assessable exposure. The tendency towards a more normal distribution with a long follow-up time in miners may be recalled in reference to the other cancer forms.

Radon progeny have a tendency to attach to environmental tobacco smoke, as well as to other particles in the air (18). However, the fraction of unattached progeny in the air is reduced while there is a proportional increase of the attached fraction. The unattached fraction is usually believed to contribute considerably more than the attached fraction to the irradiation of the epithelium. However, the unattached radon progeny seems to be deposited in the nose to a considerable extent, i.e. some 50%, whereas the attached fraction is little affected by nose breathing (43, 56). To a great extent, the smoke attached progeny might be deposited further down into the respiratory tract, or in those regions of the bronchii in which the epithelium is less thick than in the upper respiratory tract so that the α-particles may penetrate to the basal cells, from which the cancer can develop (104). Taking these aspects together, the biological net effect of environmental tobacco smoke, the increased radioactivity of smoke-polluted indoor air, and the subsequent change of the proportion of unattached and attached radon progeny is not yet clear.

RISK ESTIMATION FOR MINERS AND THE GENERAL POPULATION

Risk estimates for exposure to radon progeny have been derived (79) from uranium miners in the Colorado Plateau area as followed for many years (73). The increase of the risk ratio over a 30-year working life was calculated to be 1.57 for a cumulated exposure of 30 WLM (above background). The corresponding excess of lung cancer deaths per 1000 miners was estimated to ten cases. Similarly, the risk ratio was estimated to 1.31 for a cumulative exposure of 15 WLM, and the expected excess of cases per 1000 miners was given as 4.9. In additive terms, exposures of 15 WLM, as well as of 30 WLM and some higher exposures, would result in an excess over lifetime of about 0.33 cases per WLM among 1000 individuals. The Committee on the Biological Effects of Ionizing Radiations (BEIR) IV report (17) arrived at a similar figure, namely 0.35 cases per WLM among 1000 individuals over their lifetimes.

If a corresponding figure is derived from some of the studies of indoor radon exposure (11, 38), the risk estimate will be 0.3–0.8 cases per WLM among 1000 individuals over their lifetimes (36). The small number of cases underlying this estimate makes the agreement with the figures from the miners highly uncertain, even if formally consistent.

A multiplicative model for the lung cancer risk from radon was adopted both by the National Institute for Occupational Safety and Health (79) and the BEIR IV (17) committee, whereas earlier risk assessments usually have presumed additivity. A multiplicative model implies synergistic effects with other causes of lung cancer that influence the background rate of this disease. Foremost among these causes is smoking, but in principle synergistic effects may occur for any preceeding exposure to radon progeny, both occupational and background in character.

The model proposed by the BEIR IV committee may be presented as

$$R(a)/r(a) = 1 + 0.025 \, M(a) \, (W + 0.5V)$$

where $R(a)$ is the lung cancer rate at age a among the exposed, $r(a)$ is the baseline rate (as in the 1980–1984 US population); $M(a)$ is 1.2 for ages less than 55 years, 1.0 for ages 55–64 years, and 0.4 for age 65 years or older. W is the cumulated exposure in WLM from 5 to 15 years before age a, and V is the cumulative exposure in WLM 15 years or more before age a. The expression $R(a)/r(a)$ represents the risk ratio at age a. Interestingly, the model suggests a greater role of relatively recent exposure for lung cancer development than usually assumed, i.e. exposure from the last 5 to 15 years has been given more weight than earlier exposure. The implication is that α-radiation to a great extent might operate as a late stage carcinogen, even if the animal experiments referred to also clearly indicate an early stage effect from exposure to radon decay products (23).

For one of the house studies (10), the M-factor in the BEIR IV model may be taken as 0.8 as an average because of the relatively high ages for the lung cancer cases. The recent exposure, W, might be calculated from the measured average for elevated exposure, i.e. 151 Bq/m^3 (4.08 WL). At age 60, with some 80% indoor occupancy time, 25 WLM would have been obtained for the more recent 15 years of exposure, W. For the earlier period of life, i.e. until age 45, V might be 50 WLM as accumulated at those probably somewhat lower exposure levels, which may have occurred in the past. Then, (W + 0.5V) would be 50 WLM, and the rate ratio, $R(a)/r(a)$, is obtained as 2, or just as found in the study with 151 Bq/m^3 (4.08 pCi/1) as the average level for the exposure category. Similar comparisons could be made for some other existing data and would presumably show reasonable agreements, as well. It is premature, however, to go into such further calculations at this time; the results of ongoing, larger studies might provide a more definite, quantitated risk estimation.

SOME CONCLUDING REMARKS

In view of the current interest for indoor radon as a potentially serious health hazard, it is not surprising that many studies are being performed worldwide. Because of the recognition of radon in mines as a health hazard, the results available so far from epidemiologic studies of indoor radon exposure suggest that much of the general population actually is at risk of lung cancer. The quantitative aspect of this health hazard is not yet possible to clearly assess because of a lack of sufficiently large studies with quantitated data. Therefore, it is important to look critically at the preliminary and crude comparisons made here between miners and general populations, especially because of a possible, and potentially considerable, influence from different other risk factors in mines, as well as in houses.

A tentative conclusion regarding the health hazard of indoor radon could perhaps be that the lung cancer risk per amount of exposure to radon progeny can be quantitatively similar, irrespective of whether the radiation has been obtained in mines or in homes. By now, it also is reasonable to believe that good insights are likely to be obtained into the dose-response and time relationships of radon progeny exposure and the interaction with smoking from the approximately 25 studies that are now under way in many countries. Considering the lifetime risk of lung cancer in miners, one extra death per 1000 miners has been proposed as possibly acceptable, but as a consequence only an exposure of about 0.1 WLM per year would be permissable (80). The magnitude of the indoor radon problem might then be appreciable, as the average background exposure in the US has been estimated to 0.2 WLM per year (and up to 0.4 WLM per year in the vicinity of radon emitting ore bodies). Furthermore, the exposure levels may be even considerably higher for large population sectors in many countries. Prevention with regard to exposure to radon and decay products is clearly no longer a specific matter in mining only, but rather a general environmental concern.

Literature Cited

1. Åkerblom, G., Wilson, C. 1982. *Radon—geological aspects of an environmental problem.* Rapporter och meddelanden nr 30. Uppsala: Sveriges geologiska undersökning
2. Altschuler, B., Nelson, N., Kuschner, M. 1964. Estimation of lung tissue dose from the inhalation of radon and daughters. *Health Phys.* 10:1137–61
3. Archer, V. E. 1987. Association of lung cancer mortality with precambrian granite. *Occup. Environ. Health* 42:87–91
4. Archer, V. E. 1988. Lung cancer risks of underground miners: cohort and case-control studies. *Yale J. Biol. Med.* 61:183–93
5. Archer, V. E., Wagoner, J. K., Lundin, F. E. 1973. Uranium mining and cigarette smoking effects on man. *J. Occup. Med.* 15:204–11
6. Archer, V. E., Roscoe, J., Brown, D. 1986. Is silica or radon daughters the important factor in the excess lung cancer among underground miners? In *Silica, Silicosis, and Cancer,* ed. D. F. Goldsmith, D. M. Winn, C. M. Shy, pp. 375–84. New York: Praeger
7. Archer, V. E., Saccomanno, G., Jones, J. H. 1974. Frequency of different histologic types of bronchogenic carcinoma as related to radon exposure. *Cancer* 34:2056–60
8. Arnstein, A. 1913. Über den sogenannten "Schneeberger Lungenkrebs." *Verh. Dtsch. Ges. Pathol.* 16:332–42
9. Axelson, O. 1984. Room for a role for radon in lung cancer causation? *Med. Hypotheses* 13:51–61

10. Axelson, O., Andersson, K., Desai, G., Fagerlund, I., Jansson, B., et al. 1988. A case-referent study on lung cancer, indoor radon and active and passive smoking. *Scand. J. Work Environ. Health* 14:286–92
11. Axelson, O., Edling, C., Kling, H. 1979. Lung cancer and residency—A case referent study on the possible impact of exposure to radon and its daughters in dwellings. *Scand. J. Work Environ. Health* 5:10–15
12. Axelson, O., Rehn, M. 1971. Lung cancer in miners. *Lancet* 2:706–7
13. Axelson, O., Sundell, L. 1978. Mining, lung cancer and smoking. *Scand. J. Work Environ. Health* 4:46–52
14. Band, P., Feldstein, M., Saccomanno, G., Watson, L., King, G. 1980. Potentiation of cigarette smoking and radiation. Evidence from a sputum cytology survey among uranium miners and controls. *Cancer* 45:1237–77
15. Battista, G., Belli, S., Carboncini, F., Comba, P., Levante, G., et al. 1988. Mortality among pyrite miners with low-level exposure to radon daughters. *Scand. J. Work Environ. Health* 14:280–85
16. Bean, J. A., Isacson, P., Hahne, R. M. A., Kohler, J. 1982. Drinking water and cancer incidence in Iowa. *Am. J. Epidemiol.* 116:924–32
17. BEIR IV. Comm. Biol. Effects Ionizing Radiations, US Natl. Res. Counc. 1988. *Health Risk of Radon and Other Internally Deposited Alpha-emitters.* Washington, DC: Natl. Acad. Press

18. Bergman, H., Edling, C., Axelson, O. 1986. Indoor radon daughter concentrations and passive smoking. *Environ. Int.* 12:17–19

19. Boyd, J. P., Doll, R., Faulds, J. S., Leiper, J. 1970. Cancer of the lung in iron ore (haematite) miners. *Br. J. Ind. Med.* 27:97–105

20. Burch, P. R. J. 1978. Smoking and lung cancer. The problem of inferring cause. *J. R. Stat. Soc.* 141(P4):437–77

21. Burch, P. R. J. 1982. Cigarette smoking and lung cancer. *Med. Hypotheses* 9: 293–306

22. Castren, O., Mäkeläinen, I., Winqvist, K., Voutilainen, A. 1987. Indoor radon measurements in Finland: A status report. See Ref. 49a, pp. 97–103

23. Chameaud, J., Masse, R., Morin, M., Lafuma, J. 1985. Lung cancer induction by radon daughters in rats; present state of the data in low dose exposures. See Ref. 95a, pp. 350–53

24. Chovil, A., Chir, B. 1981. The epidemiology of primary lung cancer in uranium miners in Ontario. *J. Occup. Med.* 23:417–21

25. Cross, F. T., Palmer, R. F., Filipy, R. E., Dagle, G. E., Stuart, B. O. 1982. Carcinogenic effects of radon daughters, uranium ore dust and cigarette smoke in beagle dogs. *Health Phys.* 42:33–52

26. Dahlgren, E. 1979. Lungcancer, hjärtkärlsjukdom och rökning hos en grupp gruvarbetare (Lung cancer, cardiovascular disease and smoking in a group of miners). *Läkartidningen* 76:4811–14

27. Damber, L., Larsson, L. G. 1982. Combined effects of mining and smoking in the causation of lung cancer. A case-control study. *Acta Radiol. Oncol.* 21: 305–13

28. Damber, L. A., Larsson, L. G. 1987. Lung cancer in males and type of dwelling. An epidemiological pilot study. *Acta Oncol.* 26:211–15

29. Dean, G. 1961. Lung cancer among white South Africans. *Br. Med. J.* 2: 1599–1605

30. Dean, G. 1979. The effects of air pollution and smoking on health in England, South Africa and Ireland. *J. Ir. Med. Assoc.* 72:284–89

31. de Villiers, A. J., Windish, J. P. 1964. Lung cancer in a fluorspar mining community. I. Radiation, dust and mortality experience. *Br. J. Ind. Med.* 21:94–109

32. Dickson, D. 1978. Home insulation may increase radiation hazard. *Nature* 276: 431

33. Dousset, M., Jammet, H. 1985. Comparison de la mortalitie par cancer dans le Limousin et le Poitou-Charentes. *Radioprotection* 20:61–67

34. Edling, C. 1982. Lung cancer and smoking in a group of iron ore miners. *Am. J. Ind. Med.* 3:191–99

35. Edling, C., Axelson, O. 1983. Quantitative aspects of radon daughter exposure and lung cancer in underground miners. *Br. J. Ind. Med.* 40:182–87

36. Edling, C., Axelson, O. 1987. Radon daughter exposure, smoking and lung cancer. *Clin. Ecol.* 5:59–64

37. Edling, C., Comba, P., Axelson, O., Flodin, U. 1982. Effects of low-dose radiation—A correlation study. *Scand. J. Work Environ. Health* 8 (Suppl. 1):59–64

38. Edling, C., Kling, H., Axelson, O. 1984. Radon in homes—A possible cause of lung cancer. *Scand. J. Work Environ. Health* 10:25–34

39. Fisher, R. A. 1974. *Smoking. The Cancer Controversy: Some Attempts to Assess the Evidence. In Collected Papers of R. A. Fisher, vol. V, 1948–1962*, ed. J. H. Bennett, pp. 428–31. Adelaide: Univ. of Adelaide

40. Fleischer, R. L. 1981. A possible association between lung cancer and phosphate mining and processing. *Health Phys.* 41:171–75

41. Forastiere, F., Valesini, S., Arca, M., Magiola, M. E., Michelozzi, P., Tasco, C. 1985. Lung cancer and natural radiation in an Italian province. *Sci. Total Environ.* 45:519–26

42. Fox, A. J., Goldblatt, P., Kinlen, L. J. 1981. A study of the mortality of Cornish tin miners. *Br. J. Ind. Med.* 38: 378–80

43. George, A. C., Breslin, A. J. 1969. Deposition of radon daughters in human exposed to uranium mine atmospheres. *Health Phys.* 17:115–24

44. Härting, F. H., Hesse, W. 1879. Der Lungenkrebs, die Bergkrankheit in den Schneeberger Gruben. *Vierteljahresschr. gerichtl. Med. öff. Gesundheitswes.* 30:296–309; 31:102–32, 313–37

45. Henshaw, D. L., Eatough, J. P., Richardson, R. B. 1990. Radon as a causative factor of myeloid leukaemia and other cancers. *Lancet* 335:1008–12

46. Hess, C. T., Weiffenbach, C. V., Norton, S. A. 1983. Environmental radon and cancer correlation in Maine. *Health Phys.* 45:339–48

47. Higenbottam, T., Shipley, M. J., Rose, G. 1982. Cigarettes, lung cancer, and coronary heart disease: The effects of

inhalation and tar yield. *J. Epidemiol. Community Health* 36:113–17

48. Hofmann, W., Katz, R., Zhang, C. 1985. Lung cancer incidence in a Chinese high background area—epidemiological results and theoretical interpretation. *Sci. Total Environ.* 45:527–34

49. Holaday, D. A. 1955. Digest of the proceedings of the 7-state conference on health hazards in uranium mining. *Arch. Ind. Health* 12:465–67

49a. Hopke, P. K., ed. 1987. *Radon and Its Decay Products—Occurence, Properties and Health Effects.* Washington, DC: Am. Chem. Soc.

50. Horacek, J., Placek, V., Sevc, J. 1977. Histologic types of bronchogenic cancer in relation to different conditions of radiation exposure. *Cancer* 34:832–35

51. Howe, G. R., Nair, R. C., Newcombe, H. B., Miller, A. B., Frost, S. E., Abbatt, J. D. 1986. Lung cancer mortality (1950–1980) in relation to radon daughter in a cohort of workers at the Eldorado Beaverlodge uranium mine. *J. Natl. Cancer Inst.* 77:357–62

52. Hultqvist, B. 1956. Studies on naturally occurring ionizing radiations with special reference to radiation dose in Swedish houses of various types. *K. Sven. Vetenskapsakad. Handl.* 4:e ser., band 6, Nr 3

53. IARC. 1987. *Monographs on the Evaluation of Carcinogenic Risks to Humans, Suppl.* 7. Lyon: Int. Agency Res. Cancer

54. IARC. 1988. *Monographs on the Evaluation of Carcinogenic Risks to Humans. Radon and Man-made Mineral Fibres.* Lyon: Int. Agency Res. Cancer

55. Int. Comm. Radiol. Prot. 1976. *Radiation Protection in Uranium and Other Mines.* ICRP Publ. No. 24. Oxford: Pergamon

56. James, A. C. 1987. A reconsideration of cells at risk and other key factors in radon daughter dosimetry. In See Ref. 49a, pp. 400–18

57. Jörgensen, H. S. 1973. A study of mortality from lung cancer among miners in Kiruna 1950–1970. *Work Environ. Health* 10:126–33

58. Jörgensen, H. S. 1984. Lung cancer among underground workers in the iron ore mine of Kiruna based on thirty years of observation. *Ann. Acad. Med. (Singapore)* 13:371–77

59. Jörgensen, H., Swensson, A. 1970. Undersökning av arbetare i gruva med dieseldrift, särskilt med hänsyn till lungfunktion, luftvägssymtom och rök-

vanor (Investigation of workers in a mine with diesel drift, especially regarding lung function, respiratory symptoms and smoking habits) AI report No. 16. Stockholm: Arbetarskyddsverket (English summary)

60. Kinlen, L. J., Willows, A. N. 1988. Decline in the lung cancer hazard: a prospective study of the mortality of iron ore miners in Cumbria. *Br. J. Ind. Med.* 45:219–24

61. Klotz, J. B., Petix, J. R., Zagraniski, R. T. 1989. Mortality of a residential cohort exposed to radon from industrially contaminated soil. *Am. J. Epidemiol.* 129:1179–86

62. Kunz, E., Sevc, J., Placek, V. 1978. Lung cancer in uranium miners. *Health Phys.* 35:579–80

63. Lanes, S. F. 1983. Lung cancer and environmental radon exposure: A case-control study. *Diss. Abstr. Int.* 43: 2787B–88B

64. Lanes, S. F., Talbott, E., Radford, E. 1982. Lung cancer and environmental radon. *Am. J. Epidemiol.* 116:565

65. Lawler, A. B., Mandel, J. S., Schuman, L. M., Lubin, J. H. 1985. A retrospective cohort mortality study of iron ore (hematite) miners in Minnesota. *J. Occup. Med.* 27:507–17

66. Lees, R. E. M., Steele, R., Robert, J. H. 1987. A case-control study of lung cancer relative to domestic radon exposure. *Int. J. Epidemiol.* 16:7–12

67. Letourneau, E. G., Mao, Y., McGregor, R. G., Semenciw, R., Smith, M. H., Wigle, D. T. 1983. Lung cancer mortality and indoor radon concentrations in 18 Canadian cities. *Proc. 16th Midyear Top. Meet. Health Phys. Soc. Epidemiol. Applied Health Physics,* Albuquerque, NM Jan. 9–13, pp. 470–83. Ottawa: Health Phys. Soc.

68. Loomis, D. P., Collman, G. W. 1987. A case-control study of lung cancer relative to domestic radon exposure. *Int. J. Epidemiol.* 16:622–23

69. Lorenz, E. 1944. Radioactivity and lung cancer; a critical review of lung cancer in the miners of Schneeberg and Joachimsthal. *J. Natl. Cancer Inst.* 5:1–5

70. Lubin, J. H. 1988. Models for the analysis of radon exposed population. *Yale J. Biol. Med.* 61:195–214

71. Lubin, J. H., Qiao, Y. L., Taylor, P. R., Yao, S.-X., Schatzkin, A., et al. 1990. Quantitative evaluation of the radon and lung cancer association in a case control study of Chinese tin miners. *Cancer Res.* 50:174–80

72. Ludewig, P., Lorenser, E. 1924. Untersuchung der Grubenluft in den Schneeberger Gruben auf den Gehalt und Radiumemanation. *Strahlenterapie* 17:428–35
73. Lundin, F. E. Jr., Wagoner, J. K., Archer, V. E. 1971. *Radon Daughter Exposure and Respiratory Cancer. Quantitative and Temporal Aspects.* NIOSH-NIEHS Joint Monogr. No. 1. Springfield, Va: Public Health Serv.
74. McGregor, R. G., Vasudev, P., Létourneau, E. G., McCullough, R. S., Prantl, F. A., Taniguchi, H. 1980. Background concentrations of radon and radon daughters in Canadian homes. *Health Phys.* 39:285–89
75. Morrison, H. I., Semenciw, R. M., Mao, Y., Corkill, D. A., Dory, A. B., et al. 1985. Lung cancer mortality and radiation exposure among the Newfoundland fuorspar miners. See Ref. 95a, pp. 354–64
76. Morrison, H. I., Semenciw, R. M., Mao, Y., Wigle, D. T. 1988. Cancer mortality among a group of fluorspar miners exposed to radon progeny. *Am. J. Epidemiol.* 128:1266–75
77. Muller, J., Wheeler, W. C., Gentleman, J. F., Suranvi, G., Kusiak, R. 1985. Study of mortality of Ontario miners. See Ref. 95a, pp. 335–43
78. Mur, J.-M., Meyer-Bisch, C., Pham, Q. T., Massin, N., Moulin, J.-J., et al. 1987. Risk of lung cancer among iron ore miners: A proportional mortality study of 1075 deceased miners in Lorraine, France. *J. Occup. Med.* 29:762–68
79. Natl. Inst. Occup. Safety Health (NIOSH) 1987. *A Recommended Standard for Occupational Exposure to Radon Progeny in Underground Mines.* Washington, DC: US Dep. Health Hum. Serv.
80. Nero, A. V., Schwehr, M. B., Nazaroff, W. W., Revzan, K. L. 1986. Distribution of airborne radon-222 concentrations in US homes. *Science* 234:992–97
81. Passey, R. D. 1962. Some problems of lung cancer. *Lancet* 2:107–12
82. Pershagen, G., Damber, L., Falk, R. 1984. Exposure to radon in dwellings and lung cancer: A pilot study. In *Indoor Air. Radon, Passive Smoking, Particulates and Housing Epidemiology,* ed. B. Berglund, T. Lindvall, J. Sundell, 2:73–78. Stockholm: Swed. Counc. Build. Res.
83. Placek, V., Smid, A., Sevc, J., Tomasek, L., Vernerova, P. 1983. Late

effects at high and very low exposure levels of the radon daughters. In *Radiation Research—Somatic and Genetic Effects. Proc. 70th Int. Congr. Radiat. Res,* ed. J. J. Broerse, G. W. Barendsen, H. B. Kal, A. J. Vanderkogel. Amsterdam: Martinus Nijhoff
84. Qiao, Y. L., Taylor, P. R., Yao, S.-X., Schatzkin, A., Mao, B.-L., et al. 1989. Relation of radon exposure and tobacco use to lung cancer among tin miners in Yunnan Province, China. *Am. J. Ind. Med.* 16:511–21
85. Radford, E. P., Renard, K. G. St. C. 1984. Lung cancer in Swedish iron miners exposed to low doses of radon daughters. *N. Engl. J. Med.* 310:1485–94
86. Roscoe, R. J., Steenland, K., Halperin, W. E., Beaumont, J. J., Waxweiler, R. J. 1989. Lung cancer mortality among nonsmoking uranium miners exposed to radon daughters. *J. Am. Med. Assoc.* 262:629–33
87. Saccomanno, G., Huth, G. C., Auerbach, O., Kuschner, M. 1988. Relationship of radioactive radon daughters and cigarette smoking in the genesis of lung cancer in uranium miners. *Cancer* 62:1402–8
88. Samet, J. M., Kutvirt, D. M., Waxweiler, R. J., Key, C. R. 1984. Uranium mining and lung cancer in Navajo men. *N. Engl. J. Med.* 310:1481–84
89. Samet, J. M., Pathak, D. R., Morgan, M. V., Marbury, M. C., Key, C. R., Valdivia, A. A. 1989. Radon progeny exposure and lung cancer risk in New Mexico U miners. *Health Phys.* 56:415–21
90. Schmier, H., Wick, A. 1985. Results from a survey of indoor radon exposures in the Federal Republic of Germany. *Sci. Total Environ.* 45:307–10
91. Schoenberg, J. B., Klotz, J. B., Wilcox, H. B., Gil-del-Real, M., Stemhagen, A., Nicholls, G. P. 1989. Lung cancer and exposure to radon in women—New Jersey. *Morbid. Mortal. Wkly. Rep.* 38:715–18
92. Sevc, J., Kunz, E., Placek, V. 1976. Lung cancer in uranium miners and longterm exposure to radon daughter products. *Health Phys.* 30:433–37
93. Sevc, J., Kunz, E., Tomasek, L., Placek, V., Horacek, J. 1988. Cancer in man after exposure to Rn daughters. *Health Phys.* 54:27–46
94. Simpson, S. G., Comstock, G. W. 1983. Lung cancer and housing characteristics. *Arch. Environ. Health* 38:248–51

95. Sluis-Cremer, G. K., Walthers, L. G., Sichel, H. F. 1967. Chronic bronchitis in miners and non-miners: An epidemiological survey of a community in the goldmining area in Transvaal. *Br. J. Ind. Med.* 24:1–12

95a. Stocker, H., ed. 1985. *Occupational Radiation Safety in Mining. Proc. Int. Conf.* Toronto: Can. Nucl. Assoc.

96. Stranden, E. 1987. Radon-222 in Norwegian dwellings. See Ref. 49a, pp. 70–83

97. Stranden, E., Berteig, L., Ugletveit, F. 1979. A study on radon in dwellings. *Health Phys.* 36:413–21

98. Svensson, C., Eklund, G., Pershagen, G. 1987. Indoor exposure to radon from the ground and bronchial cancer in women. *Int. Arch. Occup. Environ. Health* 59:123–31

99. Svensson, C., Pershagen, G., Klominek, J. 1989. Lung cancer in women and type of dwelling in relation to radon exposure. *Cancer Res.* 49:1861–65

100. Swedjemark, G. A., Buren, A., Mjönes, L. 1987. Radon levels in Swedish homes: A comparison of the 1980s with the 1950s. See Ref. 49a, pp. 85–96

101. Tirmarche, M., Brenot, J., Piechowski, J., Chameaud, J., Pradel, J. 1985. *The present state of an epidemiological study of uranium miners in France.* See Ref. 95a, pp. 344–49

102. Wagoner, J. K., Miller, R. W., Lundin, F. E. Jr., Fraumeni, J. F. Jr., Haij, M. E. 1963. Unusual mortality among a group of underground metal miners. *N. Engl. J. Med.* 269:284–89

103. Wald, N. J., Idle, M., Boreham, J., Bailey, A. 1983. Inhaling and lung cancer: an anomaly explained. *Br. Med. J.* 287:1273–75

104. Walsh, P. J. 1970. Radiation dose to the respiratory tract of uranium miners—A review of the literature. *Environ. Res.* 3:14–36

105. Waxweiler, R. J., Roscoe, R. J., Archer, V. E., Thun, M. J., Wagoner, J. K., Lundin, F. E., Jr. 1981. Mortality follow-up through 1977 of the white underground uranium miners cohort examined by the United States Public Health Service. In *Radiation Hazards in Mining: Control, Measurement and Medical Aspects,* ed. M. Gomez, pp. 823–30. New York: Soc. Min. Eng. Am. Inst. Min. Metal. Pet. Eng.

106. Waxweiler, R. J., Wagoner, J. K., Archer, V. E. 1973. Mortality of potash workers. *J. Occup. Med.* 15:486–89

107. Whittemore, A. S., McMillan, A. 1983. Lung cancer mortality among US uranium miners: A reappraisal. *J. Natl. Cancer Inst.* 71:489–99

108. WHO. 1972. *Health Hazards of the Human Environment.* Geneva: WHO

109. Wilkinson, G. S. 1985. Gastric cancer in New Mexico counties with significant deposits of uranium. *Arch. Environ. Health* 40:307–12

Annu. Rev. Publ. Health 1991. 12:257–80

EPIDEMIOLOGIC SURVEILLANCE IN DEVELOPING COUNTRIES

Ralph R. Frerichs

Department of Epidemiology, University of California at Los Angeles, Los Angeles, California 90024-1772

KEY WORDS: microcomputers, sample surveys

INTRODUCTION

Developing countries are different from technologically-developed countries in many ways. Most people are poorer, less educated, more likely to die at a young age, and less knowledgeable about factors that cause, prevent, or cure disease. Biological and physical hazards are more common, which results in greater incidence, disability, and death. Although disease is common, both the people and government have much fewer resources for prevention or medical care. Many efficacious drugs are too expensive and not readily available for those in greatest need. Salaries are so low that government physicians or nurses must work after-hours in private clinics to feed, clothe, and educate their families. The establishment and maintenance of an epidemiological surveillance system in such an environment requires a different orientation from that found in wealthier nations. The scarcity of resources is a dominant concern. Salaried time spent gathering data is lost to service activities, such as treating gastrointestinal problems or preventing childhood diseases. As a result, components in a surveillance system must be justified, as are purchases of examination tables or radiographic equipment. A costly, extensive surveillance system may cause more harm than good.

In this article I will define epidemiologic surveillance. I also will describe the various components of a surveillance program, show how microcomputers and existing software can be used to increase effectiveness, and illustrate how

257

rapid microcomputer-assisted surveys can be used to supplement existing efforts.

EPIDEMIOLOGIC SURVEILLANCE

The word "surveillance" evokes images of mystery, police, saboteurs, and intrigue. The word was adopted by the English from a French term during the Napoleonic Wars (10). The original meaning was to watch over people who supposedly had subversive or criminal tendencies so as to prevent future problems. In contrast epidemiologists use the word in a way that is now common to public health. Epidemiologists follow disease cases or deaths with the intention of preventing future harm. Thus, surveillance is "the continued scrutiny of all aspects of occurrence and spread of disease that are pertinent to effective control" (11).

An expanded definition, which has been adopted by many health professionals in the United States, was published in 1986 by the Centers for Diseases Control (CDC) (37):

> [Epidemiologic surveillance is] the on-going systematic collection, analysis, and interpretation of health data essential to the planning, implementation, and evaluation of public health practice, closely integrated with timely dissemination of these data to those who need to know. The final link in the surveillance chain is the application of these data to prevention and control. A surveillance system includes a functional capacity for data collection, analysis, and dissemination to linked public health programs.

Again, the definition emphasizes the use of systematically collected data for control of disease.

Two terms that are related to surveillance are "monitoring" and "register" (or "registry"). Monitoring and surveillance are sometimes, but not always, used synonymously (10, 30, 37). Epidemiologic surveillance is a monitoring process. Both surveillance and monitoring feature continuous scrutiny and detection of change from expected levels. A surveillance system, however, goes one step further. Because surveillance also includes feedback and control, it is actually a monitoring and control process, rather than just a monitoring process. A register is similar to a surveillance program; both feature continuous gathering of data on all disease cases in a geographically-defined area. The primary focus of a register, however, is to list cases in need of long-term treatment (e.g. tuberculosis and leprosy registers), to describe patterns and time-trends of population-based incidence or mortality rates (e.g. diabetes registers) or to provide cases or deaths for etiologic studies (e.g. cancer registers).

Monitoring and Control Process

Perhaps the best way to explain a monitoring and control process is with the analogy of a building thermostat. Assume the thermostat regulates the heating and air-conditioning system. A person sets a temperature gauge to a comfortable level. The building temperature is continuously sensed by a thermometer in the thermostat. The actual temperature is compared with the desired, previously set level. If the observed temperature differs from the expected temperature, the thermostat sends a signal to activate the heater or air-conditioner. Either one remains on until the temperature returns to the desired level. The thermostat then sends a signal to turn off the heater or air-conditioner. The process of scrutiny and control continues until either the thermostat is turned off or the system breaks down.

An epidemiologic surveillance program is similar to the temperature-regulating system. Rather than sensing temperature, the surveillance program scrutinizes the occurrence of disease in specified populations. As shown in Figure 1, such a program typically has four components: sensor, monitor, level of expectation, and controller. The sensor identifies the state of health in the population under observation and sends a reference signal, which describes the state of health. The monitor receives the reference signal and compares it with the expected level. Usually, the expectations are set based on national or local policies or standards. If the measured level of disease differs from expectation, the monitor sends an error signal to the controller. The controller, who is a person or agency with some ability to take corrective actions, acts to reduce the level of disease in the population. The effectiveness of this action is measured by the sensor, which again sends a reference signal to the monitor. If the disease incidence falls below the expected level, no

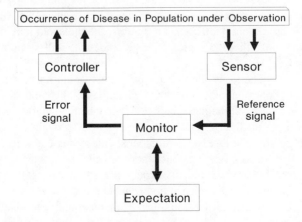

Figure 1 Components of an epidemiologic surveillance system.

further action is required. If the controller has not been successful, however, the error signal again points to the unacceptable level of disease and the process continues.

SENSOR   The sensor may take several forms. In some surveillance programs, the sensor is local physicians who are required by law to report the occurrence of notifiable diseases. In other programs, it may be health workers at a hospital or clinic. If blood is routinely screened for evidence of genetic disorders or antibodies for various infectious diseases, then the laboratory is the sensor. Teachers or school nurses may represent a sensor if they routinely report illness-associated absenteeism. Similarly, industries that routinely report absenteeism to government health agencies may be a sensor. A sensor also may be an annual interview or examination for members of the military.

MONITOR AND EXPECTATION   The monitor is usually an epidemiologist who reviews the information sent in from the field to decide if there is an acute outbreak or if the disease has reached epidemic levels. The epidemiologist compares the disease occurrence with a prior expectation and responds accordingly. For every disease, there is a threshold level of concern that might not be stated explicitly, but is there nevertheless. If a disease is uncommon, such as human rabies, or is subject to international health regulations, such as cholera, yellow fever, and plague, then the threshold to initiate action may be a single case. For more common diseases, such as malaria, influenza, and measles, the threshold may be many cases.

The level of expectation depends to a large extent on the feasibility of control and the resources of the control agency. For example, Walsh & Warren (40) note that the feasibility for malaria control in most countries is high because inexpensive drugs are available for prevention and treatment, and spraying programs work well to reduce the level of the vector. If a country has little money for control programs, the threshold may be set very high, so that only the occurrence of large epidemics will stimulate action.

CONTROLLER   The controller is the person or organization that initiates prevention or control activities. At the regional level, the controller may be a local health officer. At the national level, it may be the chief medical officer in a department of disease control. Some countries provide direct funds to epidemiology units for disease control. Most developing countries, however, maintain a tight rein on funding; the authority to allocate resources is vested in administrators, rather than epidemiologists. In such instances, the epidemiologist must explain the surveillance findings and present recommendations for action to the administrator both in a timely manner and in terms that can be understood easily.

Total Count Versus Sampling

Most surveillance programs attempt to identify all cases, deaths, or injuries in a population for the disease of interest. This type of data gathering works well in developed countries that have sufficient resources and health professionals who comply with reporting requirements. Because surveillance diseases often are rare events in wealthy countries, no single practitioner is burdened excessively by the time-demands of reporting. When the disease is more common, however, even wealthy countries revert to sampling. For example, the United States maintains an active surveillance program of pneumonia-influenza deaths. The deaths, however, are tallied each week for a sample of 121 cities, rather than for a total count of the country (5).

Samples also are commonly used in developing countries. As has been noted by the Expanded Program on Immunization (EPI) of the World Health Organization (WHO), reporting systems that require total counts are notoriously incomplete for most diseases (9). Based on EPI's experience, routine reporting is reasonably complete only when a disease is recognized as a high priority problem and when cases are less common. Thus, sampling is often the only way to obtain timely, accurate information. For example, in Myanmar (formerly Burma), hospitals are the major sources of surveillance data for several diseases. Rather than a total count of all patients, the Department of Health only requires a 10% systematic sample of hospital patients discharged alive or dead (26). Surveillance data on nutritional status in Ethiopian refugee camps are provided solely by periodic cluster surveys (42).

When routine reporting systems are not functioning properly, EPI recommends that disease-specific data be obtained in surveys of sentinel sites, such as cooperative hospitals and clinics (9). Only a few sites are selected for sentinel reporting; selection is limited to those sites that have a capable and interested staff. For common diseases, such as measles and pertussis, the EPI program recommends the use of outpatient departments of pediatric hospitals or general health centers; for less frequent diseases, such as neonatal tetanus, diphtheria, and poliomyelitis, they recommend infectious disease hospitals or rehabilitation centers. Not all researchers agree, however, that sentinel sites are effective at surveillance. Walsh (39) has presented several caveats for those researchers who plan to use sentinel surveillance, the most important of which is that the selected sites should be representative of all sites in the country.

Later in this review, I will discuss the advantage for developing countries of using occasional sample surveys to supplement a total count surveillance program. Periodic surveys are especially useful for common diseases, injuries, or other health conditions for which the burden of reporting is excessive.

Diseases Included in Surveillance Programs

Many different diseases and health conditions are included in surveillance systems. The CDC has 98 on-going systems for surveillance (3). Although many of the diseases are communicable, the list is varied and includes such conditions as ectopic pregnancies, abortions, and occupational injuries. Similar diversity was apparent in a recent text on surveillance programs, primarily in economically more developed countries (10).

For developing countries, the list of disorders is much shorter and is usually limited to infectious diseases and, possibly, nutritional disorders. Most countries attempt to gather surveillance data on cholera, yellow fever, and plague, the three diseases subject to International Health Regulations. Other conditions typically included are those under active surveillance by WHO, such as AIDS, dracunculiasis (guinea worm), poliomyelitis, influenza, and malaria. Also included are those conditions that are required to be reported at the national level by most countries, such as various forms of encephalitis and hepatitis, measles, typhoid and paratyphoid, tuberculosis, leprosy, diphtheria, pertussis, human rabies, and tetanus. Other problems occasionally reported are accidents, low weight-for-age or weight-for-height, dog bites, and snake bites.

Reporting and Feedback

In the ideal, a surveillance program receives data on a regular basis from health professionals in the field and provides them with prompt feedback on the tabulated findings. For surveillance systems that rely on multiple reporting sites, the process of reporting and feedback is shown in Figure 2. Data are systematically collected from sensors, which include hospitals, clinics, private practitioners, school nurses, and company physicians. All data are sent to

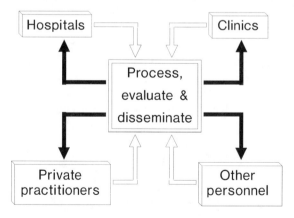

Figure 2   Reporting, processing, and feedback of surveillance data.

a central site for processing, and evaluation of disease changes over time. The information is then shared with program managers and other officials who are responsible for disease control and distributed back in summary form to the persons who initially provided the data.

The method of reporting can be either active or passive. In active surveillance, health department personnel contact sources in the field at regular intervals and requests specific data on diseases of interest. An active approach requires considerable time and effort by health department workers and is not often used in developing countries. In passive surveillance, the more common method, physicians and others in the public and private sectors complete a form for all reportable diseases. The form may be sent to the health department on a regular basis or when a disease case has been observed. Rather than relying on the salaried time of health department personnel, passive surveillance transfers part of the data acquisition cost to field professionals. Unfortunately, as noted by Evans (8), "time and lack of interest [by field personnel] greatly limit this [passive] system to a small percentage of reportable diseases." Thus, although the cost is low, so is the quality of the data.

Feedback is an extremely important component of a surveillance program. As EPI has stated, "without feedback, health workers soon realize that it makes no difference what they report or whether they report" (9). Information has value only if it is used for decision-making. If field personnel do not understand or see the results of the decision-making process, they will be less willing to contribute to future surveillance efforts.

Epidemiologic Surveillance and Health Information Systems

When a government assumes responsibility for health care, epidemiologic surveillance activities are usually included as part of the health information system. Field personnel are expected to complete reporting forms for the health information system on a regular basis and send the forms to the next highest official. At the community level, the person who delivers services also gathers data. These data are explicitly used for planning, surveillance, management, evaluation, and education. However, the implicit assumption is that the data will be used to improve health status and bring the population closer to "Health for All," the goal espoused by member nations of WHO. If health information systems did not exist, physicians and others would still deliver services and provide advice on prevention and control of various diseases. Additional knowledge should not hinder delivery; it should improve effectiveness without raising cost.

When too much time is spent gathering data, the efficiency with which a program is managed may worsen. Each health worker only has a finite amount of available time. The relationship between data-gathering time and management efficiency is shown in Figure 3. When a health worker spends little time gathering data, more time is available for the delivery of services, but not in the most efficient manner. As more data are gathered, managerial functions, such as scheduling patients, maintaining equipment, ordering supplies, arranging counseling sessions, and scheduling immunization and well-baby clinics, are improved. However, the gains in efficiency often are offset by the loss of service time. This point is labeled "threshold" in Figure 3. Once health workers have moved to the right of this threshold, too much time is spent gathering data and not enough time is spent delivering services or planning prevention or control programs. In the post-threshold situation on the right side of Figure 3, health workers become discouraged by excessive demands on their time and, as a result, no longer provide truthful information. Program administrators become overwhelmed with the volume of data and fail to review adequately the information. Finally, government health officials become cynical about quality and refuse to use the data. The cost in salary-time remains the same, but the effectiveness of the health care system is diminished.

    An example of how data gathering demands can overwhelm a health care system is taken from Myanmar in 1985 (12). Peripheral-level health workers were expected to complete more than 30 sets of forms either on a daily or monthly basis. At the rural health center level, the local staff had to submit a set of forms with 1160 variables every month. Of these variables, 72% were requested by the Division of Disease Control, the unit responsible for epidemiologic surveillance. At the next administrative level, Township Medical Officers each month had to process and review these variables, plus 786 more variables on township-level activities, for a total of 1946 variables. The surveillance needs of the Division of Disease Control accounted for nearly 1000 of the variables sent forward by the Township Medical Officer. By the time the information was received at the national level, processed and analyzed, and included in a detailed report, three years would pass. The

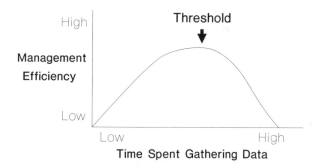

Figure 3 Effect of data gathering time on management efficiency.

information was then too dated to be used for decision-making. Although the surveillance report represented the time and effort of countless health workers, no one trusted the data.

When either too much information is requested or the local health worker does not understand the need for information, reporting quality and completeness decline. For example, in ten developing countries the estimated completeness of the existing surveillance program for poliomyelitis was 1–26%, with an average of 7–8% complete (41). Nearly 93% of poliomyelitis cases were typically unreported. In Myanmar, the best reporting system was a set of monthly forms with a 10% systematic sample of discharges from the nation's 614 hospitals (12). Unfortunately, even with this system that relied on government-funded physicians, only 38% of the hospitals submitted a complete set of 12 monthly reports.

Data, Information, Knowledge, and Action

Surveillance programs by definition are action oriented. They are intended to serve as an early warning system for both raging epidemics and small outbreaks. It is easy, however, for surveillance efforts to become too complicated and loose their focus on action. Realizing the danger of too much data, EPI has stated that disease-specific reporting forms should be simplified to include only the number of cases and be limited to those diseases for which control programs exist or for which control efforts would be initiated (9). A similar caveat is given by Walsh (39), who states that "data should be collected to provide information that is essential for making decisions."

The link between data and action is not always evident. As seen in Figure 4, the flow of information starts with data, a set of discrete observations or facts on cases, deaths, and people. When processed and analyzed by epidemiologists or statisticians, these data are converted to percentages (or proportions), incidence or mortality rates, prevalence or risk ratios, or indices, such as potential years of life lost (32) or days of healthy life lost (24). Nothing more happens, however, unless an administrator or program manager learns of the information and absorbs it as new knowledge. Action only follows if the administrator has the will and political power to act.

If data are to result in action, various requirements must be met. First, the epidemiologist can help determine a minimum data set essential for decision-making, but cannot control the quality or timeliness of data gathering. This requires highly motivated health workers and good supervisors. Once the data are collected, the epidemiologist must turn them into information that communicates clearly to the administrator. In much of the developing world, however, surveillance data are presented in complicated tables that are hard to read and do not point to any specific action. Thus, the administrator will often move on to other matters and either delay a decision or allocate the same

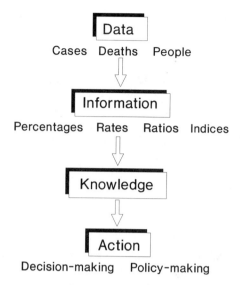

Figure 4   Link between data, information, knowledge, and action.

resources as in the past. Such decisions are especially harmful if diseases are flourishing at epidemic levels.

Graphs are the best way to present surveillance information. At minimum, every health region should have on their wall a graph showing the time trends for each disease in the surveillance system. If the disease is common, there also should be a line to distinguish epidemic levels from nonepidemic levels. Such information can easily be understood by health workers and administrators.

Action requires more than local health workers and an epidemiologist. Resources are usually scarce and there are many demands for program funds that must be satisfied by the administrator. The epidemiologist can do much, however, to guide program managers and administrators. Tugwell and colleagues have provided a framework to guide the decision-making process, which assumes that the goal is to reduce the burden that illness places on people at the community level (38).

USE OF MICROCOMPUTERS FOR SURVEILLANCE

Although much can be done in developing countries with minimal data sets, committed personnel, and active supervision, additional advances in surveillance programs can be brought about by the use of microcomputers. In the past decade, microcomputers have become increasingly important in developing countries. These small, inexpensive computers have the potential to revolutionize surveillance activities, as they have done for epidemiological research. In 1984, Frerichs & Miller (19) brought a microcomputer to Bangladesh and proved that health professionals who had never before used a computer could be taught in a short time to use this technology for epidemiologic research, data management, graphical presentations, and statistical analyses. In 1985, Gould & Frerichs (25) reported that the Bangladesh investigators were continuing to use the computer for both education applications and many research-oriented tasks. Also during the mid-1980s, Bertrand and colleagues were using microcomputers in Africa and South America for population-based surveys (1) and for management and planning purposes (2). They included an extensive surveillance program in the Sahel region of Africa to provide early warning of famine for relief projects (W. Bertrand, personal communication). Frerichs & Selwyn (20) recently have summarized many ways microcomputers serve the field of epidemiology, including data processing and analysis, program management, graphical presentations, and computer-assisted surveys.

Thacker & Berkelman (37) commented that the use of computers has increased the timeliness of data collection and analysis and has decreased the reliance of epidemiologists on programmers and statisticians for analysis and interpretation of findings. User-friendly software has allowed the epidemiologist to manipulate and analyze data for biologically- rather than statistically-significant relationships. Once, surveillance activities were hampered by lack of software; this problem no longer exists. Many types of database management programs are readily available from software vendors, along with teaching guides and reference manuals. Most of these programs, however, are costly and limited to data management. An exception is *Epi Info*.

Epi Info

Dean and colleagues at CDC have developed *Epi Info,* a multipurpose, public-domain program for word processing, database management, and statistical analysis (7). The price is minimal and includes the cost of printing the manual and preparing the computer disks for distribution. The program is used by epidemiologists around the world, including many who have been trained at CDC or by CDC personnel. The most recent version of the software was sponsored by both CDC and the Global Program on AIDS of WHO (see Ref. A). In the United States, the *Epi Info* program is of central importance to surveillance activities. Approximately 30 states use *Epi Info* to maintain, edit, and process data files containing disease reports. Every week, all 50 states send their local computer files to CDC to be merged in a standard format into a single national data file. *Epi Info* provides the standard format for the surveillance program.

For developing countries, the most recent version of the program assists with several important operations in disease surveillance. First, data from case records are entered into the computer and edited for minor errors, including duplicate entries. Second, the program processes the data and produces periodic tabulations of disease totals or disease cases. Third, frequency distributions and listings of any specified disease are produced by such variables as month, town or city, age, and sex. Fourth, the data are converted into a standard format for submission or transmission to the national reporting office. To customize the program for individual countries, CDC recommends contacting WHO representatives.

Spreadsheet Software

Among the most useful software for surveillance activities are spreadsheet programs, which resemble an accountant's ledger book with a large grid comprised of many rows and columns. The individual cells in the spreadsheet contain data, text, or formulas that relate the contents of one cell to others. The program allows health professionals to do a wide variety of functions without the assistance of professional programmers: data entry, editing, and analysis; modeling, problem solving, and decision analysis; preparing tables for annual reports; and generating many types of graphs. The following example will illustrate how a spreadsheet program can be used for surveillance purposes (see Ref. B).

Malaria has long been a problem in Southeast Asia. Cullen et al (6) have described an early warning system being used for malaria control in Northern Thailand for nearly a decade. The system is supposed to identify epidemic levels of the disease early enough so that remedial actions can prevent further spread. Following the scheme shown previously in Figure 1, the sensor is the local reporting of malaria cases (persons who are slide-positive for *Plasmodium falciparum* or *vivax*). The reference signal is the data flow from the field to the centralized processing unit at the district level. The monitor compares the observed number of malaria cases with the expected number based on nonepidemic monthly levels. Thus, the monitor attempts to determine if there are excess cases attributed to an epidemic. When the excess cases are detected, a reference signal is sent to the controller. The controller uses the information to initiate control measures, including the use of antimalarial drugs and vector control procedures.

A typical procedure for deriving excess cases is shown in Figure 5 with fourfold table common to epidemiology. The population in a given area is viewed during two time periods, when malaria is and is not at epidemic levels. During the epidemic period, persons living in the area who get malaria are listed in cell A while those who avoid the disease are in cell B. During the nonepidemic period the same two groups are cited in cells C and D. Thus, the total population in the area during the epidemic and nonepidemic periods is

A+B and C+D, respectively. All the persons in cell A had malaria. If the disease had not been epidemic, some of the persons in cell A might still have contracted malaria. These are expected or background cases. The expected cases, A_0, are derived by multiplying the malaria incidence rate during the nonepidemic period times the number of persons living in the region during the epidemic period. The excess cases, A_1, are the observed cases in cell A minus the expected cases, A_0. The excess cases represent the best estimate of cases attributed to the epidemic. By recognizing these excess cases at an early stage of the epidemic, the program manager can initiate control procedures to limit the size and duration of the epidemic.

Unfortunately, the calculation of excess cases used in actual surveillance programs is more complicated than the above-mentioned malaria example. Usually there is considerable variation from month to month in the occurrence of malaria. If the surveillance system is not very specific and identifies every increase as an epidemic, then control procedures will be initiated too frequently. That is, a nonepidemic rise will be falsely labeled as an epidemic (a false-positive epidemic). Conversely, if the surveillance program is too insensitive, then an actual epidemic will not be detected early enough (a false-negative epidemic). Cullen et al (6) also presented several, more realistic methods for determining excess malaria cases. One was favored, however, and is included here to illustrate the use of spreadsheet software (see Ref. B).

EXCESS CASES   Record keeping has been excellent in the Li District of northern Thailand for many years, which has provided Cullen et al with accurate data on the number of malaria cases. The monthly cases for nine

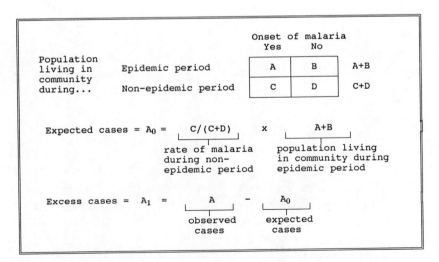

Figure 5   Determination of excess cases attributed to an epidemic.

years (1973–1981) are listed in Table 1 and shown in Figure 6. Although there was regular seasonal variation in malaria from 1973 to 1976, the peaks and valleys apparent in Figure 6 did not represent epidemic years. The data show that there were epidemics in 1977, 1978, and possibly 1981, with many more cases than expected. To derive the expected cases during 1977–1981, Cullen et al used monthly data from 1973–1976, the nonepidemic years. For each month, they determined the mean and standard deviation of cases that occurred during the four year period. Taking January as an example (see Table 1), there were 10 cases in 1973, 8 in 1974, 21 in 1975, and 24 in 1976. The mean for the four years was 15.8 cases (i.e. 63/4) with a sample standard deviation (SD) of 7.9 cases. Assuming case incidence is normally distributed, 95% of the cases per month during nonepidemic years would be expected to occur within plus or minus 1.96 SD of the mean (rounded to 2 by Cullen et al). This implies that 97.5% of the monthly malaria figures during nonepidemic months would fall below the mean plus 2 SD. Thus the mean plus 2 SD is the upper limit of monthly expected cases, which accounts for normal variation from one month to the next. Cases above this expected limit are termed excess cases.

EARLY WARNING   Using the spreadsheet program, the expected and excess cases are derived for the Li District data for the years 1973–1981 (see Figures

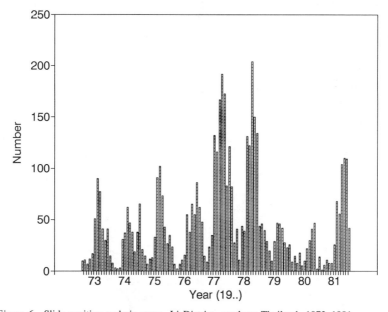

Figure 6   Slide positive malaria cases, Li District, northern Thailand, 1973–1981.

Table 1 Number of malaria cases per month for the years 1973–81 in Li district of northern Thailand (6)

Year	Jan.	Feb.	Mar.	Apr.	May	June	July	Aug.	Sep.	Oct.	Nov.	Dec.	Total
1973	10	11	7	12	17	51	90	77	41	30	41	15	402
1974	8	3	2	3	31	37	62	47	38	19	38	65	353
1975	21	15	7	12	13	33	91	102	73	43	27	35	472
1976	24	7	2	7	11	16	55	38	65	55	86	62	428
1977	48	15	9	24	35	132	116	167	192	173	83	121	1115
1978	82	28	41	11	44	39	131	122	204	150	134	44	1030
1979	46	40	29	20	10	29	47	46	42	28	23	26	386
1980	9	15	8	18	5	10	22	30	41	47	2	14	221
1981	1	6	11	8	8	26	68	56	104	110	109	42	549
Mean[a]	15.8	9.0	4.5	8.5	18.0	34.3	74.5	66.0	54.3	36.8	48.0	44.3	413.8
SD[b]	7.9	5.2	2.9	4.4	9.0	14.4	18.7	29.2	17.4	15.6	26.0	23.7	49.7
Mean + 2SD[c]	31.6	19.3	10.3	17.2	36.0	63.1	111.9	124.4	89.0	68.0	100.1	91.7	513.2

[a] Mean calculated for 1973–1978 (see text)
[b] Sample standard deviation for 1973–1978
[c] Mean plus two times the sample standard deviation for 1973–1978

A–D in the Appendix). Starting in January 1977, there were several months when observed malaria cases exceeded expection. As shown in Figure 7 there were 16 excess cases in January 1977, followed by both small and large increases in 1977–1978 and in 1981. Because the intention of a surveillance system is to provide early warning of an epidemic, a graph limited to excess cases provides a clearer reference signal for the controllers. Figure 7 shows such a graph, which includes an arrow pointing to the start of the epidemic. Figures 6 and 7 are the two graphs that would routinely be used by the malaria surveillance system.

In using this approach (although not with a spreadsheet program), Cullen et al pointed out that remedial actions could have been introduced in the first few months of 1977, rather than two years later in February 1979, as actually occurred (6). If the spreadsheet program had been available in Thailand and used to produce monthly tables and graphs, it might have been much easier to convince the local district administrator that action was needed. The ease and timeliness of producing these graphs points to the value of microcomputers for surveillance efforts.

Graphics Software

Graphics programs are another useful category of software for surveillance activities. Besides conventional line and bar graphs, which are featured in most spreadsheets programs, this software is used to display a wide variety of two- and three-dimensional graphs. The CDC uses many graphs in the

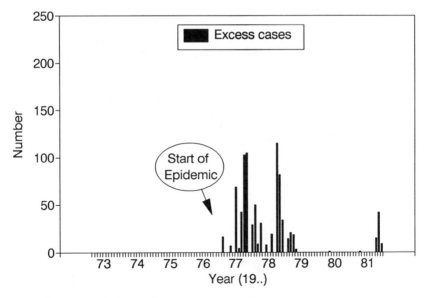

Figure 7   Excess malaria cases, Li District, northern Thailand, 1973–1981.

Morbidity and Mortality Weekly Report to notify local officials of pending health problems. Being a large agency in a wealthy country, they have computer programmers on their staff to develop specially-designed maps, graphs, and tables. Their output is generated by large computer and special graphics plotters and laser printers, none of which are available in most developing countries. Although the specific hardware and software CDC uses to display information are not readily available, commercial graphics software can often provide an acceptable substitute. Figure 8 shows a horizontal bar graph produced by one such program (see Ref. C) that is similar to the CDC surveillance graph for notifiable diseases (4). Each week, a ratio is derived of observed cases during the past four weeks to a historical average of comparable four-week periods during the prior five years. If the ratio is within normal limits, the horizontal bar for the ratio is black. If the disease has become epidemic with many excess cases, a hatched-line pattern is used to show the excess. This graph and the publication in which it appears would represent the error signal of a notifiable disease surveillance program.

A related software is the mapping program, which is used to construct and print maps of disease patterns for a given geographic area. Computer maps are a modern version of pin maps. Pins with colored heads are typically tacked in a map board to show where disease cases occurred. Different colored heads on the pins are used to designate different diseases or different groups, such as young children or males and females. Most surveillance programs in the developing world rely on both bar or line graphs and some form of pin map to show their findings. The former shows the trends over time for an entire

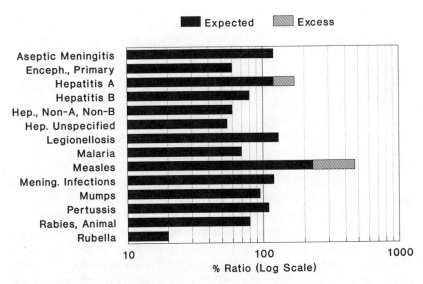

Figure 8   Expected and excess cases of notifiable diseases.

region; the latter shows the location of the individual cases. With graphics and mapping software, both figures could quickly be generated every week and shared with local decision-makers.

SAMPLE SURVEYS TO SUPPLEMENT SURVEILLANCE

Sample surveys can provide important data to supplement information derived from a surveillance system. Even when surveillance is effective, however, more information may be needed to plan and implement control efforts or to evaluate their impact on the population once the control program is in place. Surveys can provide this kind of information. Surveys may also be vital in countries that derive all their surveillance data from weekly hospital or clinic reports, rather than from a population sample. Such surveillance systems typically under-report disease cases by excluding persons who do not come to the facilities for medical assistance. Finally, surveys may provide the only source of factual information in the economically poorest countries; surveillance programs in these countries are often so inadequate that they are rarely used for decision-making. Here the governments may find that it is easier and less costly to hire and train a small survey team than to rely on a large surveillance system that cannot be effectively managed.

Large population-based surveys have been performed in many developing countries (28, 33). Examples include an extensive survey by Frerichs et al in a rural region of Bolivia (15–18), serological surveys for HIV infection in Rwanda (34), and more recently a series of demographic and health surveys being done at the national level in many developing countries by the Institute for Resource Development (27). Although these surveys do not represent surveillance efforts, they do provide useful supplementary information. Unfortunately, these large surveys of several thousand persons are costly and often require a year or more before a final report appears with the study findings.

Small, two-stage cluster surveys have been widely used by various groups in WHO to gather data on immunization coverage, diarrhea and diarrhea control procedures, neonatal tetanus, lameness (poliomyelitis), and related activities (29). These small surveys fill the information void left by limited or inadequate surveillance systems; they provide population-based data and are typically completed in a few months. The completion time was reduced even more by Frerichs and colleagues who used portable, battery-powered microcomputers to complete WHO-style surveys in a few weeks (13, 14, 21–23). Typically, they would take 3–4 days to conduct the interviews or examinations, and use a portable microcomputer to enter and edit data every afternoon or evening. On the fifth day, they present their findings in graphs and simple tables to the local medical officer and interested community members. During the following 4–5 days, they use the microcomputer and commercial software to complete the analysis, prepare tables and graphs, and produce a final written report. This form of sampling, termed "rapid survey methodology," provides yet another information source for administrators in developing countries who are faced with the time-delays and poor data quality of many surveillance programs.

UTILITY OF SURVEILLANCE PROGRAMS

For infectious disease, the early warning provided by surveillance systems allows program administrators time to start various control activities. These activities may include isolating infective cases, immunizing children, spraying pesticides, chlorinating wells, restricting food-handlers, and eliminating open sources of open water. The desired action, however, is less clear for many of the noncommunicable disease surveillance programs typically found in more developed countries.

Surveillance programs are rarely evaluated, even those programs that focus on infectious diseases. In their extensive review of surveillance in the United States, Thacker & Berkelman (37) point out that there have been no published studies on the impact of surveillance data on policies and interventions, and very few studies that relate the cost of acquiring surveillance information to any tangible benefits.

For developing countries, the need seems more apparent. However, information on the cost and usefulness of surveillance efforts is equally scarce. Smith (36) expressed this concern for surveillance programs in developing countries: "More work is . . . needed to critically evaluate the usefulness of already existing surveillance systems. If they are found not to provide useful data, then serious consideration should be given to using available resources in other ways, such as the development of sentinel sites or periodic surveys." A related concern was voiced at a recent national epidemiology conference in Chile, which concluded that the main problem with their current epidemiologic surveillance program is that it does not lead to decision-making, or else that decisions are taken too late to have an impact on the disease (31).

In the past decade, the United States Agency for International Development funded a series of methodologic studies on rapid epidemiologic assessment (REA) in developing countries. The specific intention was to develop REA methods for health planning and decision-making and to develop or validate more efficient or innovative epidemiologic methods for making timely decisions about health problems and program for health care or disease control (35).

Surveillance systems are expensive to set up and maintain. As a result, they should be evaluated along with other programs to determine if they are fulfilling their goals. This evaluation should relate the cost of the program to the effectiveness or usefulness. For most workers, timely feedback is proof enough that the system is working and that their contributions are valued. With proper graphs, they can anticipate epidemics and perceive the effects of control strategies. For administrators, program managers, and political leaders the best indication of usefulness is that epidemics are noted early and kept under control. This control is the promise of epidemiologic surveillance. However, we need to evaluate this promise.

CONCLUSION

Epidemics can devastate a population. Death and disability can drain the vitality of a community. Economic havoc follows despair as productivity decreases and even food and shelter become scarce. Surveillance systems are designed to prevent disease and empower the people by providing early warning of an epidemic. The resultant extra time can be spent battling the disease while it is still at a manageable level.

A surveillance system will be effective only if the quality of data is high, information is processed and analyzed rapidly, and the findings are clearly understood by those in power. In many developing countries, data collection and analysis are so difficult that only the most essential information should be collected: a listing of cases and deaths by cause, time of onset, and geographic area where the cases occurred. If resources are available, other related information should be considered, such as age, sex, characteristics of the agent, and circumstances leading to the disease onset. In many instances, however, the value of this additional information will not justify the added cost. When more extensive information is sought, it should be acquired in periodic community-based surveys.

Inexpensive microcomputers are being used by many national or district health departments throughout the third world. By using current computer hardware and software, surveillance data can be quickly processed and analyzed, and findings can be rapidly converted into simple, easy to understand tables and graphs. If surveillance data are believable and presented in a timely manner, administrators and program managers will be more inclined to use them to serve the community.

APPENDIX

Table 1 is entered into the spreadsheet program as numbers, text and formulas as shown in Figure A (see Ref. A). Rows 1 through 13 contain only text and numbers; rows 14 through 16 contain text and formulas. Figure B shows the same spreadsheet, but with formulae rather than calculations as shown in Figure A. The width of columns B through E was expanded to show the formulae. Elsewhere in the same spreadsheet, four long rows are created with the year in the top row, the observed malaria cases per month in the second row, the expected monthly cases in the third row, and the excess cases in the

```
 File  Edit  Style  Graph  Print  Database  Tools  Options  Window          ↑↓
A1: U [W9] 'Table 3. Number of Malaria cases per month for the years 1973-81|  ?
J       A      B      C      D      E      F      G      H      I      J      K
1    Table 1. Number of Malaria cases per month for the years 1973-81 in Li d■End
2             of northern Thailand                                             ▲
                                                                             ◄ ►
3    Year     Jan.  Feb.  Mar.  Apr.   May  June  July  Aug.  Sep.  Oct.      ▼

4       1973   10    11     7    12    17    51    90    77    41    30      Esc
5       1974    8     3     2     3    31    37    62    47    38    19
6       1975   21    15     7    12    13    33    91   102    73    43      ←┘
7       1976   24     7     2     7    11    16    55    38    65    55
8    ....................................................................    Del
9       1977   48    15     9    24    35   132   116   167   192   173
10      1978   82    28    41    11    44    39   131   122   204   150       a
11      1979   46    40    29    20    10    29    47    46    42    28
12      1980    9    15     8    18     5    10    22    30    41    47       5
13      1981    1     6    11     8     8    26    68    56   104   110
                                                                             6
14   Mean    15.8   9.0   4.5   8.5  18.0  34.3  74.5  66.0  54.3  36.8
15   SD       7.9   5.2   2.9   4.4   9.0  14.4  18.7  29.2  17.4  15.6       7
16   Mean+2SD 31.6  19.3  10.3  17.2  36.0  63.1 111.9 124.4  89.0  68.0
                                                                             ↓
LI.WQ1      [1]                            CALC                         READY
```

Figure A Image on computer monitor of spreadsheet entries.

```
 File  Edit  Style  Graph  Print  Database  Tools  Options  Window          ↑↓
A1: U [W15] 'Table 3. Number of Malaria cases per month for the years 1973-8|  ?
J       A             B              C              D              E
1    Table 3. Number of Malaria cases per month for the years 1973-81 in Li d■End
2             of northern Thailand                                             ▲
                                                                             ■◄ ►
3    Year          Jan.           Feb.           Mar.           Apr.          ▼

4       1973         10             11             7             12         Esc
5       1974          8              3             2              3
6       1975         21             15             7             12         ←┘
7       1976         24              7             2              7
8    ....................................................................    Del
9       1977         48             15             9             24
10      1978         82             28            41             11          a
11      1979         46             40            29             20
12      1980          9             15             8             18          5
13      1981          1              6            11              8
                                                                            6
14   Mean    aAVG(B4..B7)   aAVG(C4..C7)   aAVG(D4..D7)   aAVG(E4..E7)
15   SD      aSTDS(B4..B7)  aSTDS(C4..C7)  aSTDS(D4..D7)  aSTDS(E4..E7)       7
16   Mean+2SD +B14+2*B15    +C14+2*C15     +D14+2*D15     +E14+2*E15
                                                                            ↓
LI.WQ1      [1]                            CALC                         READY
```

Figure B Image on computer monitor of spreadsheet formulas.

third row (see Figure C). Excess cases are defined as 0 if the observed cases are less than the expected cases and observed cases minus expected cases if the observed cases are greater than the expected cases. The formulae for deriving the excess cases are shown in Figure D. In words the formulae read, if observed minus expected is less than 0, enter 0, otherwise enter observed minus expected.

```
                              1973
Observed    10   11    7   12    17   51    90   77   41   30   41   15   continued but
Expected  31.6 19.3 10.3 17.2 36.0 63.1 112. 124. 89.0 68.0 100. 91.7   shown on next
Excess       0    0    0    0    0    0    0    0    0    0    0    0    line


                              1974
             8    3    2    3    31   37    62   47   38   19   38   65   continued but
          31.6 19.3 10.3 17.2 36.0 63.1 112. 124. 89.0 68.0 100. 91.7   shown on next
             0    0    0    0    0    0    0    0    0    0    0    0    line


                              1975
            21   15    7   12    13   33    91  102   73   43   27   35   continued but
          31.6 19.3 10.3 17.2 36.0 63.1 112. 124. 89.0 68.0 100. 91.7   shown on next
             0    0    0    0    0    0    0    0    0    0    0    0    line


                              1976
            24    7    2    7    11   16    55   38   65   55   86   62   continued but
          31.6 19.3 10.3 17.2 36.0 63.1 112. 124. 89.0 68.0 100. 91.7   shown on next
             0    0    0    0    0    0    0    0    0    0    0    0    line


                              1977
            48   15    9   24    35  132   116  167  192  173   83  121   continued but
          31.6 19.3 10.3 17.2 36.0 63.1 112. 124. 89.0 68.0 100. 91.7   shown on next
          16.4    0    0 6.78    0 68.9 4.10 42.6 103. 105.    0 29.3   line


                              1978
            82   28   41   11    44   39   131  122  204  150  134   44   continued but
          31.6 19.3 10.3 17.2 36.0 63.1 112. 124. 89.0 68.0 100. 91.7   shown on next
          50.4 8.67 30.7    0 7.96    0 19.1    0 115. 82.0 33.9    0   line


                              1979
            46   40   29   20    10   29    47   46   42   28   23   26   continued but
          31.6 19.3 10.3 17.2 36.0 63.1 112. 124. 89.0 68.0 100. 91.7   shown on next
          14.4 20.7 18.7 2.78    0    0    0    0    0    0    0    0   line


                              1980
             9   15    8   18     5   10    22   30   41   47    2   14   continued but
          31.6 19.3 10.3 17.2 36.0 63.1 112. 124. 89.0 68.0 100. 91.7   shown on next
             0    0    0 .782    0    0    0    0    0    0    0    0   line


                              1981
             1    6   11    8    26   68    56  104  110  109   42
          31.6 19.3 10.3 17.2 36.0 63.1 112. 124. 89.0 68.0 100. 91.7
             0    0 .726    0    0    0    0    0 15.0 42.0 8.92    0
```

Figure C Spreadsheet entries for observed, expected, and excess cases (entered but not shown as four long rows).

```
 File  Edit  Style  Graph  Print  Database  Tools  Options  Window          ↑↓
P1: [W11]                                                                   | ?
 J        P              Q                         R                        ───
1                                                                          ■End
2    Observed                    10                      11                 ▲
3    Expected                  31.6                    19.3                ◄ ►
4    Excess        @IF((Q2-Q3)<0,0,Q2-Q3)  @IF((R2-R3)<0,0,R2-R3)          ▼
5
6                                                                          Esc
```

Figure D Spreadsheet formulas for observed, expected, and excess cases (entered as four long rows starting in cells P1 through P4; top row is year).

Literature Cited

1. Bertrand, W. E. 1985. Microcomputer applications in health population surveys: experience and potential in developing countries. *World Health Stat. Q.* 38(1):91–100
2. Bertrand, W. E. 1987. Use of microcomputers in health and social service applications in developing countries. *Crit. Rev. Med. Informatics* 1(3):229–40
3. Cent. Dis. Control. 1986. Comprehensive plan for epidemiologic surveillance. *General Surveillance Activities.* Atlanta: Cent. Dis. Control
4. Cent. Dis. Control. 1989. Proposed changes in format for presentation of notifiable disease report data. *Morb. Mortal. Wkly. Rep.* 38(47):805–09
5. Cent. Dis. Control. 1990. Update: Influenza—United States, 1989–90. *Morb. Mortal. Wkly. Rep.* 39:157–59
6. Cullen, J. R., Chitprarop, U., Doberstyn, E. B., Sombatwattanangkul, K. 1984. An epidemiological early warning system for malaria control in northern Thailand. *Bull. WHO.* 62:107–14
7. Dean, A. G., Dean, J. A., Burton, A. H., Dicker, R. C. 1990. Epi Info, Version 5.0: a word-processing, database, and statistics program for epidemiology on microcomputers. Atlanta: Cent. Dis. Control. 384 pp.
8. Evans, A. S. 1989. Surveillance and seroepidemiology. In *Viral Infections of Humans—Epidemiology and Control,* ed. A. S. Evans, 2:51–73. New York/London: Plenum. 829 pp.
9. Expand. Program Immun. 1987. Disease surveillance: Information for action. *WHO Update* Dec: 1–6. Geneva, Switzerland
10. Eylenbosch, W. J., Noah, N. D. 1988. The surveillance of disease. In *Surveillance in Health and Disease,* ed. W. J. Eylenbosch, N. D. Noah, 2:9–24. Oxford/New York/Tokyo: Oxford Univ. Press. 286 pp.
11. Eylenbosch, W. J., Noah, N. D. 1988. Introduction. See Ref. 10, pp. xv–xvii
12. Frerichs, R. R. 1985. Existing health information system. In *Burma Primary Health Care II Project Report.* USAID Project 482–004. West. Consort. Public Health, Berkeley, Calif.
13. Frerichs, R. R. 1988. Rapid microcomputer surveys. *J. Trop. Pediatr.* 34:147–49
14. Frerichs, R. R. 1989. Simple analytic procedures for rapid microcomputer-assisted surveys in developing countries. *Public Health Rep.* 104(1):24–35
15. Frerichs, R. R., Becht, J. N., Foxman, B. 1980. A household survey of health and illness in rural Bolivia. *Bull. Pan Am. Health Organ.* 14:343–55
16. Frerichs, R. R., Becht, J. N., Foxman, B. 1980. Prevalence and cost of illness episodes in rural Bolivia. *Int. J. Epidemiol.* 9(3):233–38
17. Frerichs, R. R., Becht, J. N., Foxman, B. 1981. Childbearing and breastfeeding in rural Bolivia—A household survey. *J. Trop. Pediatr.* 27:245–49
18. Frerichs, R. R., Becht, J. N., Foxman, B. 1981. Screening for childhood malnutrition in rural Bolivia. *J. Trop. Pediat.* 27:285–91
19. Frerichs, R. R., Miller, R. A. 1985. Introduction of a microcomputer for health research in a developing country—the Bangladesh experience. *Public Health Rep.* 100:638–64
20. Frerichs, R. R., Selwyn, B. J. 1991. Microcomputer applications in epidemiology. In *Oxford Textbook Public Health,* ed. W. W. Holland, R. Detels, E. G. Knox. Oxford/New York: Oxford Med. Publ. 2nd ed. In press
21. Frerichs, R. R., Tar, K. T. 1988. Use of rapid survey methodology to determine immunization coverage in rural Burma. *J. Trop. Pediatr.* 34:125–30
22. Frerichs, R. R., Tar, K. T. 1988. Breastfeeding, dietary intake, and weight-for-age of children in rural Burma. *Asian-Pac. J. Public Health* 2:125–30
23. Frerichs, R. R., Tar, K. T. 1989. Computer-assisted rapid surveys in developing countries. *Public Health Rep.* 104(1):14–23
24. Ghana Health Assess. Proj. Team. 1981. A quantitative method of assessing the health impact of different diseases in less developed countries. *Int. J. Epidemiol.* 10:73–80
25. Gould, J. B., Frerichs, R. R. 1986. Training faculty in Bangladesh to use a microcomputer for public health work: a follow-up report. *Public Health Rep.* 101:616–23
26. Health Inf. Serv. 1985. Hospital inpatient morbidity and mortality data, 1982. *Burma Health Stat. Rep.* Dep. Health, Minist. Health, Rangoon, Burma. 73 pp.
27. Inst. Resour. Dev. 1990. Status of demographic and health surveys as of March 1990. *Demogr. Health Surv. Newsl.* 3(1):6–7
28. Kroeger, A. 1983. Health interview surveys in developing countries: a review of the methods and results. *Int. J. Epidemiol.* 12(4):465–81

29. Lemeshow, S., Robinson, D. 1985. Surveys to measure programme coverage and impact: a review of the methodology used by the Expanded Programme on Immunization. *World Health Stat. Q.* 38:65–75

30. Lwanga, S., (Chairman). 1978. Statistical principles of monitoring and surveillance in public health. *Bull. WHO* 56:713–22

31. Pan Am. Health Organ. 1990. First Chilean meeting on epidemiology. *Epidemiol. Bull.* 10(4):1–16

32. Romeder, J-M., McWhinnie, J. R. 1977. Potential years of life lost between ages 1 and 70: an indicator of premature mortality for health planning. *Int. J. Epidemiol.* 6:143–51

33. Ross, D. A., Vaughan, J. P. 1986. Health interview surveys in developing countries: a methodological review. *Stud. Fam. Plann.* 17:78–94

34. Rwandan HIV Seroprevalence Study Group. 1989. Nationwide community-based serological survey of HIV-1 and other human retrovirus infections in a Central African Country. *Lancet* 1:941–43

35. Selwyn, B. J., Frerichs, R. R., Smith, G. S., Olson, J. 1989. Rapid epidemiologic assessment: the evolution of a new discipline—introduction. *Int. J. Epidemiol.* 18(Suppl. 2):S1

36. Smith, G. S. 1989. Development of rapid epidemiologic assessment methods to evaluate health status and delivery of health services. *Int. J. Epidemiol.* 18 (4):S2–S15

37. Thacker, S. B., Berkelman, R. L. 1988. Public health surveillance in the United States. *Epidemiol. Rev.* 10:164–90

38. Tugwell, P., Bennett, K. J., Sackett, D., Haynes, B. 1985. Relative risks, benefits, and cost of intervention. In *Tropical and Geographical Medicine,* ed. K. S. Warren, A. A. F. Mahmoud, 124:1097–13. New York: McGraw-Hill. 1175 pp.

39. Walsh, J. A. 1986. Prioritizing for primary health care: methods for data collection and analysis. In *Strategies for Primary Health Care,* ed. J. A. Walsh, K. S. Warren. Chicago/London: Univ. Chicago Press. 330 pp.

40. Walsh, J. A., Warren, K. S. 1980. Selective primary health care: an interim strategy for disease control in developing countries. *Soc. Sci. Med.* 14C:145–63

41. WHO. 1982. *Wkly. Epidemiol. Rec.* 57:361–68

42. WHO. 1990. Nutritional status of Somali refugees in Eastern Ethiopia, September 1988–May 1989. *Wkly. Epidemiol. Rec.* 65(13):93–100

SOFTWARE

A. Epi Info, Version 5. 1990. Div. Surveill. Epidemiol. Stud., Epidemiol. Program Off., Cent. Dis. Control, Atlanta, Ga. 30333

B. Quattro Pro, Version 2. 1990. Borland Int. Inc., 1800 Green Hills Road, P.O. Box 660001, Scotts Valley, Calif., 95067-0001

C. Harvard Graphics, Version 2.3. 1990. Software Publ. Corp., P.O. Box 7210, 1901 Landings Dr., Mountain View, Calif., 94039-7210

Annu. Rev. Publ. Health 1991. 12:281–307
Copyright © 1991 by Annual Reviews Inc. All rights reserved

COMPETING RISKS IN MORTALITY ANALYSIS

Chin Long Chiang

School of Public Health, University of California, Berkeley, California 94720

KEY WORDS: potential lifetimes, crude and net probabilities, independence of risks, life table, multiple decrement table

INTRODUCTION

Every human is continuously exposed to many risks of death, such as cancer, heart disease, and tuberculosis. Because death is not a repetitive event and is usually attributed to a single cause, these risks compete with one another for the life of a person. Competing risks must be considered in any cause-specific mortality analysis. In a study of cancer as a risk of death, for example, some persons might die from other causes during the study period. These persons no longer could die from cancer, but neither would they survive to the end of the study period. What, then, would be the contribution of their survival experience to the study, and what adjustment would have to be made for the competing effect of other causes in the study of cancer? If cancer were eliminated as a risk of death, what would be a person's chance of surviving a given time period? How many years in life expectancy has one lost because cancer is risk of death? As another example, the AIDS epidemic is spreading over the world population. Does the presence the AIDS virus infection in a population increase the death rate from pneumonia, or from heart disease? Are AIDS patients more likely to die from cancer than persons without AIDS? A meaningful study of these questions requires the evaluation of AIDS as a competing risk.

The basic statistical quantities that measure the effect of a risk of death are survival probability, death probability, and life expectation. To evaluate a risk

281

of death, we would ideally have the risk in question operate alone in a population to determine the probabilities and the expectation of life. Alternatively, we would remove the risk in question from a population and evaluate the changes in the probabilities and the life expectation. Rarely is the ideal situation realized, but one can estimate these probabilities and the expectation of life by using the theory of competing risks in a cause-specific mortality study.

In this paper, we present a brief review of the concept of competing risks and the statistical methods of mortality analysis, including estimation of three types of probability of dying with respect to a particular cause of death. We will describe formulas of estimates for cohort studies, medical follow-up studies, and analyses of mortality data for a current population. To illustrate this method of analysis, we will use the major cardiovascular (CV) diseases and malignant neoplasms mortality data of the United States white male and female population in 1986.

BACKGROUND

Evolution of the Concept of Competing Risks

The concept of competing risks began in April 1760, when Daniel Bernoulli read his memoir on mortality due to smallpox and the advantage of inoculation for its prevention before the French Academy of Science (5). During the early eighteenth century, there were constant debates and discussions in England, France, and other European countries over the advantage of inoculation against smallpox, because deaths occurred among those who were inoculated. Data were collected and tables were prepared to show the results of some inoculation programs, without definitive conclusions regarding the advantage of inoculation. Karn (31) gave a detailed account of the events related to this controversy.

Bernoulli had proposed a mathematical approach to the problem. He wanted to compare the mean duration of life in two differently constituted populations: a real population who were subject to death from smallpox and from other causes versus another, hypothetical population for whom smallpox was not a cause of death. Assuming that during one year one in n persons acquires smallpox, and one in m persons who had smallpox dies, Bernoulli arrived at a formula for estimating the number of persons who will die from smallpox. He then used Edmond Halley's (27) life table of the city of Breslou to illustrate numerically the advantage of eliminating smallpox as a cause of death. Bernoulli set $n = 8$ and $m = 8$ and calculated that inoculation against smallpox would lengthen the average duration of life by about three years.

An important assumption in Bernoulli's solution to the smallpox controversy was, in present-day terminology, a constant incidence rate ($1/n$) and a constant case fatality rate ($1/m$) for smallpox. D'Alembert, Trembley, and

Laplace all had considered the problem when n and m both were functions of age. It was D'Alembert who was the most critical of Bernoulli's solution, and his criticism prompted Bernoulli to write an "Introduction apologétique" to preface his memoir. Although he, too, recognized the value of inoculation, D'Alembert felt that Bernoulli had overstated the epidemic and overestimated the advantage of inoculation. In response to the question, "Of all persons alive at a given epoch, what fractional part has not been attacked by the small pox?" D'Alembert estimated the number at one-fourth, whereas Bernoulli estimated two-thirteenths, which gave the estimate of the smallpox "prevalence rate" at 75% (= 1–1/4) by D'Alembert and 85% (= 1–2/13) by Bernoulli. D'Alembert also stressed the difference between the immediate danger of inoculation and the remote benefit in the additional years gained through inoculation. He also distinguished physical life from civil life, from which may have emerged the concept of quality of life. It was this exchange between D'Alembert and Bernoulli that brought out the notion of competing risks. Todhunter (49) gave mathematical details of their discussion.

Makeham (36) formulated the theory of multiple decrement forces and explored the practical applications. Actuarial mathematicians have applied Makeham's work to develop multiple decrement tables in the study of life contingencies. Spurgeon (48) described methods of analysis that involved two or more causes of decrement. In particular, Spurgeon included "withdrawal from observation" in his formula for the probability of dying during a year. The result was the now popular "actuarial method," which was promoted by Berkson & Gage (4). Bailey & Haycocks (2) discussed some theoretical aspects of multiple decrement life tables. Hooker & Longley-Cook (28) considered life and other contingencies. In the area of vital statistics, Greville (26) analyzed mortality tables by cause of death. The concept of competing risks also has applications in survival analysis (29, 40), reliability theory and life testing (3), and other fields.

Two papers on the problem of competing risks that have aroused much interest among researchers in public health were by Fix & Neyman (24) and by Cornfield (15). Fix & Neyman introduced a stochastic model to describe recovery, relapse, death, and loss of patients in medical follow-up studies. Cornfield described problems in the estimation of the probability of the development of a disease when there were competing risks. Chiang (9) considered causes of death as competing risks and formulated relations between three types of probability of death with respect to a specific cause as a basis for mortality analysis.

Recent Developments

Recent developments in the subject of competing risks have been based mainly on the concept of potential lifetimes (41). Suppose that a system with r components fails as soon as one of the components fails. For example, a room that has r electrical lights connected in series becomes dark as soon as one of the bulbs burns out. Each component is subject to a failure risk R_i and has a potential or net lifetime X_i, for i = 1, . . ., r. The lifetime of the system, denoted by Y, is the smallest of $(X_1, . . . ,X_r)$, or

$$Y = \min (X_1, . . .,X_r). \tag{1.}$$

Generally it is assumed that the r potential lifetimes, denoted by an r-dimensional random vector,

$$\mathbf{X} = (X_1, . . ., X_r), \tag{2.}$$

has a joint distribution function

$$F_\mathbf{X}(\mathbf{x}) = F_\mathbf{X}(x_1, . . ., x_r). \tag{3.}$$

The marginal distribution of X_i,

$$F_{X_i} (x) = \Pr(X_i \leq x) = F_\mathbf{X}(\infty, ..,\infty,x,\infty, ..,\infty), \tag{4.}$$

is the net probability of failure of the i-th component before time x. Its complement, $1\text{-}F_{X_i} (x)$, is the net survival probability of the i-th component to time x. The ratio,

$$\frac{dF_{X_i} (x)/dx}{1 - F_{X_i} (x)} = \mu(x;i), \tag{5.}$$

is the failure rate (force of mortality) of the i-th component. Thus, the connection between the potential lifetimes and competing risks is clear. Although the marginal distribution (Eq. 4) can be derived from the joint distribution (Eq. 3), the converse is not necessarily true. When the random components $(X_1, . . ., X_r)$ are mutually dependent, the joint distribution (Eq. 3) cannot be derived from the marginal distribution (Eq. 4), for i = 1, . . .,r. In David & Moeschberger (19) and in Birnbaum (6), discussion on competing risks was given in sections that dealt separately with dependent lifetimes and with independent lifetimes. Elandt-Johnson & Johnson (22) offered a review of the theory of competing risks.

Using potential lifetimes, we can study competing risks within the framework of multivariate analysis (see, for example, 18, 34, 39). Most articles have used exponential distributions (38). Moeschberger & Klein (42) discussed consequences of departure from independence of exponential series systems. Boardman & Kendall (7) developed maximum likelihood estimators when there are only two causes of failure. Gail (25a) used the joint survival function to compare the actuarial method with other models. Birnbaum (6) devised a situation to illustrate the difference between the net and crude lifetimes of a system. In his discussion on the nonidentifiability of competing risks, Tsiatis (50) showed that, when potential lifetimes $(X_1, \ldots, X_r)$ are not known to be mutually independent, the crude probabilities are not of much use for identifying the joint distribution of $(X_1, \ldots, X_r)$ or the net distribution of each X_i. But, when risks are dependent, there is no simple statistical method available for the analysis of competing mortality risks in the human population. The competing risks problem is difficult indeed.

REMARK   There is a major conceptual difficulty in using the potential lifetime theory to study competing risks in the human population. The difficulty is in the definition of sample space. Generally, the sample space of a random vector X in formula 2 is an r-dimensional space. For every sample point $(x_1, \ldots, x_r)$, for $x_i \leq 0$, in the r-dimensional space, there is a density function $f(x_1, \ldots, x_r)$ and a distribution function

$$F_X(x) = \int_0^{x_1} \ldots \int_0^{x_r} f(t_1, \ldots, t_r) dt_1 \ldots dt_r. \qquad 6.$$

But what does the sample point $(x_1, \ldots, x_r)$ represent in a competing risks analysis? According to the concept of multivariate distribution, it represents the event that an individual dies from r different causes at r different times, which is an impossible event! A human being can die only once from a single cause, and no one dies more than once and at different times. Consequently, the corresponding density function $f(x_1, \ldots, x_r)$ has no meaning. The sample space of the random vector $X = (X_1, \ldots, X_r)$ is not an r-dimensional space, and neither is the domain of the distribution function $F_X(x)$ in formula 3. It is unclear what the sample space of the random vector X should be and how the distribution function $F_X(x)$ should be determined. Perhaps we need to reevaluate some of the theoretical results regarding competing mortality risks that are derived from the distribution function $F_X(x)$. This discussion of the conceptual difficulty also applies to the joint distribution of potential failure times in survival analysis.

In the following sections, competing risks of death will be discussed without the benefit of the potential lifetime concept. The lifetime of an individual will be represented by a single random variable that has a univariate distribution. The sample space is the positive real line, and competing risks affect the lifetime through the force of mortality.

Independence Assumption of Competing Risks

Competing risks of death are independent of one another if the force of mortality of each risk remains constant after one or more risks are eliminated or altered. Because there is no simple statistical method available for cause-specific mortality analysis when risks are dependent, independence of risks is generally assumed. But some researchers have questioned the validity of the assumption (see, for example, Ref. 47), which has become the focal point in the discussion of analysis methods. Perhaps there is no unique answer to the question of risk independence. The answer probably depends on the risks involved and, possibly, on the population under study. The independence assumption may not hold among closely related causes of death, but it may be true between distant disease categories. A direct approach to the problem is to either physically remove the specific risk from the human population or introduce a new risk of death, and check the change in mortality from other causes. This seemingly drastic proposal is not always unrealistic, as we have seen in two events of the recent past. The first event occurred in 1955, when the Salk vaccine and subsequently the Sabin vaccine drastically reduced the incidence of poliomyelitis in the United States and elsewhere in the world. A thorough analysis of mortality data in the United States before and after the vaccine should help to determine the effect of poliomyelitis on other causes of death operating in the population, particularly among the very young.

The second event was the AIDS epidemic in 1981, which was a completely new risk. The epidemic started rather suddenly and spread swiftly in the human population. Tens of thousands of persons have died of AIDS and millions of others are thought to be infected with the human immunodeficiency virus. This disease and the changes in mortality also provide us with an opportunity to verify the independence assumption, at least between major disease categories. Does the appearance of AIDS affect the force of mortality of other risks of death, such as cancer?

The National Cancer Institute (NCI) has published data that may help to determine if cancer is independent of AIDS. Table 1 was reproduced from *Cancer Statistics Reviews, 1973–1986,* published by the NCI (Ref. 43, especially Table IV-5). This table summarizes 14-year trends of cancer mortality from 1973 to 1986 in the United States among white males and females. For our purpose, the years 1973–1974 represent a period *before* the AIDS epidemic, and the years 1985–1986 represent a period *after* the outbreak. In addition to the age-specific cancer death rates during the *before* and *after* years, Table 1 contains percentage changes and the estimated annual percent changes from *before* to *after* for each age group among males and females. As most AIDS victims were young males and very few were females in 1985–1986, the white males may be considered "cases," and the white females, "controls." The changes in cancer mortality from *before* to *after* among males (cases) can be compared with the changes among females (controls) for each age group. If the changes in cancer mortality from *before*

Table 1 Summary of 14-year trends. Age specific cancer death rates by sex and age, US white population, 1973–1986[a]

Sex/Age	Average rate 1973–74	Average rate 85–86	Percent change	EAPC[b]
Males	202.7	212.6	4.9	0.4
0–54	37.3	33.1	−11.2	−1.0
0–14	6.2	4.0	−35.8	−3.4
15–34	11.3	9.2	−18.5	−1.8
35–44	47.5	40.7	−14.4	−1.3
45–54	172.3	160.4	−6.9	−0.6
55–64	492.5	494.9	0.5	0.1
65+	1290.0	1423.0	10.3	0.8
65–74	1018.0	1085.0	6.5	0.5
75+	1734.0	1975.0	13.9	1.1
Females	130.0	138.2	6.3	0.5
0–54	37.3	33.2	−11.1	−1.0
0–14	4.8	3.2	−33.7	−3.1
15–34	9.4	7.5	−20.3	−1.8
35–44	58.7	49.5	−15.6	−1.4
45–54	170.1	158.7	−6.7	−0.7
55–64	345.1	363.6	5.4	0.5
65+	690.8	790.3	14.4	1.2
65–74	553.8	651.1	17.6	1.4
75+	914.2	1017.0	11.3	0.9

[a]All sites combined. Rates per 100,000 and age-adjusted to the 1970 US standard population.
[b]EAPC: Estimated Annual Percent Change over the 14-year interval.
Source: Natl. Cancer Inst. May 1989. *Cancer Statistics Review,* Section IV, Table IV-5

to *after* among males are quite different from the changes among females, then cancer may be dependent on AIDS. If the changes in cancer mortality among males are similar to those among females, then cancer probably is independent of AIDS.

In the four age groups less than 55 years of age, the percentage changes in cancer death rates from *before* to *after* were very close: (−35.8, −18.5, −14.4, −6.9) for white males and (−33.7, −20.3, −15.6, −6.7) for white females. Thus, the NCI cancer mortality trends analysis seems to suggest that cancer is independent of AIDS. Although more data and statistical analysis are needed to establish, or to repudiate, the independence assumption, we use the assumption to proceed with our discussion.

COMPETING RISKS

Three Types of Probability

The concept of competing risks has been expressed in terms of probability of dying (9). In a mortality analysis without specification of cause of death, the meaning of the probability of dying (in a time interval) is clear. When competing risks are considered, the probability of dying is subject to various interpretations. Each interpretation leads to a different probability, and each probability serves a different purpose. One can select a particular type of probability to suit the needs of a mortality study. To understand the concept of competing risks, one needs to understand various types of probability. For a person alive at the exact age x_i, three types of probability are possible:

THE CRUDE PROBABILITY: The probability of dying from a specific cause in the presence of all other competing risks. In reference to age interval (x_i, x_{i+1}), the probability is:

$Q_{i\delta} = $ Pr (of dying in the interval (x_i, x_{i+1}) from cause R_δ in the presence of all other risks in the population).

THE NET PROBABILITY: The probability of dying if a specific risk is the only risk in effect in the population or, conversely, the probability of dying if a specific risk is eliminated from the population. For age interval (x_i, x_{i+1}), the probabilities are:

$q_{i\delta} = $ Pr (of dying in the interval (x_i, x_{i+1}) if risk R_δ is the only risk in effect in the population);
$q_{i.\delta} = $ Pr (of dying in the interval (x_i, x_{i+1}) if risk R_δ is eliminated as a risk of death).

THE PARTIAL CRUDE PROBABILITY: The probability of dying from a specific cause when another risk (or risks) is eliminated as a risk of death from the population. Or

$Q_{i\delta.1} = $ Pr (of dying in the interval (x_i, x_{i+1}) from R_δ when risk R_1 is eliminated as a risk of death);

and

$Q_{i\delta.12} = $ Pr (of dying in the interval (x_i, x_{i+1}) from R_δ when R_1 and R_2 are eliminated as risks of death).

When cause of death is not specified, the probabilities are:

$q_i = $ Pr (a person alive at age x_i will die in the interval (x_i, x_{i+1}))

and

$p_i = $ Pr (a person alive at age x_i will survive to the end of the interval (x_i, x_{i+1})),

with $q_i + p_i = 1$.

For example, if R_1 represents the risk of dying from cancer and the age interval is (40, 45), then the crude probability Q_{i1} is the probability that a person 40 years of age will die from cancer before reaching age 45. The net probability q_{i1} is the probability of the person dying in the interval (40, 45) if cancer were the only cause of death operating in a population, and $q_{i.1}$ is the probability that the person will die in interval (40, 45) if cancer were eliminated as a risk of death. If R_2 represents the risk of death from heart disease, then the partial crude probability $Q_{i2.1}$ is the probability of dying in the age interval (40, 45) from heart disease, if cancer were eliminated as a risk of death.

The probabilities p_i, q_i, and $Q_{i\delta}$ are real and can be estimated directly from a cause-specific mortality analysis. The net probabilities $q_{i\delta}$ and $q_{i.\delta}$ and the partial crude probabilities $Q_{i\delta.1}$ and $Q_{i\delta.12}$ are probabilities in a hypothetical situation. They cannot be estimated directly, but only through their relations with p_i, q_i and $Q_{i\delta}$. Generally, the net probability of dying $q_{i.\delta}$ and the partial crude probability $Q_{i\delta.1}$ are of particular interest in a mortality analysis, and we will use them in the following section.

The terms "risk" and "cause" need clarification, as both may refer to the same condition, but are distinguished by their position in time relative to the occurrence of death. Before death, a condition is a risk; after death the same condition is a cause. For example, cancer is risk of death to which a person is exposed, but cancer also is the cause of death if a person eventually dies from it.

Relations Between Crude, Net, and Partial Crude Probabilities

Suppose that r risks of death are acting simultaneously on each person in a population, and let these risks be denoted by $R_1, \ldots, R_r$. For each risk, R_δ, there is a corresponding force of mortality $\mu(t;\delta)$ such that

$\mu(t;\delta)dt = $ Pr (a person alive at time t will die in time element
$\qquad\qquad (t, t+dt)$ from risk R_δ),   7.

for $\delta = 1, \ldots, r$. The sum

$$\mu(t;1) + \ldots + \mu(t;r) = \mu(t) \qquad\qquad 8.$$

is the total force of mortality so that,

$$\mu(t)dt = \text{Pr (a person alive at time t will die in time}$$
$$\text{element } (t, \; t+dt)). \tag{9.}$$

The probability of dying q_i is a function of the force of mortality $\mu(t)$:

$$q_i = 1 - \exp\left\{ - \int_{x_1}^{x1+1} \mu(t)dt \right\}, \tag{10.}$$

where the limits of the integral are the limits of the interval (x_i, x_{i+1}). When the force of mortality $\mu(t) = \mu$ is constant in the interval, the formula of the probability q_i reduces to

$$q_i = 1 - e^{-n_i \mu}, \tag{11.}$$

where $n_i = x_{i+1} - x_i$ is the length of the interval.

PROPORTIONALITY ASSUMPTION   The theory of competing risks requires two assumptions: the above-mentioned independence assumption and the proportionality assumption described below. For each risk R_δ, the force of mortality $\mu(t;\delta)$ is a function of time t and of risk R_δ. Under the proportionality assumption, within the time interval (x_i, x_{i+1}) and ratio of $\mu(t;\delta)$ to the total force of mortality $\mu(t)$,

$$\frac{\mu(t;\delta)}{\mu(t)} = c_{i\delta}, \tag{12.}$$

is independent of t, but is a function of the interval (x_i, x_{i+1}) and of risk R_δ. This assumption permits the risk-specific force of mortality $\mu(t;\delta)$ to vary in absolute magnitude, but requires that it remain a constant proportion of the total force of mortality in the interval (x_i, x_{i+1}). David (17) has shown that the proportionality assumption in formula 12 can be satisfied whenever the underlying distribution of lifetime has one of three possible forms of the extreme-value distribution of the minimum. Thus, the assumption also is satisfied in the exponential and Weibull distributions.

Formula 12 can be extended immediately to the probability of dying. When the ratio of the risk-specific force of mortality to the total force of mortality is constant throughout a time interval, this constant must be equal to the ratio of the corresponding probabilities of dying over the entire interval. That is,

$$\frac{\mu(t;\delta)}{\mu(t)} = \frac{Q_{i\delta}}{q_i}, \tag{13.}$$

and hence

$$Q_{i\delta} = \frac{\mu(t;\delta)}{\mu(t)} q_i, \tag{14.}$$

for $\delta = 1, \ldots, r$. Thus, the (crude) probability of dying in an interval from risk R_δ is the proportion $\mu(t;\delta)/\mu(t)$ of the (total) probability of dying in the interval, q_i. The larger this proportion is, the greater is the probability of dying from the corresponding risk R_δ.

Taking the summation of both sides in equation 14, for $\delta = 1, \ldots, r$, yields the equation

$$Q_{i1} + \ldots + Q_{ir} = q_i . \tag{15.}$$

The sum on the left hand side of the equality in formula 15 is the probability of dying from one of the risks $(R_1, \ldots, R_r)$, and hence is equal to the probability of dying, q_i.

Using the proportionality assumption in formula 12, we find formulas that express the net probability $q_{i.\delta}$ and the partial crude probability $Q_{i\delta.1}$ in terms of the probabilities p_i, q_i and $Q_{i\delta}$. For example, when R_1 is eliminated as a risk of death, the net probability of dying in age interval (x_i, x_{i+1}) is

$$q_{i.1} = 1 - p_i^{(q_i - Q_{i1})/q_i}, \tag{16.}$$

and the partial crude probability of dying from R_δ is

$$Q_{i\delta.1} = \frac{Q_{i\delta}}{q_i - Q_{i1}} [1 - p_i^{(q_i - Q_{i1})/q_i}], \tag{17.}$$

for $\delta = 1, \ldots, r$. Formulas 16 and 17 are basic for estimating the net and the partial crude probabilities in practical applications of the theory of competing risks.

SOME OBSERVATIONS   Table 2 represents a hypothetical situation in which an individual is exposed to $r = 3$ risks of death (R_1, R_2, R_3) in two time intervals. The forces of mortality of risks R_1 and R_3 are constant with $\mu(t;1) = .10$ and $\mu(t;3) = .30$, respectively, in both intervals, but the force of mortality of R_2 changes, from $\mu(t;2) = .20$ in the first interval to $\mu(t;2) = .25$ in the second. These values and the total force of mortality $\mu(t)$ are recorded in columns 2 through 5. The probabilities of dying q_i, $Q_{i\delta}$, $q_{i.\delta}$, and $Q_{i\delta.1}$, computed from formulas 11, 14, 16, and 17 are shown in columns 6 through 14. The following points deserve some attention when studying competing risks of death, as illustrated with the numerical example in Table 2.

1. A risk that has a low force of mortality has a small crude probability of

Table 2 Force of mortality and probability of dying when three risks acting in a population

Time interval i (1)	Force of mortality				Crude probability				Net probability			Partial crude probability	
	R_1 $\mu(t;1)$ (2)	R_2 $\mu(t;2)$ (3)	R_3 $\mu(t;3)$ (4)	total $\mu(t)$ (5)	R_1 Q_{i1} (6)	R_2 Q_{i2} (7)	R_3 Q_{i3} (8)	total q_i (9)	R_1 $q_{i.1}$ (10)	R_2 $q_{i.2}$ (11)	R_3 $q_{i.3}$ (12)	R_2 $Q_{i2.1}$ (13)	R_3 $Q_{i3.1}$ (14)
1	.10	.20	.30	.60	.075	.150	.226	.451	.393	.330	.259	.157	.236
2	.10	.25	.30	.65	.073	.184	.221	.478	.424	.330	.295	.193	.231

COMPETING MORTALITY RISKS   293

dying. In Table 2, the force of mortality of R_1, R_2, and R_3 are in the order of magnitude: $\mu(t;1)<\mu(t;2)<\mu(t;3)$. The corresponding crude probabilities of dying are in the same order, $Q_{i1}<Q_{i2}<Q_{i3}$, in both time intervals. More precisely, the proportion of the probability of dying, q_i, attributable to a risk R_δ is equal to the proportion of the corresponding forces of mortality, $Q_{i\delta}/q_i = \mu(t;\delta)/\mu(t)$, as shown in formula 13.

In the first time interval, $Q_{i1}/q_i = \mu(t;1)/\mu(t) = .10/.60$ for risk R_1, $Q_{i2}/q_i = \mu(t;2)/\mu(t) = .20/.60$ for risk R_2, and $Q_{i3}/q_i = \mu(t;3)/\mu(t) = .30/.60$ for risk R_3.

2. Elimination of a risk that has a low force of mortality will cause a small reduction in the probability of dying. Therefore, when risk R_δ is eliminated as a risk of death, the net probability of dying $q_{i.\delta}$ has a reverse order of magnitude as that of the force of mortality.

In the first interval, the forces of mortality are: $[\mu(t;1)<\mu(t;2)<\mu(t;3)] = [.10<.20<.30]$, whereas the net probabilities are: $[q_{i.1}>q_{i.2}>q_{i.3}] = [.393>.330>.259]$.

3. When R_1 is eliminated as a risk of death, the net probability of dying $q_{i.1}$ equals the sum of the partial crude probabilities: $q_{i.1} = Q_{i2.1}+Q_{i3.1}$, because when R_1 is eliminated, an individual either dies from R_2 with a probability $Q_{i2.1}$ or dies from R_3 with a probability $Q_{i3.1}$. Therefore their sum equals $q_{i.1}$.

From columns 10, 13 and 14, we find the equality $.393 = .157+.236$ in the first interval and the equality $.424 = .193+.231$ in the second.

4. Although survival and death of an individual are determined by the force of mortality $\mu(t)$, the chance of dying from a specific cause is influenced by competing risks. For example, the crude probability of dying from risk R_1, Q_{i1}, is a function of the force of mortality $\mu(t;1)$, as well as the forces of mortality of R_2 and R_3, $\mu(t;2)$ and $\mu(t;3)$. The probability Q_{i1} decreases as the sum $\mu(t;2) + \mu(t;3)$ increases, even when $\mu(t;1)$ remains unchanged.

In Table 2, the crude probability of dying from R_1 decreases from $Q_{i1} = .075$ in the first interval to $Q_{i1} = .073$ in the second when $\mu(t;2)$ increases from $\mu(t;2) = .20$ to $\mu(t;2) = .25$, even though $\mu(t;1) = .10$ in both intervals.

5. Independence of competing risks is judged by the force of mortality, not by the (crude) probability of dying. In this example, risk R_1 is independent of risk R_2, because the force of mortality of R_1 $\mu(t;1)$ remains constant when $\mu(t;2)$ changes in the two intervals; however, the crude probability of dying from R_1, Q_{i1}, changes with $\mu(t;2)$. Similarly, risk R_3 also is independent of risk R_2, as $\mu(t;3) = .30$ in both intervals, although Q_{i3} changes with $\mu(t;2)$.

6. When R_1 is eliminated, only R_2 and R_3 remain as competing risks. The (partial crude) probability of dying from R_3 is affected by the magnitude of the force of mortality of R_2 $\mu(t;2)$.

When $\mu(t;2)$ increases from .20 to .25, the probability of dying from R_3

decreases from $Q_{i3.1} = .236$ in the first interval to $Q_{i3.1} = .231$ in the second.

The example in Table 2 was taken, with changes, from a table in Kimball (32). Kimball suggested a conditional probability of dying from a risk, say R_2, given not dying from another risk, R_1, or $Q_{i2}/(1-Q_{i1})$, as a substitute for the partial crude probability $Q_{i2.1}$. These two probabilities, however, are different in concept. Kimball's article has caused much discussion from Mantel & Bailer (37), Pike (46), and Chiang (13). Another substitute for the partial crude probability $Q_{i2.1}$ was proposed by Wong (51), who uses multiple causes of death information to estimate the additional number of deaths from R_2 if risk R_1 is eliminated as a risk of death.

Estimation of Probabilities

Chiang (9, 12) and David & Moeschberger (19) have reported methods of analysis and statistical inference in competing risks studies. This section briefly describes probability estimates in three types of studies: cohort, medical follow-up, and current population mortality analysis.

COHORT STUDIES   Let a cohort of l_0 newborn infants be observed from birth until the death of the last member of the cohort. For age interval (x_i, x_{i+1}), let l_i be the number of persons (out of l_0) alive at x_i, l_{i+1} who survive to age x_{i+1}, and $d_{i\delta}$ die from cause R_δ, for $\delta = 1, \ldots, r$, so that

$$d_{i1} + \ldots + d_{ir} \mid l_{i+1} = l_i . \qquad 18.$$

Each of the l_i individuals is subject to the probability $Q_{i\delta}$ of dying from R_δ in (x_i, x_{i+1}) and p_i of surviving to x_{i+1}, with

$$Q_{i1} + \ldots + Q_{ir} + p_i = 1. \qquad 19.$$

Estimates of the probabilities in formula 19 are the corresponding proportions in formula 18. Namely,

$$\hat{Q}_{i\delta} = d_{i\delta}/l_i, \quad \hat{q}_i = d_i/l_i, \text{ and } \hat{p}_i = l_{i+1}/l_i, \qquad 20.$$

for $\delta = 1, \ldots, r$; where $d_i = d_{i1} + \ldots + d_{ir}$ is the total number of deaths in the interval (x_i, x_{i+1}).

Substituting the estimates $\hat{Q}_{i\delta}$, $\hat{q}_i$ and $\hat{p}_i$ in formulas 16 and 17 yields the estimates of the net and the partial crude probabilities:

$$\hat{q}_{i.\delta} = 1 - [l_{i+1}/l_i]^{(d_i - d_{i\delta})/d_i}, \qquad 21.$$

and

$$\hat{Q}_{i\delta.1} = \frac{d_{i\delta}}{d_i - d_{i1}} \{1 - [l_{i+1}/l_i]^{(d_i - d_{i1})/d_i}\}.$$ 22.

Birnbaum (6) proved that, under the proportionality assumption 12, $\hat{q}_{i.\delta}$ in formula 21 is a consistent estimate of the probability $q_{i.\delta}$. Using Birnbaum's approach, we can show that $\hat{Q}_{i\delta.1}$ in formula 22 is a consistent estimate of the probability $Q_{i\delta.1}$.

MEDICAL FOLLOW-UP STUDIES   Consider a medical follow-up study conducted over a period of y years. A total of N_0 patients are admitted to the study at various times during the study period and observed until either their deaths or the end of the observation period (such as termination of the study), whichever comes first. The time of admission is taken as the common point of origin for all N_0 patients. For a given patient, time zero is the date of admission. Thus, if Patient A is admitted to the study on January 1, 1978, and Patient B is admitted on July 1, 1981, their points of origin are January 1, 1978 and July 1, 1981, respectively. The first anniversary of follow-up is January 1, 1979, for Patient A and July 1, 1982, for Patient B. It is customary in medical follow-up studies to use the anniversary year (the number of years since admission) as the time scale. The typical interval will be denoted by $(x, x+1)$, for $x = 0, 1, \ldots, y-1$, so that x is the exact number of years of follow-up. The symbol p_x will denote the probability that a patient alive at time x will survive to the end of the interval $(x, x+1)$; q_x, the probability of dying during the interval; and $Q_{x\delta}$, the probability of dying during the interval from cause R_δ, with $Q_{x1} + \ldots + Q_{xr} = q_x$, and $p_x + q_x = 1$. At time x, there are N_x patients alive and to be observed over the interval $(x, x+1)$. Of these patients, S_x will survive to time $x+1$ to become N_{x+1}; $D_{x\delta}$ will die from R_δ in $(x, x+1)$, for $\delta = 1, \ldots, r$. Finally, the sum $D_{x1} + \ldots + D_{xr} = D_x$ is the total number of deaths in $(x, x+1)$.

Up to this point, the follow-up study is similar to the cohort study. In a follow-up study, however, there are two categories of patients for whom the survival and mortality information will be incomplete. First, there will be patients who are admitted to the study between x and $x+1$ years before termination of study. These patients cannot be observed for the entire interval $(x, x+1)$. They are subject to withdrawal from the study during the interval. Second, there will be patients who are lost to the study because of follow-up failure in the interval $(x, x+1)$. Survival or death of these patients will be unknown to the researchers. These two groups of patients are different from a statistical viewpoint, simply because every one of the N_x patients is subject to the risk of getting lost, but only those who are admitted between x and $x+1$ years before termination of study are subject to withdrawal in $(x, x+1)$. Loss to follow-up can be treated as a competing risk, whereas withdrawal should not be. However, when the end of observation of each patient is known, the distinction between the two groups has little effect on the estimates of the probabilities.

The two sources of incomplete information have created interesting statistical problems. Many have contributed to the method of analysis of follow-up data. Spurgeon (48) proposed formulas to deal with withdrawals; Frost (25) introduced the concept of "person years." Others include Fix & Neyman (24), Armitage (1), Dorn (20), and Littel (35). Berkson & Gage (4) and Culter & Ederer (16) promoted the actuarial method to compute estimates of the probability q_x. Kaplan & Meier (30) introduced a nonparametric formula, and Elvebeck (23), Chiang (10), and Drolette (21) each proposed formulas. for estimating q_x. Kuzma (33) provided a review of some of these methods (see also 25a). Others have extended the follow-up concept in survival analysis and introduced several types of censorship (see, for example, 29, 40).

With the current easy access to computer facilities, one should collect more information so that statistical formulas will be simple in concept and require fewer assumptions. The most useful information in a follow-up study is the time of each death, the time of every withdrawal, and the time when a patient is lost for each lost case. With such information in mind, we can proceed to derive estimates of the probabilities $p_x, Q_{x1}, \ldots, Q_{xr}$. For convenience, being lost is considered as a competing risk denoted by R_0 with the "force" $\mu(t;0)$.

For time interval $(x, x+1)$, let

N_x = number of patients alive at time x;
S_x = number of patients who survive to $x+1$;
W_x = number of withdrawals;
    τ_i = the time of i-th withdrawal, $i = 1, \ldots, W_x$;
D_{x0} = number of lost patients;
    t_{0j} = the time at which j-th patients is lost, $j = 1, \ldots, D_{x0}$;
$D_{x\delta}$ = number died from R_δ, $\delta = 1, \ldots, r$;
    $t_{\delta j}$ = the time of j-th death from R_δ, $j = 1, \ldots, D_{x\delta}$.

The total length of time that the N_x patients are under observation in the interval $(x, x + 1)$ is

$$T_x = S_x + \sum_{i=1}^{W_x} \tau_i + \sum_{\delta=0}^{r} \sum_{j=1}^{D_{x\delta}} t_{\delta j}. \qquad 23.$$

The estimates of p_x, q_x, and $Q_{x\delta}$ are function of the number of deaths and the total length of observation T_x (12). Namely,

$$\hat{p}_x = \exp\{-D_x/T_x\}, \quad \hat{Q}_{x\delta} = \frac{D_{x\delta}}{D_x}[1 - \exp\{-D_x/T_x\}], \qquad 24.$$

and $\hat{q}_x = 1 - \hat{p}_x$. Using formulas 16 and 17 once again, we can find the estimates of the net and the partial crude probabilities. For example, the estimate of the net probability $q_{x.\delta}$ is

$$\hat{q}_{x.\delta} = 1 - \exp\{-(D_x - D_{x1})/T_x\} . \qquad 25.$$

CURRENT POPULATION MORTALITY ANALYSES   Mortality data of a current population, such as the United States 1989 population, are of the form of age-specific and age-cause-specific death rates. The National Center for Health Statistics publishes annual vital statistics that contains tables of age-specific death rate M_i and age-cause-specific death rate $M_{i\delta}$, for each cause R_δ and for each interval (x_i, x_{i+1}), by race and sex for the US population and for many geographical areas in the country. The rates also can be computed from $M_i = D_i/P_i$ and $M_{i\delta} = D_{i\delta}/P_i$, for $\delta = 1, \ldots, r$, and $i = 0, 1, \ldots, w$. Here, $D_{i\delta}$ is the number of deaths from cause R_δ, $D_i = D_{i1} + \ldots + D_{ir}$ is the total number of deaths, and P_i is the midyear population for age interval (x_i, x_{i+1}) during the current year. The midyear population P_i can be found in the Bureau of the Census publications (8).

Tables 3 and 4 show age-specific death rates for all causes (M_i), for malignant neoplasms (ICD# 140–209) (M_{i1}) and for major cardiovascular diseases (ICD# 390–448) (M_{i2}), for white males and white females in the United States in 1986. The last age interval is an open interval, x_w and above. In this case, $x_w = 85$ years.

These rates are used to derive estimates of the probabilities q_i and $Q_{i\delta}$ by means of formulas of conversion. Several conversion formulas from death rate M_i to the probability q_i (known as methods of life table construction) have appeared during the development of the life table. King (32a) used a gradua-tion process to derive q_i from M_i. Reed & Merrell (47a) proposed an ex-ponential function of M_i for $1 - q_i$. Greville (25b) used Euler-Maclaurin summation formula to obtain a formula for q_i. The formulas proposed by Chiang (11), Sirken (47b), and Keyfitz (31a) all use the concept of the fraction of the last age interval of life a_i. When a person dies in an age interval (x_i, x_{i+1}), he or she has lived a fraction of the interval before death. This fraction varies from one person to another; the mean (expected) value is the fraction a_i. Generally, the fraction a_i is invariant with respect to cause of death and is subject to little variation over time. For a discussion of the fraction see Chiang (12, p. 204). The average length of time lived in the interval (x_i, x_{i+1}) by those who die during the interval is $a_i n_i$, where $n_i = x_{i+1} - x_i$ is the length of the interval. We discuss one of the formulas below.

This formula of converting the age-specific death rate M_i to the correspond-ing age-specific probability of dying q_i is based on the following definition of the death rate M_i:

$$M_i = \frac{\text{expected number of deaths occurring in } (x_i,\ x_{i+1})}{\text{expected length of exposure to the risk of dying in } (x_i,\ x_{i+1})} \quad . \qquad 26.$$

The definition in formula 26 is independent of the number of persons involved. For a person alive at age x_i, the number of deaths is either one or zero. If the person dies in the interval (with a probability q_i), the number of deaths is one. If the person survives the interval (with a probability $1-q_i$), the number of deaths is zero. Therefore, the expected number of deaths is q_i, which is the numerator in formula 26. For the denominator, we realize that the person is exposed to the risk of dying in the entire interval $(x_i,\ x_{i+1})$. But this exposure to death ends as soon as death occurs. If the person dies in the interval (with a

Table 3 Population, death rate from all causes, from malignant neoplasms and from cardiovascular diseases by age group, US white males, 1986

Age interval (in years)	Midyear population[a] (in 1000s)	Death rate per 100,000[b]		
		All causes	Malignant neoplasms (140–208)	Cardio-vascular diseases (390–448)
x_i to x_{i+1}	P_i	M_i	M_{i1}	M_{i2}
0–1	1,565	976.6	3.0	29.0
1–5	5,973	52.2	4.7	2.4
5–10	7,171	25.3	4.1	1.0
10–15	6,849	34.7	3.6	1.3
15–20	7,757	124.2	5.5	3.1
20–25	8,532	165.6	7.9	4.6
25–30	9,347	157.6	10.8	7.5
30–35	8,846	180.6	16.4	16.3
35–40	8,028	212.3	25.9	38.0
40–45	6,144	295.6	53.0	85.8
45–50	5,060	452.0	107.7	162.9
50–55	4,603	746.3	214.4	306.0
55–60	4,742	1,221.5	390.8	521.7
60–65	4,548	1,939.8	622.6	864.4
65–70	3,928	2,908.7	900.9	1,338.2
70–75	2,948	4,602.1	1,279.6	2,200.9
75–80	1,982	6,988.1	1,661.6	3,485.7
80–85	1,080	10,825.7	2,130.6	5,723.5
85+	706	18,576.1	2,462.3	10,555.7

[a] Bur. of the Census. 1988. *Current Population Reports*, Ser. P-25, No. 1022
[b] Natl. Cent. for Health Stat. 1986. *Vital Statistics of the US*, Vol. II, Part A

Table 4 Population, death rate from all causes, from malignant neoplasms and from cardiovascular diseases by age group, US white females, 1986

Age interval (in years)	Midyear population[a] (in 1000s)	Death rate per 100,000[b]		
		All causes	Malignant neoplasms (140–208)	Cardio-vascular diseases (390–448)
x_i to x_{i+1}	P_i	M_i	M_{i1}	M_{i2}
0– 1	1,486	759.1	2.4	21.5
1– 5	5,674	40.7	3.4	2.3
5–10	6,803	17.4	3.2	0.9
10–15	6,493	19.9	3.0	1.1
15–20	7,448	49.1	3.8	1.7
20–25	8,413	51.6	4.6	2.9
25–30	9,150	54.1	8.2	4.8
30–35	8,702	67.0	16.2	7.3
35–40	8,031	94.2	33.0	12.8
40–45	6,266	156.0	65.8	28.3
45–50	5,213	250.1	116.7	54.7
50–55	4,826	416.9	197.7	103.5
55–60	5,161	650.4	299.7	187.0
60–65	5,190	1,055.0	438.7	357.0
65–70	4,707	1,608.2	580.0	630.3
70–75	3,950	2,536.7	752.4	1,155.8
75–80	3,111	3,995.0	879.0	2,101.2
80–85	2,055	6,794.5	1,073.5	4,002.8
85+	1,825	14,502.9	1,283.6	9,509.7

[a] Bur. of the Census. 1988. *Current Population Reports*, Ser. P-25, No. 1022
[b] Natl. Cent. for Health Stat. 1986. *Vital Statistics of the US*, Vol. II, Part A

probability q_i), the length of exposure is $a_i n_i$; if the person survives the interval (with a probability $1-q_i$), the length of exposure is the entire length of the interval n_i. Therefore the expected length of exposure is $q_i a_i n_i + (1-q_i)n_i$, and the analytic expression of the definition in formula 26 is

$$M_i = \frac{q_i}{q_i a_i n_i + (1 - q_i)n_i}. \qquad 27.$$

Solving equation 27 for q_i yields the desired formula for the probability q_i:

$$q_i = \frac{n_i M_i}{1 + (1 - a_i)n_i M_i}, \qquad 28.$$

which was given in Chiang (11). For a theoretical derivation see Chiang (14) and Elandt-Johnson & Johnson (22).

The age-cause-specific death rate $M_{i\delta}$ from cause R_δ is defined in a similar manner as M_i. For a person alive at age x_i, the death rate $M_{i\delta}$ is defined as:

$$M_{i\delta} = \frac{\text{expected number of deaths from cause } R_\delta \text{ in } (x_i,\ x_{i+1})}{\begin{array}{c}\text{expected length of exposure to the risk of dying from}\\ \text{cause } R_\delta \text{ in } (x_i,\ x_{i+1})\end{array}}.$$

29.

The corresponding analytic formula is

$$M_{i\delta} \quad \frac{Q_{i\delta}}{q_i a_i n_i + (1 - q_i)n_i}.$$

30.

The probability $Q_{i\delta}$ in the numerator is the expected number of deaths from R_δ in $(x_i,\ x_{i+1})$. The denominator is the expected length of exposure to the risk of dying from R_δ, which of course is the same as the denominator in formula 27. Equations 27 and 30 imply that the estimate of $Q_{i\delta}$ is given by

$$\hat{Q}_{i\delta} = \frac{M_{i\delta}}{M_i}\,\hat{q}_i.$$

31.

Note that formula 31 is a logical extension of formula 14, as the ratio of two death rates is equal to the ratio of the corresponding forces of mortality.

In summary, formulas 28 and 31 are used to estimate the probabilities q_i and $Q_{i\delta}$, for each age interval. Substituting these formulas in 16 and 17 gives formulas for estimating the net probability $q_{i.\delta}$ and the partial crude probability $Q_{i\delta.1}$. For example, estimate of $q_{i.\delta}$ is

$$\hat{q}_{i.\delta} = 1 - \hat{p}_i^{(M_i - M_{i\delta})/M_i}.$$

32.

where $\hat{p}_i = 1 - \hat{q}_i$.

An Application to Current Mortality Analysis

We have chosen the net probability of dying $(q_{i.\delta})$ as an example, and use the current mortality data from malignant neoplasms (ICD # 140–209) and major CV diseases (ICD# 390–448) of US white male and female populations in 1986 for illustration. Cardiovascular diseases and malignant neoplasms have been the major causes of death in the US for many years. These diseases accounted for nearly 70% of all deaths in the entire white population in 1986, including 75% of deaths among persons aged 55 or older. Cardiovascular diseases alone were responsible for 50% of all deaths among persons older than age 75. Tables 5, 6, and 7 show the impact of these diseases on the probability of dying and the expectation of life in numerical figures.

Table 5 Multiple decrement: Probability of dying, q_i, and crude probabilities of dying, Q_{i1}, Q_{i2}, and Q_{i3}, United States white male population and white female population, 1986[a]

Age Interval (in years) x_i to x_{i+1} (1)	White Males				White Females			
	All causes q_i (2)	Neoplasms neoplasms Q_{i1} (3)	Major CV diseases Q_{i2} (4)	Other causes Q_{i3} (5)	All causes q_i (6)	Neoplasms neoplasms Q_{i1} (7)	Major CV diseases Q_{i2} (8)	Other causes Q_{i3} (9)
00–01	0.0096	0.0000	0.0003	0.0093	0.0075	0.0000	0.0002	0.0073
01–05	0.0021	0.0002	0.0001	0.0018	0.0016	0.0001	0.0001	0.0014
05–10	0.0013	0.0002	0.0000	0.0010	0.0009	0.0002	0.0000	0.0007
10–15	0.0017	0.0002	0.0001	0.0015	0.0010	0.0001	0.0001	0.0008
15–20	0.0062	0.0003	0.0002	0.0058	0.0025	0.0002	0.0001	0.0022
20–25	0.0082	0.0004	0.0002	0.0076	0.0026	0.0002	0.0001	0.0022
25–30	0.0078	0.0005	0.0004	0.0069	0.0027	0.0004	0.0002	0.0021
30–35	0.0090	0.0008	0.0008	0.0074	0.0033	0.0008	0.0004	0.0022
35–40	0.0106	0.0013	0.0019	0.0074	0.0047	0.0016	0.0006	0.0024
40–45	0.0147	0.0026	0.0043	0.0078	0.0078	0.0033	0.0014	0.0031
45–50	0.0224	0.0053	0.0081	0.0090	0.0124	0.0058	0.0027	0.0039
50–55	0.0367	0.0105	0.0150	0.0111	0.0206	0.0098	0.0051	0.0057
55–60	0.0594	0.0190	0.0254	0.0150	0.0320	0.0148	0.0092	0.0081
60–65	0.0928	0.0298	0.0413	0.0217	0.0515	0.0214	0.0174	0.0127
65–70	0.1359	0.0421	0.0625	0.0313	0.0775	0.0279	0.0304	0.0192
70–75	0.2072	0.0576	0.0991	0.0505	0.1197	0.0355	0.0545	0.0297
75–80	0.2983	0.0709	0.1488	0.0786	0.1823	0.0401	0.0959	0.0463
80–85	0.4242	0.0835	0.2243	0.1164	0.2921	0.0461	0.1721	0.0739

[a] Figures had been individually rounded off in computer. Expected relations may not hold exactly.

MULTIPLE DECREMENT TABLE   In Table 5, typical multiple decrement tables show the relative importance of different risks of death and changes in the importance as age advances. In the present case, three risks are included: malignant neoplasms (R_1), major CV diseases (R_2), and other causes (R_3). The sum of the crude probabilities equals the probability of dying: $Q_{i1}+Q_{i2}+Q_{i3} = q_i$, for each age interval (x_i, x_{i+1}).

Under age 50, mortality level was low, with neither neoplasms nor CV diseases playing an important role in the probability of dying. From age 50 on, both CV diseases and neoplasms began to assert their influence. For white males, CV disease definitely was the greater risk of death. In age interval (50, 55), the probability of dying from CV diseases was about 40% the probability of dying from all causes (Q_{i2}/q_i =.40). This proportion increased steadily with age: from 45% for age interval (60, 65), to 50% for age interval (75, 80),

Table 6 Probability of dying in each age interval and the effect of eliminating major cardiovascular diseases as a risk of death, United States white male population and white female population, 1986[a]

Age Interval (in years) x_i to x_{i+1}	White Males				White Females			
	CV diseases present q_i	CV diseases eliminated $q_{i.2}$	Difference $q_i - q_{i.2}$	Percent change $\dfrac{q_i - q_{i.2}}{q_i} \times 100$	CV diseases present q_i	CV diseases eliminated $q_{i.2}$	Difference $q_i - q_{i.2}$	Percent change $\dfrac{q_i - q_{i.2}}{q_i} \times 100$
(1)	(2)	(3)	(4)	(5)	(6)	(7)	(8)	(9)
00–01	0.0097	0.0094	0.0003	2.96	0.0075	0.0073	0.0002	2.82
01–05	0.0021	0.0020	0.0001	4.59	0.0016	0.0015	0.0001	5.65
05–10	0.0013	0.0012	0.0000	3.95	0.0009	0.0008	0.0000	5.17
10–15	0.0017	0.0017	0.0001	3.74	0.0010	0.0009	0.0001	5.53
15–20	0.0062	0.0060	0.0002	2.49	0.0025	0.0024	0.0001	3.46
20–25	0.0082	0.0080	0.0002	2.77	0.0026	0.0024	0.0001	5.61
25–30	0.0078	0.0075	0.0004	4.74	0.0027	0.0025	0.0002	8.86
30–35	0.0090	0.0082	0.0008	8.99	0.0033	0.0030	0.0004	10.88
35–40	0.0106	0.0087	0.0019	17.82	0.0047	0.0041	0.0006	13.56
40–45	0.0147	0.0104	0.0042	28.87	0.0078	0.0064	0.0014	18.08
45–50	0.0224	0.0144	0.0080	35.78	0.0124	0.0097	0.0027	21.76
50–55	0.0367	0.0218	0.0149	40.55	0.0206	0.0156	0.0051	24.63
55–60	0.0594	0.0345	0.0249	41.96	0.0320	0.0229	0.0091	28.42
60–65	0.0928	0.0525	0.0402	43.36	0.0515	0.0344	0.0171	33.25
65–70	0.1359	0.0759	0.0601	44.20	0.0775	0.0479	0.0296	38.23
70–75	0.2072	0.1141	0.0931	44.93	0.1197	0.0670	0.0527	43.99
75–80	0.2983	0.1627	0.1356	45.46	0.1823	0.0910	0.0913	50.08
80–85	0.4242	0.2291	0.1951	46.00	0.2921	0.1323	0.1598	54.70
85+	1.0000	1.0000	0.0000	0.00	1.0000	1.0000	0.0000	0.00

[a] Figures had been individually rounded off in computer. Expected relations may not hold exactly.

Table 7 Expectation of life at each age x_i and the effect of eliminating major cardiovascular diseases as a risk of death, United States white male population and white female population, 1986

Age (in years) x_i	White Males				White Females			
	CV diseases present e_i	CV diseases eliminated $e_{i,2}$	Difference $e_{i,2} - e_1$	Percent change $\dfrac{e_{i,2} - e_i}{e_i} \times 100$	CV diseases present e_i	CV diseases eliminated $e_{i,2}$	Difference $e_{i,2} - e_1$	Percent change $\dfrac{e_{i,2} - e_i}{e_i} \times 100$
(1)	(2)	(3)	(4)	(5)	(6)	(7)	(8)	(9)
00	72.08	80.39	8.31	11.52	79.08	91.24	12.16	15.37
01	71.79	80.15	8.36	11.65	78.68	90.91	12.23	15.54
05	67.93	76.30	8.37	12.32	74.81	87.05	12.24	16.36
10	63.02	71.39	8.37	13.29	69.87	82.12	12.25	17.53
15	58.12	66.51	8.39	14.43	64.94	77.19	12.25	18.87
20	53.47	61.90	8.43	15.77	60.09	72.37	12.28	20.44
25	48.89	57.38	8.49	17.36	55.24	67.54	12.30	22.27
30	44.26	52.79	8.53	19.28	50.38	62.70	12.32	24.45
35	39.63	48.20	8.57	21.62	45.54	57.88	12.34	27.09
40	35.03	43.60	8.57	24.47	40.74	53.11	12.37	30.34
45	30.51	39.03	8.52	27.93	36.04	48.43	12.39	34.37
50	26.15	34.56	8.41	32.18	31.46	43.88	12.42	39.46
55	22.04	30.27	8.23	37.35	27.07	39.53	12.46	46.03
60	18.27	26.26	7.99	43.77	22.88	35.39	12.52	54.73
65	14.86	22.57	7.71	51.86	18.97	31.56	12.59	66.34
70	11.79	19.21	7.42	62.90	15.34	28.01	12.67	82.56
75	9.19	16.35	7.16	77.81	12.07	24.83	12.76	105.76
80	7.02	14.03	7.01	99.89	9.18	22.06	12.88	140.30
85	5.38	12.47	7.09	131.61	6.90	20.03	13.13	190.45

and 53% for age interval (80, 85). Thus, from age 75 on, about one in every two white male deaths was attributable to CV diseases.

The absolute value of the probability of dying from CV diseases also increased with age. For white males, the probability was $Q_{i2} = 150$ per 10,000 for age interval (50, 55), to $Q_{i2} = 2243$ per 10,000 for age interval (80, 85)—a 1400% increase over 35 years of life, or 40% per year!

Malignant neoplasms are the second most important risk of death. During 1986, for white males, the probability of dying from malignant neoplasms also increased with age: from $Q_{i1} = 105$ per 10,000 for age interval (50, 55) to $Q_{i1} = 835$ per 10,000 for age interval (80, 85), which is nearly a 700% increase over the 35 years. For white males, the risk of dying from neoplasms was about 70% as high as major CV diseases in the age interval 50–65 years. Beyond age 65, the relative importance of neoplasms decreases with age, because CV diseases became the dominant risk of death.

The mortality pattern among white females differs from that among white males. Table 5 confirms the general impression that females live longer. Between ages 45 and 75, the sex ratio of the probability of dying, $q_i(f):q_i(m)$, was consistently lower than 60%. Also, CV diseases were not as overwhelming a risk of death among white females as among white males. Below age 65, the probability of dying from CV diseases was lower than that from neoplasms. Beyond age 65, CV diseases overtook neoplasms and assumed the role of the major risk of death among white females.

IMPACT OF CARDIOVASCULAR DISEASES ON HUMAN MORTALITY AND HUMAN LONGEVITY   Major cardiovascular diseases, as illustrated in Tables 5–7, have caused more deaths in the human population than has any other diseases. To evaluate the impact of the CV diseases on human longevity, we can compare the mortality and survival experience of the current population with the hypothetical experience of the same population under the conditions that would exist if major CV diseases were removed as a risk of death. The basic quantities needed for this purpose are the probability q_i and the net probability $q_{i.2}$ that a person alive at age x_i will die in age interval (x_i, x_{i+1}) if CV diseases (R_2) were eliminated as a risk of death.

The required data are age-specific death rate M_i and age-cause-specific death rate M_{i2} for each age interval (x_i, x_{i+1}), given in Table 3 for white males and in Table 4 for white females. Using a procedure described in Chiang (12), two life tables had been constructed for each group: one based on the probability q_i using formula 28, and other based on the net probability $q_{i.2}$ computed from formula 32. The probabilities and the corresponding expectations of life shown in Tables 6 and 7 reflect in different ways the effect of the CV diseases on human mortality.

Table 6 gives a comparison between the probabilities q_i and $q_{i.2}$. The difference $q_i - q_{i.2}$ is the reduction in probability of dying if CV diseases were eliminated, or alternatively, the excess probability of dying because of the presence of CV diseases. The difference was not pronounced before age 40 because the disease then is quite rare, but advances with age at an accelerated rate. If CV diseases were removed, the reduction in the probability of dying in age interval (40, 45) would be 28.8% for white males and 18% for white females. For age interval (50, 55), the reduction in the probability of dying would be over 40% for white males and nearly 25% for white females. At age 70 or older, the reduction would be about 45% for both white males and females.

The impact of the major CV diseases on the expectation of life are shown in Table 7, where e_i is the "real" expectation of life in the current population under the normal condition with the presence of all causes of death, whereas $e_{i.2}$ is the (hypothetical) expectation of life if CV diseases were eliminated as a cause of death. The difference $e_{i.2} - e_i$ is the increase in the life expectancy if CV diseases were eliminated, or the number of years lost because the presence of CV diseases as a risk of death. The nearly constant difference $e_{i.2} - e_i$ under age 50 was because CV diseases cause death mainly among older persons and the reduction in the expectation of life because of CV diseases occurred almost entirely in persons older than age 50.

As the CV diseases became an increasingly dominant cause of death in older ages, the expectations of life $e_{i.2}$ became much greater than the expectation e_i. At age 60, the expectation of life for white males was $e_{i.2} = 26.2$ years and $e_i = 18.2$ years, with a difference of $e_{i.2} - e_i = 8$ years, a 43% reduction because of the presence of CV diseases. The corresponding reduction for white females was 54.7%. At age 70, the expectations were $e_{i.2} = 19.2$ and $e_i = 11.7$ for white males with a relative reduction of 62%, and $e_{i.2} = 28$ and $e_i = 15.3$ for white females with a relative reduction of 82.6%. Thus, if the major CV diseases were eliminated as a cause of death, a white male could expect an additional 8 years of life at age 60, and nearly 7½ additional years of life at age 70. For white females, the increase in the life expectancy would be even more impressive. If CV diseases were eliminated, a white female could enjoy an additional 12½ years of life at age 60 and at age 70.

ACKNOWLEDGMENTS

A computer program and Tables 5–7 have been prepared by C. Y. Liu. Copies of the program, which are not included because of the length of the paper, are available for distribution to interested readers. I wish to thank L. Le Cam for a helpful comment, B. J. van den Berg and M. White for reading the manuscript, and Mr. Liu for his help in the computations.

Literature Cited

1. Armitage, P. 1959. The comparison of survival curves. *J. R. Stat. Soc. A.* 122:279–300
2. Bailey, W. G., Haycocks, H. W. 1946. *Some Theoretical Aspects of Multiple Decrement Life Table.* Edinburgh: Inst. Actuar., London Fac. Actuar. 40 pp.
3. Barlow, R. E., Prochan, F. 1975. *Statistical Theory of Reliability and Life Testing.* New York: Holt, Rinehart & Winston. 290 pp.
4. Berkson, J., Gage, R. P. 1952. Survival curve for cancer patients following treatment. *J. Am. Stat. Assoc.* 47:501–15
5. Bernoulli, D. 1760. Essai d'une nouvelle analyse de la mortalité causée par la petite verole et des avantages de l'inoculation pour la prévenir. *Historie avec les Memoire,* pp. 1–45. Paris: Acad. Sci.
6. Birnbaum, Z. W. 1979. On the mathematics of competing risks. *Natl. Cent. Health Stat. Vital Health Stat.* Ser. 2, No. 77:1–58
7. Boardman, T. J., Kendall, P. J. 1970. Estimation in compound exponential failure models. *Technometrics* 12:891–900
8. Bur. Census. 1987. *United States Population Estimates, by Age, Sex, and Race:* 1980 to 1987
9. Chiang, C. L. 1961. On the probability of death from specific causes in the presence of competing risks. *Proc. 4th Berkley Symp. Math. Stat. Prob.* J. Neyman ed., IV:169–180
10. Chiang, C. L. 1961a. A stochastic study of the life table and its applications: III. The follow-up study with the consideration of competing risks. *Biometrics* 17:57–78
11. Chiang, C. L. 1961b. Standard error of the age-adjusted death rate. *Natl. Cent. Health Stat. Vital Stat. Spec. Rep.* 47:273–85
12. Chiang, C. L. 1968. *Introduction to Stochastic Processes in Biostatistics.* New York: Wiley. 313 pp.
13. Chiang, C. L. 1970. Competing risks and conditional probabilities. *Biometrics* 26:767–76
14. Chiang, C. L. 1972. On constructing current life tables. *J. Am. Stat. Assoc.* 67:538–41
15. Cornfield, J. 1957. The estimation of the probabilities of developing a disease in the presence of competing risks. *Am. J. Public Health* 47:601–7
16. Cutler, S. J., Ederer, F. 1958. Maximum utilization of the life table method in analysing survival. *J. Chron. Dis.* 8:699–712
17. David, H. A. 1970. On Chiang's proportionality assumption in the theory of competing risks. *Biometrics* 26:336–39
18. David, H. A. 1974. Parametric approaches to the theory of competing risks. *Reliab. Bio.* 275–90
19. David, H. A., Moeschberger, M. L. 1978. *The Theory of Competing Risks.* London: Griffin. 103 pp.
20. Dorn, H. 1950. Methods of analysis for follow-up studies. *Hum. Biol.* 22:238–48
21. Drolette, M. E. 1975. The effect of incomplete follow-up. *Biometrics* 31:135–44
22. Elandt-Johnson, R. C., Johnson, N. L. 1980. *Survival Models and Data Analysis.* New York: Wiley. 457 pp.
23. Elveback, L. 1958. Estimation of survivalship in chronic disease. *J. Am. Stat. Assoc.* 53:420–40
24. Fix, E., Neyman, J. 1951. A simple stochastic model of recovery, relapse, death and loss of patients. *Hum. Biol.* 23:205–41
25. Frost, W. H. 1933. Risk of persons in familiar contact with pulmonary tuberculosis. *Am. J. Public Health* 23:426–32
25a. Gail, M. 1975. A review and critique of some models in competing risk analysis. *Biometrics* 31:209–22
25b. Greville, T. N. E. 1943. Short methods of constructing abridged life table. *Rec. Am. Inst. Actuar.* 32:29–43
26. Greville, T. N. E. 1948. Mortality tables analysis by cause of death. *Rec. Am. Inst. Actuar.* 37:283–94
27. Halley, E. 1693. An estimate of the degrees of the mortality of mankind, drawn from curious tables of the births and funerals at the city of Breslau. *Philos. Trans. R. Soc. London* 17:569–610
28. Hooker, P. F., Longley-Cook, L. H. 1957. *Life and Other Contingencies,* Vol. II. Cambridge: Cambridge Univ. Press. 256 pp.
29. Kalbfleisch, J. D., Prentice, R. L. 1980. *The Statistical Analysis of Failure Time Data.* New York: Wiley. 321 pp.
30. Kaplan, E. L., Meier, P. 1958. Nonparametric estimation from incomplete observations. *J. Am. Stat. Assoc.* 53:457–81
31. Karn, N. M. 1931. An inquiry into various death rates and the comparative influence of certain diseases on the duration of life. *Ann. Eugen.* 4:279–326
31a. Keyfits, N. 1966. A life table that

agrees with the data. *J. Am. Stat. Assoc.* 61:305–12

32. Kimball, A. W. 1969. Models for the estimation of competing risks from grouped data. *Biometrics* 25:329–37

32a. King, G. 1914. On a short method of constructing an abridged mortality table. *J. Inst. Actuar.* 48:294–303

33. Kuzma, J. W. 1967. A comparison of two life table methods. *Biometrics* 23:51–64

34. Lee, L., Thompson, W. A. 1974. Results on failure time and pattern for the series system. *Reliab. Bio.* Phila. Soc. Ind. Appl. Math, pp. 291–302

35. Littel, A. S. 1952. Estimation of T-year survival rate from follow-up studies over a limited period of time. *Hum. Biol.* 24:87–116

36. Makeham, W. M. 1874. On an application of the theory of the composition of decremental forces. *J. Inst. Actuar.* 18: 317–22

37. Mantel, N., Bailer, J. C. 1970. Letter to the editor. *Biometrics* 26:861–63

38. Marshall, A. W., Olkin, I. 1967. A multivariate exponential distribution. *J. Am. Stat. Assoc.* 62:30–44

39. Miller, D. R. 1977. A note on independence of multivariate lifetimes in competing risks models. *Ann. Stat.* 5:576–79

40. Miller, R. G. 1981. *Survival Analysis.* New York: Wiley. 238 pp.

41. Moeschberger, M. L., David, H. A. 1971. Life tests under competing causes of failure and the theory of competing risks. *Biometrics* 27:909–33

42. Moeschberger, M. L., Klein, J. P. 1984. Consequence of departure from independence in exponential series system. *Technometrics* 262:277–84

43. Natl. Cancer Inst., Div. Cancer Prev. Control Surveill. Program. 1989. *Cancer Statistics Review, 1973–1986.* US Dep. Health Hum. Serv. PHS, NIH Publ. No. 89–2789

44. Natl. Cent. Health Stat. 1986. *Vital Stat. of the US*, Vol. II, Part A

45. Natl. Cent. for Health Stat. 1987. *Life Table. Vital Stat. of the US*, 1987. Vol. II, Sec. 6:1–19

46. Pike, M. C. 1970. A note on Kimball's paper "Models for the estimation of competing risks from grouped data." *Biometrics* 26:579–81

47. Prentice, R. L., Kalbfleisch, J. D., Peterson, A. V., Jr., Flournoy, N., Farewell, V. T., Breslow, N. E. 1978. The analysis of failure times in the presence of competing risks. *Biometrics* 34:541–54

47a. Reed, L. H., Merrell, M. 1939. A short method of constructing an abridged life table. *Am. J. Hyg.* 30:33–62

47b. Sirken, M. G. 1964. Comparisons of two methods of constructing abridged life tables by reference to a "standard" table. *Vital Health Stat.*, Ser. 2, No. 4 1–11. Natl. Cent. Health Stat., US Dep. Health Educ. Welf.

48. Spurgeon, E. F. 1922. *Life Contingencies.* Cambridge: Cambridge Univ. Press. 479 pp.

49. Todhunter, I. 1865. *A History of the Mathematical Theory of Probability.* New York: Chelsea. 624 pp.

50. Tsiatis, A. 1975. A nonidentifiability aspect of the problem of competing risks. *Proc. Natl. Acad. Sci. USA* 72: 20–22

51. Wong, O. 1977. A competing risks model based on the life table procedure in epidemiological studies. *Int. J. Epidemiol.* 6:153–59

Annu. Rev. Publ. Health 1991. 12:309–33

NUTRITION AND EXERCISE: EFFECTS ON ADOLESCENT HEALTH

Carol N. Meredith and Johanna T. Dwyer

Division of Clinical Nutrition, School of Medicine, University of California, Davis, California; Department of Medicine and Community Health, Tufts University Medical School, New England Medical Center Hospitals, Boston, Massachusetts

KEY WORDS: growth, teenagers

INTRODUCTION

This century has seen a marked improvement in the health of American adolescents, but currently the trend is being reversed; today's teenagers are in poorer health than their parents were at the same age. Mortality is mostly related to crime, drugs, and suicide, but there also are nonfatal health problems, which have immediate and long-term consequences that require the attention and financial support of our society (19). Good nutrition and adequate physical activity must be recognized as cost-effective means for normal growth and development during adolescence and for decreased risk of future chronic diseases.

In the past, undernutrition and overwork in unsanitary environments stunted the growth of many American children. Today, inadequate nutrition ranges from excesses that lead to obesity, to deficits that produce anemia or low weight babies born to teenagers. At the same time, physical exercise paradoxically has become a "leisure activity" that is more accessible to the rich than to the poor. Many of these problems could be solved by better support for adolescents at high risk and greater education about adolescents' needs for food and exercise.

309

0163-7525/91/0501-0309$02.00

NUTRIENT NEEDS AND EATING HABITS DURING ADOLESCENCE

Adolescents need diets of higher quality and greater quantity, compared with children or adults (86). The growth spurt requires a greater supply of energy and structural materials. Puberty-related changes in physiological function alter nutrient needs, such as the greater requirement for iron after menarche (142). Special physiological conditions, such as pregnancy or lactation, can further increase requirements (136). Pathological conditions, such as chronic disease or disability, can alter nutrient needs by affecting absorption, metabolism, or excretion.

Energy Substrates: Carbohydrates, Fats, and Proteins

Recent surveys of American adolescents show energy intakes below the Recommended Dietary Allowances (RDA) (30). The National Health and Nutrition Examination Surveys (NHANES) and the National Food Consumption Survey show low energy intakes among girls aged 12–17, boys a few years older, blacks, and adolescents from poor families (96, 145). Despite low reported energy intakes, several studies suggest that American adolescents are actually becoming fatter (31). In late adolescence, energy intake tends to be inversely related to fatness; for example, low income girls who eat less are more likely to be obese than more affluent girls (53). Adolescents apparently are becoming increasingly sedentary, but there are no solid data to prove this suggestion.

The energy intake of adolescents should be increased, together with an increase in energy expenditure through physical exercise. A larger total intake of food can better provide necessary substrates, vitamins, and minerals. For an adolescent who eats less than about 1800 kcal per day, it is difficult to consume enough vitamin B_6, copper, magnesium, and iron, which are present in low concentrations in most foods. Higher energy intakes, especially together with physical exercise, increase the utilization of dietary protein (24) and improve skeletal development (71). Energy expended in regular, prolonged exercise of low intensity can reduce body fat in obese adolescents, but has a more marked effect on the risk factors for heart disease: it lowers insulin response to glucose, increases HDL-cholesterol/total cholesterol, and lowers blood pressure (35, 116).

The need for protein rises during adolescence, but national surveys show that median intakes are satisfactory.

The diet consumed by American adolescents provides more fat than the recommended 30% of total calories (29, 97). National surveys and longitudinal studies show diets high in total fat, saturated fat, and cholesterol (31, 41, 47, 97), which are risk factors for coronary artery disease. Indeed, among young Americans killed in Vietnam, 45% showed evidence of early athero-sclerosis (92).

Alcohol also can be considered an energy substrate. However, the con-sumption of alcohol is illegal for adolescents, and impairs health and nutri-tional status.

Vitamins, Minerals, Water, and Fiber

The need for most vitamins and minerals rises markedly during adolescence. Inadequate intake is most likely for iron, calcium, and vitamin A (146). The low iron content of adolescent diets leads to anemia in certain subgroups, as discussed in the next section.

Calcium tends to be low in adolescent diets. The new RDA for calcium, 1200 mg per day, is intended to cover the needs for the most rapidly growing adolescents, based on evidence that high bone mass achieved during adoles-cence and young adulthood decreases the risk of osteoporosis in old age (90). Although calcium intake is especially important for women, the median calcium intake of adolescent girls is about 400 mg below the RDA, whereas boys tend to consume a more satisfactory amount (147). Blacks have a lower intake of dairy products and thus consume less calcium, but their genetically determined large bone and muscle mass makes them less susceptible to osteoporosis (78). In young women, pregnancy and lactation place a further demand on calcium stores (33).

Intakes of vitamins A, C, folic acid, thiamin, and riboflavin also fall below recommended levels in 10- to 20-year-olds. However, the clinical signifi-cance of this is uncertain (113).

Water homeostasis becomes more efficient after puberty, but the im-portance of water for temperature regulation in hot environments and during exercise is often underestimated (10). The need for water is usually 1 ml/kcal of energy expended under normal circumstances (30).

Intake of dietary fiber among adolescents is not well documented, but it is probably lower than recommended. Increased dietary fiber in the diet of adolescents may help reduce risks for future chronic diseases and conditions (29).

Effects of Puberty on Nutrient Needs and Dietary Habits

Adolescent nutrient needs differ by sex, change rapidly with biological development during adolescence, and vary between individuals (131). Girls reach their full height about two years before boys. The timing of the pubertal growth spurt within each sex has a range of about 3.5 years. The difference in timing of development for different individuals and for each sex contributes to the variable nutrient needs of adolescents of the same age. Nutrient needs correlate with biological maturity, rather than with chronological age (40). Sexual maturity ratings or other clinical indices for assessing biological age are useful in making nutritional recommendations (142).

Chronic undernutrition and some chronic illnesses slow height growth during childhood, reduce cortical bone growth, and slightly delay puberty (79, 141). Other adverse conditions associated with poverty reduce the chance of attaining full growth potential. In most societies, children from affluent families grow faster and attain greater adult height (141). Differences in adolescent growth also exist between different ethnic groups, but these are often confounded by socioeconomic and cultural differences. Until the early twentieth century, blacks matured later and attained lower adult height than whites; today, black girls reach menarche some three months earlier than white girls (142). Childhood malnutrition and infectious diseases, which were more common in blacks, were probably the cause of impaired growth. Ethnic differences in the US today are much smaller than those associated with sex and normal variation (59).

The foods chosen voluntarily by adolescents define their nutrient intakes. Foods can be divided into those that provide most of the essential nutrients and those that provide primarily kilocalories, also termed "junk" food. About a quarter of the energy intake of adolescents comes from foods that are low in protein, vitamins, and minerals, such as desserts, nondiet soft drinks, candy, cookies, pies, cakes, salad dressing, french fries, and other deep-fried foods. Boys who are poor or black are especially likely to consume junk food (41).

American adolescents tend to have erratic patterns of eating snacks and meals (137). About 5% of adolescents, especially older girls, regularly skip meals. The omission of certain meals, such as breakfast, can decrease total daily intake of several nutrients. Erratic meals become a problem if the total diet is impaired, i.e. if low nutrient-density snacks make up most of the diet (41).

Fast foods, convenience foods, and snacks are increasingly popular (25). Nearly all fast foods are high in total and saturated fat, cholesterol, and sodium (88). Few items from fast food restaurants provide less than 50% of calories as fat, although menus are gradually offering a healthier choice of foods. Adolescents can choose better quality snacks and use a daily food guide to attain a balanced diet (41). The US Department of Agriculture has developed a food guide for adolescents that fulfills both the RDA and the Dietary Guidelines for Americans (Table 1). The food guide ensures nutrient adequacy, variety, balance, and moderation.

Table 1 Food guide for adolescents

Food group	Recommended daily servings

Fruits
   Citrus, melon, berries
   Other fruits
	2–4

Vegetables
   Dark green and deep yellow
   Starchy, including dry beans, peas
   (include dark green and dry beans and peas
   several times per week)
Other vegetables
	3–5

Meat, fish, poultry, eggs (total of 5–7 oz. daily from lean choices)	2–3
Milk, yogurt, cheese	3–4 (4 for pregnant or nursing)

Grains, breads, cereals
   Whole grain and enriched
   (include several servings of whole grain pro-
   ducts daily)
	6–11

Fats, sweets, alcohol	In moderation; alcohol is not recommended for teenagers

ACTIVITY PATTERNS AND FITNESS IN ADOLESCENCE

Effects of Puberty on Body Composition, Physical Capacity, and Exercise Habits

During adolescence, nutrition and physical activity influence growth and development of skeletal bone, muscle, and fat. They also may affect future susceptibility to chronic diseases. Activity patterns developed during these years carry over to later life and affect morbidity and longevity (103).

The capacity for physical exercise increases with puberty, as strength, skill, and endurance increase. These changes involve increased linear growth, body mass, and physiological changes, such as greater control of body temperature, that improve athletic ability. Boys increase their aerobic power (VO_2 max) during adolescence and peak between 18 and 20 years of age. In adolescent girls after puberty, VO_2 max per unit of body weight declines as body fat increases, hemoglobin tends to decline (14, 93), and voluntary activity decreases (140, 151). Aerobic capacity measured on a treadmill in adolescent boys and girls in different countries, expressed as ml O_2 kg min, is about 45 to 55 in boys, and about 36 to 46 in girls (125).

Age of puberty and aerobic power are inversely related. Early maturers are fatter, especially girls, and remain fatter, taller, and less aerobically fit as adults (54, 74). A late menarche is common among athletic, thin girls. The capacity to improve aerobic power through training is greater in adolescents than children; it peaks at the age of fastest linear growth (12).

There is greater efficiency of movement after puberty. Even as aerobic capacity declines, performance in a given sport may peak a few years after adolescence, because of better coordination, economy of movement, and strategy (2). Strength peaks at about age 20 in boys, and at about age 17 in girls. It is mainly determined by muscle mass, with a constant relationship between maximum strength and cross-sectional area of muscle (2). Anaerobic power, typical of sprinting, is greater after puberty (68) and is a linear function of fat-free mass (18).

Tolerance to environmental conditions changes with puberty. The pre-pubescent child has a low tolerance for exercise in the heat because of a high surface/mass ratio, a lower production of sweat per sweat gland, a higher core temperature at the onset of sweating, slower acclimation to exercise in the heat, a high thirst threshold, and a greater increase in core temperature for a given degree of water loss (10). Those adolescents who have not yet undergone puberty and are fat, not acclimated to heat, and physically untrained have a greater need for ensuring adequate water intake before exercise to avoid heat-related illness. Risk increases in sports that use dehydration to "make weight," such as in wrestling or judo. Obese adolescents are at greater risk because of the difficulty in dissipating heat. They make up the greatest proportion of heatstroke victims in military or police training academies and among football players, usually during the first two days of training (8, 10).

Tolerance for exercise in the cold increases after puberty. Swimming in cool water, which leads to rapid heat loss, is poorly tolerated by prepubescent and thin adolescents, but is easily tolerated by obese adolescents (133). Thin, young adolescents are more susceptible to hypothermia (152).

The duration and intensity of voluntary exercise change after childhood. Detailed, accurate studies of physical activity patterns among children and adolescents have not been carried out in the United States. However, longitudinal studies in Europe show that behavior changes after puberty in ways that affect fitness. Spontaneous activity decreases about 50% from age 12 to 18, with boys being consistently more active than girls. The decline is observed for walking and for vigorous exercising (151, 152). Lower activity is related to lower aerobic power per unit of weight (73). In the United States, physical activity throughout adolescence has been studied through cross-sectional surveys and semi-quantitative measures of fitness. Participation in physical education classes declines from about 98% at age 10 to about 50% at age 17 (119). These percentages did not change between 1974 and 1986 (110). The time devoted to moderate or vigorous activity during a physical education class is only 20%, with most time devoted to competitive sports (basketball, volleyball, baseball), rather than activities and skills (jogging, swimming) that can be carried over to later years (13). The National Children and Youth Fitness Study, a cross-sectional survey of 8800 children aged 10 to 18 years, showed that cardiorespiratory endurance (minutes to run one mile) and abdominal strength (number of situps per minute) increase or stay constant between the ages of 12 to 18 (119). However, these figures have not been corrected for age-related increases in muscle mass and running efficiency (12).

Opportunities for Activity

Among adults, women of low socioeconomic class spend less time being physically active than men or women of a higher socioeconomic class (49), and black women are less physically active than white women (154). As physical activity patterns tend to be similar for members of the same family (46), the adolescent children of poorer families are less likely to exercise regularly, and, in the case of girls, are likely to be fatter (52).

Activity outside the school environment probably has declined in the United States. Transportation to school is often in a bus or a car. Recreation involves hours in front of the television set, and the time adolescents spend watching TV has increased from 18.8 h/wk in 1968–1970 to 23.3 h/wk in 1976–1980 (58). Spontaneous play and sports, organized by children themselves, is difficult in geographic areas with a harsh climate or unsafe playgrounds and streets, and in cultures in which vigorous physical exercise is not socially acceptable, especially for girls. An exception to the trend is the greater participation of high school girls in interscholastic sports, because of the implementation in 1972 of Title IX of the Education Amendments (26).

WIDESPREAD NUTRITIONAL PROBLEMS IN ADOLESCENTS

The most prevalent nutritional problems among today's adolescents are obesity, anemia, and eating disorders. Strong & Dennison (138) have reviewed the role of diet in childhood as a risk for later atherosclerosis and coronary heart disease.

Obesity

The prevalence of obesity among adolescents is high, ranging from 10% to 30% of the population (36). A comparison of skinfold thicknesses in three National Health Examination Surveys between 1960 and 1980 showed a 30% increase in obesity and a 64% increase in very pronounced obesity among adolescents 10–17 years old (58). However, another recent analysis of the same national health surveys, which used body mass indicators to assess obesity, showed no consistent secular trends among 12–17-year-old adolescents or among 18–34-year-old males, although fatness has tended to become more prevalent in adult females (63). Inconsistent conclusions may be due to the different indices of obesity employed, and differences in age distributions and sample designs. However, no study suggests that the prevalence of obesity is decreasing among adolescents.

Activity has an important role in the genesis and treatment of obesity. The spontaneous physical activity of babies tends to be lower among those who later become fat (115). In an adult population with a high genetic risk of obesity, such as the Pima Indians, low total daily energy expenditure is a predictor of body weight gain in the subsequent two years (112). However, it has been difficult to demonstrate lower energy expenditure in children who are already obese. Recorded activity patterns in overweight schoolgirls have shown lower physical exercise compared with lean children (39), and obese adolescents tend to exercise less vigorously (22). Parents rate their obese adolescent offspring as less active than the nonobese siblings, but physical fitness per unit of fat-free mass is not different (45). Studies of young children have shown lower physical activity in the obese (17), but an accurate and objective measurement of daily energy expenditure showed similar values for overweight and normal-weight adolescents (6).

Exercise helps weight loss in obese adolescents, especially on a long-term basis. Adding exercise to a hypocaloric diet in obese adolescents may not accelerate fat loss, but reduces risk factors, such as systolic blood pressure and heart rate (16, 35, 116).

A surfeit of energy due to excess intake and low energy expenditure may be particularly detrimental to certain racial groups, as has become evident over the past 50 years (87). Obesity is less prevalent among adolescents of African ancestry compared with Caucasian adolescents, and it is more prevalent among adolescents of Native American or Pacific Islander heritage (143, 158), including Hispanics of Mexican and Central American origin (60, 117). Adolescent Mexican Americans tend to have a higher weight for height than Caucasians or blacks (117), higher skinfold measurements (120), and a more central distribution of fat. Obesity and extreme obesity are more prevalent among Mexican Americans from an early age, especially in women (117, 121). This group is a rapidly growing segment of the population, particularly in the Western United States. Obesity with an accumulation of fat in the abdomen and upper body is associated with greater risk of future diabetes, hypertension, and gallbladder disease (121) and may be a genetic trait called the "New World Syndrome." The syndrome occurs at highest frequency among Native Americans, with familial aggregation and prevalence proportional to the amount of Amerindian admixture. It is absent in Hispanic groups of similar socioeconomic status but different racial background, such as Cubans or Puerto Ricans (155). A confounding factor is that Amerindian admixture, measured by genetic markers, is associated with lower socioeconomic status (114), in which fatness, sedentary habits and ill-health also are more prevalent (53). Thus, the interaction between obesity and the environment, including physical activity patterns and dietary habits, is not only determined by culture, but also by genetic background.

Obesity has immediate and delayed effects on social development and health (70). American society prizes leanness, especially in girls (55). Distortions of body image and low self-esteem are common in obese adolescents. American girls tend to feel guilty after eating, to be uncomfortable eating with others, and to cope with emotional distress by eating (95). At the same time, the American food supply is inexpensive, abundant, tasty, and readily available, which increases temptation and opportunities for overindulgence.

Many adolescents try to lose weight by using methods that may be unhealthy. A survey of eighth and tenth grade students showed that in the past year, 61% of the girls and 28% of the boys had tried to lose weight by dieting (147). Strategies included food restriction, fasting, diet pills, self-induced vomiting, and laxatives. The desire to lose weight can lead to a nutrient-deficient intake, a tendency to develop a chaotic eating pattern that can result in bulimia, and distorted attitudes about eating and the body. Retardation of growth and puberty has been reported with chronic dieting that begins in later childhood and continues into adolescence (79, 111).

Most obese children are not predestined to become obese adults, unless they are already very obese as children (70). Children may become obese transiently in early adolescence, before the growth spurt, but this is a physiological phenomenon and not a cause for treatment. Obese adolescents who are poor and/or from certain minority groups, such as blacks, Mexican Americans, and American Indians, may be more likely to maintain obesity as adults (148, 149). During and after adolescence, females from poor families become fatter than those of more affluent families (52, 53). The stigma associated with obesity is greater among the upwardly mobile (51, 89, 118), as obese children might feel that they are social misfits (43).

Obesity further encourages the tendency towards physical inactivity. Children in obese families expend less energy than those in lean families, even as early as the preschool years, possibly because they copy sedentary family habits (3). The parents of lean children are leaner and more active and exercise more frequently with their children than do the parents of obese children (106). For children with orthopedic problems, obesity increases the pain and difficulty of movement.

Signs of future health problems are present in obese adolescents. The main predictors of later ill-health are high blood pressure and high blood insulin levels, with a weaker association with aerobic capacity and high serum cholesterol (70). Overt disease may be absent in obese adolescents, but the risk of future health problems must be addressed by health educators and counselors, especially if family members are obese (51, 159). Obesity that persists throughout childhood and adolescence is likely to be associated with increased risks of later hypertension, high serum cholesterol and coronary artery disease, adult onset diabetes, gall bladder disease, certain forms of hormone dependent cancer, and other medical problems. The importance of improving the way children and adolescents eat and exercise in the United States is indicated by the apparent decline in the physical activity of all adolescents, the prevalence of obesity, and the rapid increase of a population that is genetically prone to maturity onset diseases that are exacerbated by obesity and inactivity.

Anemia

Iron deficiency is the most prevalent dietary deficiency among adolescents today (34). The 1976–1978 NHANES II survey found the highest prevalence of iron deficiency (7.2% average) in older adolescent girls. This prevalence is due to increased iron need, low dietary intakes (especially of the more bioavailable iron in meat), and, in high risk groups, lack of iron supplements. Few older adolescent boys showed iron deficiency. In young adolescents, aged 11 to 14 years, iron deficiency was 4.1% in boys and 2.8% in girls. Impaired iron status was defined by using the average estimates of three hematological and biochemical measures (146). Iron deficiency is more common among the poor, especially at high risk ages and during pregnancy (82).

Iron deficiency is less frequent today than it was in years gone by, although it still is a problem among some teenagers, such as those mentioned above (34). Its lower prevalence may be due to higher iron fortification of cereals, greater use of oral contraceptives that lead to lower losses of menstrual blood, and perhaps a greater awareness on the part of the public that iron deficiency is a problem.

Iron deficiency during adolescence is partly due to rapid growth. Lean body mass, blood volume, and red cell mass all increase sharply during puberty, which then increases iron needs for myoglobin in muscle and hemoglobin in blood. Because of the rapid growth of boys during puberty, anemia is more likely during the growth spurt.

In later adolescence, the greater iron reserves in the large lean body mass of boys and the menstrual losses of iron in girls account for high iron needs. Among older adolescents, girls are more likely to become anemic, because their iron losses are greater and intake is usually lower. In contrast to oral contraceptives, intrauterine devices increase menstrual blood loss and can further increase iron needs. Pregnancy sharply increases the iron requirement, as it depletes the iron stores of the adolescent mother and, in severe cases, of the fetus. Adolescents who consume low amounts of a vegetarian diet are at greater risk for anemia, as the iron in plant foods has a lower bioavailability. Female athletes, especially runners, risk iron deficiency because of low intake and increased losses (100).

Anemia decreases the capacity for exercise. Impaired body temperature regulation, lower resistance to infection, and alterations in behavior and intellectual performance also may occur, although evidence in adolescents is limited (34).

Adolescents should be encouraged to eat iron-fortified or whole grain breads and cereals, lean red meats, and other iron-rich animal foods. When plant foods are eaten together with vitamin C-rich foods, such as citrus fruits, the bioavailability of non-heme iron increases. The National School Lunch and Breakfast programs ensure that iron-rich meals are provided in school menus, and adolescents should be encouraged to eat them. Pregnant adolescents need iron supplements.

Eating Behavior Problems

Eating disorders severe enough to disturb mental and physical health are more common in adolescence than at any other time of life. These disorders, which include anorexia nervosa, bulimia, bulimarexia, self-induced vomiting, and laxative abuse, have been described as psychological disorders with nutritional complications. They are about nine times more common among females than among males (104). Occasional disorganized eating behavior and dieting, if present without psychological disturbance, is not necessarily a sign of an eating disorder. Laxative abuse, diuretic abuse, and self-induced vomiting may occur without related bulimia for weight control in females and for competitive weights in adolescent athletes of both sexes. True eating disorders are present when disorganized eating behavior and dieting appear together with other signs, such as frequent vomiting, laxative abuse, regular diet misuse, constant and continued eating problems, extreme weight loss, amenorrhea, and other signs of physiological disturbance.

Eating disorders impair growth, development, and mental health. They are strongly associated with affective disorders, particularly depression, which can persist after nutritional treatment (80).

Bulimia is diagnosed if two or more episodes of binge eating occur per week for at least three months, accompanied by the feeling of lack of control and excessive rapid eating of large amounts of food in a short amount of time (94). Later, the individual may resort to vomiting or using laxatives or diuretics, with more frequent binging and purging (94). This behavior is secret and difficult to discover. Bulimics may have normal weight, especially early in their disorder. Bulimic episodes may follow a period of excessive dieting or restrained eating (75) and often are associated with other impulse disorders, such as substance abuse and alcohol abuse (80).

The rarest and most dangerous eating disorder is anorexia nervosa. This is a psychiatric condition that involves a disorder of eating, body image, and thought processes and leads to life-threatening emaciation. There are at least two forms of anorexia nervosa. Classical anorexia, also referred to as starver-restrictor anorexia, involves constant and compulsive limitation of food intake and fasting with accompanying emaciation. Bulimarexia, or bulimic anorexia nervosa, alternates fasting with binge eating, which is followed by self-induced vomiting or laxative abuse to rid the body of the food. Both result in emaciation if untreated (72).

The prevalence of bulimia is 2%, based on binging and coupled with self-induced vomiting or laxative abuse, but less rigorous definitions suggest that it is as high as 3% to 19% (94). It usually occurs among girls in later adolescence (80). It is most prevalent in high-achieving but unassertive young women from high-achieving but disorganized families. The prevalence of anorexia nervosa is 0.3% for females, with a rate of 0.5% in one recent survey of girls aged 15 to 19 years (83). Eating disorders have become more prevalent, particularly among affluent white girls (64, 111).

Eating disorders can produce clinical complications that require hospitalization, especially in the case of anorexia (104). Binge eating leads to acute gastric dilatation. Repeated vomiting causes electrolyte disturbances, cardiac arrhythmias, enlarged parotid glands, esophageal inflammation, and eventually eroded dental enamel. Laxative abuse causes electrolyte abnormalities, dehydration, metabolic changes, and gastrointestinal complications, including cathartic colon and increased dependence on laxatives to induce elimination. Anorexia nervosa leads to protein calorie malnutrition, anemia, amenorrhea, and lower bone mineral content. Endocrine changes and low calcium intake may prevent the achievement of high peak bone mass during the period of rapid skeletal growth. Death rates from anorexia are 2% to 8%. Treatment of these adolescents is difficult and requires the cooperation of psychiatrists, nutritionists, counselors, and family therapists.

SPECIAL GROUPS AT RISK FOR MALNUTRITION

Certain groups of adolescents are at high risk of malnutrition. They include pregnant teenagers, physically and socially disabled adolescents, and highly trained athletes.

Pregnant Adolescents

Rates of adolescent pregnancy and childbirth, especially in girls under 15 years of age, and rates of abortion in adolescence, are higher in the United

States than in most other Western countries (156). More than one million American teenagers become pregnant each year; about half give birth to a live infant. Most pregnancies are unintended and unwanted (61), and they are more prevalent among the poor.

The nutrient needs of pregnant adolescents are greatly increased, but dietary quality does not necessarily improve, and intakes are often lower than recommended. Nutritional risk increases because of higher energy and nutrient needs, especially if the pregnancy occurs in very young women who are still growing. Teenagers often enter pregnancy at lower weights, and gain weight less efficiently than mature women (50).

Early childbearing is a threat to the well-being of the adolescent mother and her child. Additional problems, such as substance abuse, venereal disease, absent or delayed prenatal care, and expulsion from the family home, can lead to an extraordinarily high risk of health problems, including poor nutrition, in the mother and infant. Dietary intakes can be inadequate in energy, calcium, and iron. Poor health care and poor nutrition can lead to iron deficiency anemia, acetonuria, inadequate or limited weight gain, pre-eclampsia, eclampsia, pregnancy-induced hypertension, cephalopelvic disproportion, cervical trauma, prolonged and difficult labor, premature delivery, low birth weight, and increased perinatal and infant mortality. These risks are especially common in young girls who become pregnant within one or two years of menarche (136). Lactation adds to the nutritional needs of the new mother (33), but breastfeeding is rare in adolescents, especially among poor, black, and very young inner-city adolescents (5).

The health risks of pregnancy are lower in older adolescents, but poor outcome is still more prevalent than for mature women (96). Poor nutrition is less of a problem, as older adolescents have completed their rapid growth period. Older adolescents also are more physically, socially, and emotionally mature, have more education, and are more likely to be married. All adolescent mothers require the social, psychological, and financial support to ensure adequate nutrition and care for their babies and themselves.

Family planning, contraceptive services, and prenatal services all must emphasize the importance of nutrition. Public programs, such as the WIC program (the US Department of Agriculture's Special Supplemental Program for Women, Infants, and Children, which supplies food, education, and some health assessment for pregnant women and their infants), must seek out and care for pregnant adolescents, especially those at highest risk. Comprehensive prenatal care using a team approach, social support, and an individualized case management system decreases perinatal mortality rates and pregnancy complications (62).

It is most important to gain 30–35 pounds or more during pregnancy. Weight gains during pregnancy should be higher in the adolescent, especially if weight is low before pregnancy. The young woman must understand why her nutrient needs increase during pregnancy and learn to adjust her diet to meet these needs. First priority must be given to ending the use of substances that are directly toxic and/or impair the intake and utilization of nutrients (i.e., alcohol, cocaine, cigarettes). Given the possible social, economic, and psychologic problems, food and eating may seem unimportant. Programs such as WIC can help ensure that food is available and teach the pregnant adolescent which nutrients to obtain from a good diet and which to obtain by supplements. She must learn that energy and most minerals and vitamins are provided by a varied and abundant diet. Iron supplements of 30–60 mg per day usually are necessary, as it is difficult to meet the increased needs for iron during pregnancy from food sources alone. Folic acid supplements often are recommended, as needs rise steeply during pregnancy, and it is difficult to supply an adequate amount from food alone. Multivitamin supplements at levels that approximate the RDA for pregnant adolescents may be advisable.

Highly Trained Athletes

Athletes may not always consume a good diet, especially if they are young and do not know much about good nutrition. The diet should be appropriate for the type of body composition required by the sport or activity, for the type of physical performance required, and for short-term and long-term health.

Energy needs increase with vigorous training, yet athletes who require a lean physique for aesthetic reasons, weight classification, or performance may reduce food intake to the point of undernutrition. Among young girls, the combination of early training and undernutrition, which leads to delayed menarche and amenorrhea, is most common among dancers, gymnasts, skaters, and runners. Even in the absence of amenorrhea, the levels of reproductive hormones may be below normal (124). Reducing food intake can lead to abnormal attitudes towards food. Low levels of reproductive hormones, with or without amenorrhea, are associated with an energy deficit because of excessive exercise or inadequate intake (98). In runners, the prevalence of amenorrhea or shortened luteal phase increases with weekly mileage (122, 123). In young women who are beginning a rigorous training program, delayed menstruation and loss of luteal hormone surge was more prevalent among those who restrict food intake (23). Delayed menarche or amenorrhea impair skeletal health, with a higher prevalence of scoliosis (153), stress fractures (15), and low mineral density of the lumbar spine (37).

The quality of the diet is important, especially with low energy intake. Many young athletes are vegetarian or they restrict meat intake (132). The high fiber, low fat, low energy nature of vegetarian diets may reduce estrogens by increasing their fecal elimination and by favoring metabolism to less active products (57, 66). A vegetarian hypocaloric diet has a greater effect on luteal phase levels of luteinizing hormone, estradiol, and progesterone than an omniverous, hypocaloric diet (108).

Adolescent women who are active and amenorrheic should receive dietary counseling. Although they may not be concerned about the long-term risk of osteoporosis, they may be persuaded by the increased risk of bone fracture and the problem of hypothermia while exercising in cold (14, 15). The resumption of normal menstruation increases bone mineral density (38). Qualitative and quantitative changes in the diet of adolescent athletes with amenorrhea are an initial treatment that should be preferred to the prescription of hormone therapy. The possibility of eating disorders should be explored, as vigorous athletic activity is a common feature of anorexia nervosa (76, 81).

The effects of vigorous activity and low food intake on the hormonal development of boys have not been extensively studied. A vegetarian diet is associated with lower levels of testosterone, which together with a low energy, low fat, high fiber diet and other life-style changes may affect the rate of development in vegetarian boys (66). The metabolic effects of sporadic fasting and dieting have not been extensively studied in adolescent athletes. About 83% of young male wrestlers regularly try to lose weight by reducing food intake, although low weight gain during puberty can affect strength (65). Adolescent wrestlers who repeatedly diet and regain weight show a 14% lower resting metabolic rate per unit of lean body mass (135), which may be an adaptation to repeated bouts of undernutrition. Repeated dieting and intermittent fasting likely impair growth. The levels of insulin-like growth factor I are three times higher during normal puberty than during the average adult level (84). Intermittent periods of negative nitrogen balance and lower growth factors induced by dietary restriction may lead to delayed growth and development (27).

Dehydration can be used to reduce weight acutely, by excessive sweating, limited fluid intake, and diuretics. When athletes compete according to weight categories, repeated bouts of dehydration and rehydration are common and may eventually be harmful to the kidneys (134). In strength-trained athletes, the desire to increase muscle mass and strength may lead to the use of illegal anabolic steroids. Some 7% of high school adolescents have used anabolic steroids to improve athletic performance or appearance (21). Users were older, more athletic, and of lower socioeconomic class. They believed themselves "stronger than average" (21, 69). The American Academy of Pediatrics has condemned the use of anabolic steroids because of the known toxic effects and because of the unfair enhancement of athletic performance (44). However, the National Strength and Conditioning Association has concluded that their use is unethical, but not harmful (157). Anabolic steroids impair glucose utilization (28, 56), diminish triglyceride clearance, lower HDL-cholesterol, and increase LDL-cholesterol (67), but favor net accretion of body protein, especially as muscle mass (48). The higher risk of eventual cardiovascular disease may not deter an adolescent athlete, but immediate effects, such as acne, baldness, reduced libido, breast growth, impaired sexual function (157), and affective and psychotic symptoms (109) may provide more persuasive arguments against the use of these illegal drugs.

Faddism and ignorance are evident among many young athletes and their trainers. Many believe that additional vitamins and protein supplements will improve performance (77, 105); however, multivitamin and mineral supplements have no effect on performance (9). Athletes who eat a large amount of food will almost certainly consume adequate levels of vitamins, minerals, and protein. Of a group of university football players who consumed an average 5270 kcal/day, which provides about 200 g protein per day, 20% took protein supplements and 93% took vitamins (127). Most protein supplements in specialty stores are mixtures of good quality proteins, but they are expensive and have no proven effect on athletic performance. Pure single amino acids are expensive and unlikely to have any nutritional value and do not improve muscle mass or strength.

Physically Disabled Adolescents

Physical handicaps and chronic diseases afflict 1% to 20% of adolescents and can change nutritional needs (99). The highest figure includes mild functional impairments, such as uncomplicated asthma, minimal sensory deficits, or emotional disturbances.

Nutritional problems vary among handicapped adolescents (4), but they complicate the difficult transition from dependence on parents for food and feeding to independent eating (91). The transition ranges from special help with managing food and feeding, to the provision of therapeutic diets for control of the disease, to the prevention of secondary malnutrition, to improved well-being.

Chronically ill adolescents are at higher risks of malnutrition and psychological distress related to food. Many chronically ill adolescents are now treated in outpatient settings and live at home, so that good nutrition is mainly the responsibility of the family.

Growth may be affected by the disease itself, as well as by malnutrition secondary to the condition, which leads to delayed puberty or stunting. Nutrition counseling and interventions can prevent poor growth. Special feeding or eating devices or forms of food may be helpful in certain disorders, such as cerebral palsy and muscular dystrophy. Therapeutic diets for diseases, such as diabetes, renal disease, gastrointestinal disorders, and severe allergies, can be adapted to the tastes of adolescents, which helps them develop a sense of control (107, 129). Although lapses are expected, it is important to keep nonadherence low enough for it not to become a medical issue and a source of family conflict (32, 128). Interdisciplinary clinics with dietitians or nutritionists who have special expertise in disabilities must be included on the health team. When nutritionists are not present on site in such clinics, nutritional care may be overlooked.

Disability or disease can dramatically reduce physical activity. Hypoactivity occurs in crippling conditions, such as muscular dystrophy, paralysis, respiratory failure, or cardiac failure. Low activity also has been documented for massive obesity, asthma, diabetes, blindness, Down's syndrome, or mental retardation of other types (11, 126, 139).

Down's syndrome patients make up the largest proportion of mentally retarded persons. They tend to be short, obese, and physically unfit. Inactivity is due to poor motor skills, social isolation, and inadequate programs or facilities for exercise. Vigorous exercise training of adolescent boys with Down's syndrome reduces subcutaneous fat, increases strength and aerobic power, and provides beneficial psychological effects (130). In the United States, the first "Special Olympics" in 1968 heightened interest in creating exercise programs for retarded children and adults. Today, Special Olympics includes over one million members.

Blind adolescents also tend to be shorter, fatter, and less physically fit (126, 139). Lower aerobic capacity in the blind is apparent by 8 years of age, possibly because of low physical activity throughout childhood. With adequate physical education and special facilities, blind students attain nearly normal aerobic fitness (126).

Adolescents with spina bifida, some forms of cerebral palsy, quadriplegia, or other disabilities that preclude walking tend to be fatter and less active than nondisabled adolescents. The effort involved in getting around, especially with crutches, can be very great (1). Movement cannot be sustained for long if the metabolic cost is greater than 40% of the person's aerobic capacity. Adolescents who are confined to a wheelchair need upper-body strength to propel the wheelchair and sufficient aerobic power so that movement is not an exhausting effort. Disabled adolescents who are obese also must overcome the high metabolic cost of ventilation. Circuit training improves the strength and capacity of disabled children to propel a wheelchair and can help prevent obesity (101). Intermittent crutch-walking should be encouraged to increase aerobic power, prevent joint contractures of the lower limbs, and prevent bone atrophy (1).

Socially Disabled Adolescents

Interactions between psychological, social, and economic factors have produced new conditions of disability, which have nutrition and fitness implications. These conditions include the problems of runaway and "throwaway" teenagers who are no longer welcome in their own homes, juvenile delinquents, abusers of mood altering drugs or alcohol, and adolescents living in extreme poverty. Today, their problems are not being adequately identified, prevented, or treated.

Americans living in poverty comprise 13%–14% of the population today (102), a figure that has not changed over the last ten years. Approximately 16% of individuals 14–21 years of age are poor, and the poverty rate among people under 18 years of age is among the highest in society.

Poverty is prevalent among ethnic minorities, especially blacks and Hispanics. Poverty is high in rural areas, especially in the Southeast, Appalachia, and some parts of the Southwest, where social and public welfare programs are poorly funded. Rural, nonfarm families are more likely to be poor and lack the means for home food production. Access to food stores, health services, and food stamps is more difficult in rural areas (7). Salaries earned by adolescents usually are not enough to lift them out of poverty and allow them to support themselves or a family (102). The number of homeless, runaways, or cast-out adolescents is not known with certainty, but has been estimated to be as high as 1 million.

Substance abuse is a major cause of sickness and death in adolescents. In a survey of high school seniors, the proportion that reported daily use was 4% for alcohol, 2.7% for marijuana, and 0.2% for cocaine (M. Story et al, unpublished findings). Alcohol is high in calories, but lacks other nutrients. Coupled with its mood altering effects, alcohol tends to "crowd out" nutritious foods from the diet. Alcohol impairs digestion and absorption of nutrients. Alcohol consumption during pregnancy greatly increases risks to the mother and the fetus, including fetal alcohol syndrome, low birth weight, and complications of pregnancy. Mood-altering drugs may be toxic in themselves and also decrease interest in food. In the throes of addiction to cocaine, heroin, or other drugs, food is a minor concern, and any available money is spent to support the habit.

Adolescents living in poor families or on their own are more likely to be malnourished and have fewer opportunities for sports or other physical activities. Lack of food is not the only dietary problem that afflicts poor adolescents. Dietary imbalances, lack of variety, and overnutrition also are often present. Voluntary physical activity tends to be low in poor families, especially in women. Because of their high nutrient needs, children and adolescents among the poor are especially vulnerable (20). The presence of disease or disability increases nutritional risk.

In adults, aerobic exercise is believed to improve psychosocial status. Positive psychological effects of aerobic training have been described in male juvenile delinquents, measured as self-concept and depression score (85).

Steps to alleviate malnutrition in poor adolescents include setting a federal floor for Aid to Families with Dependent Children (AFDC) benefits, strengthening federal standards in poverty programs, improving state "safety net" programs for the poor, especially poor families, and placing the emergency food programs on a more permanent basis (20).

Many of the homeless and other patrons of emergency food programs are families with children and teenagers (7). Little is known about the nutritional status of homeless and runaway adolescents, but there is reason to suspect that it is precarious, and that undernutrition and malnutrition are common.

STRATEGIES TO IMPROVE ADOLESCENT HEALTH THROUGH BETTER NUTRITION AND EXERCISE

If our national goals of productive and satisfying lives, with good nutrition and good health, are to be realized for all adolescents, the problems mentioned above and many others must be addressed. One useful approach is to follow the goals and objectives set out in the *Year 2000 Objectives for the Nation,* recently published by the US Department of Health and Human Services and the US Public Health Service (USDHHS 1990). Additional measures for improving adolescent health have recently been summarized by the Office of Technology Assessment, US Congress (144) (Table 2).

The *Year 2000* goals cannot be implemented by federally funded efforts alone. However, federally funded programs, such as food stamps, WIC, the Child Nutrition programs, the Nutrition Education and Training program, health and education, and public welfare programs, such as AFDC and

Table 2   Goals for adolescent nutrition and fitness

---

1. Nutrition
    —Prevent overweight, especially in minorities
    —Improve knowledge of factors involved in weight loss and sensible dieting practices
    —Reduce anemia in low income pregnant adolescents
    —Increase use of Dietary Guidelines for Americans in school meals
    —Include nutrition education in school health education
    —Increase intakes of calcium and iron
    —Reduce dietary fat to no more than 30% of total kilocalories, and saturated fat to no more than 10% of kilocalories
    —Increase those in the population who are able to identify diet related risk factors for heart disease, hypertension, cancer, and osteoporosis
    —Increase the proportion of those who can identify the major food sources of fat
    —Require nutrition education from preschool to grade 12 as part of comprehensive health education

2. Fitness
    —More than 60% should participate in daily physical education classes
    —More than 70% should participate in assessments of physical fitness

---

Medicaid, are critical elements of success, especially for the most disadvantaged teenagers. State and local government, as well as the private and voluntary sectors, must also contribute efforts and money (144).

By the year 2000, with political will and continued implementation of preventive medicine, education, and social welfare programs, which include nutritional elements, many of the difficulties described in this review can be overcome. Adults who care for adolescents, such as teachers, coaches, social workers, and health providers, need to learn about their nutritional needs and how best to meet them (42, 137). But, education of adolescents themselves on nutrition and fitness is equally important (40). The schools, the mass media, and special programs must be recruited to improve adolescents' awareness and knowledge of their own health, nutrition, and fitness.

ACKNOWLEDGEMENTS

Partial support was provided to Dr. Dwyer by MCJ 9120 from the Maternal and Child Health Service USDHHS and to Dr. Meredith through USPHS DK-35747 for the preparation of this manuscript.

The assistance of Anne Bourgeois and secretarial work of Diane Hardy are gratefully acknowledged.

Literature Cited

1. Agre, J. C., Findley, T. W., McNally, C., Habeck, R., Leon, A. S., et al. 1987. Physical activity capacity in children with myelomeningocele. *Arch. Phys. Med. Rehabil.* 68:372–77

2. Astrand, P. O., Rodahl, K. 1986. Physical performance. In *Textbook of Work Physiology*, pp. 295–353. New York: McGraw-Hill, 3rd ed.

3. Avons, P., James, W. P. 1986. Energy expenditure of young men from obese and nonobese families. *Hum. Nutr. Clin. Nutr.* 10:259–70

4. Baer, M. T. 1987. Nutrition services. In *Handicapped Children and Youth: A Comprehensive Community and Clinical Approach*, eds. H. M. Wallace, R. F. Biehl, A. C. Ogelsby, pp. 134–50. New York: Human Sciences

5. Baisch, M. J., Fox, R. A., Goldberg, B. D. 1989. Breast-feeding attitudes and practices among adolescents. *J. Adolesc. Health Care* 10:41–45

6. Bandini, L. G., Schoeller, D. A., Dietz, W. H. 1990. Energy expenditure in obese and nonobese adolescents. *Pediatr. Res.* 27:198–203

7. Barancik, S. 1990. The rural disadvantage: growing income disparities between rural and urban areas. Washington, DC: Cent. Budget Policy Prior.

8. Barcenas, C., Hoeffler, H., Lie, J. T. 1976. Obesity, football, dog days, and siriasis: a deadly combination. *Am. Heart J.* 92:237–44

9. Barnett, D. W., Conlee, R. K. 1984. The effects of a commercial dietary supplement on human performance. *Am. J. Clin. Nutr.* 40:586–90

10. Bar-Or, O. 1980. Climate and the exercising child: a review. *Int. J. Sports Med.* 1:53–65

11. Bar-Or, O. 1986. Pathophysiological factors which limit the exercise capacity of the sick child. *Med. Sci. Sports Exerc.* 18:276–82

12. Bar-Or, O. 1987. Importance of differences between children and adults for exercise testing and exercise prescription. In *Exercise Testing and Exercise Prescription for Special Cases*, ed. J. S. Skinner, pp. 49–65. Philadelphia: Lea & Febiger

13. Bar-Or, O. 1987. A commentary to children and fitness: a public health perspective. *Res. Q. Exerc. Sport* 58:304–7

14. Bar-Or, O. 1988. The prepubescent female. In *Women and Exercise: Physiology and Sports Medicine*, eds. M. M. Shangold, G. Mirkin, pp. 109–19. Philadelphia: Davis

15. Barrow, G. W., Saha, S. 1988. Men-

strual irregularity and stress fractures in collegiate female distance runners. *Am. J. Sports Med.* 16:209–15

16. Becque, M. D., Katch, V. L., Rocchini, A. L., Marks, C. R., Moorehead, C. 1988. Coronary risk incidence of obese adolescents: reduction by exercise plus diet intervention. *Pediatrics* 81:605–12

17. Berkowitz, R. I., Agras, J. A., Korner, A. F., et al. 1985. Physical activity and adiposity: a longitudinal study from birth to childhood. *J. Pediatr.* 106:734–38

18. Blimkie, C. J., Roache, P., Hay, J. T., Bar-Or, O. 1988. Anaerobic power of arms in teenage boys and girls: relationship to lean tissue. Eur. J. Appl. Physiol. 57:677–83

19. Blum, R. 1987. Contemporary threats to adolescent health in the United States. *J. Am. Med. Assoc.* 257:3390–95

20. Brown, J., Allen, D. 1988. Hunger in America. *Annu. Rev. Public Health* 9:503–26

21. Buckley, W. E., Yesalis, C. E., Friedl, K. E., Anderson, W. A., Streit, A. L. et al. 1988. Estimated prevalence of anabolic steroid use among male high school seniors. *J. Am. Med. Assoc.* 260:3441–45

22. Bullen, B. A., Reed, R. B., Mayer, J. 1970. Physical activity of obese and nonobese adolescent females as appraised by motion picture sampling. *Am. J. Clin. Nutr.* 14:211–18

23. Bullen, B. A., Skrinar, G. S., Beitins, I. Z., Mering, G., Turnbull, B. A., et al. 1985. Induction of menstrual disorders by strenuous exercise in untrained women. *N. Engl. J. Med.* 312:1349–53

24. Butterfield, G. E., Calloway, D. H. 1984. Physical activity improves protein utilization in young men. *Brit. J. Nutr.* 51:171–84

25. Cassell, J. A. 1989. Commentary: American food habits in the 1980s. *Topics Clin. Nutr.* 4:47–58

26. Clement, A. 1987. Legal theory and sex discrimination in sport. *Med. Sport Sci.* 24:138–53

27. Clemmons, D. R., Klibanski, A., Underwood, L. E., McArthur, J. W., Ridgway, E. C., et al. 1981. Reduction of plasma immunoreactive somatomedin C during fasting in humans. *J. Clin. Endocrinol. Metab.* 53:1247–50

28. Cohen, J. C., Hickman, R. 1987. Insulin resistance and diminished glucose tolerance in powerlifters ingesting anabolic steroids. *J. Clin. Endocrin. Metab.* 64:960–63

29. Comm. Diet Health. 1989. Food Nutr. Board, Comm. Life Sci., Natl. Res. Counc. *Diet and Health: Implications for Reducing Chronic Disease Risk.* Washington, DC: Natl. Acad. Press

30. Comm. Diet. Allowances. 1989. Food Nutr. Board, Comm. Life Sci., Natl. Res. Counc. *Recommended Dietary Allowances.* Washington, DC: Natl. Acad. Press, 10th ed.

31. Cresanta, J. L., Burke, G. L., Downey, A. M., Freedman, D. S., Berenson, S. S. 1986. Prevention of atherosclerosis in childhood. *Pediatr. Clin. N. Am.* 33:835–58

32. Crummette, B. 1983. Assessing the impact of illness upon an adolescent and family. *Matern. Child Nurs. J.* 12:155–67

33. Cunningham, A. 1983. Bone mineral loss in lactating adolescents. *J. Pediatr.* 102:1016–17

34. Dallman, P. R. 1986. Biochemical basis for the manifestations of iron deficiency. *Annu. Rev. Nutr.* 6:13–40

35. Despres, J. P., Bouchard, C., Malina, R. M. 1990. Physical activity and coronary heart disease risk factors during childhood and adolescence. *Exerc. Sport Sci. Rev.* 18:243–61

36. Dietz, W. H., Gortmaker, S. L., Sobol, A. M. 1985. Trends in the prevalence of childhood and adolescent obesity in the United States. *Pediatr. Res.* 19:198A:203A

37. Drinkwater, B. L., Nilson, K., Chestnut, C. H., Bremner, W. J., Shainholtz, S., et al. 1984. Bone mineral content of amenorrheic and eumenorrheic athletes. *N. Engl. J. Med.* 311:277–81

38. Drinkwater, B. L., Nilson, K., Ott, S., Chestnut, C. H. 1986. Bone mineral density after resumption of menses in amenorrheic athletes. *J. Am. Med. Assoc.* 256:380–82

39. Durnin, J. V. 1966. Age, physical activity and energy expenditure. *Proc. Nutr. Soc.* 25:107–13

40. Dwyer, J. T. 1980. Diets for children and adolescents that meet the dietary goals. *Am. J. Dis. Child.* 134:1073–80

41. Dwyer, J. T. 1986. Nutrition education. In *What is America Eating: Proceedings of a Symposium.* Comm. Diet. Allowances, Food Nutr. Board. Washington, DC: Natl. Acad. Press

42. Dwyer, J. T., Bourgeois, A. 1991. Nutrition and school health services. In *School Health Services,* ed. H. Wallace. Oakland: Third Party. In press

43. Dwyer, J. T., Mayer, J. 1973. Psychosexual aspects of weight control and dieting behavior in adolescents. *Med. Asp. Hum. Sex.* 7:82–114

44. Dyment, P. G., Goldberg, B., Haefele, S. B., Rissler, W. L., et al. 1989. An-

abolic steroids and the adolescent athlete. *Pediatrics* 83:127–28

45. Elliot, D. L., Goldberg, L., Kuehl, K., Hanna, C. 1989. Metabolic evaluation of obese and nonobese siblings. *J. Pediatr.* 114:957–62

46. Everson, S. K., Freedson, P. S. 1989. Familial aggregation and physical activity. *Med. Sci. Sports Exerc.* 21:S94

47. Ferris, R. P., Cresanta, J. L., Frank, G. C., Webber, L. S., Berenson, G. S. 1986. Dietary studies of children from a biracial population: intakes of fat and fatty acids in 10- and 13-year-olds. *Am. J. Clin. Nutr.* 39:114–28

48. Forbes, G. B. 1985. The effect of anabolic steroids on lean body mass: the dose response curve. *Metabolism* 34: 571–73

49. Ford, E., Heath, G., Merritt, R., Washburn, R., Kriska, A. 1989. Physical activity and socio-economic status. *Med. Sci. Sports Exerc.* 21:S94

50. Frisancho, A. R., Matos, J., Leonard, W. R., Yaroch, L. A. 1985. Developmental and nutritional determinants of pregnancy outcome among teenagers. *Am. J. Phys. Anthropol.* 66:247–61

51. Garn, S. M. 1985. Two decades of followup of fatness in early childhood. *Am. J. Dis. Child.* 139:181–85

52. Garn, S. M., Bailey, S., Cole, P. E., Higgins, I. T. 1977. Level of education, level of income, and level of fatness in adults. *Am. J. Clin. Nutr.* 30:721–25

53. Garn, S. M., Clark, D. C. 1976. Trends in fatness and the origins of obesity. *Pediatrics* 57:443–56

54. Garn, S. M., LaVelle, M., Rosenberg, K. R., Hawthorne, V. M. 1986. Maturational timing as a factor in female fatness and obesity. *Am. J. Clin. Nutr.* 43:879–83

55. Garner, D. M., Garfinkel, P. E., Schwartz, D., Thompson, M. 1980. Cultural expectations of thinness in women. *Psychol. Rep.* 47:483–91

56. Godsland, I. F., Shennan, N. M., Wynn, V. 1986. Insulin action and dynamics modelled in patients taking the anabolic steroid methandienone (Dianabol). *Clin. Sci.* 71:665–73

57. Gorbach, S. L., Goldin, B. R. 1987. Diet and the excretion and enterohepatic cycling of estrogens. *Prev. Med.* 16: 525–31

58. Gortmaker, S. L., Dietz, W. H., Sobol, A. M., Wehler, C. A. 1987. Increasing pediatric obesity in the United States. *Am. J. Dis. Child.* 141:535–40

59. Hamill, P. V., Drizd, T. A., Johnson, C. L. 1979. Physical growth: National

Center for Health Statistics Percentiles. *Am. J. Clin. Nutr.* 32:607–29

60. Hanis, C. L., Ferrell, R. E., Barton, S. A., Aguilar, L., Garza, A., et al. 1983. Diabetes among Mexican-Americans in Starr County, Texas. *Am. J. Epidemiol.* 118:659–72

61. Hardy, J. B. 1988. Teenage pregnancy: an American dilemma. In *Maternal and Child Health Practices*, eds. H. M. Wallace, G. Ryan, A. C. Oglesby, pp. 539–54. Oakland: Third Party

62. Hardy, J. B., King, T. M., Repke, J. T. 1987. The Johns Hopkins Adolescent Pregnancy Program: an evaluation. *Obstet. Gynecol.* 69:300–5

63. Harlan, W. M., Landis, J. R., Flegal, K. M., Davis, C. S., Miller, M. E. 1988. Secular trends in body mass in the United States, 1960–1980. *Am. J. Epidemiol.* 128:1065–74

64. Herzog, D. 1982. Bulimia in the adolescent. *Am. J. Dis. Child.* 136:985–89

65. Housh, T. J., Johnson, G. O., Hughes, R. A., Housh, D. J., Hughes, R. J., et al. 1989. Isokinetic strength and body composition of high school wrestlers across age. *Med. Sci. Sports Exerc.* 21:105–9

66. Howie, B. J., Schultz, T. D. 1985. Dietary and hormonal interrelationships among vegetarian Seventh-Day Adventists and non-vegetarian men. *Am. J. Clin. Nutr.* 42:127–34

67. Hurley, B. F., Seals, D. R., Hagberg, J. M., Goldberg, A. C., Ostrove, S. M., et al. 1984. High-density lipoprotein cholesterol in bodybuilders v powerlifters: negative effects of androgen use. *J. Am. Med. Assoc.* 252:507–13

68. Inbar, O., Bar-Or, O. 1986. Anaerobic characteristics in male children and adolescents. *Med. Sci. Sports Exerc.* 18:264–69

69. Johnson, M. D., Jay, M. S., Shoup, B., Rickert, V. I. 1989. Anabolic steroid use by male adolescents. *Pediatrics* 83:921–24

70. Johnston, F. E. 1985. Health implications of childhood obesity. *Ann. Intern. Med.* 103:1068–72

71. Kanders, B., Dempster, D. W., Lindsay, R. 1988. Interaction of calcium nutrition and physical activity on bone mass in young women. *J. Bone Min. Res.* 3:145–49

72. Kaye, W., Gwirtsman, H., Obarzanek, E., George, T., Jimerson, D. C., et al. 1986. Caloric intake necessary for weight maintenance in anorexia nervosa: nonbulimics require greater caloric intake than bulimics. *Am. J. Clin. Nutr.* 44:435–43

73. Kemper, H. C., Verschuur, R., Essen, L. S., van Aalst, R. 1986. Longitudinal study of maximal aerobic power in boys and girls from 12 to 23 years of age. *Child. Exerc.* 12:203–11

74. Kemper, H. C., Verschuur, R., Ritmeester, J. W. 1986. Maximal aerobic power in early and late maturing teenagers. *Child. Exerc.* 12:213–25

75. Kirkley, B. 1986. Bulimia: clinical characteristics, development, and etiology. 1986. *J. Am. Diet. Assoc.* 86:468–75

76. Kron, L., Katz, J. L., Gorzynski, G., Weiner, H. 1978. Hyperactivity in anorexia nervosa: a fundamental clinical feature. *Compr. Psychiat.* 19:433–40

77. Krowchuk, D. P., Anglin, T. M., Goodfellow, D. B., Stancin, T., Williams, P., et al. 1989. High school athletes and the use of ergogenic aids. *Am. J. Dis. Child.* 143:486–89

78. Liel, Y., Edwards, J., Shary, J., Spicer, K. M., Gordon, L., et al. 1988. The effects of race and body habitus on bone mineral density of the radius, hip, and spine in premenopausal women. *J. Clin. Endocrinol. Metab.* 66:1247–54

79. Lifschitz, F., Moses, N., Cervantes, C. 1987. Nutritional dwarfing in adolescents. *Sem. Adolesc. Med.* 3:255–66

80. Lipscomb, P. A. 1987. Bulimia: diagnosis and management in the primary care setting. *J. Fam. Prac.* 24:187–94

81. Litt, I. F., Glader, L. 1986. Anorexia nervosa, athletics, and amenorrhea. *J. Pediatr.* 109:150–53

82. Looker, A. C., Sempos, C. T., Johnson, C. L., Yetley, E. Q. 1987. Comparison of dietary intakes and iron status of vitamin-mineral supplement users and nonusers aged 1–19 years. *Am. J. Clin. Nutr.* 46:655–72

83. Lucas, A. R. 1989. Update and review of anorexia nervosa. *Contemp. Nutr.* 14(9):1–2

84. Luna, A. M., Wilson, D. M., Wibbelsman, C. J., Brown, R. C., Nagashima, R. J., et al. 1983. Somatomedins in adolescence: a cross-sectional study of the effect of puberty on plasma insulin-like growth factor I and II levels. *J. Clin. Endocrin. Metab.* 57:268–71

85. MacMahon, J. R., Gross, R. T. 1988. Physical and psychological effects of aerobic exercise in delinquent adolescent males. *Am. J. Dis. Child.* 142:1361–66

86. Mahan, L. K. 1985. Nutrition in adolescent pregnancy. In *Nutrition in Adolescence*, eds. L. K. Mahan, J. M. Rees. St. Louis: Times Mirror/Mosby

87. Malina, R. M., Martorell, R., Mendoza, F. 1986. Growth status of Mexican American children and youths: historical trends and contemporary issues. *Yearb. Phys. Anthr.* 29:45–79

88. Mass. Med. Soc. Comm. Nutr. 1989. Fast food fare. *N. Engl. J. Med.* 321:752–56

89. Massara, E. B. 1980. Obesity and cultural weight evaluations. *Appetite* 1:291–98

90. Matkovic, V., Kostial, K., Simonovic, I., Buzina, R., Brodarec, A., et al. 1979. Bone status and fracture rates in two regions of Yugoslavia. *Am. J. Clin. Nutr.* 32:540–49

91. McArneney, E. 1985. Social maturation: a challenge for handicapped and chronically ill adolescents. *J. Adolesc. Health Care* 6:90–101

92. McNamara, J. J., Molot, M. A., Stremple, J. F., Cutting, R. T. 1971. Coronary artery disease in combat casualties in Vietnam. *J. Am. Med. Assoc.* 216:1185–87

93. Micheli, L. J., LaChabrier, L. 1984. The young female athlete. In *Pediatric and Adolescent Sports Medicine*, ed. L. Micheli, pp. 167–78. Boston: Little, Brown

94. Mitchell, J. E. 1989. Bulimia nervosa. *Contemp. Nutr.* 14(10):1–2

95. Moses, N., Banilivy, N. M., Lifschitz, E. 1989. Fear of obesity among adolescent girls. *Pediatrics* 83:393–98

96. Natl. Cent. Health Stat. 1987. *Advance Report of Final Natality Statistics for 1985.* Month. Vital Stat. Rep. 36, PHS Publ. No. 87-1120, Hyattsville, Md: Dept. Health Hum. Serv.

97. Natl. Cholesterol Educ. Program. 1990. *Report of the Expert Panel on Population Strategies for Blood Cholesterol Reduction.* Bethesda, Md: Natl. Inst. Health, Natl. Heart Lung Blood Inst.

98. Nelson, M. E., Fisher, E. C., Catsos, P., Meredith, C. N., Turksoy, N., et al. 1986. Diet and bone health in amenorrheic runners. *Am. J. Clin. Nutr.* 43:910–16

99. Newacheck, P., Budetti, P., McManus, P. 1984. Trends in childhood disability. *J. Public Health* 74:232–36

100. Nickerson, H. J., Holubets, M., Weiler, B. R., Haas, R. G., Schwartz, S., et al. 1989. Causes of iron deficiency in adolescent athletes. *J. Pediatr.* 114:657–63

101. O'Connell, D. G., Barnhart, R. C., Parks, L. 1989. Strength training in disabled children: improvements in strength and wheelchair propulsion. *Med. Sci. Sports Exerc.* 21:S95

102. O'Hare, W. P. 1987. *Poverty in America: Trends and New Patterns.* Washington, DC: Popul. Ref. Bur.

103. Paffenbarger, R. S., Hyde, R. T., Wing, A. L., Hsieh, C. C. 1986. Physical activity, all-cause mortality, and longevity of college alumni. *N. Engl. J. Med.* 314:605–13
104. Palla, B., Litt, I. F. 1988. Medical complications of eating disorders in adolescents. *Pediatrics* 81:613–23
105. Parr, R. B., Porter, M. A., Hodgson, S. C. 1984. Nutrition knowledge and practice of coaches, trainers, and athletes. *Phys. Sportsmed.* 12:127–38
106. Pate, R. R., Ross, J. 1987. Factors associated with health related fitness. *J. Phys. Educ. Rec. Dance* 48:93–98
107. Perrin, E., Ramsey, B., Sandler, H. 1987. Competent kids: children and adolescents with chronic illness. *Child Care Health Dev.* 13:13–32
108. Pirke, K. M., Schweigger, V., Laessle, R., Dickhant, B., Schweigger, M., et al. 1986. Dieting influences the menstrual cycle: vegetarian vs nonvegetarian diet. *Fertil. Steril.* 46:1083–88
109. Pope, H. G., Katz, D. L. 1988. Affective and psychotic symptoms associated with anabolic steroid use. *Am. J. Psychiatr.* 145:487–90
110. Powell, K. E., Spain, K. G., Christenson, G. M., Mollenkamp, M. P. 1986. The status of the 1990 objectives for physical fitness and exercise. *Public Health Rep.* 101:18–21
111. Pugliese, M. T., Lifschitz, F., Grad, G. 1983. A cause of short stature and delayed puberty. *New Engl. J. Med.* 309:513–18
112. Ravussin, E., Lillioja, S., Knowler, W. C., Christin, L., Freymond, D., et al. 1988. Reduced rate of energy expenditure as a risk factor for body weight gain. *N. Engl. J. Med.* 318:467–72
113. Rees, J. M. 1988. *Nutritional Issues in Adolescent Health: Information Bulletin, Youth 2000.* Dep. Health Hum. Serv., Bur. Matern. Child Health Resourc. Dev. Rockville, Md: US Dep. Health Hum. Serv.
114. Relethford, J. H., Stern, M. P., Gaskill, S. P., Hazuda, H. P. 1983. Social class, admixture, and skin color variation in Mexican-Americans and Anglo-Americans living in San Antonio, Texas. *Am. J. Phys. Anthropol.* 61:97–102
115. Roberts, S., Savage, J., Coward, W. A., Chew, B., Lucas, A. 1988. Energy expenditure and intake in infants born to lean and overweight mothers. *N. Engl. J. Med.* 318:461–66
116. Rocchini, A. P., Katch, V., Anderson, J., Hinderliter, J., Becque, D., et al. 1988. Blood pressure in obese adolescents: effect of weight loss. *Pediatrics* 82:16–23
117. Roche, A. F., Guo, S., Baumgartner, R. N., Chumlea, W. C., Ryan, A. S., et al. 1990. Reference data for weight, stature, and weight/stature^{2}2^{in} Mexican-Americans from the Hispanic Health and Nutrition Examination survey (HHANES 1982–1984). *Am. J. Clin. Nutr.* 51:917S–24S
118. Ross, C. E., Mirowsky, J. 1983. The social epidemiology of overweight: a substantive and methodological investigation. *J. Health Soc. Behav.* 24:288–98
119. Ross, J. G., Gilbert, G. G. 1985. The National Youth and Fitness Study: a summary of findings. *J. Phys. Educ.* 1:45–50
120. Deleted in proof
121. Samet, J. M., Coultas, D. B., Howard, C. A., Skipper, B. J., Hanis, C. L. 1988. Diabetes, gallbladder disease, obesity, and hypertension among Hispanics in New Mexico. *Am. J. Epidemiol.* 128:1302–11
122. Sanborn, C. F., Maratin, B. J., Wagner, W. W. 1982. Is athletic amenorrhea specific to runners? *Am. J. Obstet. Gynecol.* 143:859–61
123. Schweiger, U., Laessle, R., Schweiger, M., Herrmann, F., Riedel, W., et al. 1988. Caloric intake, stress, and menstrual function in athletes. *Fertil. Steril.* 49:447–50
124. Shangold, M. 1985. Causes, evaluation, and management of athletic oligoamenorrhea. *Med. Clin. N. Am.* 69:83–95
125. Shephard, R. F. 1986. *Fitness of a Nation: Lessons from the Canada Fitness Study,* pp. 94–97. New York: Karger
126. Shephard, R. J., Ward, G. R., Lee, M. 1986. Physical ability of deaf and blind children. *Child. Exerc.* 12:355–62
127. Short, S. H., Short, W. R. 1983. Four-year study of university athletes' dietary intake. *J. Am. Diet. Assoc.* 82:632–45
128. Siegel, D. Adolescents and chronic illness. 1987. *J. Am. Med. Assoc.* 257:3396–99
129. Sillanpaa, M. 1987. Social adjustment and functioning of chronically ill and impaired children and adolescents. *Acta Pediatr. Scand.* 310S:1–70
130. Skrobak-Kaczynski, J., Vavik, T. 1980. Physical fitness and trainability of young male patients with Down Syndrome. *Child. Exerc.* 9:300–16
131. Slap, G. 1986. Normal physiological and psychological growth in the adolescent. *J. Adolesc. Health Care* 7:13S–23S

132. Slavin, J., Lutter, J., Cushman, S. 1984. Amenorrhea in vegetaria athletes. *Lancet* 1:1474–75
133. Sloan, R. E., Keatinge, W. R. 1973. Cooling rates of young people swimming in cold water. *J. Appl. Physiol.* 35:371–75
134. Steen, S. N., McKinney, S. 1986. Nutrition assessment of college wrestlers. *Phys. Sportsmed.* 14:100–16
135. Steen, S. N., Oppliger, R. A., Brownell, K. D. 1988. Metabolic effects of repeated weight loss and regain in adolescent wrestlers. *J. Am. Med. Assoc.* 260:47–50
136. Story, M., Alton, I. 1987. Nutrition issues and adolescent pregnancy. *Contemp. Nutr.* 12:7–12
137. Story, M., Blum, R. W. 1988. Adolescent nutrition: self-perceived deficiencies and needs of practitioners working with youth. *J. Am. Diet. Assoc.* 88:591–94
138. Strong, W. B., Dennison, B. A. 1988. Pediatric preventive cardiology: atherosclerosis and coronary heart disease. *Pediatr. Rev.* 9:303–14
139. Sundberg, S. 1982. Maximal oxygen uptake in relation to age in blind and normal boys and girls. *Acta Pediatr. Scand.* 71:603–8
140. Sunnegardh, J., Bratteby, L. E., Sjolin, S., Hagman, U., Hoffstedt, A. 1985. The relation between physical activity and energy intake of 8- and 13-year old children in Sweden. *Child. Exerc.* 11:194–202
141. Tanner, J. W. 1981. Catchup growth in man. *Br. Med. J.* 37:233–38
142. Tanner, J. W. 1981. *Fetus into Man: Physical Growth from Conception to Maturity.* Cambridge, Mass: Harvard Univ. Press
143. Taylor, R., Ram, P., Raper, L. R., Ringrose, H. 1984. Physical activity and prevalence of diabetes in Melanesian and Indian men in Fiji. *Diabetologia* 27:578–82
144. US Congr., Office Technol. Assess. 1990. Nutrition and fitness problems. In *Adolescent Health.* Washington, DC: US Congr.
145. US Dep. Agric., Hum. Nutr. Inf. Serv. 1984. *Nationwide Food Consumption Survey, Nutrient Intakes: Individuals in 48 States, Year 1977–1978.* report No. I-2. Hyattsville, Md: USDA

146. US Dep. Health Hum. Serv. 1988. *The Surgeon General's Report on Nutrition and Health.* Washington, DC: GPO
147. US Dep. Health Hum. Serv. Am. Sch. Health Assoc., Assoc. Adv. Health Educ., Soc. Public Health Educ., Inc. 1989. *The National Adolescent Student Health Survey: A Report on the Health of America's Youth.* Oakland: Third Party
148. Van Itallie, T. B. 1985. Health implications of overweight and obesity in the United States. *Ann. Int. Med.* 103:983–88
149. Van Itallie, T. B., Abraham, S. 1985. Some hazards of obesity and its treatment. *Obes. Res.* 4:1–19
150. Deleted in proof
151. Verschuur, R., Kemper, H. C. 1985. Habitual physical activity in Dutch teenagers measured by heart rate. *Child. Exerc.* 11:194–202
152. Wakeling, A., Russell, G. F. 1970. Disturbances in the regulation of body temperature in anorexia nervosa. *Psychol. Med.* 1:30–39
153. Warren, M. P., Brooks-Gunn, J., Hamilton, L. H., Warren, L. F., Hamilton, W. G. 1986. Scoliosis and fractures in young ballet dancers. *N. Engl. J. Med.* 314:1348–53
154. Washburn, R. A., Kline, G., Lackland, D. T., Wheeler, F. C. 1989. Leisure time physical activity: are there black-white differences? *Med. Sci. Sports Exerc.* 21:S94
155. Weiss, K. M., Ferrell, R. E., Hanis, C. L. 1984. A New World syndrome of metabolic diseases with a genetic and evolutionary basis. *Yearb. Phys. Anthropol.* 27:153–78
156. Westoff, C. F., Calot, G., Foster, A. D. 1983. Teenage fertility in developed nations. *Fam. Plann. Perspect.* 14:105–10
157. Wright, J. E., Stone, M. H. 1985. NSCA statement on anabolic drug use. *NSCA J.* 7:45–59
158. Young, T. K., Sevenhuysen, G. 1989. Obesity in Northern Canadian Indians: patterns, determinants, and consequences. *Am. J. Clin. Nutr.* 49:786–93
159. Zack, P., Harlan, W., Leaverton, P., et al. 1979. A longitudinal study of body fatness in childhood and adolescence. *J. Pediatr.* 95:126–30

Annu. Rev. Publ. Health. 1991. 12:335–360

BIOETHICS AND PUBLIC HEALTH IN THE 1980s: RESOURCE ALLOCATION AND AIDS

R. R. Faden

Program in Law, Ethics, and Health, Department of Health Policy and Management, The Johns Hopkins School of Hygiene and Public Health, Baltimore, Maryland 21205; The Kennedy Institute of Ethics, Georgetown University, Washington, DC 20057

N. E. Kass

The Kennedy Institute of Ethics, Georgetown University, Washington, DC 20057

KEY WORDS: access to medical care, justice and health policy, ethics and the HIV epidemic

INTRODUCTION

Bioethics is an interdisciplinary field concerned with moral issues in the biomedical sciences, medical care, and health policy. Before 1980, the interests of bioethics focused primarily on such topics as the nature of the doctor-patient relationship, death and dying, and the ethics of human experimentation. In the 1980s, however, there was a discernible increase in questions of social ethics and community and, thus, in public health.

The sheer volume of bioethics literature is showcased in Table 1. Using BIOETHICSLINE, a computerized information retrieval system, we collapsed the bioethics literature of the 1980s into 17 categories by grouping database keywords. BIOETHICSLINE includes articles published in public health, medical, social science, and legal journals, as well as the specialty bioethics publications. This range reflects both the interdisciplinary character of bioethics and the frequency with which relevant normative issues are addressed by authors who are not bioethicists or who do not write primarily for a bioethics audience.

335

0163-7525/91/0501-0335$02.00

Table 1   Bioethics literature in the 1980s

Topic	Number of Citations[a]		
	1980–1982	1983–1986	1987–1989
Bioethics (general)	581	882	554
Codes of ethics	168	148	93
Professional-patient relationship	1430	1597	925
Health care	596	1190	926
AIDS	none	214	666
Public health	89	226	245
Resource allocation	197	472	389
Contraception	151	174	78
Abortion	551	466	306
Reproduction and reproductive technologies	429	818	606
Genetic intervention	484	579	311
Mental health therapies	249	240	99
Research ethics	738	984	552
Organ donation and transplantation	94	514	357
Death and dying	806	1417	881
Biomedicine and violence	107	189	55
Animal experimentation	21	221	114

[a] Citations can be assigned to more than one category.

Traditional topics, such as death and dying, organ transplantation, and the professional-patient relationship, continued to command significant attention in the literature throughout the decade. However, there also was considerable interest in topics of central concern to public health, such as health care, contraception, abortion, resource allocation, and AIDS. Indeed, from 1987 through 1989, the number of citations for AIDS alone—666—was not far behind the number of citations for death and dying, which includes allowing to die, determination of death, brain death, euthanasia, living wills, advanced directives, resuscitation, wrongful life, and terminal care.

The growing interest in the normative dimensions of public health was reflected in several professional developments. The 1980s saw the establishment of the first professional organization specifically focused on the intersection of bioethics and public health: the Forum on Bioethics, a Special Primary Interest Group of the American Public Health Association. The percentage of schools of public health that offered at least one course in bioethics or the ethical dimensions of public health increased from about 60% at the beginning of the decade to about 90% by the end.

However, normative dimensions of several key issues (and areas) in public health remained relatively unexplored at the close of the decade. The heading of public health (Table 1) comprised a comparatively modest 560 citations. More than 60% were articles or books about AIDS, and another 20% were about immunization or mass screening for other infectious or genetic diseases. The next most common subject was ethical issues in primary prevention, in particular, how to reconcile respect for individual liberty with the goals of health promotion and disease and injury prevention (8, 19, 29, 34, 44, 55, 64, 79, 115, 124, 138, 141, 142, 147, 149, 151). Only a few citations addressed such central topics in public health as justice and smoking policy (9, 40, 84); fair distribution of risks to health in the workplace, the environment, and the marketplace (52, 77, 82, 105, 155); and the ethics, meaning, and goals of public health itself (14–16, 96–98, 117).[1]

In this paper we review the issues and arguments of the 1980s for two central topics in public health about which a substantial literature on ethical issues did emerge—resource allocation and AIDS. As we shall see, at the close of the decade most of the normative issues raised by these topics were far from resolved.

RESOURCE ALLOCATION

Broadly construed, resource allocation asks: How much of society's resources should be allocated to health, as compared with other socially valued goods, like education, defense, or preservation of natural and historical treasures? Also included is the question of how to allocate resources within the category of health between those interventions that can reduce risks to health in the environment, food supply, and workplace and those that are delivered through the health care system, which themselves have diverse purposes and effects.

To date, most of the literature on resource allocation and health policy has failed to address such foundational issues. Given the political intractability and seemingly reason-defying character of these "guns versus butter" questions, this failure is not surprising. The literature of the 1980s concentrated on problems of allocation of resources within the health care system, i.e. the fair or just allocation of resources devoted to the delivery of health care services.

Access

In the first part of the decade, much of the literature concerned with ethics and resource allocation focused on access to health care and whether and to what extent moral rights or entitlements to health care services exist. Much of this literature was stimulated by the President's Commission for the Study of Ethical Problems in Medicine and Biomedical and Behavioral Research (131). Their 1983 report, *Securing Access to Health Care,* drew on numerous analyses by writers in bioethics, several of which were commissioned specifi-

---

[1]Here, as throughout the article, it is not possible to cite every relevant reference. The articles cited should be taken as representative of the literature, but by no means necessarily exhaustive.

cally for the report. Many perspectives on justice and health policy were brought to bear on the problem of access and moral entitlement, with varying degrees of success. Some of the more notable efforts include Green's (71) and Daniels' (36, 37) examinations of access from a Rawlsian perspective, Gibbard's (61, 62) analysis from within a utilitarian framework, Brody's (21) "quasilibertarian" analysis, and Buchanan's (24) pluralistic, "enforced beneficence" account.

Given this diversity of perspectives, it is perhaps surprising how much consensus emerged, particularly about minimal entitlements. Despite disagreements about the moral justification for access to health care, the relevance of rights language, and the rightness of redistributing income rather than distributing vouchers or in-kind services, there was near universal agreement that all individuals should have access to at least an "adequate level" or "decent minimum" of health care services (48, 108). However, despite several serious attempts, this literature failed to provide a useful, principled, or procedural mechanism for determining what this adequate level would look like or how it would be implemented. The important question of which, if any, services could be excluded without violating the demands of justice remained essentially unanswered. Thus, the programs fell far short of being able to guide concrete policy decisions.

Rationing

In the latter part of the decade, the focus of the literature shifted from access to health services to allocation and rationing (17, 26, 30, 126, 153). The interest in rationing can be traced to several factors, particularly the continued escalation of health care costs and the concomitant focus in health policy on cost containment. Indeed, cost containment policies generated their own bioethics literature. Numerous articles examined what was arguably the most significant cost containment policy to be instituted in the 1980s—prospective hospital reimbursement based on diagnostic related groups (DRGs) (2, 23, 49, 53, 76, 116, 140, 144). Another factor behind this interest was the increasing recognition of the role of rationing in the National Health Service of Great Britain, which was a central observation in the influential book, *The Painful Prescription* (1). Increasingly, there was a call to recognize both the implicit rationing inherent in the American system and the need for a morally acceptable, explicit rationing policy.

Perhaps the most controversial issue to have emerged thus far is the proposal to ration by age (139). Intergenerational justice and the claims of the aged on social resources have taken on new significance as costs escalate, resources diminish, and the population ages. Two major works on this subject are Callahan's *Setting Limits* (25) and Daniels' *Am I My Parents' Keeper?* (38). Both books defend the view that it is not necessarily unjust to ration life-extending health care resources purely by age; however, Callahan and Daniels use very different arguments. As Brock (20) has noted, Daniels approaches the age-group problem from within the tradition of Rawlsian political liberalism. Daniels assumes that there is no single substantive account of the good life against which allocation decisions for the elderly can be made. In Daniels' "prudential lifespan account," prudent persons choose selected age-rationing plans for health care allocations because such allocation patterns foster equality of opportunity and the ability to pursue one's own visions of the good life over the course of a lifetime.

Callahan rejects central elements of the tradition of political liberalism and defends the view that allocation decisions that affect the elderly should be based on a communal consensus about the proper purpose and meaning of aging and old age. Central to Callahan's account is the notion of a "tolerable death"—a death free of degrading pain that occurs after one has largely exhausted life's possibilities and discharged one's obligations to others, a death after the "normal lifespan" of roughly 80 years. Callahan argues that the proper goals for health care are to secure a normal lifespan for all and to provide relief of suffering for those who live beyond that lifespan. Long-term care and other supportive services to the elderly need to be dramatically expanded, but those living beyond the normal lifespan have no entitlement to life-extending health care services. Not surprisingly, others in the literature have rejected the arguments put forward in both books, finding any pure age-rationing policy to be morally objectionable (10, 89).

Whether any form of age-rationing is either morally justifiable or politically feasible remains unresolved. Nor do all commentators agree that rationing in general is either necessary or morally appropriate. Underlying any call for rationing is what Brody (22) has called the emerging standard view of American health care policy. This view asserts that rationing is inevitable because none of the traditional and, perhaps, more desirable approaches to solving the problems of escalating costs—better regulation, more encouragement of competition, and an emphasis on prevention—can solve the problem. Because of shifting demographics and the ever-increasing development of expensive medical advances, even a country as wealthy as the United States has no choice but rationing. Brody resists this emerging view on moral grounds. Emphasizing respect for individual choice, rather than collective social choices, Brody proposes several alternatives to rationing policies. He argues that costs can be saved by systematically eliciting the preferences of patients and their families and withholding care from patients who are terminally ill or have very low quality of life whenever this is requested. Rationing care to the poor is to be avoided by providing all Americans with a fair and adequate level of income, thus empowering the poor to select from among alternative insurance schemes the package of health care services to which they will be entitled.

Other critics reject rationing on different grounds. They argue that the United States can afford to provide all its citizens with the best of medical care, if only the political will to redistribute public expenditures at the macro level is present. Pellegrino & Thomasma (128) have stated that all alternatives to rationing have not yet been exhausted. They argue that any proposals to save costs by rationing expensive forms of medical care must be compared against massive national expenditures in other areas, such as the $65 billion spent on cosmetics and the $30 billion spent on alcohol.

Both proponents and critics of rationing believe that the problems and contradictions of the American health care system are fundamentally moral in character. Insofar as rationing is inevitable, rationing and access essentially are two sides of the same coin. If, as most commentators agree, society is obligated to assure all Americans access to an adequate level of health care and not to all the health care from which they can benefit, then the problem of deciding which health care to provide is the problem of determining a principled or procedural basis for rationing care.[2]

From a public health perspective, it is noteworthy that, despite the absence of consensus regarding a principled or procedural basis for rationing, the literature on access sees prevention and primary care as paradigmatic of the interventions that should fall under the decent or adequate level of health care to which all should be entitled. Indeed, prenatal care and immunizations often are cited as among the most obvious, least controversial services to be included within this basic or adequate package (30, 131). At the same time, a subtheme in the literature defends a moral priority on "medical treatment" over "prevention." According to this view, the efficiency arguments that favor prevention are outweighed by a combination of other moral considerations, including the claims of identifiable versus statistical lives, the expressive or symbolic value of acts of rescue in medical care, and the difficulties in turning away persons in acute need (58, 108).

This apparent confusion about the relative moral priority of prevention compared with treatment can be attributed to several difficulties, including a failure to recognize that the two concepts are much too broad and far too overlapping to serve as useful categories for determining the fair allocation of resources. Another problem is the implicit assumption that the only argument for prevention is efficiency.

Contrast the apparent first principle of the British health care system, which assures universal access to primary care, with the American system, which fails to provide any assured level of access to significant numbers of individuals. Is it more just to provide universal access to primary care, while

---

[2]Alternatively, following Brody's suggestion, the problem is determining and assuring fair income shares and allowing individuals to choose.

rationing x-ray film, medical management of metastatic cancers, and renal dialysis, or to engage in the extensive use of these diagnostic and therapeutic services, while "rationing" or failing to provide millions with prenatal care and immunizations (110)?

Underlying one answer to this question is a distinctive position on justice and health care policy: In the distribution of limited health care resources, primary care, including basic preventive services, ought to be provided to everyone before any allocations are made to provide subsets of the population with more sophisticated medical care. This position, specific to the use of public subsidies, is embedded in the report, *Securing Access*, but has received surprisingly little attention (131). Adhering to this proposition would require a radical rehauling of the American health care system.

Looking Ahead

As we move further into the 1990s, the issues of access and rationing are likely to become even more hotly debated, and the question of priority in allocation on universal access to primary care is likely to be a central theme (27). One foretaste of this debate is currently showcased in Oregon. The Oregon legislature is experimenting with a new proposal to finance the expansion of Medicaid coverage to all Oregonians at or below the poverty line by rationing the services covered under Medicaid (122). An 11-member Health Services Commission has been charged with rank ordering medical interventions from most to least important; the state legislature is to determine how far down the list Medicaid coverage will extend based on available funding. The tradeoff is simple—for more of the state's poor to have access to basic health care, the extent of medical services to current Medicaid beneficiaries will be reduced.

The preliminary list of 1600 procedures prepared by the Oregon Health Services Commission gives high priority to many preventive and primary care services. The Commission held 50 public hearings across the state. Overwhelmingly, persons who attended the hearings favored preventive interventions over expensive life-saving surgical interventions.

In addition to public input, the Commission's rankings were based on a formal analytic method for comparing interventions. Interventions were assigned a rating on a Quality of Well Being scale; these ratings were based on the responses of 1000 Oregonians to a telephone survey in which they were asked to rate how they would feel about their quality of life if they were compromised in numerous ways. The cost of each intervention was divided by the number of years the average person could be expected to live after treatment and adjusted for the intervention's rating on the Quality of Well Being scale (45).

This methodology is sure to spark renewed criticism of the role of formal methods, such as cost-benefit and cost-utility analysis in the setting of health policy. At this juncture, efficiency and cost containment clearly will continue to be defining elements of the health policy agenda. As a result, formal methods for maximizing efficiency are likely to be employed increasingly in allocation policy. At the same time, perhaps even more so than in the 1980s, these methods will be criticized for introducing systematic injustices in access and allocation patterns (47).

In the field of risk assessment there already exists a lively debate concerning the normative dimensions of risk-cost-benefit analysis and the extent to which such analyses should be permitted to either define or influence risk policy (82, 105, 136). More work is needed to explore the parallel questions in health policy; indeed, the social issues engaged in justly distributing health services and justly distributing risks to health are remarkably similar. Particularly useful would be an examination of the implications of the interconnections of moral and economic utilitarian theories for distributional problems in both fields.

As suggested in the Oregon methodology, one area that is likely to prove contentious in the 1990s is whether and how to take account of quality of life in setting health policy goals and defining allocational patterns. It is widely felt that, at least at the extreme, an intervention that leaves a person in a persistent, vegetative state should be "devalued" in any policy comparison with an intervention that leaves a person fully functional. Also widely held, however, is the opposing view that it is morally wrong to attach less value to the lives of those with disabilities.

As a general rule, the elderly and persons with disabilities tend to fair poorly in allocation policies that formally adjust for years of life saved and "quality of life" (93). Perhaps for that reason, in the Oregon experiment, Medicaid benefits to the elderly and those with disabilities will not be ranked or assigned priorities; rather, the structure for these groups will remain unaltered. The extension of health care coverage to all poor Oregonians is thus not at the expense of all of the state's current Medicaid beneficiaries, but de facto at the expense of women and children only. This is itself ethically suspect.

The interests of both the elderly and persons with disabilities tend to be represented by strong, politically significant advocacy and lobbying groups; the interests of poor women and children usually are not. Other than political influence, are there any relevant differences between beneficiaries who are elderly or have disabilities from (other) women and children that could justify retaining their benefits structure? One distinction that may have relevance has to do with the services provided under Medicaid to the different groups. For the elderly and those with disabilities, Medicaid generally pays for long-term and home care services. Because these services are not "medical care," and indeed function to reduce the need for medical care, they arguably should be exempted from the rationing plan. However, if it is a characteristic of a service and not a recipient that determines protection from rationing cuts, then the Oregon policy, at least in principle, should be designed differently.

The Oregon experiment attempts to merge a straightforwardly utilitarian methodology with a democratic political process. Whether the procedures employed to determine whose services should be rationed and to rank health care services were fair and democratic is as much open to question as the utilitarian methodology itself. In clinical medical ethics, there is a substantive literature about just procedures for making decisions in a context of conflict, for example, the roles of hospital ethics committees and the courts. By contrast, there has been almost no analysis of the analogous issue of just procedures for policy decisions about health care allocations in the context of cultural and ethical pluralism. The 1980s did see the development of the grassroots bioethics movement that has sought to create mechanisms for involving the community in health policy debates (35, 81, 87). The 1990s are likely to see an increased focus on the problem of just procedures: Who should make rationing policy—experts, legislators, the courts, the public—and which combination of mechanisms should they use—referenda, public health regulation, governmental commissions, legislation (27)?

Just procedures will not eliminate the problem of substantive criteria for rationing policies, however. At the very least, individuals or groups that are designated through procedural mechanisms to make health policy will have to use some criteria for making rationing decisions. In Oregon, for example, a fiscal analysis will determine how far down the list of health services the money will stretch and, thus, which services will be covered under Medicaid, given existing resources for the program. However, this fiscal analysis will not determine whether that which falls within the pay line constitutes a decent level of health care.

At this writing, it is unknown whether the Oregon experiment will be implemented. Oregon cannot proceed without a specific waiver from the federal government. Whether a waiver will be granted depends on numerous considerations, including the adequacy of the health care services provided, the propriety of rationing by disease-specific medical interventions, and the propriety of exempting elderly persons and those with disabilities from the rationing plan.

Perhaps the most fundamental issue for the 1990s, as illustrated by the Oregon experiment, is the moral and political viability of a "two-tiered system" of medical care embedded in a patchwork of multiple private and public insurers and third-party payers. At first, the Oregon plan seems to be a straightforward application of the plan adopted by Great Britain and other countries in which the moral priority of a just health care system is to provide access to all, even if this requires rationing more advanced forms of medical therapy or restoration. But, there is a crucial difference between the two plans. In Great Britain, all citizens are subject to the country's prioritization process, as all citizens may enroll in the National Health Service. In Oregon, only persons enrolled in health programs administered by the state are subject to rationing. It is estimated that just over half of those in Oregon who are subject to rationing are Medicaid recipients and are poor; most of the remainder are part of the state's small employer insurance fund (Paige Sipes-Metzler, Health Services Commission, state of Oregon, personal communication). There is nothing inherent in the position that access to primary care should have priority that justifies denying to the poor efficacious and conventional medical interventions that are available widely to the bulk of the nonpoor (whose health care programs are not administered by the state). Admittedly, there also is no justification for a system that says that services should be provided to some of those who cannot afford them, but not to others.

In the 1980s most commentators, in rallying around the concept of guaranteed access to a decent or adequate level of health care, endorsed the concept of a two-tiered system of medical care. That is, it seemed proper that the nonpoor should remain free to purchase with personal resources services not available to the poor under the decent minimum (131). This position is easy to support in the abstract, as a compromise between egalitarian impulses to assure access and libertarian impulses to respect liberty and property rights. The problems with this compromise are emerging now, as concrete proposals, such as the Oregon plan, attempt to stipulate both the content of the decent minimum and its financial structure. Increasingly it appears that as long as proposals for expanding access to medical care in the context of rationing work within the current structure of Medicaid, Medicare, and employment-based medical insurance, the decent minimum for the poor runs the risk of falling far short of any ordinary understanding of decency. At the same time, restricting rationing policies to government entitlement programs makes questionable ethical and economic sense. Already there are signs that the 1990s may see a resurgence of interest in a more unified system of medical care. For example, a recent, provocative position paper of the American College of Physicians put forward for discussion the potential desirability of establishing universal access to health care through a national health insurance program (3, 72).

The 1990s are likely to see a continuation of the tension between egalitarian and libertarian impulses in health care policy. However, as the debate becomes more concrete and practical, the actual implications of continuing with starkly different programs and systems of financing for the poor and the nonpoor are likely to come under increasing ethical and public health scrutiny.

AIDS AND BIOETHICS

Few diseases have brought to light as many ethical questions as AIDS. Unlike the topic of resource allocation, which could neatly be divided into the twin concerns of access and rationing, AIDS raises widely different moral considerations that involve many, if not most, of the central issues in contemporary bioethics. This broad range of concerns is due to a unique combination of factors that characterize this disease: it has affected certain populations disproportionately, it is infectious and fatal, it is new and unpredictable, it is a costly condition, and it has affected a large number of individuals.

AIDS first was recognized only a decade ago, but the response to the disease has changed even in this short period of time. At first, little action was seen. Indeed, one of the fundamental questions about the HIV epidemic is whether the initial response of government and the public health and medical communities was "too little, too late" (114, 137) or, alternatively, understandable and acceptable given the unusual circumstances. Strategies early in the epidemic were most likely to originate from the already well-organized gay community, although some approaches were proposed by government officials and by private individuals.

One of the first instances in which AIDS was addressed in the bioethics literature was in 1983 in reference to the Public Health Service's recommendation that gay men be discouraged from donating blood (11). However, as more proposals for combating the epidemic appeared in the public arena, more articles appeared in the bioethics literature, as well. Some of the early public proposals, such as quarantine, were more restrictive than are most current proposals. Other restrictive strategies that now are on the rise include targeted HIV screening or screening as a mandatory condition for receiving a desired or needed benefit, such as prenatal care or a marriage license.

It is not surprising that we have witnessed changes in approach to the epidemic. There was even more panic initially than there is today concerning the contagiousness of the infection. The virus had not been identified, routes of transmission were not understood, and no treatments were available. At the same time, the early epidemiologic evidence suggested that AIDS would develop in only a fraction of infected individuals, which led some researchers and policymakers to argue for a less aggressive response.

Questions of ethics and AIDS have received considerable attention, not only from bioethicists and lawyers, but also from the broader medical community. Indeed, the importance of moral issues is highlighted in the two most significant overall reports on the epidemic, the Institute of Medicine's volumes *Confronting AIDS* (85, 86) and the *Report of the Presidential Commission on the Human Immunodeficiency Virus Epidemic* (132). Both of these reports included significant discussion of the ethical issues raised by the disease.

In this section we review ethical issues about AIDS that arose in the 1980s, which are organized under three broad headings: public health measures, health care delivery, and research. We conclude the section with a discussion of the moral issues we might expect to see as we enter the 1990s.

Public Health Measures

QUARANTINE AND ISOLATION   When the AIDS epidemic began, fear and uncertainty led some persons to argue for the isolation of infected individuals or of persons with AIDS (46, 74, 133). In a 1986 report, the Institute of Medicine described proposals from the public, which ranged from tattooing seropositive individuals to isolating all HIV-infected persons. Also in 1986, 46% of respondents to a poll conducted by *The Los Angeles Times* favored isolation of persons with AIDS (106).

There was an immediate and almost uniform rejection of quarantine and widespread isolation measures from the legal, ethics, and public health communities (69, 92, 104, 118, 130). Arguments included the infrequency with which infected individuals purposely harm others, the impracticality of isolating 1–2 million individuals for, conceivably, an average of 15 years each, a concern about how such a policy would undermine trust in the medical and public health communities, and fundamental criticisms of justice.

There also was little support in academic circles for proposals to exclude infected persons from schools, employment, or housing. The now famous case of Ryan White, who was barred from attending his public school, publicized this issue perhaps more than any other. Challenges to such exclusions have been based on the federal Rehabilitation Act and the federal Education for All Handicapped Children Act (42, 68), as well as numerous state laws. However, this legal patchwork is far from adequate, and many commentators have called for more comprehensive antidiscrimination protections (39, 68).

However, the isolation of "recalcitrant" or "noncompliant" individuals has received greater public and professional support, and, in certain circumstances such isolation has been implemented (68, 69). One early such case involved a Florida prostitute who was required to wear an electronic monitor and to stay within 200 feet of her phone (111). Although legally restricting individuals who knowingly transmit the virus to others has been considered to be justifiable for certain individual cases, there has been some argument against isolation, as HIV is transmitted primarily through voluntary behaviors, and it is difficult to determine purposeful spreading of the disease.

SCREENING   Perhaps the liveliest debates in the 1980s concerned HIV screening. Initially, many commentators framed this as a classic case of the tension between individual civil liberties and protection of the public health

(60, 65, 83). However, more recently it has been argued that this conflict was overdrawn and that it may be in the interests of the public's health to have screening policies that are respectful of civil liberties.

Normative criteria for evaluating screening programs have been proposed by several authors, including Childress (28) and Bayer and colleagues (12, 13). Whether the screening program under consideration is to be voluntary or mandatory, targeted or universal, it is critical to justify the purpose of screening and to know whether the screening program is likely to achieve that purpose. Although widespread screening was proposed on the heels of the ELISA test's 1985 licensure, treatments were unavailable to those who tested positive. Therefore, because screening could not be justified in terms of identifying individuals to whom health benefits could be provided, it was encouraged with the hope that it could facilitate the wider societal benefit of preventing transmission to others. However, whether widespread screening actually would lead to a reduction in transmission often was not included in debates. Rather, this was taken as a given, and public policy discussions jumped immediately into whether the assumed benefit of preventing transmission outweighed the infringement of personal privacy imposed by screening. Indeed, research conducted to determine behavior changes based on HIV antibody results has generated somewhat contradictory findings (33, 43, 56, 107, 143). In many instances, screening seems to be promoted because it permits a forum for conveying other messages, typically educational ones. Again, we need empirical evidence to evaluate a screening program for this purpose. Is education in the context of screening any more effective than education separate from screening? If not, the public health benefits from education could be provided without risking compromise of individual rights or interests.

Within the bioethics and public health communities, the dominant appeals have been for voluntary screening. This position has been defended on numerous grounds: screening is most likely to identify persons already at risk of social and economic discrimination in our society; identification may lead to denial of rights and benefits to which one otherwise would be entitled—not only in the health care arena but also in employment, housing, and insurance; and because adequate protections against discrimination are not in place, we cannot demand that persons undergo these risks (39, 60, 88). Mandatory screening is defensible only when therapeutic intervention is available, when the condition for which citizens are being screened is sufficiently infectious to put others at risk via casual contact, and when no less restrictive measure is available to achieve the same benefit (13, 69, 70, 83).

As treatments become more readily available, there is renewed interest in more aggressive screening policies (57, 78). However, treatments that help infected persons by alleviating symptoms or improving prognosis must be distinguished from treatments that prevent transmission and thereby benefit others. At present, there is no drug available that prevents transmission. Therefore, screening can be justified only because it is in the best interests of persons with HIV to initiate treatment as early in the course of the disease as possible. Indeed, the interventions currently available do change the harm-to-benefit ratio of testing, but only as they reduce or delay morbidity among those already infected. These interventions do not reduce transmission or prevent harm to others.

Targeting populations for screening raises additional ethical concerns, which have been discussed by Nolan (119) and Mitchell (113). Clearly, there are both advantages and disadvantages to selective or targeted screening. Resources are used more efficiently if tests are not performed in low prevalence populations, and the predictive value of a positive result is considerably higher in high prevalence populations. However, screening only in high prevalence populations conveys the message that only certain people are at risk for infection, which constitutes a public health concern and risks the perpetuation of invidious stereotypes. More fundamentally, targeted screening is potentially socially divisive. In particular, if screening is targeted to minority communities, it raises important questions of social justice, eugenics, and exploitation.

MANDATORY REPORTING   Whether by participation in a screening program or in the context of clinical care, once a person's HIV antibody status is known to be positive, should the state be notified of the test result? In 1985, Colorado became the first state to require that positive ELISA and western blot results be reported to state and local health departments (145). Advocates of reporting suggested that more accurate understanding of the disease could be achieved with mandatory reporting and that education and potential treatments could be targeted to known infected individuals. At the same time, critics argued that such a policy was an unjustified invasion of privacy. They warned that without strict antidiscrimination protections, this measure would drive at risk persons from being tested for the virus. As with screening policies, the advent of treatments for asymptomatic HIV-positive persons has shifted the momentum somewhat in favor of mandatory reporting. As of July 1989, 28 states require health care providers to report cases of persons infected with HIV (66).

PARTNER NOTIFICATION/CONTACT TRACING   In a 1986 article that examined legal and social issues raised by the epidemic, Gostin & Curran (68) distinguish partner notification from contact tracing. They define partner notification as the "voluntary notification by the client" of his or her sexual or needle-sharing partners, whereas contact tracing is "medical surveillance in which public health officials [have] a statutory power or duty to inquire about [an infected] person's previous and current sexual partners." This latter category has met with mixed response. Gostin & Curran believe that, in the instance of HIV, the public health benefits from contact tracing would be marginal and could undermine other public health efforts already in place to contain the spread of the disease. There has been support in the medical community for contact tracing, however. Commentators, such as Francis & Chin (57) argue that contact tracing will assist materially the public health goal of containing the epidemic. Dimas & Richland (41) report that every state health department counsels seropositive persons to notify their partners, and 37 state health departments offer provider referral services, through which the health department or a health care provider may notify partners on behalf of the index patient without revealing his or her identity.

EDUCATION   Given that worthwhile treatments were not available early in the epidemic and a cure remains to be discovered, there is near universal agreement that education currently is the most effective strategy for fighting AIDS. In the 1986 report *Confronting AIDS,* the Institute of Medicine called the level of AIDS-related education "woefully inadequate." The Institute's 1988 report cited increased efforts to educate the public on the local, state, and federal level.

Because specific information about routes of transmission is available, education campaigns can explicitly address how to avoid infection. However, the precise content of educational messages remains a source of debate. Some persons believe that candid education programs are offensive or likely to foster immoral or illegal behaviors; others argue that messages that are not explicit are too ambiguous to truly guide anyone away from potentially fatal situations (18, 51, 86). The Presidential Commission on the Human Immunodeficiency Virus Epidemic (132) raised its concern that, "in the promotion of the personal moral and political values of those from both ends of the political spectrum, the consistent distribution of clear, factual information about HIV transmission has suffered."

In addition, the issue of who should be targeted for education campaigns remains a source of controversy. Clearly, specific behaviors, rather than membership in any particular group, place a person at risk. Certain groups, however, have higher seroprevalence rates than others; thus, it may be efficient and efficacious for resources and messages to be directed disproportionately toward members of those groups (146).

A major ethical concern in providing education messages is the degree to which recommendations should be given. There is little argument with recommending that persons engage in safe sex and do not share unsterilized needles. The case is not so clear in recommending that HIV-positive women avoid pregnancy, and advising women to terminate existing pregnancies is particularly controversial. Nevertheless, such recommendations are widespread (7, 57, 73, 112).

Health Care Delivery Issues

DUTY TO WARN AND MEDICAL CONFIDENTIALITY   In some respects, the so-called professional "duty to warn" is the flip side of partner notification and contact tracing. The central questions are whether and under which circumstances a health professional is not only permitted but obligated to inform the sexual or needle-sharing partners of a seropositive individual. In discussions of duty to warn and HIV infection, much has been made of the landmark legal case, Tarasoff v. Regents of the University of California. In this case, the California Supreme Court ruled that therapists who know that a patient poses a threat to an identifiable third person have an obligation to take reasonable steps to protect that person. However, as Winston (154) points out, Tarasoff does not create a duty to warn; it creates a duty to protect, and this responsibility can be discharged in many ways.

In 1988, the American Medical Association (AMA), "breaking with the centuries-old tradition of confidentiality," adopted a policy, which recommended that doctors inform infected patients' spouses and sexual partners of the index patient's seropositivity if the patient cannot be relied upon to do so (150). Several authors have granted that there may be exceptional circumstances in which such a disclosure would be justifiable, but fear that policies advocating a duty to warn might lead to a tendency to overnotify (Thomas D. Stoddard, Executive Director of the Lambda Legal Defense and Education Fund, as cited in Ref. 150). Other commentators similarly argue that a policy of duty to warn often is unnecessary. It can be counterproductive to public health goals, as it may discourage individuals from being tested (63, 92), and it is unlikely to be implemented fairly in terms of which partners would be informed (95).

The duty to warn debate focuses on justified exceptions to obligations of medical confidentiality. A related question is how far health care professionals and health care institutions can and should go to protect the confidentiality of HIV-related information. For example, some proposed policies have suggested that serostatus should not be part of the patient's medical record, because many individuals have access to that document who, arguably, do not need to know that information. Alternatively, it has been argued that it is virtually impossible to conceal the HIV status of patients in hospital settings and that the focus properly should be on adequate anti-discrimination protections for persons whose seropositivity inevitably will be revealed.

DUTY TO TREAT AND OCCUPATIONAL RISK   There has been concern that persons infected with HIV have been denied health care in a way not seen with other diseases. In a 1988 study, 25% of the physicians interviewed believed it would be ethical to refuse treatment to a person with AIDS (101). Some members of the medical community have offered that this hesitation is motivated by a fear of contagion. It also has been speculated that discrimination is based on those who comprise the groups at highest risk for the disease. Loewy (103), in one of the early articles on this subject, suggested that with mere contagion, physicians, although fearful, probably would treat. However, when patients have additional qualities, which are perceived by physicians as repulsive, physicians might avoid providing care.

Among writers in bioethics, there always has been near unanimity that health professionals have a moral duty to care for persons with HIV infection (63, 90, 109, 125, 127). The major professional organizations also hold this position. For example, both the AMA and the American Nurses Association (ANA) have released statements that address duty to treat (4–6). The first statement by the AMA, issued in 1986, acknowledged that "not everyone is emotionally able to care for patients with AIDS." A physician who cannot care for these patients, the charge read, should find alternative arrangements for the patient. A 1987 revision of the statement, which was stronger, affirmed that a physician "may not ethically refuse to treat a patient whose condition is within the physician's current realm of competence" solely because the patient has AIDS or is infected with HIV. The ANA position similarly states that nurses have a moral obligation to care for a person with AIDS.

Thus, more than most other ethical issues of the HIV epidemic, the question of a professional's moral duty to treat appeared resolved by the end of the decade. However, despite this broad consensus, a few voices continue to defend the right of health professionals to refuse to treat persons with HIV infection (75, 129). The degree to which refusals occur remains undocumented. Another undocumented concern is the extent to which young health professionals are making geographic and specialty choices based on a desire to avoid HIV-positive patients.

It is increasingly apparent that any comprehensive policy regarding professional duties will have to include mechanisms for compensating persons who do contract the virus from an occupational exposure. Also related is the controversial issue of mandatory HIV antibody screening of patients. The key question here is whether such screening offers sufficient additional protection over a policy of "universal precautions" to warrant the attendant invasion of privacy and risk to patients, particularly when universal precautions also help in the prevention of hepatitis B virus, a far more infectious virus than HIV

(31). It also has been argued that if health care workers have a "right to know," so, too, do patients. Whether or under which circumstances patients should be informed that a health care provider is HIV-positive remains unresolved.

ACCESS AND FINANCING   It often is said that AIDS not only has highlighted the problems in our health care delivery system, but also that it may serve as the impetus for change. The issues of access to care and rationing of care have been major problems for persons with HIV infection. Seventeen percent of the American population has no health insurance, but among persons with AIDS the problem is even more severe. The Presidential Commission on the HIV Epidemic estimates that 20% of persons with AIDS have no coverage. Of persons with AIDS, an estimated 40% have Medicaid coverage, compared with 9% of the general population. In certain areas of the country, such as New York and New Jersey, the proportion of persons with AIDS covered by Medicaid is estimated to be 65%–70% (86).

Underlying this complex situation are fundamental questions about how to finance the costs of caring for persons with HIV infection justly (134). Initially, the main ethics and public policy question raised was whether insurance companies should be permitted to test applicants for the antibody to HIV. Schatz (135) was one of the early opponents of such a policy. He argued that testing would inevitably discriminate against gay men, that it would encourage employers to discriminate, and that it would undermine public health efforts that advocate testing. Schatz's concerns were echoed by other commentators (80, 121). Clifford & Iuculano (32), representatives of the insurance industry, presented an opposite commentary. They argued that HIV testing is completely in line with the sort of risk assessment typically conducted by insurance companies and that adverse selection will occur if companies are forbidden from performing HIV antibody tests.

States have changed their policies concerning HIV testing by insurance companies. At one point, up to nine states prohibited health insurance companies from testing applicants for HIV (50, 123). Currently, California is the only state that forbids companies from doing so under any circumstances.

More recently, attention has turned to the questions of whether and to what degree AIDS should be singled out as the focus of new financing programs (94). On the one hand, HIV disease is not the only illness or health risk for which there are problems of access to adequate care. On the other hand, the new and extreme disruptions that HIV disease has created within the health care system, particularly in areas such as New York City, as well as the disproportionately high numbers of persons affected by the disease who have no private health insurance, may justify such an approach.

There also have been concerns about access to specific therapies (67). State

Medicaid policies and other state programs vary widely regarding coverage for zidovudine [also known as retrovir or azidothymidine (AZT)] treatment, for example. These policies of rationing, as well as gaps in eligibility for Medicaid and shortages of treatment facilities, all contribute to the problems of inadequate and inequitable access to treatment. Recent data have suggested that among those who are HIV positive, gay men may have greater access to AZT than intravenous drug users. At the end of the 1980s, the actual incidence of AIDS cases among gay men was lower than had been projected by modeling techniques conducted earlier in the decade, whereas the incidence of AIDS was in keeping with the projections for drug users. Gail (59), a biostatistician who has developed and analyzed several of these models, believes that a difference in access to therapy is the most likely explanation.

Research

The HIV epidemic has posed perhaps as many challenges to established research ethics as it has to traditional health care delivery and financing issues. One of the first research ethics issues to be raised by the HIV epidemic was whether subjects in studies that are performing HIV antibody testing have a moral obligation to receive their test results (99, 120). In 1988, the US Public Health Service (PHS), which oversees both the National Institutes of Health and the Centers for Disease Control, settled the issue by instituting a policy that required individuals who participate in activities funded by the PHS to be informed of their test results if these results are associated with personal identifiers (152). The wisdom of the PHS policy remains unclear. In addition to making it plain that the federal government believes individuals should know their HIV antibody status, such a policy perhaps biases results of research in terms of limiting research protocols to those willing to know their HIV antibody status.

The research issue that received the most public attention in the 1980s was whether the traditional protocol for approval of new drugs is appropriate in the context of this fatal disease. The central issue is how to balance the government's obligation to protect individuals from potentially unsafe and inefficacious treatments with the obligation to facilitate access to therapies considered by some to be their "last chance" for survival. Should therapies be tested against either placebos or existing therapies before being approved, and should the process for drug approval be altered so that treatments can be made available to anyone who wants them (100, 102)?

Protests by AIDS activists struck at the core of the Food and Drug Administration's (FDA) investigational drug policies and doubtlessly influenced the government to revise its procedures. On May 22, 1987, new FDA regulations went into effect (54, 148), which permitted the use of investigational drugs outside of clinical trials:

if . . . (1) the proposed use is intended for a serious disease condition in patients for whom no satisfactory approved drug or other therapy is available; (2) the potential benefits of the drug's use outweigh the potential risks; and (3) there is sufficient evidence of the drug's safety and effectiveness to justify its intended treatment use.

Some commentators were not satisfied by the FDA response; on autonomy (91) or privacy (148) grounds, they continue to argue for greater access to investigational new drugs for HIV.

Attention recently has turned to another important issue in research ethics: how to select subjects for HIV-related clinical trials justly. Traditionally, certain groups, such as intravenous drug users and pregnant women, have been excluded from trials: They were thought to have other characteristics that might confound the findings; they were considered to be noncompliant; or they (or their fetuses) were considered to be at greater risk for harm from the intervention. The problem is that significant numbers of individuals in both of these groups are HIV infected. They are denied access to experimental treatments, and the effectiveness of therapies in the populations to which they belong will not be tested by the research.

Looking Ahead

Many of the moral issues about AIDS and HIV infection that dominated the 1980s will be with us as well in the 1990s. Undoubtedly, screening for HIV will remain a controversial issue. With the advent of new treatments and of new screening tests, there will be the call for more testing and for routine or mandatory screening. However, until an intervention is available that would render those treated no longer infectious, a justification for expanded testing on traditional public health grounds of infection control will remain difficult to sustain.

Integrally related to moral issues about the HIV epidemic are policies related to the use of illegal drugs. Among the normative questions expected are whether there should be more coercive measures for users of illegal substances and whether, given limited resources for treatment, HIV infection should be either an inclusionary or exclusionary criterion for access to drug treatment programs. Debates also can be expected to continue about such controversial policies as needle-exchange programs and the decriminalization of drug use.

Reproductive issues also are raised by the HIV epidemic and are destined to receive more attention in the 1990s with the advent of new therapies and screening tests. Looming on the horizon is the issue of intervention policies for HIV-positive pregnant women for the benefit of their fetuses. Will the availability of interventions beneficial to fetuses justify mandatory prenatal HIV screening or mandatory acceptance of treatment? A related question is

BIOETHICS AND PUBLIC HEALTH   355

whether pregnant women who are seropositive are being unjustly denied efficacious treatment for their HIV infection because of misguided fetal protection policies.

The question of how seropositive pregnant women should be counseled already has been the subject of intense debate, which is unlikely to diminish. Some groups advocate discouraging seropositive women from becoming pregnant or from carrying pregnancies to term. Others consider such a policy to be a threat to reproductive freedoms and the status of women generally. The ethical issues regarding choice of policies for seropositive pregnant women or for at risk women of reproductive age are heightened by the demographic realities of which women thus far have been most likely to be infected with the virus. African-American and Hispanic women have been disproportionately affected by this epidemic, and any policy that advocates control of reproduction will inevitably raise concerns regarding ethnic discrimination and genocide, as well as gender discrimination.

Finally, ethical questions are likely to be even more arduously debated in the realm of alternative financing mechanisms, rationing, and access to care. It already is tragic that many persons with HIV infection have no meaningful access to either regular medical care or efficacious interventions, such as zidovudine and prophylaxis for pneumocystis. Related social and drug rehabilitation services also are inadequate. In the 1990s, more persons will require care who never had insurance in the first place; others who always had maintained health insurance policies will find themselves unable to afford them because of lost income resulting from their illness. Certain geographic areas will continue to be hit particularly hard, as the demand simply will overwhelm existing resources and service programs.

Whether AIDS does become the proverbial straw that breaks the back of the existing American health care system remains to be seen. Insofar as the future is mirrored in the Oregon policy experiment, persons with HIV infection may fare well in rationing schemes. At present, it appears likely that outpatient care for persons in the early stages of HIV infection, including treatment with zidovudine, and palliative treatment for persons at the end stages of AIDS, receive a high ranking by the Oregon Health Services Commission. Treatments for other HIV-related conditions are expected to be ranked somewhere in the middle; where these treatments will fall with respect to the "payline" remains to be seen (Paige Sipes-Metzler, personal communication).

Barring the identification of another new and unanticipated threat to the public's health, the ethical issues for public health in the 1990s will not differ sharply in many respects from those of the 1980s. Difficult questions will continue to be raised concerning access to care and decision-making in the context of rising costs and conflicting priorities. AIDS has served as a springboard to examine these issues, as well as other taxing questions in all areas of health care delivery and research. The 1990s promise to be a decade in which the interface of public health and bioethics will continue to expand at an ever-increasing pace. In the upcoming decade, this expansion hopefully will include more attention to topics other than AIDS and resource allocation, such as policies for the control of risks and hazards to health, that also loom large on the public health agenda.

Literature Cited

1. Aaron, H. J., Schwartz, W. B. 1984. *The Painful Prescription: Rationing Hospital Care* Washington, DC: Brookings Inst. 161 pp.
2. Agich, G. J. 1987. Incentive and obligations under prospective payment. *J. Med. Philos.* 12(2):123–44
3. Am. Coll. Phys. 1990. Access to health care. *Ann. Int. Med.* 112(9):641–44
4. Am. Med. Assoc., Counc. Ethical Judic. Aff. 1986. Statement on AIDS
5. Am. Med. Assoc., Counc. Ethical Judic. Aff. 1988. Ethical issues involved in the growing AIDS crisis. *J. Am. Med. Assoc.* 259:1360–61
6. Am. Nurses' Assoc. Comm. Ethics. 1986. Statements regarding risk v. responsibility in providing nursing care.
7. Arras, J. 1989. *HIV infection and reproductive decisions: An ethical analysis.* Presented at Int. Conf. AIDS, 4th, Montreal
8. Baker, S. P., Teret, S. P. 1981. Freedom and protection: A balancing of interests. *Am. J. Public Health* 71(3):295–97
9. Barth, J. M. 1986. The public smoking controversy: Constitutional protection v. common courtesy—comment. *J. Contemp. Health Law Policy* 2:215–29
10. Battlin, M. P. 1987. Age rationing and the just distribution of health care: Is there a duty to die? *Ethics* 97(2):317–40
11. Bayer, R. 1983. Gays and the stigma of bad blood. *Hastings Cent. Rep.* 13:5–7
12. Bayer, R. 1989. Ethical and social policy issues raised by HIV screening: The epidemic evolves and so do the challenges. *AIDS* 3:119–24
13. Bayer, R., Levine, C., Wolf, S. M. 1986. HIV antibody screening: An ethical framework for evaluating proposed programs. *J. Am. Med. Assoc.* 256: 1768–74
14. Beauchamp, D. E. 1980. Public health and individual liberty. *Annu. Rev. Public Health* 1:121–36
15. Beauchamp, D. E. 1985. Community: The neglected tradition of public health. *Hastings Cent. Rep.* 15(6):28–36
16. Beauchamp, D. E. 1988. *The Health of the Republic: Epidemics, Medicine, and Moralism as Challenges to Democracy* Philadelphia: Temple Univ. Press. 290 pp.
17. Blank, R. H. 1988. *Rationing Medicine.* New York: Columbia Univ. Press. 290 pp.
18. Booth, W. 1987. The odyssey of a brochure on AIDS. *Science* 237:1410
19. Boughton, B. J., Downic, R. S. 1984. Compulsory health and safety in a free society. *J. Med. Ethics* 10(4):186–90
20. Brock, D. W. 1989. Justice, health care, and the elderly. *Philos. Public Aff.* 18(3):297–312
21. Brody, B. 1981. Health care for the haves and have nots: Toward a just basis of distribution. In *Justice and Health Care,* ed. E. E. Shelp, pp. 151–59. Boston: Reidel
22. Brody, B. A. 1988. The macroallocation of health care resources. In *Health Care Systems: Moral Conflicts in European and American Public Policy,* ed. H. Sass, R. U. Massey, pp. 213–368. Boston: Kluwer Acad. 368 pp.
23. Brown, E. R. 1987. DRGs and the rationing of hospital care. In *Health Care Ethics: A Guide for Decision Makers,* ed. G. R. Anderson, V. A. Glesnes-Anderson, pp. 69–90. Rockville, Md: Aspen. 365 pp.
24. Buchanan, A. E. 1984. The right to a decent minimum of health care. *Philos. Public Aff.* 13(1):55–78
25. Callahan, D. 1987. *Setting Limits: Medical Goals in an Aging Society.* New York: Simon & Schuster. 256 pp.
26. Callahan, D. 1988. Meeting needs and rationing care. *Law Med. Health Care* 16(3 4):261–66
27. Callahan, D. 1990. *What Kind of Life: The Limits of Medical Progress.* New York: Simon & Schuster. 318 pp.
28. Childress, J. F., 1987. An ethical framework for assessing policies to screen for antibodies to HIV. *AIDS Public Policy J.* 2:28–31
29. Christoffel, T. 1985. Fluorides, facts

and fanatics: Public health advocacy shouldn't stop at the courthouse door. *Am. J. Public Health* 75(8):888–91

30. Churchill, L. 1987. *Rationing Health Care in America.* Notre Dame, Ind: Univ. Notre Dame Press. 180 pp.

31. Clever, L. H., Omenn, G. S. 1988. Hazards for health care workers. *Annu. Rev. Public Health* 9:273–303

32. Clifford, K. A., Iuculano, R. P. 1987. AIDS and insurance: The rationale for AIDS-related testing. *Harv. Law Rev.* 100:1806–25

33. Coates, T. J., Stall, R. D., Kegeles, S. M., Lo, B., Morin, S. F., McKusick, L. 1988. AIDS antibody testing. *Am. Psychol.* 43:859–64

34. Coopersmith, H. G., Korner-Bitensky, N. A., Mayo, N. E. 1989. Determining medical fitness to drive: Physicians' responsibilities in Canada. *Can. Med. Assoc. J.* 140(4):375–78

35. Crawshaw, R., Garland, M. J., Hines, B., Lobritz, C. 1985. Oregon health decisions: An experiment with informed community consent. *J. Amer. Med. Assoc.* 254(22):3213–16

36. Daniels, N. 1985. *Just Health Care.* New York: Cambridge. 245 pp.

37. Daniels, N. 1985. Fair equality of opportunity and decent minimum: a reply to Buchanan. *Philos. Public Aff.* 14(1):106–10

38. Daniels, N. 1988. *Am I My Parent's Keeper? An Essay on Justice Between the Young and the Old.* New York: Oxford Univ. Press. 194 pp.

39. Dickens, B. M. 1988. Legal rights and duties in the AIDS epidemic. *Science* 239:580–86

40. DiFranza, J. R., Norwood, B. D., Garner, D. W., Tye, J. B. 1987. Legislative efforts to protect children from tobacco. *J. Am. Med. Assoc.* 257(24):3387–89

41. Dimas, J. T., Richland, J. H. 1989. Partner notification and HIV infection: Misconceptions and recommendations. *AIDS Public Policy J.* 4:206–11

42. *Dist. 27 Community School Board v. Board Educ. City of New York,* 502 NYS 2d 325 (US Supreme Court 1986)

43. Doll, L. S., Darrow, W., O'Malley, P., Bodecker, T., Jaffe, H. 1987. *Self-reported behavioral change in homosexual men in the San Francisco City Clinic Cohort.* Presented at Int. AIDS Conf., 3rd, Washington, DC

44. Doxiadis, S. 1985. *Ethical Issues in Preventive Medicine.* Boston: Martinus Nijhoff. 108 pp.

45. Egan, T. May 6, 1990. New health test: The Oregon plan. *NY Times*

46. Eisenberg, L. 1986. The genesis of fear: AIDS and the public's response to science. *Law Med. Health Care* 14:243–49

47. Emery, D. D., Schneiderman, L. J. 1989. Cost-effectiveness analysis in health care. *Hastings Cent. Rep.* 19(4): 8–13

48. Engelhardt, H. T., 1986. Rights to health care. In *The Foundations of Bioethics,* pp. 337–74. New York: Oxford Univ. Press. 398 pp.

49. Erde, E. L. 1987. Efficiency, ethics and indigent care: A review of the proceedings of the conference, The all-payers DRG system: Has New Jersey found an efficient and ethical way to provide indigent care? *J. Med. Philos.* 12(2):197–201

50. Faden, R. R., Kass, N. E. 1988. Health insurance and AIDS: The status of state regulatory activity. *Am. J. Public Health* 78:437–38

51. Fineberg, H. V. 1988. Education to prevent AIDS: Prospects and obstacles. *Science* 239:592–96

52. Fischoff, B., Lichtenstein, S., Slovic, P., Derby, S. L., Keeney, R. L. 1981. *Acceptable Risk.* New York: Cambridge Univ. Press. 185 pp.

53. Fleck, L. H. 1987. DRGs: justice and the invisible rationing of health care resources. *J. Med. Philos.* 12(2):165–96

54. Food Drug Admin. May 22, 1987. Investigational New Drug, Antibiotic and Biological Drug Product Regulations; Treatment Use and Sale: Final Rule. *Fed. Regist.* 52:19466–77

55. Forster, J. L. 1982. A communitarian ethical model for public health interventions: an alternative to individual behavior change strategies. *J. Public Health Policy* 3(2):150–63

56. Fox, R., Odaka, N. J., Brookmeyer, R., Polk, B. F. 1987. Effect of HIV antibody disclosure on subsequent sexual activity in homosexual men. *AIDS* 1: 241–46

57. Francis, D. P., Chin, J. F. 1987. The prevention of Acquired Immunodeficiency Syndrome in the United States. *J. Am. Med. Assoc.* 257:1357–66

58. Freedman, B. 1977. The case for medical care: Inefficient or not. *Hastings Cent. Rep.* 7:31–39

59. Gail, M. H., Rosenberg, P. S., Goedert, J. J. 1990. Therapy may explain recent deficits in AIDS incidence. *J. Acquired Immun. Defic. Syndr.* 3:296–306

60. Gevers, J. K. M., 1987. AIDS: Screening of possible carriers and human rights. *Health Policy* 7:13–19

61. Gibbard, A. 1982. The prospective Pareto principle and equity of access to

health care. *Milb. Mem. Fund Q./Health Soc.* 60(3):399–428

62. Gibbard, A. 1984. Health care and the prospective Pareto principle. *Ethics* 94(2):261–82

63. Gillon, R. 1987. Refusal to treat AIDS and HIV positive patients. *Br. Med. J.* 294:1675

64. Goodman, L. E., Goodman, M. J. 1986. Prevention—how misuse of a concept undercuts its worth. *Hastings Cent. Rep.* 16(2):26–38

65. Gostin, L. 1986. The future of communicable disease control: Toward a new concept in public health law. *Milb. Mem. Fund Q.* 64(Suppl.):79–98

66. Gostin, L. O. 1990. The AIDS Litigation Project: A national review of court and human rights commission decisions/ Part I: The social impact of AIDS. *J. Am. Med. Assoc.* 263:1961–70

67. Gostin, L. O. 1990. The AIDS Litigation Project: A national review of court and human rights commission decisions/ Part II: Discrimination. *J. Am. Med. Assoc.* 263:2086–93

68. Gostin, L., Curran, W. J. 1986. The limit of compulsion in controlling AIDS. *Hastings Cent. Rep.* (Suppl.) 24–29

69. Gostin, L., Curran, W. J. 1987. Legal control measures for AIDS: Reporting requirements, surveillance, quarantine, and regulation of public meeting places. *Am. J. Public Health* 77:214–18

70. Gostin, L. O., Curran, W. J., Clark, M. E. 1987. The case against compulsory casefinding in controlling AIDS— testing, screening and reporting. *Am. J. Law Med.* 12:7–53

71. Green, R. M. 1983. The priority of health care. *J. Med. Philos.* 8(4):373–80

72. Greenberger, N. J., Davies, N. E., Maynard, E. P., Wallerstein, R. O. 1990. Unusual access to health care in America: A moral and medical imperative. *Ann. Int. Med.* 112(9):637–38

73. Grossman, M. 1987. Human immunodeficiency virus infection in children: Public health and public policy issues. *Pediatr. Infect. Dis. J.* 6:113–16

74. Grutsch, J., Robertson, A. D. 1986. The coming of AIDS: It didn't start with homosexuals and it won't end with them. *Am. Spect.* 19:12–15

75. Guy, P. J. 1987. AIDS: A doctor's duty. *Br. Med. J.* 294:445

76. Halper, T. DRGs and the idea of a just price. *J. Med. Philos.* (122):155–64

77. Harrison, D. 1981. Distributional objectives in health and safety regulation. In *The Benefits of Health and Safety Regulation*, ed., A. R. Ferguson, E. P. LeVeen, pp. 177–201. Cambrige: Ballinger. 270 pp.

78. Health Public Policy Comm., Am. Coll. Phys. Infect. Dis. Soc. Am. 1988. The Acquired Immunodeficiency Syndrome (AIDS) and infection with the Human Immunodeficiency Virus (HIV). *Ann. Intern. Med.* 108:460–69

79. Hedner, T., Hansson, L. 1988. A utilitarian or deontological approach toward primary prevention of cardiovascular disease? *Acta Med. Scand.* 2244:293–302

80. Hiam, P. 1987/88. Insurers, consumers and testing: The AIDS experience. *Law Med. Health Care* 15:212–22

81. Hines, B. 1986. Health policy on the town meeting agenda. *Hastings Cent. Rep.* 16(2):5–7

82. Humber, J. M., Almeder, R. F. 1987. *Biomedical Ethics Reviews, 1986: Quantitative Risk Assessment.* Clifton NJ: Humana. 278 pp.

83. Hunter, N. D. 1987. AIDS prevention and civil liberties: The false security of mandatory testing. *AIDS Public Policy J.* 2:1–10

84. Iglehart, J. K. 1984. Smoking and public policy. *N. Engl. J. Med.* 310(8):539–44

85. Inst. Med., Natl. Acad. Sciences. 1986. *Confronting AIDS,* Washington, DC: Natl. Acad. 374 pp.

86. Inst. Med., Natl. Acad. Sciences. 1988. *Confronting AIDS Update 1988,* Washington, DC: Natl. Acad. 239 pp.

87. Jennings, B. 1988. A grassroots movement in bioethics: Community health decisions. *Hastings Cent. Rep.* 18(3):S1–S16

88. Juengst, E. T., Koenig, B. A. eds. 1989. *The Meaning of AIDS: Implications for Medical Science, Clinical Practice, and Public Health Policy.* New York: Praeger. 198 pp.

89. Kilner, J. F. 1988. Age as a basis for allocating lifesaving medical resources: an ethical analysis. *J. Health Polit. Policy Law* 13(3):405–23

90. Kim, J. H., Perfect, J. R. 1988. To help the sick: An historical and ethical essay concerning the refusal to care for patients with AIDS. *Am. J. Med.* 84:135–38

91. Krim, M. 1987. Making experimental drugs available for AIDS treatment. *AIDS Public Policy J.* 2:1–5

92. Koop, C. E. 1986. Surgeon General's report on Acquired Immune Deficiency Syndrome. *J. Am. Med. Assoc.* 256:278–89

93. Kuhse, H., Singer, P. 1988. Age and the

allocation of medical resources. *J. Med. Philos.* 13:101–16

94. Lamm, R. D. 1989. Who pays for AZT: Commentary. *Hastings Cent. Rep.* 19: 32

95. Landesman, S. February 1987. AIDS and a duty to protect: Commentary. *Hastings Cent. Rep.* 17:23

96. Lappe, M. 1983. Values and public health: value considerations in setting health policy. *Theor. Med.* 4(1):71–92

97. Lappe, M. 1985. Virtue and public health; societal obligation and individual need. In *Virtue and Medicine: Explorations in the Character of Medicine,* ed. E. E. Shelp, pp. 289–303. Boston: Reidel

98. Lappe, M. 1986. Ethics and public health. In *Maxcy-Rosenau Public Health and Preventive Medicine,* ed. J. M. Last, pp. 1867–77. Norwalk, Conn: Appleton-Century-Crofts. 1958 pp. 12th ed.

99. Levine, C. 1988. Has AIDS changed the ethics of human subjects research? *Law Med. Health Care* 16:167–73

100. Levine, R. J. 1987. AIDS treatment drugs: Clinical trials and compassionate use. *AIDS Public Policy J.* 2(2):6–8

101. Link, R. N., Feingold, A. R., Charap, M. H., Freeman, K., Shelov, S. P. 1988. Concerns of medical and pediatric house officers about acquiring AIDS from their patients. *Am. J. Public Health* 78:455–59

102. Lo, B. 1990. Clinical ethics and HIV-related illnesses: Issues in treatment and health services research. *Med. Care Rev.* 47:15–32

103. Loewy, E. H. 1986. Duties, fears and physicians. *Soc. Sci. Med.* 12:1363–66

104. Macklin, R. 1986. Predicting dangerousness and the public health response to AIDS. *Hastings Cent. Rep.* 16(Suppl.):16–23

105. MacLean, D. 1986. *Values at Risk.* Totowa, NJ: Rowman & Allanheld. 178 pp.

106. Mayo, D. J. 1988. AIDS, quarantines, and noncompliant positives. In *AIDS, Ethics and Public Policy,* ed. C. Pierce, D. Van DeVeer. pp. 113–23. Belmont, Calif: Wadsworth. 241 pp.

107. McCusker, J., Stoddard, A. M., Mayer, K. H., Zapka, J., Morrison, C., Saltzman, S. P. 1988. Effects of HIV antibody test knowledge on subsequent sexual behaviors in a cohort of homosexually active men. *Am. J. Public Health* 78:462–67

108. Menzel, P. T. 1983. *Medical costs, moral choices: A philosophy of health care economics in America.* New

Haven, Conn: Yale Univ. Press. 260 pp.

109. Miles, S. H. 1988. The medical profession's duty to HIV-infected persons. *J. Med. Educ.* 63:573

110. Miller, F. H., Miller, G. A. H. 1986. The painful prescription: A procrustean perspective. *N. Engl. J. Med.* 314(21): 1383–86

111. Mills, M., Wofsy, C., Mills, J. 1984. Special Report: The Acquired Immunodeficiency Syndrome: Infection control and public health law. *N. Engl. J. Med.* 314:934

112. Minkoff, H. L., Schwarz, R. H. 1986. AIDS: Time for obstetricians to get involved. *Obstet. Gynecol.* 68:267–68

113. Mitchell, J. L. 1988. Women, AIDS, and public policy. *AIDS Public Policy J.* 3:50–52

114. Mohr, R. 1987. AIDS, gays, and state coercion. *Bioethics* 1:35–50

115. Moreno, J. D., Bayer, R. 1985. The limits of the ledger in public health promotion. *Hastings Cent. Rep.* 15(6):37–41

116. Morreim, E. H. 1985. The limits of the ledger in public health promotion. *Hastings Cent. Rep.* 153):30–38

117. Muller, C. 1985. A window on the past: the position of the client in twentieth century public health thought and practice. *Am. J. Public Health* 75(5):470–76

118. Musto, D. F. 1986. Quarantine and the Problem of AIDS. *Milb. Mem. Fund Q.* 64(Suppl.):113

119. Nolan, K. 1989. Ethical Issues in caring for pregnant women and newborns at risk for human immunodeficiency virus infection. *Semin. Perinatol.* 13:55–65

120. Novick, A., Dubler, N. N., Landesman, S. M. 1986. Do research subjects have the right not to know their HIV antibody status? *IRB: Rev. Hum. Subj. Res.* 8: 6–9

121. Oppenheimer, G. M., Padgug, R. A. 1986. AIDS: The risks to insurers, the threat to equity. *Hastings Cent. Rep.* 16:18–22

122. Oregon Legis. Assem., 1989 Regul. Sess., Senate Bill 27

123. Pascal, A., Cvitanic, M., Bennett, C., Gorman, M., Serrator, C. A. 1989. State policies and the financing of Acquired Immunodeficiency Syndrome. *Health Care Fin. Rev.* 11:91–104

124. Pellegrino, E. D. 1981. Health promotion as public policy: the need for moral groundings. *Prev. Med.* 10(3):371–78

125. Pellegrino, E. D. 1987. Altruism, self-interest and medical ethics. *J. Am. Med. Assoc.* 258:1939–40

126. Pellegrino, E. D. 1988. Rationing health

care: The ethics of medical gatekeeping. In *Medical Ethics: A Guide for Health Professionals,* ed. J. F. Monagle, D. C. Thomasma, pp. 261–70. Rockville, Md: Aspen. 522 pp.

127. Pellegrino, E. D. 1989. HIV infection and the ethics of clinical care. *J. Leg. Med.* 10:29–46

128. Pellegrino, E. D., Thomasma, D. C. 1988. *For the Patient's Own Good.* New York: Oxford Univ. Press. 240 pp.

129. Pogash, C. Jan. 15, 1989. Bad blood. *San Franc. Examiner Image Mag.,* pp. 8–17

130. Porter, R. 1986. History says no to the policeman's response to AIDS. *Br. Med. J.* 293:1589–90

131. President's Commission for the Study of Ethical Problems in Medicine and Biomedical Behavioral Research Securing Access to Health Care: The Ethical Implications of Differences in the Availability of Health Services. Volume One: Report. 1983. Washington, DC: GPO. 223 pp.

132. *Report of the Presidential Commission on the Human Immunodeficiency Virus Epidemic.* 1988. Washington, DC: GPO. 201 pp.

133. Restak, R. 1986. Worry about survival of society first: Then about AIDS victims rights. *J. Public Health Dent.* 46:77–79

134. Ross, J. W. 1988. AIDS, rationing of care, and ethics. *Fam. Comm. Health* 12:24–33

135. Schatz, B. 1987. The AIDS insurance crisis: Underwriting or overreaching? *Harv. Law Rev.* 100:1782–1805

136. Schrader-Frechette, K. 1987. Values, scientific objectivity and risk analysis. In *Quantitative Risk Assessment,* ed. J. M. Humber, R. F., Slesmeder, pp. 149–68. Clifton, NJ: Humana. 278 pp.

137. Shilts, R. *And the Band Played On.* 1987. New York: St. Martin's. 630 pp.

138. Skrabanek, P. 1986. Preventive medicine and morality. *Lancet* 1:143–44

139. Smeeding, T. M., Battlin, M. P., Francis, L. P. Landesman, B. M. 1987. *Should medical care be rationed by age?* Ottawa, NJ: Rowman & Littlefield. 172 pp.

140. Spicker, S. F. 1987. Introduction to the theme of prospective payment. *J. Med. Philos.* 12(2):101–6

141. Tesh, S. N. 1988. *Hidden Arguments: Political Ideology and Disease Preven-tion Policy.* New Brunswick, NJ: Rutgers Univ. Press. 215 pp.

142. Trent, B. 1989. Attempts to improve rail safety run head on into CMA concerns. *Can. Med. Assoc. J.* 140(4):430,432–34

143. Van Griesven, G. J. P., De Vroome, E. M. M., Tielman, R. A. P., Goudsmit, J., Van Der Noordaa, J., et al. 1988. Impact of HIV antibody testing on changes in sexual behavior among homosexual men in the Netherlands. *Am. J. Public Health* 78:1575–77

144. Veatch, R. M. 1986. DRGs and the ethical reallocation of resources. *Hastings Cent. Rep.* 16(3):32–40

145. Vernon, T. 1987. The HIV epidemic: Colorado's traditional approach to disease control. *AIDS Public Policy J.* 2:33–36

146. Walters, L. 1988. Ethical issues in the prevention and treatment of HIV infection and AIDS. *Science* 238:597–603

147. Weale, A. 1983. Invisible hand or fatherly hand? Problems of paternalism in the new perspective on health. *J. Health Polit. Policy Law* 7(4):784–807

148. Weitzman, S. A., Marcy, T. 1987. FDA treatment use regulations: A compassionate response. *AIDS Public Policy J.* 2:22–32

149. Wikler, D. 1987. Personal responsibility for illness. In *Health Care Ethics: An Introduction,* ed. D. VanDeVeer, T. Regan, pp. 326–85. Philadelphia: Temple Univ. Press. 464 pp.

150. Wilkerson, I. July 1, 1988. AMA urges breach of privacy to warn potential AIDS victims. *NY Times*

151. Williams, G. 1984. Health promotion—caring concern or slick salesmanship? *J. Med. Ethics* 10(4):191–95

152. Windom, R. E. May 9, 1988. Assist. Secr. Health, Policy on informing those tested about HIV serostatus, letter to PHS agency heads. Washington, DC.

153. Winslow, G. R. 1986. Rationing and publicity. In *The Price of Health,* ed. G. J. Agich, C. E. Begley, pp. 199–215. Boston: Reidel. 280 pp.

154. Winston, M. February 1987. AIDS and a duty to protect: Commentary. *Hastings Cent. Rep.* 17:22–23

155. Zeckhauser, R., Shepard, D. S. 1981. Principles for saving and valuing lives. In *The Benefits of Health and Safety Regulation,* ed. A. R. Ferguson, E. P. LeVeen, pp. 91–130. Cambridge: Ballinger. 270 pp.

Annu. Rev. Publ. Health 1991. 12:361–82

ABORTION: A LEGAL AND PUBLIC HEALTH PERSPECTIVE

Hillary Kunins and Allan Rosenfield

Columbia School of Public Health, New York, NY 10032

KEY WORDS: history of abortion, abortion laws, RU 486, abortion morbidity and mortality

INTRODUCTION

No single health-related issue today engenders more controversy, debate, and even violence, than does abortion. Recent policy and legal changes, developments in medical technologies, and maternal deaths from illegal abortions are some of the indicators of the centrality of abortion as an issue in women's reproductive lives. Since the 1973 landmark US Supreme Court decision on abortion, Roe v. Wade, the issue of abortion has generated vast literature, which spans many disciplines. In this article, we will summarize the history of abortion in the United States and discuss key recent legal and legislative developments. We also will review relevant recent research generated from the field of public health and several other related disciplines on such topics as the safety of abortion, the new "abortion" pill (RU 486), and abortion in the developing world.

CRIMINALIZATION OF ABORTION IN NINETEENTH-CENTURY UNITED STATES

In the midst of the current debates regarding abortion, an historical analysis lends insight into the contemporary discussion. The decriminalization of abortion in the United States, which began in the late 1950s and culminated with the Roe v. Wade decision in 1973, is well known. The forces that helped lead to legalization include health professionals' concerns about the dangers of illegal abortions, the woman's movement, changing social morays, and,

361

0163-7525/91/0501-0361$02.00

for some groups, concerns about overpopulation (52, 58, 69). These forces coalesced in the 1960s to form a powerful social movement to decriminalize abortion. A major concern of health professionals today, however, is the possibility of the recriminalization. Thus, in reviewing the current legal and public health status of abortion, it is particularly useful to examine the origins of the criminalization of abortion in the US.

In the latter half of the nineteenth century, the practice of abortion in the US shifted from one governed by earlier British common law to a heavily regulated, and criminalized, medical procedure. This period matched our own for the amount of controversy and debate surrounding abortion. Many of the themes that characterize the current controversy emerged from the controversy and debate that occurred in this earlier period.

Before the nineteenth century, no legislation had been passed in the US regarding the legality of abortion. Thus, American courts relied on British common law doctrine to hand down decisions (52). Under common law, abortion was a criminal act only after the pregnant woman felt fetal movement (quickening). Before quickening, however, abortion was not criminal; at that time, it was medically impossible to confirm a pregnancy before quickening had occurred (52).

During the first half of the nineteenth century, many state legislatures began to pass laws that regulated the practice of abortion. These laws largely preserved the common law doctrine of quickening; however, they set precedents for the practice of abortion to be subjected to statutory, rather than common law, regulation (520).

From 1860 to 1880, state legislatures again intervened in the issue of abortion. As several historians point out, the legal status of abortion for most of the twentieth century was largely formulated by the legislative actions during this period of the nineteenth century (50, 52). The enacted statutes overturned the quickening doctrine, and abortion was made illegal at any point during the pregnancy. Some of the state laws, however, made an exception for abortions to preserve the life of the mother (50, 52). In addition, many of the laws held the woman, as well as the abortionist, criminally liable.

The major advocates for criminalization of abortion were an emerging group of organized doctors primarily associated with the American Medical Association (AMA) and anti-obscenity crusaders led by Anthony Comstock. Surprisingly, feminists supported doctors in their anti-abortion stance, whereas religious groups were virtually absent from the debates. A review of the major arguments and individual motivations is helpful in attempting to understand both the basis of these groups' positions and the construction of abortion debates.

Physicians associated with the AMA, which had been formed in 1847, were a dominant, if not major, force in criminalizing abortion in the United

States. Through their writings, lectures, and, perhaps most importantly, their successful lobbying of state legislators to pass anti-abortion statutes, these doctors galvanized efforts to restrict the practice of abortion. (52, 58, 72) Historians attribute a variety of motivations to the physicians' anti-abortion position, which ranged from the explicit concerns for maternal health and issues of morality to the more subtle, and often unstated, designs for professional power and control over women's fertility.

The doctors themselves put forward powerful rationales for the stringent regulation of abortion based on a moral interpretation of scientific knowledge of fetal development. They argued that abortion was immoral at any point during a pregnancy, thus disagreeing with the common law doctrine, under which the fetus was worthy of legal protection only after quickening. Instead, they concurred with the new scientific evidence that fetal development was a continuum. This scientific evidence led them to conclude that abortion at any time was wrong, as they did not believe that the fetus became alive only when fetal movement was first perceived. (50, 72)

Another concern expressed by these physicians was that of maternal health. They argued that the abortion procedure was harmful, as one physician noted in a lecture to medical students: "Many physicians . . . have regarded abortions . . . as far more dangerous to life than natural labor at the full period of gestation" (36). Even during the anti-abortion campaign, however, the doctors believed that abortion was acceptable to preserve the woman's life (50, 52).

Some historians suggest that the physicians who opposed abortion were motivated by more than moral and health concerns. They argue that doctors also were attempting to gain economic power and professional consolidation (50, 72). The work of these scholars depends upon an understanding of the position of the loosely organized medical field in the 1880s. As the historian James Mohr notes, ". . . physicians in America had fallen into low repute during the period of democratized and wide-open medicine that characterized the first half of the nineteenth century" (52). Instead of one dominant and standardized practice characterized by current alleopathic medicine as we know it, there was a variety of practitioners. Folk healers, midwives, and homeopaths, for example, had healing practices that competed with those of the "professional" doctors who were university-educated, alleopathic practitioners.

One characteristic of the professional doctors was their adherence to the Hippocratic Oath, which they interpreted as forbidding the practice of abortion. Because, historians suggest, they could not perform abortions and still uphold their standards of medical practice, they stood to lose patients to other practitioners who would be willing to perform abortions, as well as other health care services. Apparently, their economic concerns were borne out by the number of nonprofessional practitioners who were able to support their practices by performing abortions (52).

Interestingly, the anti-abortion regulation for which they fought allowed for therapeutic abortions to save a woman's life. Thus, when a doctor deemed a women's life to be endangered by the pregnancy, abortion was acceptable. The caveat was that the doctor be a qualified one, i.e. a practitioner of alleopathic medicine (50). The abortion regulations conferred upon these physicians the power to decide when abortion was permissible. Thus, it has been suggested, their professional power increased by controlling women's access to abortion.

Historians identify yet another explanation for the physicians anti-abortion stance. They argue that the physicians were interested in having more control over women's fertility (52, 58, 72). Resistant to changing sex roles, the primarily male doctors saw abortion as a means by which women could avoid their traditional familial responsibility to raise children. In addition, falling birthrates among American-born middle and upper class women posed a perceived threat to the continuation of the doctors' own social and economic class. Historians suggest that by limiting, or even preventing, women's recourse to abortion as a means of fertility control, physicians believed they could promote more traditional sex roles.

Nineteenth-century feminists, as expected, were opposed to requiring women to conform to traditional sex roles. Surprisingly, however, they supported the doctors' campaign to criminalize abortion (in contrast to the position their twentieth-century successors would take). In their writings, these feminists advocated the concept of "voluntary motherhood," by which women would have a choice about whether to become mothers. They believed that by limiting their fertility, women would have more freedom to participate in spheres other than the domestic one. But here their argument parts ways with those of contemporary feminists: The method of fertility control that they generally advocated was abstinence. Feminists argued that the availability of abortion allowed male sensualism to go unchecked and created a situation in which a woman had to comply with her husband's sexual demands (25, 52). The nineteenth-century feminists' assumption was that male and female sexuality was innately different; men were inherently sexual beings, and women were asexual. Engaging in sexual activity as often as men would have liked would compromise women's inherently asexual nature. The availability of abortion meant women would no longer have a convenient excuse to limit the number of children or to avoid sexual activity.

Religious leaders comprised another group that had a considerably different stance than their twentieth-century counterparts. Before the 1860s, the clergy, including Catholics, were generally unwilling to speak out against the practice of abortion. In 1869, for the first time, a council of American bishops condemned abortion; later that year, the Pope reiterated the condemnation. According to one historian, the pronouncements received little public attention (52). Unlike its role in current debates, the Church was hardly a leader in the nineteenth-century campaign to criminalize abortion in the United States.

Anti-obsenity crusaders were a second group crucial to the success of the campaign to criminalize abortion. The most well-known among this group was Anthony Comstock. He began his anti-obscenity career in 1872 as a member of the Committee for the Suppression of Vice (under the auspices of the Young Men's Christian Association of New York City). Comstock successfully lobbied at the federal level for the passage of "An Act for the Suppression of Trade in, and Circulation of, Obscene Literature and Articles of Immoral Use." Among its provisions, the Comstock Law, as it came to be known, prohibited the advertising of abortion by mail, as well as the distribution of drugs or instruments used for abortion purposes through the postal system. It also made it a federal crime to sell or advertise abortion services if the person who provided such services was not a physician acting "in good faith" (43, 52).

Although the Comstock Law was stringent, it held little power without diligent enforcement. Appointed as a "special agent" of the Post Office, Comstock himself became the primary enforcer. Endowed with a badge and the authority to issue warrants for arrest, he helped to indict 55 persons for their activity as abortionists between 1872 and 1880 (52). His entrapment of perhaps the most infamous New York City abortionist, Madame Resell, is said to have led to her suicide in 1878 (43). After she died, Comstock supposedly "boasted that she was the fifteenth malefactor he had driven to suicide, in less than five years on the job" (43).

Comstock's vigilance in enforcing the provisions of the anti-obscenity law helped secure the success of the anti-abortion campaign. By involving the federal government in the suppression of abortion advertising and services, the state lobbying conducted by the doctors gained credibility. The anti-obscenity campaign also decreased the public visibility of abortion services by criminalizing its advertisement (52).

By 1900, the criminalization of abortion was completed. Virtually all states and territories had passed restrictive abortion statutes. Courts were more willing to mete out stricter fines and sentences to convicted abortionists (52). Although the criminalization process itself was successful, the doctors' goals of achieving greater maternal health was undermined by that very process. Because, by 1890, doctors regularly used antiseptic procedures, "at the very time abortion might theoretically have become a safer procedure than it had been earlier in the century, it came instead to be perceived as more dangerous than ever" (52). The consequence of criminalization was to force the practice underground, where less reputable practitioners could not or would not avail themselves of the safer methods. The legacy of the nineteenth century, which increased the physical health risks associated with abortion, would persist into the twentieth century until legal and legislative actions in the 1960s and 1970s reversed it.

Abortion in the nineteenth century was a battleground for conflicting ideas about fetal life, as well as women's health, fertility and sexuality, and physicians' professional position in society. The historical literature reveals the complexity of the raging debates. Although the actors and some of the issues were different from those involved in the debate today, the intensity and amount of societal disruption that took place in the nineteenth century is similar to that of the late twentieth century. The nineteenth century example shows us that there are no simple resolutions to the conflict surrounding abortion; the conflict stems from the tangled interplay of social, economic, and moral concerns.

LEGAL AND POLICY ISSUES IN THE TWENTIETH CENTURY

Two Supreme Court cases in the latter half of this century marked the end of outright legal bars to abortion in the United States. In the 1965 case of Griswold v. Connecticut, the Supreme Court articulated a constitutional right of privacy that would ultimately lead to a successful challenge of the constitutionality of anti-abortion laws (27). Connecticut's law prohibited the use and distribution of contraceptives. Griswold, the executive director of Connecticut's Planned Parenthood, opened a center to distribute birth control educational materials and contraceptives to test the law's constitutionality. The Supreme Court upheld Griswold's right to distribute contraception, as well as married peoples' right to use contraception, based on a constitutionally guaranteed right of privacy. Because no single amendment was cited by the justices who wrote the plurality opinion, many groups felt that the constitutional basis for the Court's right to privacy decision was not very firm. The Griswold decision, nevertheless, was crucial in elucidating the right of privacy.

In 1973, the Roe v. Wade decision established a woman's constitutional right to an abortion (64). A Texan, Jane Roe (alias), sued to obtain an abortion although her life was not threatened by the pregnancy. Her claim was that a Texas statute prohibiting abortion infringed on her right of privacy. Justice Blackmun delivered the landmark decision that upheld Roe's right of privacy to terminate an unwanted pregnancy. The ruling established a trimester framework by which the state's interest in potential life of the fetus and in women's health becomes more compelling as the pregnancy progresses. Blackmun argued that the right of privacy, although not explicitly stated in the text of the constitution, is "broad enough to encompass a woman's decision whether or not to terminate her pregnancy" (64). This right of personal privacy, however, is not "absolute . . . a state may properly assert important interests in safeguarding health, in maintaining medical standards, and in protecting potential life. At some point in pregnancy, these respective interests become sufficiently compelling to sustain regulation of the factors that govern the abortion decision" (64). The Court's task was to balance a woman's right to an abortion and the protection of health.

Under the trimester framework, abortion is not regulable by the State during the first trimester. At this stage, the State lacks a compelling interest in either the health of the mother or the potential life of the fetus. Blackmun accorded formal responsibility to the medical doctor by stating that for first trimester abortions, "the abortion decision and its effectuation must be left to the medical judgment of the pregnant woman's attending physician" (64). In the second trimester, the State's interest in the woman's health becomes compelling; therefore, the State may regulate abortion to protect women's health. Blackmun argued that the State's interest in potential life becomes compelling at the point in the pregnancy when the fetus becomes viable. From Roe, we implicitly understand viability to be at the beginning of the third trimester, at which time the State may "regulate, and even proscribe, abortion except where it is necessary, in appropriate medical judgment, for the preservation of the life or health of the mother" (64).

Blackmun's denial of judicial responsibility for the decision regarding the point at which life begins created an important model for federal involvement in that problematic question: "We need not resolve the difficult question of when life begins. When those trained in the respective disciplines of medicine, philosophy, and theology are unable to arrive at any consensus, the judiciary, at this point in the development of man's [sic] knowledge, is not in a position to speculate as to the answer" (64). However, Blackmun noted that fetuses have never been regarded in the law as full persons. Thus, according to Blackmun, the State interest in protecting life becomes compelling when the fetus is able to exist outside the mother's womb as a separate and full person. This is the viability point during the pregnancy, when the State may regulate or proscribe abortion to protect its interest. Blackmun stated that viability occurs at the earliest at 24 weeks.

Using viability as a criterion has created much controversy. Some legal scholars and members of the judiciary claim that this concept lacks a constitutional basis. They argue that the determination of State interest should be part of the legislative process (21, 79). Other scholars have suggested that newer, technological advances will lower the date of viability. Most obstetrical and pediatric expert opinion suggests, however, that viability less than 500 grams (about 25–26 weeks) is highly unlikely, because the lungs at earlier ages are not at a stage of development that will allow expansion (80). Significantly different types of technology will have to be developed to lower the age of viability. Such technological advances are not now in sight, nor, one can argue, given the extraordinary costs, should they be the subject of research.

Abortion laws were liberalized in several states a few years before the Roe v. Wade decision, but only four states, Alaska, Hawaii, New York and Washington, had abortion laws that were compatible with Roe. Fifteen other states had somewhat liberalized abortion laws that needed modification after the Roe decision. All other states needed to completely reform their state laws 23).

After Roe was decided, many other abortion cases came before the Supreme Court. One recurring theme was the challenge to federal funding and, later, state funding of abortions. The challenges shifted the debate from one about a woman's abstract right to an abortion at all to one about the right of poor women to receive economic support from the federal government to enable them to exercise that right. In 1976, the federal government decided the issue by passing the Hyde Amendment, which prohibited the use of federal funds (in this case, primarily Medicaid) or abortions except when the mother's life was endangered.

The constitutionality of the Hyde Amendment was challenged in court and finally reached the Supreme Court on appeal in 1980. In Harris v. McRae, the Court held that not only was the Hyde Amendment constitutional, but that individual states participating in the Medicaid program, funded by Title XIX of the Social Security Act, were not required to pay for Medicaid recipients' abortions (28). In another case, Williams v. Zbaraz, which was decided at the same time as Harris, the Court held again "that a participating State is not obligated under Title XIX to pay for those medically necessary abortions for which federal reimbursement is unavailable under the Hyde Amendment" (81). Thus, by 1980, elective abortion was no longer federally financed. In the wake of these cases, however, several state legislatures have passed laws that provide state Medicaid coverage for abortions for indigent women. As of June 1990, however, Medicaid paid for abortion in only 13 states.

Medicaid restrictions against abortion unfairly discriminate against the poor, who rely on Medicaid support for their medical needs. The Hyde Amendment, therefore, compromises the health status and reproductive choices of poor women by restricting their normal source of funding for medical care. Researchers have found that 18%–35% of Medicaid-eligible women who would choose to terminate their pregancies are unable to do so because of lack of funds (70, 78). Some of these women essentially are forced to undergo child bearing simply because of their economic status. Poor women who manage to obtain abortions often delay the procedure while collecting sufficient funds (35). Because abortion after the first eight weeks is associated with somewhat higher health risks, which increase with each additional week of gestation, poor women's health can be compromised because of the Hyde Amendment (10).

Consent and notification are two related issues about which there has continued to be much legal debate (41). In 1976, the Supreme Court held that states that require minors to obtain parental consent must also provide them with an alternate process to obtain consent (6). One common alternative system is the judicial bypass system, by which the minor must apply to the court to obtain consent if she is unwilling or unable to obtain parental consent. The judicial bypass option has been criticized on grounds that it is a lengthy procedure, which places undue stress on the minor. It also often fails to preserve the anonymity or privacy of the minor (74). This issue is one of significant current controversy based on two recent (mid-1990) Supreme Court decisions, Hodgson v. Minnesota and Akron Center for Reproductive Health v. Ohio. In essence, these decisions approved parental consent laws, with a required judicial bypass option, at least when both biologic parents' permission is required.

A second area of contention has been spousal consent. In 1976, the Supreme Court ruled that it was unconstitutional to require a woman to obtain consent from her husband to have an abortion (59). Despite this decision, federal judges in the lower courts have issued more than 11 injunctions at the request of husbands or boyfriends to prevent women from obtaining abortions (R. Holt 1988, unpublished paper). The implicit challenge to the 1976 decision has yet to be litigated in front of the Supreme Court.

In July 1989, the Webster v. Reproductive Health Services decision represented the greatest challenge to Roe thus far. Though leaving the Roe decision formally intact, it further opened the door to a broad range of possible state restrictions on abortion services. The Supreme Court ruling held that a Missouri law, which prohibited the use of public employees and facilities in performing abortions, was constitutional. Further, the Supreme Court upheld the provisions of Missouri's law, which required a physician to test for fetal viability at 20 or more weeks' gestation. Finally, the court held that the preamble to the Missouri statute, which said that life begins at conception and that unborn children have the same rights as all other people, was constitutional (79).

In the Webster decision, Chief Justice Rehnquist clearly stated that the Court should dismantle Roe's trimester framework:

Roe's rigid trimester analysis has proved to be unsound in principle and unworkable in practice . . . The Roe framework is hardly consistent with the notion of a Constitution like ours that is cast in general terms and usually speaks in general principles. The framework's key elements—trimesters and viability—are not found in the Constitution's text . . . [T]he result has been a web of legal rules that have become increasingly intricate, resembling a code of regulations rather than a body of constitutional doctrine. There is . . . no reason why the State's compelling interest in protecting potential human life should not extend throughout pregnancy rather than coming into existence only at the point of viability. Thus, the Roe trimester framework should be abandoned (79).

Abandoning the trimester framework might result in the nullification of a woman's constitutional right to an abortion.

Because Rehnquist did not gain the support of a majority of the Court for this part of his opinion, the basic constitutional right to abortion still holds. The Court's opinion stated that Webster "affords us no occasion to revisit the holding of Roe . . . and we leave it undisturbed" (79). Justice Scalia's separate opinion, which indicated that he is prepared to overturn Roe, and Rehnquist's harsh criticism suggest that Roe's framework eventually may be overturned.

By limiting access to public facilities and personnel for the purposes of abortion the Webster ruling will particularly affect low-income women (2, 3, 15). Wealthier women can afford to pay the cost of an abortion at a private medical institution or travel to distant abortion facilities; however, poorer women may not be able to do so. Further, Webster's requirement that physicians test for fetal viability after 20 weeks since the last menstrual period (LMP) may constrain sound medical practice. This requirment involves invasive, unnecessary testing, such as amniocentesis, in an effort to ascertain fetal lung maturity at a point in pregnancy in which such testing is not reliable (15).

Another potential consequence of Webster may be the limitation of training in the techniques of abortion in obstetrics-gynecology residency programs (at least for those who are training in public facilities). The resultant decrease in surgical skill in this area could lead to complications from abortion procedures as the number of experienced personnel decreases (15).

Since the Webster decision was issued, legislative and judicial actions have taken place in different states and territories, which both restrict and protect the accessibility of abortion. Legal experts have commented that much activity can be expected at the state level, as new laws and referenda challenge and protect the right to abortion (R. Holt 1990, personal communication). Examples of such state activity are the 1990 vetoes of restrictive abortion laws by the governors of Idaho and Louisiana. Both laws would have prohibited abortion except in very narrow circumstances. In another instance, the territory of Guam has passed a restrictive statute, which prohibits abortion except when the woman's life is endangered. In response to a lawsuit filed against this statute, however, a Federal district judge in Guam has issued a restraining order, which prevents the statute from being enforced at present. This decision has been appealed by the governor of Guam.

Activity at the state level to protect the right of abortion also is occurring. In 1988, pro-choice groups in Michigan and Colorado attempted to pass referenda to restore state funding for poor women. Although both these referenda were defeated, this type of activity at the state level is likely to continue (20). The recent passage of a Connecticut abortion statute is an example of a successful state effort to ensure a woman's right to abortion should Roe v. Wade be overturned. The law, passed in April 1990 by the Connecticut state legislature, would preserve the legal status of abortion in Connecticut, even if the Surpreme Court were to reverse the federal constitutional guarantees.

An important case, which was argued before the Supreme Court in October 1990, deals with a federal regulation that prohibits providers who receive federal money under Title X from counseling or informing women about abortion. Pro-choice advocates believe that this example of state regulation violates both free speech and proper medical practice. The regulations were overturned by the First Circuit Court of Appeals, but upheld by the Second Circuit Court. Because of the conflicting decisions at two different courts at the same judicial level, the Supreme Court agreed to hear the case (61). If the Court upholds the regulations, discussion of abortion in Title X-funded clinics will be eliminated. The effect will be to severely limit access to abortion for women who use these facilities and compromise the quality of care they receive.

PUBLIC HEALTH AND MEDICAL ASPECTS OF ABORTION

Since in 1973, the subject of abortion has generated vast amounts of research on public health and medical issues. Researchers' interests have ranged from descriptive studies of demographic characteristics and morbidity and mortality rates to studies of how those rates and characteristics change over time (4, 10, 32, 60, 73). The US Government's Centers for Disease Control in Atlanta and the private Alan Guttmacher Institute collect, on an ongoing basis, the most comprehensive data on demographic information about abortion seekers, incidence, complication rates, mortality rates, availability of abortion services, and other statistical information. Other researchers have examined the physical and emotional sequelae of abortion (37, 49, 56). Still others have carried out social science studies on the reasons women choose to abort and on contraceptive attitudes and practices regarding contraception (34, 77). Due to the abundance of studies, Willard Cates, a prominent researcher in the field, has stated, "we have come to know more about [abortion] than any other surgical operation" (10).

Abortion-Related Complications and Mortality

Abortions have been among the most commonly performed surgical procedures since the Roe v. Wade decision. When performed by properly trained personnel, they are also among the safest. Before the federal legalization (or, for several states, before state liberalization of abortion laws preceding 1973) abortion was not the relatively risk-free procedure it is today. It is impossible to know with certainty the number of induced abortions that took place before the liberalization of the abortion laws. Because the total number of abortions would be the denominator for constructing both morbidity and mortality rates, it also is difficult to make comparisons between these rates before and after legalization. However, many researchers have been concerned with precisely these issues, and their estimates and calculations are considered valuable approximations.

The difficulty of estimating the incidence of abortion before legalization is exemplified by the large range presented in the 1958 published report of the first medical conference devoted to illegal and therapeutic abortion. The statistics committee of that conference reported that "a plausible estimate of the frequency of induced abortion in the United States could be as low as 200,000 and as high as 1,200,000 per year" (8).

Estimates for the death-to-case ration in 1972 were 30–40 deaths per 100,000 abortions (12, 75). These ratios are similar to the maternal mortality ratios in the United States in the 1950s. Writing in 1975, Tietze (75) calculated the risk of mortality from illegal abortion to be eight times greater than the risk from legal abortions. Since his writing, the mortality ratio for legal abortions has further decreased because of improved surgical techniques and experience (10).

Health care providers who practiced before 1973 report many anecdotes about women with hemorrhage, fever, shock, or a foreign object in the uterus as a result of attempted induced abortion by either an incompetent abortionist or by the individual herself (8, 24). In 1975, an Institute of Medicine report stated that "medical complications associated with illegal (nonmedical or self-induced) abortion appear to have declined markedly since abortion legalization, based on hospital admissions due to septic and incomplete abortion, two adverse consequences of the illegal procedure" (49). Clearly, the federal legalization of abortion has resulted in the availability of safer abortions, thus promoting the health of women of child-bearing age.

A slow decline in abortion-related mortality began as early as 1940, when the abortion mortality ratio (abortion-related deaths to live births) decreased at a rate of 11% per year until 1950 (13). Researchers have speculated that this decline resulted from the utilization of antibiotics. From 1951 to 1965, the ratio continued to decline, albeit at the greatly reduced rate of 1.7% per year. But from 1965 to 1976, which represents the legalization period, the mortality ratio dropped at a rate of 25% per year. This rapid rate of decline has been attributed to the availability of legal abortion, as well as to the availability of effective contraceptives (13).

The decline in the actual number of abortion-related deaths further demonstrates the effect of federal legalization on public health. From 1958 to 1962, approximately 290 deaths occurred annually in the United States because of "other-than-legal" abortions, which include spontaneous, criminal, and undetermined abortions (75). That number dropped to 142 deaths in 1969, when abortion had become available in a number of states; in 1973, the number dropped to 27 deaths.

After the federal legalization of abortion in 1973, abortion-related mortality continued to decrease. Abortion-related mortality in 1973 was an estimated 3.4 deaths per 100,000 legal abortions. In 1980, the figure was 0.5 deaths per 100,000 legal abortions—an 85% decrease (76). The same study estimates the mortality due to childbirth to be 11 deaths per 100,000 births. Although the denominators are different, it appears that legal abortion is much safer than childbirth (76).

The continued decrease in abortion-related mortality may be attributed to several causes. The shift from the riskier, later abortions to safer, earlier ones certainly helped to reduce mortality. For example, in 1974, 10% of abortions were performed on women with gestations of more than 15 weeks; 43% were in gestations of less than 8 weeks. In 1985, however, only 5% of abortions occurred in women with gestation of more than 16 weeks, and slightly more than 50% of all abortions took place when the woman was less than 8 weeks LMP (14). Because the earliest abortions are least risky, the shift to earlier abortions contributed to the decrease in mortality (4). Increases in the use of local, rather than general, anaesthesia also made the typical abortion procedure safer (76). Finally, the physicians who provided abortions received better training and gained experience. Their skill further enhanced the safety of abortion (4, 76).

The change in the techniques used to perform both first and second trimester abortions since 1973 has contributed significantly to the increased safety of abortion procedures. As of 1985, more than 97% of all abortions were primarily performed using instrumental evacuation, which includes vacuum aspiration (or suction curettage), dilation and evacuation, and sharp curettage (14). In the first trimester, most instrumental evacuations are now performed using suction curettage. Many studies have demonstrated the decreased morbidity and mortality rates associated with its use compared with the use of dilatation and sharp curettage (42). In 1985, approximately 95% of all abortion procedures were performed using suction curettage (14).

The percentage of abortions performed by intrauterine instillation has decreased over time. In 1975, 6% of abortions were performed using this method; in 1985, only 2% used this method (14). Correspondingly, the number of second trimester abortions performed using dilatation and evacuation, which is safer than medical instillation when carried out by experienced practitioners, has increased (11, 26). In 1985, slightly more than 50% of abortions at more than 21 weeks LMP were performed using dilatation and evacuation; and nearly two thirds of abortions between 16 and 20 weeks LMP were performed with this method.

Hysterectomies and hysterotomies, as methods of abortion, had virtually disappeared in 1982 (14). These two methods were the only ones that required major abdominal surgery, which conferred on the woman all the attendant risks of major surgery. The disappearance of these methods contributes to the current level of safety of the abortion procedure.

Demographic and Other Characteristics of Abortion Patients

Nearly two decades after Roe, we are able to construct a picture of abortion rates and ratios in an environment in which the procedure is safe and legal. Official abortion rates increased from 1973 to 1981, at which time the annual rate stabilized at approximately 28–29 abortions per 1000 women (aged 15–44), or about 1.6 million abortions annually (33).

According to 1987 data, approximately one quarter of the women who obtained abortions were teenagers, more than 80% of whom were unmarried. More than 50% of the women did not have a previous live birth, and about 43% had at least one prior abortion (24). Poorer women, with family incomes of less than $11,000 per year, were more likely to have abortions than were women with higher income levels (34). Younger women had higher abortion rates than older women, with 18–19-year-olds having the highest rate of all age groups. Hispanics had higher rates than nonhispanics; nonwhites had higher rates than whites (34).

The relationship between contraceptive use and abortion is another question that has been recently studied. According to data from 1987, the vast majority (91%) of abortion patients reported that they had used a birth control method at some point in their lives. Slightly more than half reported using a method in the month before they became pregnant (24). Among 1987 abortion patients, students and working women were more likely to be in the group of recent users of birth control. The same study found that the women seeking abortion who were younger, had less income, fewer years of education, or who were black or hispanic were more likely to report not having used contraceptives (34).

Consequences of Abortion

The physical and psychological sequelae of abortion have been the subject of many studies. Although research on the physical consequences of abortion conclusively demonstrates a very low rate of morbidity and essentially no long-term physical sequelae, the results of studies of the psychological sequelae are somewhat less firm.

In one of the most comprehensive reviews of the physical consequences of abortion, Hogue and colleagues (37) examined over 150 studies regarding the association between induced abortion and subsequent reproductive outcomes. They concluded that the weight of evidence shows no association between induced abortion and subsequent infertility, midtrimester spontaneous abortion, shortened gestation, or ectopic pregnancy. [Two later studies confirm this finding with regard to ectopic pregnancy (7, 39)]. However, Hogue and colleagues note that the effects of repeated, induced abortions remain unknown. The studies they reviewed contained contradictory findings, many of which may have shown effects only because of the failure to control for confounding variables. Some evidence, however, indicates that procedures that require wider dilatation of the cervix may be associated with negative outcomes, such as increased risk of subsequent spontaneous abortion. The introduction of laminaria to dilate the cervix slowly helped to avoid this risk. Hogue and colleagues call for future studies to examine the "technical subtleties" of various abortion methods to understand the effect, if any, on subsequent reproductive function (37).

Findings on the psychological effects of abortion have been politicized by those on both sides of the abortion debate. As Rogers and colleagues (65) note, "both advocates and opponents of abortion can prove their points by judiciously referencing only articles supporting their political agenda." These researchers find that many studies of psychological sequelae suffer from methodological flaws, such as inadequate sample size, lack of an appropriate comparison group, and the use of data collecting instruments that do not have known reliability or validity.

A more recent examination of the medical and psychological sequelae of abortion was conducted in 1987 by former US Surgeon General C. Everett Koop, at the direction of Ronald Reagan (46). The implicit agenda behind Reagan's directive was for the Surgeon General to accumulate evidence to support the overturning of Roe v. Wade (40). Koop interviewed members of 27 groups with interests in abortion (both anti-abortion and pro-choice) and reviewed over 250 scientific articles to complete his project. Although his full report was never released, a congressional subcommittee gained access to it and then heard testimony from some of the groups and individuals with whom Koop had consulted. These hearings were made public in 1989. The information gleaned from them indicates that Koop, despite his admitted anti-abortion stance, had essentially concluded that there are no negative medical or psychological consequences for women who undergo abortion. The subcommittee found that Koop had "expressed doubts about the existence of Postabortion Stress Syndrome," the condition often cited by anti-abortion groups to argue the deleterious aftereffects of abortion (40).

The subcommittee also reported that the American Psychological Association had submitted a review paper to Koop, which concluded that "despite the flaws in the research, there is so little evidence of psychiatric problems following abortion, and so much evidence of relief, that therefore abortion does not cause more psychiatric problems than unwanted pregnancy" (40). The subcommittee report made public that Koop had failed to uncover serious medical or psychological consequences for women who have had abortions.

Medical Termination of Pregnancy: RU 486

For many years, researchers have sought agents that would function as an anti-progesterone and interfere with the critically important role played by progesterone, particularly in early pregnancy (5). With the discovery by scientists at the Roussel-UCLAF Company in France of the anti-progestin RU 486 (commercially marketed as Mifepristone), for the first time the possibility of the medical termination of pregnancy became a reality. The "abortion pill," as RU 486 is known in the mass media (45), holds great promise as an alternative to surgical first trimester abortions. When RU 486 is used in combination with a prostaglandin within the first 49 days of a pregnancy, a successful and safe termination of pregnancy occurs in 96% of cases (63, 71).

As of mid-1990, however, the drug only was available in France. Although there are discussions about introducing the drug in England and the Scandinavian countries, the Roussel-UCLAF Company and its parent company, Hoechst, have been unwilling to have the drug introduced into the United States, apparently because of fear of controversy and protest by anti-abortion groups.

RU 486 also generated much controversy in France, with public protests by anti-abortion activists. Soon after the French government approved the marketing of RU 486 on September 23, 1988, Roussel announced that it was abandoning plans to distribute the drug in France. Their announcement made clear that their decision was in response to public pressure. Two days later, however, the French Health minister offered a powerful statement that RU 486 was "the moral property of women, not just the property of the drug company," and ordered Roussel to make the drug available in France (44). In taking such action, the Health Minister made use of a French law that gave him the authority to withdraw a company's license to a drug if the company refuses to make it available and then offer it to another company to distribute.

Although the development of RU 486 poses difficult moral questions, there is clear medical evidence that suggests the drug is safe and efficacious for early abortion when used in combination with a prostaglandin (5, 9, 63). The prostaglandin used in conjunction with the RU 486 encourages uterine contractions, thereby increasing the probability of expulsion of the contents of the uterus. A recent clinical study of more than 2000 women reported an overall efficacy rate of 96%, with efficacy defined as the complete expulsion of the products of conception without the need for additional procedures (71). The study was conducted on women who were no more than eight weeks from their last menstrual period.

The most obvious advantage of the RU 486 is that it avoids surgery and anesthesia and their attendant risks. In addition, greater privacy is afforded to the patient. One disadvantage of RU 486 is the number of visits to a medical facility that is required in France. Currently, four visits are needed in conjunction wih use of RU 486, three of which are medically necessary. Fewer visits are generally required for the surgical procedure in the United States. Thus, abortion using RU 486 may pose problems of access for women who must travel a distance to a medical facility. In France, the first visit is to actually request the abortion, because, according to French law, the applicant must then wait one week to be sure of her decision. She then returns to the clinic a second time to take the RU 486. On the third visit, two days later, she is given the prostaglandin analogue. At that time, she remains in the clinic to be monitored for four hours. Finally, on the fourth visit, she returns 8–12 days after the administration of the RU 486 for follow up (17, 71).

Other applications of RU 486, both for contraceptive and noncontraceptive indications, are the subject of current research. One potential use is as a once-a-month contraceptive pill taken late in the menstrual cycle (51, 53). Other potential uses include treatment for breast cancer (66), Cushing's Syndrome (48), and glaucoma (16). RU 486 also may be useful in inducing labor after fetal death (57).

Although the future for RU 486 in the US is unclear, its development is a remarkable advance from a scientific, as well as a societal, point of view. Clearly, with a woman's right to an abortion still constitutionally protected in the US, women should have the option to choose a medical procedure, once this new agent has been reviewed by the Food and Drug Administration (FDA). Unfortunately, an FDA review only can be initiated at the request of the drug company and, at least for the present, Roussel has been unwilling to do so. Were the company to reverse its present stance, anti-abortion advocates in Congress and in the Bush Administration may attempt to prevent the FDA from undertaking its normal review process for a new drug, an action, if taken, that is unprecedented in the US.

Abortion in an International Context

The worldwide trend in the last decade is toward the liberalization of abortion laws (18, 31). As of 1990, approximately three quarters of the world's population lives in countries in which abortion is available for health reasons, but only about 40% live in countries where is is available on demand (29). The most restrictive abortion policies exist in Latin America, sub-Saharan Africa, and some of the fundamentalist Arab nations. Abortion policies in Western, Central, and Eastern Europe are generally nonrestrictive, with the exception of Ireland and Malta (30).

Approximately 33 million legal abortions are performed every year. Once the number of illegal abortions is added, that number rises to an estimated 40 to 60 million (30). Fourteen million and 11 million abortions are performed each year in China and the Soviet Union, respectively. The Soviet Union, with an approximate abortion rate of 181 abortions per 1000 women of reproductive age, has the highest rate among all developed countries (30).

Romania provides an often quoted example of the effect of changing abortion policy on population fertility rates and abortion-related mortality rates. Abortion policies were first liberalized in 1957 and were followed by a decline in the birth rate (82). In 1966, abortion laws were tightened in the first pronatalist policy changes. The birth rate rose from 14.3 per 1000 population in 1966 to 26.7 in 1968, which suggests that women were no longer terminating pregnancies at the same rate (19). By 1983, however, the birthrate had again dropped to its original rate (61), mainly because of both an increase in the practice of contraception and illegal abortion.

Increased abortion-related mortality rates accompanied the restrictive abortion policies—the rates increased from 19 per 1 million women (aged 15–45) in 1966 to 69 per 1 million in 1970 (82). The pronatalist policies of the Ceaucescu Government were so onerous that liberalization of the abortion policy was one of the very first actions of the new Government in December 1989, after Ceaucescu was overthrown. This most recent change should be followed by a fall in the maternal mortality rate, which is much higher than in the rest of Europe, probably as a result of the high rate of illegal abortion.

In many developing countries, complications of illegal abortion are one of the five leading causes of maternal mortality (68). The absence of good data in the developing world, however, makes it difficult to assess quantitatively the relationship between abortion and health status. Much of the information about maternal deaths is based on hospital studies, which include only a self-selected group of patients who actually come to a hospital (67).

Studies of maternal deaths show a range in the proportion attributed to abortion. In sub-Saharan Africa, accurate data on abortion-related mortality have been difficult to obtain, and there have been varying estimates of its prevalence in different settings. (54). A well-designed study, conducted in a large, urban community in the early 1980s in Addis-Ababa, Ethiopia, however, found that 54% of maternal deaths in that city were due to illegal abortion complications (47). Similar high rates of maternal deaths due to illegal abortion have been estimated in many other recent African studies, and the rates are particularly high in urban areas (67). In Latin America, despite the lack of reliable data, abortion-related complications may be the leading cause of maternal mortality in many of the countries of the region (67).

The cost of treating complications from illegal abortions is a substantial burden in poor developing countries. In Nigeria, for example, women with abortion-related complications are said to occupy approximately 60% of acute gynecological beds (1). Similarly, a study in Latin America found that septic abortion accounts for a disproportionate share of expenditures for transfusions, operating room costs, and total bed-nights (22).

Overall, the World Health Organization has estimated that 20%–40% of all maternal deaths in developing countries are due to complications of illegal and/or unsafely performed abortion procedures (68). Thus, an estimated 100,000–200,000 women die each year from these unsafe abortions, a public health tragedy of immense proportion. Because the public health and obstetrical communities, policy makers, and the media have not provided effective programming, planning, or detailed discussion (until very recently) about abortion, maternal mortality, and women's overall reproductive health abortion is considered one of the great neglected "diseases" of the tropics (67).

ACKNOWLEDGMENTS

We wish to express our thanks to Renee Holt for sharing information with us while we prepared the legal section, and Marc Schachter, Amy Shire, and Daniel Weitzner for their helpful editorial suggestions.

Literature Cited

1. Aggarwal, V. P., Mati, J. K. G. 1982. Epidemiology of induced abortions in Nairobi, Kenya. *J. Obstet. Gynecol. East Cent. Afr.* 31:67–70
2. Allen, A. E., Pearse, W. H. 1989. The implications of Webster for Practicing Physicians. *J. Am. Med. Assoc.* 262:1510–11
3. Annas, G. J. 1989. The Supreme Court, Privacy, and Abortion. *J. Am. Med. Assoc.* 321:1200–3
4. Atrash, H. K., MacKay, T., Binkin, N. J., Hogue, C. J. R. 1987. Legal abortion mortality in the United States: 1972 to 1982. *Am. J. Obstet. Gynecol.* 156:605–12
5. Baulieu, E. E. 1989. RU-486 as an Anti-progesterone Steroid: From Receptor to Contragestion and Beyond. *J. Am. Med. Assoc.* 262:1808–14
6. *Bellotti v. Baird,* 443 US 622 (US Supreme Court, 1979)
7. Burkman, R. T., Mason, K. J., Gold, E. B. 1988. Ectopic pregnancy and prior induced abortion. *Contraception* 37(1):21–27
8. Calderone, M. S., ed. 1958. *Abortion in the United States.* New York: Hoeber-Harper. 224 pp.
9. Cameron, I. T., Baird, D. T. 1988. Early pregnancy termination: a comparison between vacuum aspiration and medical

abortion using prostaglandin (16,16 dimethyl-trans 2-PGE1 methyl ester) or the antiprogestogen RU-486. *Br. J. Obstet. Gynecol.* 95:271–76

10. Cates, W. 1982. Legal abortion: The public health record. *Science* 215:1586–90

11. Cates, W., Grimes, D. A. 1981. Deaths from second trimester abortion by dilation and evacuation: causes, prevention, facilities. *Obstet. Gynecol.* 58:401–8

12. Cates, W., Rochat, R. W. 1976. Illegal abortions in the United States: 1972–1974. *Fam. Plann. Perspect.* 8(2):86–92

13. Cates, W., Rochat, R. W., Grimes, D. A., Tyler, C. W. 1978. Legalized abortion: effect on national trends of maternal and abortion related mortality (1940–1976). *Am. J. Obstet. Gynecol.* 132:211–14

14. Cent. Dis. Control. 1989. Abortion Surveillance, United States, 1984–1985. *Morbid. Mortal. Wkly. Rep.* 38(SS–2):11–15

15. Chavkin, W., Rosenfield, A. 1990. A chill wind blows: Webster, obstetrics and the health of women. *Am. J. Obstet. Gynecol.* 163:450–52

16. Cheeks, L., Green, K. 1986. Distribution of a steroid antagonist in the eye following topical administration. *Curr. Eye Res.* 5:705–9

17. Cook, R. 1989. Antiprogestin drugs: Medical and legal issues. *Fam. Plann. Perspect.* 21:267–72

18. Cook, R., Dickens, B. M. 1988. International developments in abortions laws: 1977–78. *Am. J. Public Health.* 78:1305–11

19. David, H. P. 1982. Eastern Europe: pronatalist policies and private behavior. *Popul. Bull.* 36(6):1–48

20. Donovan, P. 1989. The 1988 Abortion Referenda: Lessons for the future. *Fam. Plann. Perspect.* 21(5):218–23

21. Ely, J. H. 1973. The wages of crying wolf: A comment on Roe v. Wade. *Yale Law J.* 82:920–44

22. Fortney, J. A. 1981. The use of hospital resources to treat incomplete abortions: examples from Latin America. *Public Health Rep.* 96:574–79

23. Fujita, B., Wagner, N. N. 1973. Referendum 20—Abortion reform. See Ref. 55, pp. 232–60

24. Furth, P. 1989. A piece of my mind: Roe v. Wade. *J. Am. Med. Assoc.* 262:1519

25. Gordon, L. 1977. *Woman's Body, Woman's Right.* New York: Penguin. 479 pp.

26. Grimes, D. A., Schulz, K. F. 1985. The comparative safety of second-trimester abortion methods. In *Abortion: Medical Progress and Social Implications,* ed. R. Porter, M. O'Conner, pp. 83–96. London: Pitman. 285 pp.

27. *Griswold v. Connecticut,* 381 US 479 (US Supreme Court, 1965)

28. *Harris v. McRae,* 100 Supreme Court 2671 (1980)

29. Henshaw, S. K. 1986. Induced abortion: a worldwide perspective. *Fam. Plann. Perspect.* 18(6):250–54

30. Henshaw, S. K. 1986. *Induced Abortion: A World Review.* New York: Alan Guttmacher Inst. 143 pp., 6th ed.

31. Henshaw, S. K. 1990. Induced abortion: A world review, 1990. *Fam. Plann. Perspect.* 22(2):76–89

32. Henshaw, S. K., Binkin, N. J., Blaine, E., Smith, J. C. 1985. A portrait of American women who obtain abortions. *Fam. Plann. Perspect.* 17(2):90–96

33. Henshaw, S. K., Forrest, J. D., Van Vort, J. 1987. Abortion services in the United States, 1984 and 1985. *Fam. Plann. Perspect.* 19(2):63–69

34. Henshaw, S. K., Silverman, J. 1988. The characteristics and prior contraceptive use of United States abortion patients. *Fam. Plann. Perspect.* 20(4):158–68

35. Henshaw, S. K., Wallisch, 1984. The medicaid cutoff and abortion services for the poor. *Fam. Plann. Perspect.* 16(4):170–80

36. Hodge, H. L. 1869. Foeticide, or Criminal Abortion: A Lecture Introductory to the course on Obstetrics, and Diseases of Women and Children. Reprinted 1974. in *Abortion in Nineteenth-Century America.* New York: Arno

37. Hogue, C. J. R., Cates, W., Tietze, C. 1982. The effects of induced abortion on subsequent reproduction. *Epidemiol. Rev.* 4:66–94

38. Deleted in proof

39. Holt, V. L., Daling, J. R., Voigt, L. F., McKnight, B., Stergachis, A., et al. 1989. Induced abortion and the risk of subsequent ectopic pregnancy. *Am. J. Public. Health* 79:1234–38

40. Hum. Resour. Intergov. Relat. Subcomm. 1989. Report: *The Federal Role in Determining the Medical and Psychological Impact of Abortion on Women.* Excerpted in *Fam. Plann. Perspect.* 22(1):36–39

41. Isaacs, S. L. 1981. *Population Law and Policy: Source Book and Related Materials.* New York: Human Science. 431 pp.

42. Joint Program Study Abortion/Cent. Dis. Control. 1976. CDC abortion sur-

vey, 1974. *Fam. Plann. Perspect.* 8(2): 70–72

43. Kendrick, W. 1987. *The Secret Museum: Pornography in Modern Culture.* New York: Viking Penguin. 288 pp.

44. Kiltsch, M. 1989. *RU 486: The Science and the Politics.* New York: Alan Guttmacher Inst. 21 pp.

45. Kolata, G. 1990. After large study of abortion pill, French maker considers wider sale. *NY Times*, March 8

46. Koop, C. E. 1989. A measured response: koop on abortion. *Fam. Plann. Perspect.* 21(1):31–32

47. Kwast, B. E., Rochat, R. W., Kidane-Mariam, W. 1986. Maternal mortality in Addis Ababa, Ethiopia. *Stud. Fam. Plann.* 17:288–301

48. Laue, L., Chrousos, G. P., Loriaux, D. L., Barnes, K., Munson, P., et al. 1988. The antiglucocorticoid and antiprogestin steroid RU 486 suppresses the adrenocorticotropin response to ovine corticotropin relasing hormone in man. *J. Clin. Endocrin. Metab.* 66:290–93

49. Lincoln, R. 1975. The Institute of Medicine reports on legalized abortion and the public health. *Fam. Plann. Perspect.* 7(4):185–88

50. Luker, K. 1984. *Abortion and the Politics of Motherhood.* Berkeley: Univ. Calif. Press. 324 pp.

51. Luukkainen, T., Heikinheimo, U., Haukkanaa, M., Lahteenmaki, P. 1988. Inhibition of folliculogenesis and ovulation by the antiprogesterone RU 486. *Fertil. Steril.* 49:961–62

52. Mohr, J. 1978. *Abortion in America: The Origins and Evolution of National Policy.* New York: Oxford Univ. Press. 331 pp.

53. Nieman, L. K., Choate, T. M., Chrousos, G. P., Healy, D. L., Morin, M., et al. 1987. The progesterone antagonist RU 486: A potential new contraceptive agent. *N. Engl. J. Med.* 316:187–91

54. Ono, O. A., Savage, V. Y. 1974. A ten year review of maternal mortality rates in the University College Hospital Ibadan, Nigeria. *Am. J. Obstet. Gynecol.* 118:317–22

55. Deleted in proof

56. Osofsky, J. D., Osofsky, H. J., Rajan, R. R. 1973. Psychological effects of abortion with emphasis upon immediate reactions and followup. See Ref. 55, pp. 188–205

57. Padayachi, T., Norman, R. J., Moodley, J., Heyns, A. 1988. Mifepristone and Induction of labor in second half of pregnancy. *Lancet* 1:647

58. Petchesky, R. P. 1984. *Abortion and*

Women's Choice. Boston: Northeastern Univ. Press. 404 pp.

59. *Planned Parenthood of Central Missouri v Danforth*, 428 US 52 (US Supreme Court, 1976)

60. Powell-Griner, E., Trent, K. 1987. Sociodemographic determinants of abortion in the United States. *Demography* 24(4):553–61

61. Reproductive Freedom Project. 1990. First circuit finds Title X gag rules unconstitutional. *Reprod. Rights Update,* ACLU 2(7):3

62. Roberts, M. (Transl.). 1984. Romanian population policy. *Popul. Dev. Rev.* 10(3):570–73

63. Rodger, M. W., Baird, D. T. 1987. Induction of therapeutic abortion in early pregnancy with Mifepristone in combination with prostaglandin pessary. *Lancet* 2:1415–18

64. *Roe v. Wade*, 410 US 113 (US Supreme Court, 1973)

65. Rogers, J. L., Stoms, G. B., Phifer, J. L. 1989. Psychological impact of abortion: methodological and outcomes summary of empirical research between 1966 and 1988. *Health Care Women Int.* 10:347–76

66. Romieu, G., Maudelonde, T., Ulmann, A., Pujol, H., Grenier, J., et al. 1987. The antiprogestin RU 486 in advanced breast cancer: preliminary clinical trial. *Bull. Cancer* 74:455–61

67. Rosenfield, A. 1989. Maternal mortality in developing countries: an ongoing but neglected "epidemic". *J. Am. Med. Assoc.* 262:376–79

68. Rosenfield, A., Maine, D. 1985. Maternal mortality—A neglected tragedy: Where's the M in MCH? *Lancet* 2:83–85

69. Rosse, A. S., Sitarnon, B. 1988. Abortion in context: historical trends and future changes. *Fam. Plann. Perspect.* 20(6):273–81, 301

70. Rubin, G. L., Gold, J., Cates, W. 1979. Response of low-income women and abortion facilities to restriction of public funds for abortion: a study of a large metropolitan area. *Am. J. Public Health* 69:948–50

71. Silvestre, L., Dubois, C., Renault, M., Rezvani, Y., Baulieu, E. E., Ulmann, A. 1990. Voluntary interruption of pregnancy with Mifepristone (RU486) and prostaglandin analogue: A large-scale French experience. *N. Engl. J. Med.* 322:645–48

72. Smith-Rosenberg, C. 1985. *The Abortion Movement and the AMA, 1850–1880.* In *Disorderly Conduct: Visions of Gender in Victorian America*, pp. 217–

44. New York: Oxford Univ. Press. 357 pp.

73. Stewart, G. K., Hance, F. 1974. Legal abortion: Influences upon mortality, morbidity and population. *Adv. Plann. Parent.* 9:1–7

74. The Cent. Popul. Options. 1989. *Adolescent Abortion and Parental Involvement Laws: Encouraging Communication or Conflict?* Washington, DC

75. Tietze, C. 1975. The effect of legalization of abortion on population growth and public health. *Fam. Plann. Perspect.* 7(3):123–27

76. Tietze, C. 1984. The public health effects of legal abortion in the United States. *Fam. Plann. Perspect.* 16(1):26–28

77. Torres, A., Forrest, J. D. 1988. Why do women have abortions? *Fam. Plann. Perspect.* 20(4):169–76

78. Trussell, J., Menken, J., Lindheim, B. L., Vaughan, 1980. The impact of restricting medicaid financing for abortion. *Fam. Plann. Perspect.* 12(3):120–30

79. *Webster v. Reprod. Health Serv.,* 109 (US Supreme Court 3040, 1989)

80. Wigglesworth, J. S., Desai, R. 1982. Is fetal respiratory function a major determinant of perinatal survival? *Lancet* 1:264–67

81. *Williams v. Zbaraz,* 100 (US Supreme Court 2694, 1980)

82. Wright, N. H. 1975. Restricting legal abortion: some maternal and child health effect in Romania. *Am. J. Obstet. Gynecol.* 121:246–56

Annu. Rev. Publ. Health. 1991. 12:383–400

PROGRESS AND PROBLEMS IN INTERNATIONAL PUBLIC HEALTH EFFORTS TO REDUCE TOBACCO USAGE

John P. Pierce

University of California, San Diego, Cancer Center, San Diego, California 92103

KEY WORDS: smoking, prevalence, consumption, interventions, strategies

BACKGROUND

Tobacco or Health

The use of tobacco, whether by smoking, chewing, or sniffing, has been shown to cause untimely death and disability from cancer, heart disease, and pulmonary disease, not only in the user, but also in those who are exposed to environmental tobacco smoke (50, 53). The total amount of death and disease caused by smoking is considerable. In the United States, there were an estimated 390,000 smoking-attributable deaths in 1985 (40), which makes up almost 25% of all deaths among men and over 10% of all deaths among women.

If tobacco were discovered today, it is hard to imagine a single country in which it would be legal to grow it, refine it, advertise it, or sell it. Nevertheless, with the exception of advertising in a few countries, it is legal to do all these things in every country of the world. Why has the public health movement in every country failed to make tobacco illegal and thus protect the public from such a potent carcinogen?

How Behaviors Change in Societies

The study of the way that populations adopt new behaviors and then discard them has come to be known as diffusion research. The pattern of change in

383

0163-7525/91/0501-0383$02.00

Table 1   Indices of trends in per capita consumption of tobacco products (gram equivalent) in selected OECD countries[a]

Country	1960 consumption in grams	Peak consumption (year)	1986 consumption in grams	Reduction from peak
United States	4655	4700 (1964)	3275	30.4%
New Zealand	3294	3325 (1966)	2303	30.7%
Canada	4011	4301 (1966)	3305	23.2%
Australia	3329	3338 (1969)	2308	31.0%
United Kingdom	3258	3403 (1972)	2417	29.0%
Germany (FDR)	2411	3198 (1972)	2779	13.1%
Denmark	3055	3250 (1973)	2703	16.8%
Finland	2189	2505 (1974)	2012	19.7%
Japan	1939	3440 (1975)	3334	3.1%
Iceland	1982	3982 (1976)	2718	31.0%
Sweden	1517	2104 (1976)	1893	10.0%
Netherlands	3860	4708 (1979)	3264	30.3%
Norway	1759	2118 (1980)	1927	9.1%
Italy	1462	2327 (1982)	2291	5.5%
Portugal	1114	2087 (1983)	1963	6.0%
France	1901	2468 (1985)	2383	3.5%
Greece	2024	3780 (1985)	3777	0.2%
Spain	1591	3055 (1985)	2885	5.6%

[a] Source: Laugesen & Meads (27)

such situations as infectious disease epidemics (6, 44), health practices (42), and adoption of agricultural innovations (41) can be described by an S-shaped curve.

New behaviors, such as smoking, usually are adopted slowly, as new ways are unfamiliar and the immediate consequences of use are uncertain. As the first people to smoke convey information about the potential benefits of the behavior, and the product is more extensively promoted, smoking is adopted at a much faster rate within the population. Then, the diffusion rate slows down and the maximum penetration (or peak consumption) of tobacco in that society is reached. Both the time to this peak and its height may vary considerably for different subgroups in society. Once the peak has been reached, the behavior may diffuse out of the society. This pattern of decline is an inverse S-shaped curve. The decline off the peak starts slowly, then quickens to a linear trend before slowing down to approach an asymptote, which may (or may not) be zero (39).

In this review, I present tobacco usage data from different countries and discuss the data in the above diffusion framework. Key questions relate to factors that have facilitated diffusion, peak use rates, and recent trends. I review effective antismoking campaign strategies and emphasize the need for further worldwide cooperation between public health professionals.

The rapid phase of the diffusion curve for the uptake (17, 37, 38, 53) of cigarette smoking in developed countries, such as the United States and the United Kingdom, appears to have occurred in the first half of the twentieth century (20). Concerns about the health consequences of tobacco were strongly expressed in the 1950s and were firmly established in major public health reports in the United Kingdom in 1962 (43) and in the United States in 1964 (51). Thus, the early 1960s can be considered the start of the official public health campaign against tobacco use in these countries.

The data available to study the tobacco diffusion curve since the 1960s in different countries include tobacco consumption estimates from excise tax data (53) and population surveys (36). The consumption estimate includes changes in the number of persons who smoke, as well as changes in the amount they smoke. A real change in community prevalence will be reflected in a higher percentage change in consumption than in actual prevalence.

Consumption Estimates from Taxation of Tobacco Products

Most countries have an excise tax levy on tobacco, which is collected at the wholesale level and for which good statistics are available (31, 48), from which changes in tobacco consumption can be estimated. Total tobacco is used for comparative purposes, because there is considerable variability across countries in the proportion that manufactured cigarettes make up of total tobacco used.

Tobacco usage in various developed countries has been compared by many investigators, including Laugesen & Meads (27), from whose paper the data in Table 1 are adapted. Total tobacco consumption figures were obtained from excise tax data published for countries in the Organization for Economic Cooperation and Development (OECD), which used weight in grams of each tobacco product consumed (a cigarette contains approximately 1 g of tobacco). These data are then divided by the estimated population over age 15 to obtain an estimated per capita consumption.

In 1960, per capita consumption of tobacco products was highest in the United States, followed by Canada and the Netherlands; Greece and Spain consumed less than half the level of the United States. The rank order of consumption in these countries may reflect the development of consumerism in those societies, rather than factors specifically related to tobacco use (45). Although the peak consumption occurred after 1960 in all countries presented, the year that it was achieved varied from 1964 in the United States to the mid-1980s for the latin countries of Europe. It is tempting to attribute the timing of the peak to the strength of the antismoking movement in the country. However, proponents of this hypothesis need to reconcile the closeness in the publication dates for the first reports on the health consequences of smoking in the United Kingdom and the United States with the ten-year difference in their peak per capita consumption. The maximum tobacco penetration level ranged from the mid-4000 g equivalents (United States, Canada) to about 2000 (Norway, Portugal, Sweden). This major difference in peak level may reflect different peak prevalence levels or major differences in the pattern of use of tobacco in individuals in differing countries.

The diffusion of tobacco out of a society is measured by both the rate and the amount of decline in tobacco consumption since the peak year. In the 22 years after the peak in the United States, consumption declined by 30% (mean rate of 1.4% per year). Many other countries also have experienced declines of 30%, irrespective of the year in which their consumption peaked. These countries include Australia, Iceland, New Zealand, Netherlands, and the United Kingdom. This reduction occurred quickest in the Netherlands (seven years) and Iceland (ten years). The hypothesis that these differences in the rates of change reflect different influences for and against smoking behavior needs to be investigated further.

The quality of the data from non-OECD countries does not match that for OECD countries. Per capita consumption of cigarettes from non-OECD countries in 1988 has been categorized into broad groups (3, 13). The highest group of consumers (>2000 cigarettes per capita per year) includes Cuba, Hungary, Libya, and Malaysia. China is in the second highest category (1500–2000). The lowest categories are comprised of the African nations and India (less than 500). By comparison, there were five OECD countries that consumed over 3000 g equivalents of tobacco per capita in 1986 (Table 1).

PREDICTIONS OF FUTURE WORLDWIDE USE OF TOBACCO

Projections of tobacco usage worldwide have been undertaken by the Food and Agricultural Organization of the United Nations in conjunction with the United States Department of Agriculture (18, 46, 48). Figure 1 presents the estimates of actual and projected demand in developed and developing countries around the world. There are two important points in this figure: Consumption of tobacco in developed countries is decreasing, but at a slow rate; and strong growth in tobacco consumption is projected for the developing world. If these estimates are correct, world consumption of tobacco probably will double before the turn of the century (46). Of this projected growth in demand, 60% is expected to come from Asia (particularly China), and another 25% will come from the Far East countries; only 10% will come from Africa and Latin America (Figure 2).

These figures clearly indicate that the worldwide epidemic of tobacco-related deaths is still in its upward phase. Assuming that smokers in develop-

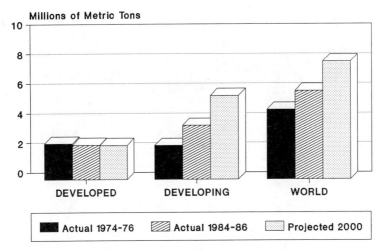

Figure 1   Actual and projected demand for tobacco in the world from 1974 to 2000.

ing countries will have the same mortality rates from smoking as those from developed countries, Peto & Lopez (35) estimate that there could be 2 million tobacco-related deaths worldwide annually by the year 1995. They emphasize the importance of China because of the sheer size of its population of smokers and potential smokers. Per capita cigarette consumption in China has increased rapidly and shows no apparent tendency to peak in the short-term future (59). Thus, future increases in consumption in China are expected to come partly from population growth and partly from measured per capita consumption. China alone may have as many as 2 million smoking-related deaths by the year 2025 (26).

COMPARISON OF ADULT SMOKING BEHAVIOR

Many developed countries undertake regular data collection of tobacco usage among nationally representative samples of their populations. Frequently, these data are obtained by adding questions to other population-based surveys, such as the National Health Interview Survey in the United States, the Labor Force survey in Canada, and commercially run market surveys in Australia (36). The accepted indicator of tobacco usage in a particular country is the point prevalence estimate of current behavior. There currently is no worldwide accepted standard question to measure the frequency of tobacco usage. To undertake cross-cultural comparisons, we need to assume that the variation in responses to the differing questions is minimal. However, it is the internal consistency in the data collected in each country that is important for

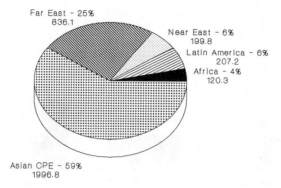

Figure 2   1974–1976 to 2000 projected change in demand for tobacco in developing countries (18).

calculating the rate of change in its point prevalence. Trends in point prevalence are used in predicting future trends.

Smoking Prevalence in Men

Table 2 presents the most recent smoking prevalence data available from several countries with regular data collection systems. Where possible, a crude mean yearly change in prevalence has been calculated for each of these countries for the decade before the last year of available data. Among these countries, smoking prevalence in men was highest in the three non-Scandinavian European countries (Poland, 55%; France, 48%; Spain, 58%) and in China (61%). There was little apparent difference in smoking prevalence in the United States, the United Kingdom, Australia, Canada, or Finland, where approximately one third of adult men smoke. The much lower figure in Sweden is supported by the earlier consumption data. However, substitution of snuff use for cigarette use in that country may be partly responsible for the much lower levels of smoking prevalence (36).

In the United States, the United Kingdom, Canada, and Australia, the decline in the proportion of male smokers has been rapid at about 1 percentage point per year, and the current proportion of smokers is relatively low. However, for most of Europe and the developing countries the decline in smoking is, at best, a very recent phenomenon and is progressing more slowly.

Smoking Prevalence in Women

The highest levels of smoking prevalence in women occur in Norway and France (33%). As of 1984, very low levels of prevalence were seen in China

Table 2   Adult smoking behavior in selected countries by sex

	Latest year data available	Men prevalence (%)	Percent change/ year	Women prevalence (%)	Percent change/ year
Australia[a]	1986	32.9	−0.7	30.6	−0.1
Canada[a]	1986	32.3	−1.2	26.6	−0.5
China[b]	1984	61.0	—	07.0	—
Finland[c]	1987	33.2	−0.2	21.1	+0.3
France[d]	1989	48.2	−0.2	32.8	+0.3
Norway[a]	1987	41.3	−0.8	33.3	+0.02
Poland[e]	1985	54.8	−0.4	27.9	+0.08
Sweden[a]	1987	24.0	−1.0	27.0	−0.6
United Kingdom[a]	1986	35.0	−1.4	31.0	−0.8
United States[a]	1987	31.7	−0.9	26.8	−0.3
Catalonia, Spain[f]	1982	58.0	—	19.8	—

Source: [a] Pierce (36)
[b] Yu (59)
[c] T. Piha (personal communication)
[d] A. Hirsch (personal communication)
[e] T. Gorski (personal communication)
[f] Department of Health and Social Security, the Autonomous Government of Catalonia (personal communication)

(12%). The data from the OECD countries suggest that the diffusion curve peaked in women at a later stage than it did in men. This might explain the slower recent rate of change as the outward diffusion curve for women may not have progressed as far into its downward linear phase as it has for men.

However, the delayed onset of the diffusion curve does not explain why the peak prevalence of smoking in women has been so much lower than in men. In the United States, the peak prevalences of male smokers occurred in the 1950s, compared with the mid-1970s for women (20). The diffusion curve for smoking among women occurred at the same time as another major social change, the movement toward social equality with men. Much of the early tobacco advertising promoted cigarettes to women by using the equality theme (e.g. Virginia Slims) (45). The lower peak seen in women smokers in the United States reflects the degree to which male smoking rates had declined before equality in smoking patterns was attained in the younger birth cohorts.

If we generalize from the diffusion patterns of tobacco in developed countries, we can anticipate that, barring successful antismoking initiatives, there will be a large increase in tobacco consumption in China and other Asian countries, which will occur partly because of marked increases in the recruitment of women to smoking. Mackay (29, 30) has documented that tobacco company advertising in these countries is clearly targeting women.

Uptake of Smoking in the Young

The issue of recruitment of young people to smoking is critical to the maintenance of a high demand for tobacco around the world. In the United States, the rate of the current decline in smoking is blunted by a daily influx of 3000 young people who become regular smokers (39). The age at which women become regular smokers has declined consistently with each birth cohort since those born in 1930. By 1985, 85% of regular smokers started before age 21, with less than 3% starting after age 25 (53). Women and blacks, who had more recent tobacco diffusion curves, had delayed onset curves in earlier years, compared with white men. However, by the 1980s, both white women and blacks had uptake rates similar to white men (53). Thus, in the United States, smoking prevalence among 20–24-year-olds can be used as a reasonable indicator of the proportion of a particular cohort who will become regular smokers (17, 39, 53).

Table 3 compares the differential rates of uptake of smoking behavior in selected countries by using this measure of uptake. In developed countries, there is little difference in the rate of smoking uptake between the sexes; however, the uptake rate among men has been declining at a faster rate than among women over the past ten years. The single exception is Sweden; smoking is not a sufficient indicator of tobacco use because of the prevalence of snuff use among men (36). As indicated earlier, Australia, Canada, the United Kingdom, and the United States had equivalent overall smoking prevalence levels. However, Australia and the United Kingdom have much higher uptake rates (around 40%) than either Canada or the United States (around 30%). This suggests that the overall prevalence rates between these two groups of countries will diverge in the near future.

In China, although over half of young men have become regular smokers, uptake among young women is almost nonexistent, which is contrary to the experience of Western societies. Reasons could be the different roles that women have in Asian societies compared with Western societies and the cultural pressures that women are under not to smoke. Tobacco companies have overcome some of these issues previously in Western countries with the help of advertising (45). With tobacco advertising at young women recently introduced into Asia (30), an enormous increase in the prevalence of smoking among women is anticipated.

Differences in Smoking by Educational Level

Diffusion both into and out of a society frequently starts among those individuals who are more educated (although this does not appear to be a function of knowledge or years of formal education) (42). The early adoption of smoking in the United States began with the higher educated (45), and they maintained a gap in prevalence through the early half of this century. Sim-

Table 3 Smoking behavior in young adults in selected countries by sex

	Latest year data available	Male smokers (%)	Percent change/ year	Female smokers (%)	Percent change/ year
Australia[a]	1986	39.8	−0.7	40.6	+0.2
Canada[a]	1986	32.0	−1.2	31.3	−1.4
China[a]	1984	54.0	—	12.0	—
Finland[b]	1987	28.0	−0.4	23.3	+0.05
France[c]	1988	33.0	−1.3	32.0	−0.9
Norway[a]	1989	26.0	−0.8	32.0	−0.4
Sweden[c]	1987	14.0	−1.7	27.0	−1.3
United Kingdom[a]	1986	41.0	−0.9	38.0	−0.7
United States[a]	1987	31.1	−1.0	28.1	−0.1
Catalonia, Spain	1982	62.8	—	60.1	—

[a] 20–24 years of age
[b] 15–24 years of age
[c] 12–18 years of age
[d] 18–24 years of age
Source: See Table 2

ilarly, the diffusion of tobacco out of a society started with the highest educated group in the United States (38, 53), Norway, Canada, and Australia (36). Hence, when smoking prevalence among the higher educated in a society is lower than prevalence in the lower educated, it probably indicates that the nation already has achieved (or is about to achieve) its peak consumption level. In all countries presented in Table 4, smoking prevalence was greater among the lower, rather than the higher, educated. In almost all of these countries, except France, a decline in overall smoking prevalence has been established. Furthermore, among the higher educated, smoking prevalence had declined to around 20%, except among Polish men and women and among French men. If we assume that smoking prevalence among men in these societies peaked at a level over 50%, then smoking prevalence also has been declining among the lower educated men in several countries, except those in Poland, France, and the United Kingdom.

Large educational discrepancies in smoking behavior may indicate a higher level of social tension in the society with respect to smoking. This discrepancy is considerably greater in the United Kingdom, the United States, and Norway (ratio over 2.0) than it is in Finland or Sweden (ratio 1.3 or lower). Another explanation could be that a large discrepancy may reflect differences in the relative effectiveness of antismoking campaigns between the education levels in these countries. In countries with a widening educational gap in smoking, the antismoking campaign may need to be reevaluated to make sure that it is not being conducted "by the better educated, for the better educated."

Table 4 Differences in smoking prevalence by education level in selected countries

Country		Latest year available	Highest education level	Lowest education level	Ratio
Australia		1986	20	36	1.8
Canada		1986	20	32	1.6
China		1984	57	64	1.1
Finland	- men	1987	29	35	1.2
	women	1987	22	26	1.2
France	- men	1989	34	52	1.5
	women	1989	18	25	1.4
Norway		1987	22	44	2.0
Poland	- men	1985	43	72	1.7
	women	1985	36	35	1.0
Sweden		1987	26	34	1.3
United Kingdom	- men	1986	17	49	2.9
	women	1986	15	38	2.5
United States		1987	16	36	2.3

Source: See Table 2

Smoking Measures Among Physicians

Among the highest educated in any society are those persons in the medical profession. In countries where it is not possible to get population smoking data by educational group, smoking prevalence among this profession is an indicator of diffusion. In addition, the medical profession is charged by society with the responsibility for the treatment and prevention of disease. Medical practitioners have been in the vanguard of the antismoking movement in most countries. When, as a group, they aggressively counsel patients to quit smoking, it is an effective population strategy to reduce smoking prevalence (25). Accordingly, the prevalence of smoking in the medical profession can be used as an indicator of the strength of a society's willingness to accept the health consequences of smoking.

Over the last 30 years, there have been more than 100 physician surveys in different countries (1, 2). As expected, the countries previously identified as having large decreases in tobacco consumption also are the ones with the lowest prevalence of smoking among physicians. Physicians in the US and Canada had the lowest level (around 10%). However, in Spain, Egypt, and the USSR, almost half of male physicians still smoke. In China, 57% of physicians smoked in 1984 (59).

Smoking among medical students can be considered the uptake rate for the profession. Starting to smoke is not an addictive behavior; hence, it may be expected to change more rapidly than quitting. Accordingly, the proportion of medical students who smoke when they enter medical school may be a more sensitive measure of the strength of the antismoking health beliefs in a society than is smoking prevalence in physicians. There are marked differences in the smoking prevalence of medical students (47). In the United States, less than 5% of medical students now smoke (T. Pearson, personal communication 1990). In the United Kingdom and Finland, smoking prevalence among medical students has been reduced to 10%-15%. However, it is much higher in Germany and France (approximately 30%) and higher still in Poland and Austria (approximately 40%).

Overview of Patterns of Tobacco Use

Smoking behavior became widespread in Western societies in the twentieth century. The first group to adopt the addiction in these societies was higher educated white men. Over time, the behavior diffused through the lower educated men and women (higher educated before lower educated). By 1960, the United States led the world in the per capita consumption of tobacco, and consumption everywhere was growing. Antismoking campaigns received public health legitimacy in the early 1960s and were associated with a leveling off and then a drop in per capita consumption, first in the United States, then in other Western nations. Marked differences in the maximum per capita consumption attained might relate to the proportion of tobacco use that comes from manufactured cigarettes (issues of ease of use and accessibility). Alternatively, these differences may relate to the amount of unfettered advertising and promotion undertaken by the tobacco companies before the increase in general knowledge of the health consequences of smoking. Tobacco use is still being adopted at a very rapid rate around the world, especially in developing nations, which are in the upward phase of a major worldwide epidemic of smoking related death and disease. The world is far from being smoke-free by the year 2000.

EFFECTIVE STRATEGIES FOR PROMOTING A DECLINE IN TOBACCO CONSUMPTION

The history of tobacco control in countries that have reduced tobacco exposure in their populations suggests that there are five main public health strategies, which are used to effectively reduce tobacco prevalence (44). I will briefly review the evidence for the effectiveness of each of these approaches.

1. Raising the Excise Tax on Tobacco

Numerous studies in the United States (53), Europe (16, 28), and New Zealand (21) indicate that an increase in the price of cigarettes is associated with a drop in consumption. A price elasticity of -0.5 implies that a 10% increase in price of a product will be associated with a 5% decrease in the quantity consumed. The short term price elasticity for tobacco is between -0.3 and -0.5 in these populations.

As teenagers who are starting to smoke may be more price sensitive than adults, many studies have analyzed the effect of price increases on the uptake of smoking (53). The United States Government Accounting Office (49) reviewed the evidence and suggested that a conservative estimate for price elasticity in this group would be -0.76. Using this figure, they projected that a 21-cent increase in the 1990 price of cigarettes would result in a reduction of over a half million teenage smokers in the United States. As there has been a recent increase in the California excise tax of this magnitude (12), this estimate can be evaluated in the near future.

The published studies have had only moderate price changes from which to calculate their price elasticities. Recently, several countries, notably Canada (15, 26), have dramatically increased the price of cigarettes so that the excise tax alone accounts for more than $2 per pack (compared with the highest tax in the United States in 1990 of 51 cents per pack). The law of diminishing returns probably applies to the effect on consumption of increasing price of cigarettes. The effect of price on consumption of an addictive product also must take into account the extent of the addiction and the perceived functional utility of smoking to the individual smoker. Over the next few years, the effect of very large increases in excise tax may lead to a reassessment of the above price elasticities across a wide range of prices. In addition, the effect of price on consumption may be influenced markedly by the amount of anti-smoking publicity associated with the increase in price (M. Laugesen 1990, personal communication).

2. Regulation of Tobacco Advertisements and Promotions

Over the last 30 years, most OECD countries have increasingly restricted tobacco advertising and promotion. They have banned it on the electronic media and mandated health warnings on cigarette packets and in print media advertising (9, 55). In all cases, the tobacco industry has vigorously opposed any new restrictions, by arguing that such restrictions are an infringement of corporate freedom regarding a product that is legal to manufacture and sell, as well as by suggesting that such restrictions are ineffective in reducing tobacco consumption (10).

Econometric analyses of tobacco consumption in OECD countries between 1962 and 1980, however, showed that tobacco legislation was associated with a decline in consumption, after price and income effects were controlled (21, 27). Tobacco legislation in each country was obtained from the International Digest of Health Legislation 1960–1988 (56), supplemented by information from health agencies. The maximum score of ten points was given when there was a total ban on tobacco advertising and sponsorship with strong and varied warnings on cigarette packs. A maximum score was achieved by Finland in 1979, Iceland in 1984, Norway in 1985, and Canada in 1989 (15, 26). One point was given for each media from which cigarette advertising was banned and up to two points for the strength of the health warnings on cigarette packets. The United States scored five points in 1986. Laugesen & Meads (27) conducted a multivariate time series analysis on per capita tobacco consumption that included the following variables: the advertising restriction score, real price of tobacco, gross domestic product, the proportion of the population who were elderly, the fraction of the workforce who were female, and the proportion of tobacco consumed from manufactured cigarettes. This model explained 99.5% of the variance in the average annual level of tobacco consumption across these countries. Estimates from this analysis suggest that should a country introduce a total ban on advertising, tobacco consumption would decrease by a permanent 5% in the following year. This model, however, did not estimate whether there was a continued effect in later years.

3. Using Mass Media in a Coordinated Antismoking Campaign

The most definitive long-term evaluation of the use of the mass media studied a coordinated mass media-led antismoking campaign in Australia beginning in the early 1980s (40). In the ten years before the campaign, smoking prevalence in men and women was stable in that country's two largest cities, Sydney and Melbourne. The antismoking campaign started in Sydney in 1983, with eight weeks of paid multimedia advertising that achieved "saturation" exposure of the population to vivid messages on the health consequences of smoking. With the start of the campaign, there was a −2.5 percentage point "jump-shift" in smoking prevalence for both men and women. This effect was replicated for each sex in Melbourne in the following year. Continuing the campaign led to an estimated 1.4 percentage point decline per year for men, a rate 40% higher than the current rate of decline for men in the United States (53). Among women, after the jump-shift in smoking prevalence at the start of the campaign, no further trend over time was identified. Important questions that still need to be answered are whether the male decline will level off as the population becomes accustomed to the campaign and why there was no continued effect identified for women. These campaigns were sufficiently successful that they have been replicated in other Australian states and in New Zealand. A major natural experiment is currently underway in California (7), the evaluation of which should be able to address many of the unanswered questions in this field.

4. Regulation of Smoking Behavior in Public Places and Worksites

The stated purpose of regulation of smoking behavior in public places and worksites is the protection of the rights and the health of the nonsmoker (50). The effect of smoking bans in public places has been difficult to isolate, as these bans generally are part of a package that includes advertising restrictions. In the largest prospective study currently reported, the effect of a smoking ban across the entire Australian Civil Service was to reduce the number of cigarettes consumed by smokers by an estimated 5.2 cigarettes per day, although there was no significant effect on the prevalence of smokers (11). This conclusion has been supported by another study in the United States (8).

5. Health Education Programs in Schools

The National Cancer Institute has conducted a major research program to identify effective school health education programs to reduce the uptake of smoking. These studies have sought to optimize the focus, the content, and the length of the program; the age group to whom it should be delivered; and the role that peers and parents may have in the program. Most school programs have had some positive effects. However, when unaccompanied by community interventions, they appear to delay the onset of tobacco use, but are not powerful enough to have a long-term effect on the uptake rate (19, 32).

Summary of Effective Interventions

There is now considerable evidence that tobacco use in a society can be affected by public health action. Increasing the price of tobacco, implementing smoking bans, limiting the type and amount of advertising that tobacco companies can undertake, and conducting coordinated campaigns all appear to have an effect on tobacco consumption. The research on school education programs strongly supports the notion that this strategy should not be used alone. However, these strategies rarely are used in isolation, and it is now the prevailing wisdom that the most effective approach is to use as many strategies as are possible concurrently (58). The Laugesen & Meads (27) analysis demonstrated that combining a price increase and a total advertising ban would have a much greater effect in a society than either would alone. They estimated that, in 1986, a permanent 30% increase in the real tobacco price, in conjunction with a total ban on total advertising, would produce twice the effect on tobacco consumption of either one alone.

An Additional Problem: Transnational Companies and US Trade Policies

The manufacture of cigarettes is increasingly becoming an oligopoly controlled by four large transnational companies and the government of China (54). In 1986, four companies controlled 31% of the world's cigarette output, and the Chinese government controlled another 26%. The four Western transnational companies are making enormous inroads into the distribution of tobacco because of their efficient manufacturing procedures and the pervasiveness of their advertising and promotion. These companies are able to overcome trade barriers by manufacturing cigarettes in foreign factories, owning all or part of local tobacco companies, licensing their brand names, and exporting their manufactured brands (54).

In addition, the United States Trade Representative and senior members of the United States Senate have threatened to impose trade sanctions against a number of Asian countries unless those countries allow the marketing and promotion of United States tobacco products (14, 29, 30). With this considerable coercive power, companies have been able to reverse national tobacco control initiatives that have not allowed advertising of cigarettes, thereby doubling the total overseas market for American cigarettes from 1986 to 1989. Such action poses a serious threat to public health action against tobacco around the world.

However, public health professionals in the United States have started to respond to requests for help from countries subject to this coercion (G. S. Omenn, personal communication, Letter to the Honorable George Bush, July 16, 1990). In his final official act, at a public hearing on a congressional investigation initiated under section 302 of the trade act of 1974, former Surgeon-General, C. Everett Koop (24) said:

> It is the height of hypocrisy for the United States, in our war against drugs, to demand that foreign nations take steps to stop the export of cocaine to our country while at the same time we export nicotine, a drug just as addictive as cocaine, to the rest of the world.

Since then, the American Cancer Society has focused on the need for advocacy on this problem. This advocacy pits the trade goals of the Bush Administration in Washington against its public health goals (5), which is the latest in a series of developments in which the international public health community has started to rally against and coordinate the fight with the transnational tobacco companies (57). In the forefront of these developments is the biannual World Conference on Smoking and Health. The 1992 meeting will be in Buenos Aires, Argentina. The International Union Against Cancer program on tobacco is proactive; its uses a regional approach with site visits and workshops to build locally based tobacco control activities worldwide. For example, the Latin American Coordinating Committee was created in the mid 1980s. It has met annually ever since to promote and report on smoking control activities in the member countries (4). Recently, the American Cancer Society has developed "Globalink," a computer-based communications network whereby tobacco control leaders from around the world can seek international help in coordinating tobacco control strategies, as well as share information and experiences. The Office on Smoking and Health, which is part of the Centers for Disease Control, is focusing on smoking in the Americas for its 1992 Congressionally-mandated Surgeon-General's Report (R. Davis 1990, personal communication).

Literature Cited

1. Adriaanse, H., Van Reek, J. 1986. *Physicians' Smoking Worldwide. A Review of 100 Surveys on Physicians' Tobacco Consumption in 27 Countries in the Period 1951–1983*. Presented at Int. Symp. Tobacco Smoking Among Health Professionals. Venice, May 30–31

2. Adriaanse, H., Van Reek, J. 1989. Physicians' smoking and its exemplary effect. *Scand. J. Prim. Health Care* 7:193–96

3. Allen, T. A. 1989. Global per capita consumption of manufactured cigarettes. *Chron. Dis. Can.* 10(3):51–53

4. Am. Cancer Soc. 1989. *Lating American Coordinating Committee on Smoking Control—Smoking Control in Latin American*. Rep. 5th annu. meet.

5. Am. Cancer Soc. 1990. Rep. of Trade for Life Summit: Washington, DC January 6–8, Atlanta

6. Armenian, H. K., Lilienfeld, A. 1983. Incubation period of disease. *Epidemiology* 5:1–15

7. Bal, D. G., Kizer, K. W., Felton, P. G., Mozar, H. N., Neimeyer, D. 1990. Reducing tobacco consumption in California: The development of a statewide anti-tobacco use campaign. *J. Am. Med. Assoc.* 264(12):1570–74

8. Beiner, L., Abrams, D. B., Follick, M. J., Dean L. 1989. A comparative evaluation of a restrictive smoking policy in a general hospital. *Am. J. Public Health* 79:192–95

9. Bjartveit, K. 1990. *Fifteen Years of Comprehensive Legislation: Results and Conclusions*. Presented at 7th World Conf. Tobacco Health, Perth West. Aust.

10. Boddewyn, J. J., ed. 1986. *Tobacco Advertising Bans and Consumption in 16 Countries*. Int. Advert. Assoc.

11. Borland, R., Chapman, S., Owen, N., Hill, D. 1990. Effects of workplace smoking bans on cigarette consumption. *Am. J. Public Health* 80(2):178–80

12. Calif. State Board of Equalization. 1990. *Annual Report 1988–1989* No. A40–41

13. Chapman, S., Weng, W. W. 1990. *Tobacco Control in the Third World—A Resource Atlas*. Penang, Malaysia: Int. Organ. Consum. Unions (IOCU). 242 pp.

14. Chen, T. T. L., Winder, A. E. 1990. The Opium wars revisited as US forces tobacco exports in Asia. *Am. J. Public Health* 80(6):659–62

15. Collishaw, N. E., Kaiserman, M. J., Rogers, B. 1990. *Monitoring Effectiveness of Canada's Health-oriented Tobacco Policies*. Presented at 7th World Conf. Tobacco Health 1990. Perth, West. Aust.

16. Cox, H., Smith, R. 1984. Political approaches to smoking control: a comparative analysis. *Appl. Econ.* 16:569–82

17. Fiore, M. F., Novotny, T. E., Pierce, J. P., Hatziandreu, E., Davis, R. 1989.

Trends in cigarette smoking in the United States: The influence of gender and race. *J. Am. Med. Assoc.* 261:49–55

18. Food Agric. Organ. (FAO). 1990. Tobacco: Supply, Demand and Trade Projections, 1995 and 2000. Rome, Italy

19. Glynn, T. J. 1989. Essential elements of school-based smoking prevention programs. *J. Sch. Health* 59(5):181–88

20. Harris, J. E. 1983. Cigarette smoking among successive birth cohorts of men and women in the United States during 1900–80. *J. Natl. Cancer Inst.* 73(3):473–79

21. Harrison, R. 1990. *The Impact of Advertising on Aggregate Demand for Cigarettes in New Zealand.* Presented at 7th World Conf. Tobacco Health, Perth, West. Aust.

22. Deleted in proof

23. Deleted in proof

24. Koop, C. E. 1990. *Tobacco Economic Grip on the World: Setting the Stage.* Presented at World Conf. Lung Health, Boston, May 20–24

25. Kottke, T. E., Battista, R. N., DeFriese, G. H., Brekke, M. L. 1988. Attributes of successful smoking cessation intervention in medical practice. *J. Am. Med. Assoc.* 259(19):2883–89

26. Kyle, K. 1990. Canada's tobacco legislation: A victory for the health lobby. *Ottawa Health Welf. Can. Health Promot.* 28(4):8–12

27. Laugesen, M., Meads, C. 1990. *Tobacco Advertising Restrictions, Price, Income and Tobacco Consumption in OECD Countries, 1960–86.* Presented at 7th World Conf. Tobacco Health, Perth, West. Aust.

28. Leeflang, P. S. H., Reuijl, J. C. 1985. Advertising and industry sales: An empirical study of the West German cigarette market. *J. Mark.* 49:92–98

29. Mackay, J. 1989. Battlefield for the tobacco war. *J. Am. Med. Assoc.* 261:28–29

30. Mackay, J. 1990. *The Tobacco Economic Grip on the World: Asian Experience.* Presented at World Conf. Lung Health, Boston, May 20–24

31. Masironi, R., Rothwell, K. 1988. Tendences et effects du tabagisme dans le monde. *Rapp. Trimest. Statist. Sanit. Mond.* 41:228–41

32. Murray, D. M., Pirie, P., Luepker, R. V., Pallonen, U. 1989. Five and six-year follow-up results from seventh-grade smoking prevention strategies. *J. Behav. Med.* 12(2) 207–18

33. Deleted in proof

34. Deleted in proof

35. Peto, R., Lopez, A. D. 1990. *The Fu-*

ture of Worldwide Health Effects of Current Smoking Patterns: 3 Million Deaths/Year in the 1990's but Over 10 Million/Year Eventually. Presented at 7th World Conf. Tobacco Health, Perth, West. Aust.

36. Pierce, J. P. 1989. International comparisons of trends in cigarette smoking prevalence. *Am. J. Public Health* 79(2):152–57

37. Pierce, J. P., Aldrich, R., Hanratty, S., Dwyer, T., Hill, D. 1987. Trends in smoking uptake and quitting in Australia: 1974–1984. *Prev. Med.* 16:252–260

38. Pierce, J. P., Fiore, M. C., Novotny, T. E., Hatziandreu, E., David, R. 1989. Trends in cigarette consumption in the United States: Educational differences are increasing. *J. Am. Med. Assoc.* 261:56–60

39. Pierce, J. P., Fiore, M. C., Novotny, T. E., Hatziandreu, E., Davis, R. 1989. Trends in cigarette smoking in the United States: Projections to the Year 2000. *J. Am. Med Assoc.* 261:61–65

40. Pierce, J. P., Macaskill, P., Hill, D. 1990. Long term effectiveness of mass media anti-smoking campaigns in Australia. *Am. J. Public Health,* 80(5):565–659

41. Rogers, E. M. 1983. *Diffusion of Innovations.* New York: Free Press. 3rd ed.

42. Rogers, E. M., Shoemaker, F. 1971. *Communication of Innovations: A Cross-cultural Approach.* New York: Free Press. 2nd ed.

43. R. Coll. Phys. 1962. *Smoking and Health. Summary and Report of the Royal College of Physicians of London on Smoking in Relation to Cancer of the Lung and Other Diseases.* New York: Pitman

44. Sartwell, P. E. 1966. The incubation period and the dynamics of infectious disease. *Am. J. Epidemiol.* 83:204–16

45. Schudson, M. 1986. *Advertising, The Uneasy Persuasion,* p. 288. New York: Basic Books

46. Stevens, D. J. 1990. Tobacco in the Year 2000. *Tobacco J. Int.* May/June 16–22

47. Tessier, J. F., Freour, P., Crofton, J., Kombou, L. 1989. Smoking habits and attitudes of medical students towards smoking and antismoking campaigns in fourteen European countries. *Eur. J. Epidemiol.* 5(3):311–21

48. US Dep. Agric. 1988. *World Tobacco Situation Report.* Publ. No. FT8-88. Washington, DC:USDA

49. US Gen. Account. Off. 1989. *Teenage Smoking. Higher Excise Tax Should Sig-*

nificantly Reduce the Number of Smokers. Publ. No. HRD-89-119. Washington, DC: US Gen. Account. Off.

50. US Dep. Health Hum. Serv. 1986. *The Health Consequences of Involuntary Smoking. A Report of the Surgeon General*. DHHS Publ. No. (CDC) 87-8398. US DHHS, Public Health Serv., Off. Smoking Health

51. US Public Health Service. 1964. *Smoking and Health. Report of the Advisory Committee to the Surgeon General of the Public Health Service*. PHS Publ. No. 1103, US Dept. Health, Educ. Welf., Public Health Serv., Cent. Dis. Control

52. Deleted in proof

53. US Public Health Serv. 1989. *Reducing the Health Consequences of Smoking: 25 Years of Progress. A Report of the Surgeon General*. DHHS Publ. No. (CDC) 89-8411. Washington, DC: US Dept. Health Hum. Serv., Public Health Serv.

54. US Public Health Serv. 1989. *Smoking Tobacco and Health: A Fact Book.*

DHHS Publ. No. (CDC) 87-8397. Washington, DC: US Dept. Health Hum. Serv., Public Health Serv.

55. Warner, K. E. 1986. *Selling Smoke: Cigarette Advertising and Public Health*. Washington, DC: Am. Public Health Assoc.

56. World Health Organization. 1960–1988. *International Digest of Health Legislation*. Geneva: WHO

57. World Health Organization. 1989. *Report of the Meeting of the WHO Technical Advisory Group on Tobacco or Health*. Geneva: WHO

58. World Health Organization. 1990. *It Can Be Done: A Smokefree Europe*. Copenhagen: WHO

59. Yu, J. J., Mattson, M. E., Boyd, G. M., Mueller, M., Shopland, D. R., et al. 1990. A comparison of smoking patterns in the People's Republic of China and the United States: an impending health catastrophe in the middle kingdom. *J. Am. Med. Assoc.* 264:1575–79

Annu. Rev. Publ. Health 1991. 12:401–24

TRAUMA SYSTEMS AND PUBLIC POLICY

John M. Mendeloff

Department of Health Policy and Management, School of Public Health, University at Albany, State University of New York, Albany, New York 12203

C. Gene Cayten

Institute for Trauma and Emergency Care, New York Medical College, Valhalla, New York 10595

KEY WORDS: emergency medical services, injuries, cost-effectiveness

INTRODUCTION

Because of high death rates in the United States due to motor vehicle (MV) accidents and violence—causes of death that disproportionately strike the young—the problem of premature death is truly an American tragedy. These two causes of death also are the major causes of the injuries that trauma centers were established to treat.

Some 20% of the deaths among injury victims who were treated at community hospitals could have been prevented if those patients had been taken to trauma centers instead. A trauma center offers the round-the-clock presence of an experienced trauma surgeon and the immediate availability of the key specialists—anesthesiologists and neurosurgeons—needed to provide definitive surgical treatment. But, the establishment of trauma centers does little good unless severely injured patients are brought to them instead of to other hospitals. The concept of a trauma system refers to the integration of prehospital emergency medical services (EMS), hospital care, and posthospitalization rehabilitation programs.

Hundreds of self-styled trauma centers have been established in the United States, and most states have at least initiated plans to develop trauma systems.

401

0163-7525/91/0501-0401$02.00

Currently, however, there are few full-fledged systems in operation. In some cases, it has been difficult to exert control over prehospital EMS providers to make sure they follow the protocols for transporting patients. More generally, such systems do not arise easily in highly competitive hospital markets, as each institution is reluctant to let others have more prestige and more patients. The result can be either no trauma system or too many. Having too many trauma centers may be as bad as having too few. Not only is there unnecessary duplication and excess costs, but none of the centers may have a large enough volume of cases to keep their staffs' skills sharp.

At the same time, reimbursements often are inadequate to pay the costs. In some cities, including Los Angeles, Chicago, and Miami, trauma systems have eroded. Hospitals that were designated trauma centers withdrew when they discovered how much money they were losing in treating serious injury victims.

Among medical technologies, the trauma system is distinctive, as it requires direct government involvement in its diffusion. Without a public authority to designate trauma centers and to require that seriously injured patients be taken there, trauma care in a region falls far short of the optimal level. Once public authorities choose to concentrate serious trauma patients at only a few selected hospitals, they then must address the added financial burdens that those institutions will bear.

The growth in payment policies that reimburse hospitals prospectively on the basis of the average costs incurred for treating fairly broad diagnostic-related groups (DRGs) poses hardships for centers that disproportionately treat the most serious and costly trauma cases. These hospitals usually have large amounts of uncompensated care, a problem that a heavy trauma load often exacerbates.

Trauma systems clearly can make a difference for some major trauma victims. But, public policymakers who are faced with the decision of how vigorously to press for their establishment must ask specific questions: Under which circumstances are trauma systems good investments in the public's health? How great are the health benefits and what does it cost to get them? As usual, the answers to these important questions are not readily at hand.

In this chapter we review the evidence on the effectiveness and costs of trauma centers; examine some of the public policy issues and options for trauma system planning and financing; and point out areas where the knowledge needed for informed policymaking is especially deficient and suggest a research agenda to address those gaps.

BACKGROUND

In 1986, more than 150,000 persons died because of injuries, and more than 2 million others were hospitalized (9). Of those injured, 6000 became paraple-

Table 1   Causes of death among trauma center patients[a]

Rank	Injury mechanism	Injury site	Percent of Deaths
1	Vehicle occupant	Head	22.8
2	Gunshot	Non-head	13.6
3	Gunshot	Head	10.5
4	Vehicle occupant	Non-head	10.0
5	Pedestrian	Head	8.5
6	Fall	Head	7.3
7	Motorcyclist	Head	6.0
8	Assault[b]	Head	5.0
9	Stab	Non-head	4.9
10	Pedestrian	Non-head	3.4
11	Fall	Non-head	2.9
12	Assault	Non-head	2.7
13	Motorcyclist	Non-head	2.1
14	Stab	Head	0.3
			100.0

[a] Adapted from Gennarelli (23). Because the death rate among the 49,000 patients in the sample was almost exactly 10%, the number of deaths in a given cohort can easily be calculated. For example, for the number of deaths among 10,000 patients, multiply the percent figure by 10.
[b] The "Assault" category is a residual, which also includes sports injuries and others.

gics or quadriplegics. Injuries were the leading cause of death before age 45 and the leading cause of life-years lost before age 65.

The leading causes of injury deaths were MV accidents (32%), firearms (22%), falls (9%), poisonings (8%), fires and burns (4%), and drownings (4%). At least half of deaths due to motor vehicles and assaults occur before arrival at a hospital, mostly at the scene of the injury.

Based on 1982–1986 data from a nonrandom sample of 95 trauma centers that participated in the Major Trauma Outcome Study, MV-related injuries accounted for almost 50% of trauma center admissions, gunshots/stabbings accounted for about 23%, and falls accounted for 15% (23). Ten percent of the trauma center patients died. Over 60% of the deaths occurred among head-injured patients, although they comprised only one third of the patients. As Table 1 shows, the causes of death varied with the nature of injury. Gunshots and stabbings caused 47% of the deaths among those without head injuries, but only 18% among those with head injuries. Motor vehicles caused 60% of the head injury deaths, but 39% of the others.

Although there is no consensus on exactly which patients should be sent to trauma centers, a common assumption is that there will be about one case of major trauma annually per 1000 population. This figure contrasts sharply with an estimate that hospital emergency department visits for injuries in 1977 totalled about 200 per 1000 (19). One Los Angeles County study that used a fairly restrictive measure of need for trauma center care estimated that only about 12% of the injury victims transported by ambulance should have been sent to trauma centers (27). By any standard, trauma centers are appropriate for only a small percentage of all injuries.

Networks of trauma care were established in a few states in the early 1970s. A few, like the one in Maryland, developed into well-coordinated trauma systems by the 1980s; others, like the one in Illinois, disintegrated rapidly.

In general, however, there was little public action to designate trauma centers or plan trauma systems until the 1980s. By that time, a substantial literature (11, 38) suggested that a sizable fraction of trauma deaths could have been prevented by improved prehospital or hospital care. A 1979 seminal article by West et al (49) demonstrated that there were far fewer "preventable deaths" in San Francisco, where all major trauma victims were brought to a single teaching hospital, than in Orange County, where patients went to the nearest hospital. In the late 1970s, the Committee on Trauma of the American College of Surgeons (ACS) became active in promulgating standards for trauma care, both in-hospital and for other elements of trauma care (2). These standards, which are continually revised by the ACS, have provided a starting point for most states that have begun to develop their own standards.

ISSUES IN EFFICACY AND EFFECTIVENESS

Tools and Methods

Several tools and methods have been developed to aid in studies of trauma care quality. Such studies can serve several purposes: assessing the magnitude of the problem of inadequate care; measuring the effectiveness of different types of prehospital or hospital care; and identifying individual cases in need of quality of care review.

A substantial literature (11) has developed, which reviews cases of trauma deaths to ascertain what percentage were "preventable," "salvageable," or represented "inappropriate outcomes." This preventable death literature raises many methodological issues (38). The studies often are not strictly comparable. Ramenofsky et al (35) required that all five judges agree to sustain a judgment of nonpreventable. For Neumann et al (34), five of six judges had to agree to sustain a judgment of preventable. Usually, the studies either never explain the decision rules or only state that a consensus had to emerge. Most of the studies rely on a comparison of outcomes with "optimal" care, but some (14, 21) asked which deaths were due to mistakes, accepting as given the existing level of trauma care resources. Fitts et al (20) included deaths following hospitalization for hip fractures (usually among the very elderly), which gave an unusually low preventability rate. Detmer et al (17), gave a figure for deaths with mistakes, but their study failed to indicate the percentage of deaths that can actually be attributed to the errors. The Detmer study also showed that the judgments of a group of specialists with experience in trauma (neurosurgeons) found twice as many cases with errors as did a group of primary care physicians. For all of these reasons, comparisons of the findings across studies must be done with caution.

Many of the preventable death studies utilize hospital records, but some rely only on autopsy findings, which provide much less detail about patient care but can be reviewed much more quickly. The only study (47) that compared the two found that all of the deaths found preventable using the autopsy method also were found preventable using clinical records, but that an additional 10%–15% of deaths were found preventable with the latter. Assessments of head injuries are especially difficult using only autopsy data, so studies using that method often exclude central nervous system (CNS) injuries.

Another problem with preventable death studies is that the ratings are subjective and the reviewers are not blinded to the hospital in which care was given. Thus, there is considerable room for investigator bias. The authors of these studies often undertake them either to demonstrate that a problem exists or to show that the system they have developed is working well.

The Injury Severity Score (ISS), developed by Baker et al (4), is the most widely used method for scoring the severity of injuries. The ISS, which is derived from scoring the severity of injuries to each of six body parts (scores ranging from 1 for minor injuries to 5 for critical injuries), takes the three most serious in three different parts and squares them. Thus, the maximum ISS score is 75. The ISS has been found to correlate well with mortality, although less well for penetrating injuries, like gunshot and knife wounds, than for blunt trauma. In general, if patients at one hospital are dying with much lower ISS scores than at another, it raises the suspicion that more of the deaths at the first are preventable.

Building on the ISS, Champion et al (8, 16) developed a tool for predicting trauma patient mortality called TRISS, which involves a logistic regression model that predicts survival for each patient. Predictions are based upon the ISS score, the patient's age (over or under 55), and a set of physiological measures used to calculate a "revised trauma score"—blood pressure, respiratory rate, and the Glasgow Coma Scale, which assesses brain injury. Each of these measurements is weighted by a formula derived from a large data base of patients in trauma centers, the Major Trauma Outcome Study (MTOS). Different weights have been developed for blunt and penetrating injuries, although further differentiations might be justified both for types of injuries (13) and for the presence of comorbidities (33). TRISS does a reasonably good job in predicting mortality among MTOS patients. About 82% of those predicted to die with blunt trauma did die; for penetrating trauma, the figure was 89% (14a). Although improvements can be made, TRISS appears to provide more objective assessments of trauma care, i.e. by comparing predicted with actual deaths at each hospital, than the preventable death approach can provide.

Unfortunately, only trauma centers, and not all of them, collect the data needed to calculate TRISS scores. Therefore, it usually is not possible to use TRISS to compare outcomes at trauma centers with those at other hospitals. And, although the data from the almost 100 hospitals in the MTOS could potentially be used to understand why some trauma centers have better outcomes than others, the data have not been used in that way. That omission appears to reflect both concerns about the comparability of data across hospitals and the politically sensitive issue of identifying good and bad performers.

Insights from Preventable Death Studies

Despite the concerns noted above, these studies may provide insights into four important questions in trauma care:

First, what percentages of all trauma deaths or of the subset of MV deaths are preventable? When studies of preventable deaths are population-based, e.g. all MV deaths that occur in a county, it is possible to estimate the fraction of all deaths that are preventable by better medical care. Table 2 presents the estimates for studies that appear to have used similar methods and criteria. One inference, which can be drawn from these studies, is that in the late 1970s, in major urban centers that lacked trauma systems, approximately 9%–12% of the MV deaths were preventable. (Because over 50% of these deaths occur prehospital, the preventable percentage for deaths that occur after arrival at a hospital would be about twice as large.) Today, a general diffusion of improved techniques would somewhat lower this figure. In rural areas the percentage of preventable deaths is probably higher, at least as judged by the standards of good urban trauma care. However, the percentage of deaths that are preventable at a reasonable cost may be lower in rural areas.

Second, are there differences between the preventability of CNS and nonCNS deaths? Every study that attempts to address both types of injuries has concluded that CNS deaths are substantially less preventable, as shown in Table 3. (All the denominators in the Table are limited to persons brought alive to the hospital; sometimes further limitations are made.) The highest figure for preventable CNS deaths comes from a 1974 autopsy study (49) in Orange County, which found 73% preventable deaths among the nonCNS cases, and 28% among the CNS. Another Orange County study before regionalization (10), which used clinical records, found rates of 86% for nonCNS and 5% for CNS in 1978–1979. The use of clinical data adds to the

Table 2 Preventable deaths as a percentage of all (or all MV) trauma deaths[a]

Region	Year	# Preventable	Total # Deaths	% Preventable
Washtenaw County, Mich. (22)	1962–1967	28	159 MV	18%
San Francisco (43)	1972	19	425 all	4%
Orange County (10)	1978–1979	37	317 MV	12%
Portland area (30)	1979	34	278 MV	12%
Orange County (10)	1980–1981	16	320 MV	5%
Vermont (21)	1969–1974	11 nonCNS MV	127 nonCNS MV	9%
			270 all MV	4%
Orange County (49)	1974	22 nonCNS MV	218 all MV	10%

[a] The denominator is the total number of trauma deaths or motor vehicle (MV) deaths occurring in the area, not the number brought alive to hospitals.

accuracy of judgments about preventability. Because no evidence showed that care for CNS victims improved dramatically from 1974 to 1978, the 28% figure for CNS is highly suspect. The other two studies with the highest figures for CNS deaths used somewhat looser definitions than the others. The figures in the Oregon study (30) refer to the percentage of inappropriate outcomes, rather than to preventable deaths. The Washington figures (37) refer almost wholly to possibly preventable deaths, whereas the other studies include mostly preventable or probably preventable deaths.

It is noteworthy that the "before-after" studies (10, 40, 48) in Orange and San Diego Counties did not claim that the introduction of trauma systems had had an impact on CNS deaths. In the former case, West et al (48) explained that the County had not developed triage criteria for CNS deaths and, thus, they remained essentially unregionalized. In San Diego, Schackford et al (40) reported that neurosurgeons already had regionalized trauma care for head injury; thus, there was no additional impact. The identical 5% figures for the

Table 3 Preventable deaths by site of injury

Region	Year	Percent of Hospital Deaths Found Preventable	
		NonCNS Deaths	CNS Deaths
Washtenaw County, Mich. (22)	1962–1967	38	2
Orange County (49)	1974	73	28
Orange County (10)	1978–1979	86	5
San Diego County (34)	1979	19	5
Portland region[a] (30)	1979	41	17
Orange County (10)	1980–1981	40	3
Seattle region (37)	1984–1985	44	14

[a] The Portland figures refer to inappropriate outcomes rather than to preventable deaths.

preregionalization percentage of preventable CNS deaths in both counties make it hard to believe that both explanations could be correct.

A balanced assessment (7) on the evidence about trauma care for the brain-injured is that "although early aggressive therapy . . . would logically be expected to affect outcome favorably, and a number of studies strongly suggest that it does, it is not possible to support such a contention conclusively from the evidence at hand. Indeed some of the evidence would indicate the opposite." Thus, although a conclusion that trauma systems have little, if any, impact on brain-injured patients is conservative, it is not unreasonable. This issue is important because CNS deaths comprise more than 60% of the deaths that now occur in trauma centers, and the percentage is probably greater among prehospital deaths.

Third, are there differences among different types of hospitals? Within a region, the university teaching hospitals (24), the trauma centers (12, 28, 29, 44, 48), and the larger hospitals (30) all had a substantially smaller percentage of deaths that were judged preventable. Not all studies reach this conclusion, however. Goldberg (25), employing a case control method with National Hospital Discharge Survey data, found no effect of trauma volumes on mortality. Cayten used TRISS in New York and found no difference in outcomes between patients treated at three Level I trauma centers and five community hospitals.

In interpreting these studies, there is undoubtedly considerable within-group variation in performance among trauma and nontrauma centers. This variation highlights the desirability of basing designation decisions on outcome data, rather than relying solely on information about the resources devoted to trauma care.

Fourth, what is the impact of trauma systems on the prevention of deaths? The most powerful evidence on the impact of good trauma care on outcomes comes from the 1979 study by West et al (49), which documented the differences in 1974 between outcomes in San Francisco, where almost all patients went to a major trauma center, and Orange County, where patients were taken to the nearest hospital. Of 90 deaths in Orange County, 39 were judged preventable or potentially preventable, compared with 1 of 92 deaths in San Francisco. For nonCNS deaths, the study found that the appropriate operation was performed 94% of the time in San Francisco, but only 20% of the time in Orange County. In San Francisco, only 1 of 16 deaths in that category occurred because of hemorrhage in a patient who was not operated on, compared with 17 of 30 deaths in Orange. These striking differences make a powerful case for the value of trauma systems, despite the obvious problems of ensuring the comparability of the cases in the two regions.

Full-fledged before-after evaluations, which use the preventable death approach, have been conducted to assess the impact of creating a trauma system in only two regions (10, 40, 48). Among nonCNS hospital deaths in Orange County, the percentages judged preventable were 73% in 1974, 71% in 1978–1979, and 19% after regionalization in 1980–1981 (48). The introduction of the trauma system also witnessed a major jump in the number of patients with the appropriate operation and a major drop in hemorrhagic deaths.

One puzzle in the assessment in Orange County (10) is that although the number of preventable nonCNS deaths fell to 6 in 1980–1981, from 22 in 1974 and 27 in 1978–1979, the number of nonCNS deaths that were judged not preventable jumped to 23, from 8 in 1974 and 11 in 1978–1979. Although this jump could have been real, it does raise questions in light of the study's method—nonblinded judging carried out by the doctors responsible for implementing the trauma system.

If the authors' conclusions are accepted, however, the trauma system could claim credit for reducing the MV death rate by about 7%–8% (about 20–25 deaths), a gain accomplished almost solely by reducing nonCNS deaths. It also is possible that nonMV deaths were prevented, but no data were presented on this.

The San Diego County assessment (40) took as its baseline a 1982 study of all hospitals in the County. It found 90 hospital deaths had occurred among what it categorized as major trauma patients. Twelve (13.6%) of these deaths were judged frankly preventable, and another seven (7.9%), potentially salvageable. The posttrauma system study, carried out by a different set of authors who used a different method, examined 112 deaths. They found only three (2.7%) frankly preventable deaths and eight (7.1) potentially salvageable. A problem with drawing inferences from this comparison is that the average ISS in the preventable group presystem was 46, compared with 37 postsystem. This finding is not consistent with the argument that trauma care improved. It suggests that judgments of preventability may not have been as demanding for the deaths studied after establishment of the trauma system.

Although these anomalies again undermine our ability to quantify the gains with any precision, the study's finding that outcomes at trauma centers in 1984 were superior to outcomes at the average hospital in 1982 is hard to question. No data were presented on deaths at nontrauma centers in 1984. Another report identifies four of them (38a). Even if all were preventable, extrapolating the results of these series to a full year would lead to a reduction of about 37 preventable deaths with the introduction of the trauma system. This figure includes essentially all types of emergency trauma (e.g., omitting hip fractures in the elderly). Part of the improvement may have been associated with increased helicopter use. The number of aeromedical transports doubled in the first year of the system (138a) and several reports suggest that those patients had lower mortality than those transported by ground (6).

The number of deaths that would be prevented with nationwide coverage of trauma systems is hard to estimate. Because San Diego and Orange Counties each have almost 1% of the nation's population, a crude first step would be to multiply their results by 100, which produces numbers of 2500 to 3700. However, in 1990, the percentage of major trauma victims who go to trauma centers is probably higher in many regions than it was in those counties before regionalization. In those regions, the added benefits would not be as great. And, the gains from feasible improvements in rural areas probably won't match those achievable in urban areas. Studies in rural Vermont (14, 21) have been much less sanguine about the number of deaths that could have been prevented if patients had quicker access to trauma centers. Thus, the potential for further reductions in hospital deaths from extensions of trauma systems will fall considerably short of the figures based on simple extrapolation.

TRAUMA SYSTEM COSTS

Intelligent planning for trauma policy is difficult to undertake without some understanding of the likely costs and effects of the programs. Although many articles (39) have been written about the costs of trauma centers to hospitals, almost no analysis has focused on the costs of trauma care to society. The former studies focus on the costs and revenues to hospitals and are relevant to understanding their incentive to serve trauma victims. The latter focus on the incremental resources that society expends to provide better trauma care and are relevant to understanding which type of trauma care is worth providing, i.e. how the social cost per unit of benefit (e.g. life-years added) compares with other health programs.

What are the social costs of a trauma system? They fall into the following categories:

1. Costs of administering the system.
2. Costs for communications equipment or upgrading a 911 system.
3. Costs to add to and upgrade the equipment and the personnel used to transport patients, possibly including helicopters.
4. Costs to upgrade the facilities and personnel at trauma centers. In some cases, the largest incremental staff costs will be attributable to keeping staff, especially surgeons and anesthesiologists, in-house or on-call around the clock.
5. Costs of treating patients. Patients whose lives are saved usually will incur higher hospital bills. In cases in which patients survive severe brain injury, treatment, rehabilitation, and maintenance costs can be more than $1 million. In other cases, improved trauma care may reduce costs by reducing complications and shortening lengths of stay.

Even when survival is not affected, costs for a given patient are likely to be higher when that patient is treated in a trauma center, rather than a community hospital. The number of surgical interventions is likely to be greater, and the level of nursing care, higher. Data from Maryland (Table 4) show that, in the same ISS groupings, trauma centers had much higher costs. Although this result partly reflects differences in the types of cases at the different hospitals, which the ISS fails to capture, it probably also indicates real cost differences among hospitals.

This itemization suggests that the costs of establishing a trauma system can vary widely depending upon the existing level of resource commitment. At one extreme, if a region has enough trauma centers but is failing to bypass community hospitals, the costs of improved outcomes could be close to zero. At the other extreme, an attempt to create a first-rate trauma system in an area that lacks even a 24-hour emergency room would be very expensive. Using cost data from the mid-1970s, Teufel & Trunkey (42) estimated that, assuming one had to hire staff physicians, the ACS optimal trauma center would cost almost $3.5 million in annual staffing costs. In 1990 dollars, the figure almost triples.

Unfortunately, the studies of the effects of implementing trauma systems in California were not accompanied by estimates of the incremental costs associ-

Table 4   Charges and length of stay (LOS) by injury severity group and hospital type—all Maryland hospital discharges for trauma, 1986[a]

ISS Group[b]	Hospital type	# Patients	Mean LOS	Mean Charges ($)
1–8	Non-TC[c]	13,202	4.3	2,100
	AWTC[d]	6,208	4.8	3,100
	MIEMS[e]	463	4.4	6,000
9–12	Non-TC	5,689	12.1	5,500
	AWTC	2,763	12.1	7,600
	MIEMS	232	14.6	18,600
13–15	Non-TC	441	12.1	4,400
	AWTC	645	13.1	10,800
	MIEMS	137	13.9	16,700
16–19	Non-TC	415	9.9	5,500
	AWTC	563	13.3	12,700
	MIEMS	172	18.0	24,200
20–75	Non-TC	146	11.4	7,800
	AWTC	528	20.2	21,800
	MIEMS	218	27.0	40,800

[a] Source is discharge data submitted to Maryland Health Services Cost Review Commission (E. J. MacKenzie, personal communication)
[b] Injury severity score group
[c] Non-trauma center hospital
[d] Area-wide trauma center (regional trauma center)
[e] Maryland Institute for Emergency Medical Systems

ated with those steps. The best study of trauma system costs was carried out in Florida (41). Researchers asked the 29 hospitals with trauma centers in 1986 to identify the costs "associated with creating and maintaining the capacity to deliver the specialized services which constitute a trauma center," rather than the specific charges or costs for treating trauma patients. The estimates given varied markedly, which reflected either real differences or difficulties in isolating trauma center costs from those related to general emergency department activities.

For the four Level I hospitals in Florida start-up costs ranged from $40,000 to $1,250,000 (in 1988 dollars) with an average of $420,000. For the 12 Level II trauma centers still operating in 1989, the average was almost $800,000, with a range of zero to $3,500,000. The Level I centers had a lower average because, as teaching hospitals, they usually had established relatively high levels of trauma care before the period studied.

For operating expenses attributable to the trauma center, the Level I centers averaged almost $1,900,000 a year, compared with $550,000 for the Level II centers. Most of these costs were for patient care, and over half were for physician specialists and nursing staff. (Payment policies for physicians vary, but Trunkey [43] notes that fees "are often in addition to patient fees." He cites figures for Phoenix and calculates that the five trauma centers paid annual on-call fees to physicians exceeding $5.5 million.) The Florida study also reported that helicopters cost $1–$2 million, with operating costs of about $650,000 (assuming 300–500 transports a year).

What might costs have been in San Diego and Orange Counties? If we estimate start up costs for each county's five trauma centers at $400,000–$800,000 and add $500,000 for equipment in Orange and $2 million for San Diego (including a helicopter), we get annualized start-up costs (discounting at 10% with a ten-year life) of $400,000–$700,000 in Orange and $650,000–$960,000 in San Diego. If the five trauma centers in each county had added operating expenses of $500,000 to $1 million per year, the extra costs per county would be $2.5–$5 million.

Adding in the annualized capital expenses and $650,000 for operation of a helicopter would lead to total costs of $2.9–$5.7 million in Orange and $3.8–$6.61 million in San Diego. Administrative expenses probably do not exceed a few hundred thousand dollars. This total does, however, exclude additional incremental costs for patient treatment beyond those counted in the fixed costs of maintaining a trauma center. If, in each county, the care of about 1000 patients were shifted to trauma centers from community hospitals (about 25% of those brought to trauma centers), we could develop very crude estimates of extra medical care costs. If they averaged an extra $1000–$5000 per patient, the extra costs would be $1–$5 million a year. Thus, total added trauma costs would be $3.9–$10.7 million in Orange and $4.8–$11.61 million in San Diego. Again, we emphasize the crudeness of these estimates.

COST-EFFECTIVENESS

As noted above, the published evaluations of the Orange County and San Diego trauma systems claim first year reductions in preventable deaths of about 20–25 and 30–37 deaths respectively. Both of these, especially the latter, are likely to be overstated. These estimates can be converted into life-years added, at 37 years per case; 740–925 life-years in Orange and 1110–1369 life-years in San Diego. Without discounting, each added life-year costs $4200 to $14,500 in Orange and $3500–$10,500 in San Diego. If life-years accruing in the future are discounted, a common though controversial practice, the costs rise. At a 5% discount, the costs per discounted life-year roughly double. However, these costs are still at the low end of the range of health programs that have been assessed in this manner (32). The costs per premature death prevented are $116,000–$280,000 in Orange and $100,000–$213,000 in San Diego. All of these numbers are far below the value of about $2 million per premature death prevented that many economists think roughly measures the value that individuals are willing to pay to reduce risk (36). Thus, even if the true number of deaths prevented were only half as large, these programs would still appear to have been worthwhile.

The generalizability of the specific estimates is uncertain. It seems likely that any urbanized region in which a substantial number of severely injured patients are not being taken to an accessible trauma center will yield potential net benefits from shifting triage patterns, even if a moderate increase in trauma resources are required.

In rural areas, the costs per death prevented will almost certainly be higher. The smaller number of trauma patients makes it harder to justify the fixed expenses of maintaining a trauma center. Alternatively, other strategies, like upgrading the trauma skills of emergency room staff or expanding the use of helicopters, may prove superior. Which strategy is worthwhile will depend on better assessments of the effects and costs of different measures and on the value placed on those effects.

DEVELOPING TRAUMA SYSTEMS: PROGRESS AND PROBLEMS

Current Status of Trauma Systems

What percentage of the population is currently served by a trauma system that, at a minimum, ensures that individuals identified as major trauma victims are taken to hospitals that meet ACS standards for a Level I or Level II trauma center? It is difficult to answer this question for several reasons.

1. The most recent surveys (1, 3, 50), taken in 1986 and 1987, showed that about 20 states, mostly along the coasts, had implemented a process to verify that hospitals meet those standards or for designating them as trauma centers.

However, the status of trauma systems can change rapidly enough to vitiate these surveys. For example, in 1990, Florida had 12 trauma centers, down from a high of 33 in 1986 (P. Ronde, personal communication). And, New York State began a formal process of designation in 1990. A 1989 study (45) reports that three quarters of the states have developed or are in the process of developing trauma center designation regulations.

2. The same surveys show that several of the states that had designation procedures either had not used them very much (e.g. West Virginia had designated only one trauma center) or had used them so indiscriminately that the purpose of designation was vitiated (e.g. 60 centers in Missouri).

3. Virginia and Maryland usually are cited as having the most developed statewide system. In Maryland in 1986, 90% of the most seriously injured hospitalized patients (with ISS above 25) were treated at a designated trauma center (31). The comparable figure for New York City, which has 13 formally designated trauma centers, was 73% in 1988. For the rest of New York, in parts of which regionalization was only beginning, the figure was 54%.

4. The regions that appear to come closest to the model of a trauma system often are found where strong public controls over the designation process and over EMS providers exists, e.g. Maryland, Virginia, New York City, San Francisco, San Diego County, Orange County, and Salt Lake City.

Obstacles to Trauma System Development

Despite enthusiastic support for trauma systems among groups like the ACS, the development of trauma systems has been slow. What are some of the most important obstacles?

1. Trauma systems need the backing of public authority. Many states have lacked a statutory framework; many more lack strong regional EMS agencies that are capable of overseeing the ongoing implementation process.

2. The failure of states and regions to act reflects, in part, lack of leadership in this area. But it also reflects political opposition. As one study (1) concluded, most hospitals "endure the existence of a publicly-funded trauma center (because it treats the uninsured and indigent and is not seen as attractive to insured patients), but they do not support the expansion into a full-fledged trauma *system*." If other hospitals become trauma centers, then the excluded hospitals may lose patients and whatever prestige accompanies the trauma center designation. In addition, there are professional rivalries involved. Surgeons stress that "trauma is a surgical disease," and trauma centers are invariably led by surgeons. The American College of Emergency Physicians (ACEP) speaks for emergency room doctors who are pushed into a subordinate role. Although ACEP has endorsed the trauma center concept and developed its own proposed standards, tensions remain.

3. Hospitals often have been reluctant to expand their role in trauma care because they fear losing money. There are several reasons why reimburse-

ments may not meet the costs: trauma patients, at least in urban settings, often are poorly insured; Medicare DRGs fail to reimburse serious trauma adequately; and trauma patients fill up the operating rooms and intensive care units, which forces the cancellation of more lucrative elective surgeries.

Trauma center designation also can have positive features, both nonfinancial and financial. Trauma staff are likely to seek the imprimatur of designation as a matter of professional pride, as a tactic to increase their own program's resources, and, at teaching hospitals, as a method to attract residents and fellows. Administrators may see several advantages: empty beds may be filled; quality of care may improve in all critical care areas; and prestige may rise, which attracts not only patients, but also nurses and doctors. Some of these incentives may vary by regions. In states like New York, where hospital occupancy rates approach 90%, the prospect of filling empty beds has much less appeal than it does in states with rates of 50%.

4. Efforts to ensure that prehospital EMS staff are properly trained and follow the proper protocol for patient triage also can encounter political obstacles. There are over 12,000 ambulance services in the United States. The more than 2 million persons in San Diego County are served by two ambulance firms, one under contract to the City and one to the rest of the County. The same number of persons in Suffolk County, New York, are served by over 100 providers, who are sponsored by different towns and villages, and who often are staffed by volunteers. Sheriffs, fire chiefs, and local volunteer organizations often are potent players in local politics and they often look askance at measures to undermine their independence. For example, in one New England state, a proposal to set up a central dispatch for 19 ambulance services was defeated by the fire chiefs who wanted to maintain control over emergency dispatches in their districts (45). In rural areas, perhaps three fourths of EMS staff are volunteers. A central EMS office has a much harder time controlling the behavior of volunteers than the behavior of contracted ambulance services.

ISSUES IN MANAGING TRAUMA SYSTEMS

Trauma Reimbursement

The more appropriate a patient is for a trauma center, the more money the hospital is likely to lose on the patient. The first reason is that, especially in urban areas, many trauma patients are uninsured. In 1986, Florida (41) found that the uninsured comprised a larger percentage of trauma patients (32%) than of total patients (24%). For uninsured trauma patients, the percentage of estimated costs covered by collections was only 51%, compared with 79% for trauma patients with Medicare and Medicaid, and over 133% for those covered by private insurers. At a major trauma center in Washington DC,

41% of the trauma patients were uninsured in 1989 (15). Those patients paid the hospital about 15% of its expenses for their care (10% of charges), which generated more than half of the hospital's total loss of $5.8 million on trauma care. One estimate (15) is that about 12% of the more than $8 billion claimed by all hospitals in 1988 for uncompensated care arose from trauma care.

A second factor is that many payors—Medicare, 14 Medicaid programs, and all other payors in New York, New Jersey, and some other states—use a DRG system for reimbursement, mostly modeled on the Medicare system. The handful of trauma DRGs used by Medicare include injuries of widely varying severity. In Florida, Medicare collections came to 87% of costs for injuries with an ISS less than 16, but only 65% for those with an ISS greater than 15. For a New Jersey trauma center, the ratio of reimbursements to costs was relatively constant for injuries up to an ISS of about 40, but the absolute size of the losses per case increased sharply with the more severe, and thus usually more expensive, injuries (39). The small number of cases with an ISS greater than 25 accounted for 55% of the losses.

Although treatment costs do tend to rise with ISS scores, adjusting reimbursement for ISS does not markedly increase payments to trauma centers. Mackenzie et al (31) estimated that a shift to Medicare DRGs for all Baltimore area hospitals would result in an $11.4 million loss for trauma centers; modification of the DRGs by using the ISS reduced this loss only to $9.8 million, because ISS explains only a small share of the variance in length of stay. The data from Maryland (see Table 4) show that patients who were treated at trauma centers had longer lengths of stay and higher costs than patients in the same ISS categories who were treated at community hospitals. Some of this difference probably reflects higher costs of treating a given patient at a trauma center, but much of it reflects the limitations of the ISS in differentiating cases.

For example, Cayten et al (13) compared blunt trauma from MV with penetrating injuries and found that, although the two groups had the same average ISS, the former used 80% more hospital days than the latter.

Who Should Be Served: Triage Criteria

Decisions about how many injury victims should be sent to trauma centers can have important implications for the politics, effectiveness, and costs of trauma systems. Of course, not all injury victims who use ambulance transport need to go to a trauma center. For example, one study (27), which used an ISS score of 16 or more as the chief basis to (retrospectively) determine whether patients needed to go to a trauma center, found that only about 12% of all of the injury victims transported by ambulance met the score. The assumption is that the rest would have done as well at the nearest hospital.

Triage criteria determine which and how many patients are sent to trauma

Table 5 Changes in overtriage and undertriage as the indications for transport to a trauma center (TC) are expanded[a]

Indications	Undertriage cases (%)	Overtriage cases (%)	% to TC
5	20 (38)	31 (47)	11
6	18 (33)	42 (54)	13
7	17 (31)	52 (58)	15
8	15 (27)	62 (61)	17
9	11 (20)	110 (71)	26
10	8 (15)	314 (87)	60
11	7 (13)	315 (87)	61

[a] Adapted from Kane et al (24), who developed a checklist of possible indications that could be used to justify transport of patients to trauma centers from among a sample (N = 595) of all injury patients transported by paramedics. The chief criterion for judging whether a patient needed to be sent to a trauma center was an ISS above 15. The undertriage rate is one minus the sensitivity of the protocol. The overtriage rate used here is the percentage of all cases sent to trauma centers who should not have been (one minus the predictive accuracy of the protocol).

centers and, thus, also determine the pattern of overtriage and undertriage errors. For any given set of measures used in a triage protocol, the rate of overtriage can be reduced only by raising the rate of undertriage. Table 5, adapted from Kane et al (27), illustrates the trade-offs for a set of proposed triage rules by examining their impact on a sample of all patients transported by ambulance. The authors developed a checklist of indications for paramedics to use to determine whether transport to a trauma center was needed. Table 5 shows that as the number of possible indications is increased, overtriage increases and undertriage drops, and the percentage of all patients who are taken to trauma centers increases.

Unfortunately, there is a dearth of research that identifies which patients benefit from trauma care. Therefore, any baseline (e.g. an ISS above 15) from which to measure overtriage or undertriage remains somewhat arbitrary. The ideal triage rule would minimize the sum of the losses to society from errors due to undertriage and errors due to overtriage. The former include possible deaths resulting from inadequate care at nontrauma centers or from delays in care caused by the need for additional transfers. For the same reasons, there may be added morbidity, as well. Large-scale undertriage also may cut the flow of patients so sharply that the skills of staff at trauma centers atrophy. Depending on reimbursement patterns, fewer cases also may make it harder to justify the fixed costs of providing trauma care.

What are the costs of overtriage? There will be added travel cost, which causes inconvenience for patients and requires more resources for the transport system. Taking more patients to trauma centers may require adding resources there even while resources at other hospitals are underutilized. There also may be higher costs of treating patients at trauma centers. Overtriage may increase hostility to the trauma system among other hospitals, even though the total volume of shifted patients is not likely to be large.

Once expected error costs have been estimated, they could be inserted into various triage protocols to find the cut-off point that has the lowest error costs, e.g. are the expected costs lower if the threshold for the Trauma Score method is reduced from 15 to 14? Intuitively, it seems plausible that the costs of an average undertriage error are likely to be higher than of an overtriage error and, thus, that we should be willing to accept more than one added case of overtriage to prevent a case of undertriage. Without better estimates of the error costs, however, the optimal error rates and triage policy cannot be identified.

Even with a better understanding of these error costs, however, the development of a good triage policy is hindered by the basic difficulty of trying to predict an injury victim's trauma care needs. Triage protocols have employed measures of patient physiology, of the nature of the injury (e.g. penetration of head), and of the mechanism of injury (e.g. fall from over 15 feet), but Eastman et al (18) observe that we still lack a protocol that "could be applied quickly and easily under field conditions, give consistent results under different observers, and have a high rate of accuracy." Baxt et al (5) argue that because we have poor markers for disease, there are inherent limitations on the predictive value of the data that can be collected in the field.

Reported overtriage and undertriage rates vary with the population being studied. For example, if the population includes many injuries so minor that they should not be taken to trauma centers, then the overtriage rate will be reduced. For any given set of error rates, the predictive ability of a triage protocol, i.e. the percentage of patients taken to trauma centers who really belong there, depends upon the fraction of the patients in the sample who need trauma center care. For these reasons, comparisons among protocols in different samples must be made with caution.

THE FEDERAL ROLE IN TRAUMA SYSTEMS

Since 1987, legislation has been introduced regularly in Congress to provide funds (about $50–$100 million a year) to states for the development of EMS/trauma plans. State policies for the designation of trauma centers, for triage, transfer, and transportation would all have to be based on specified standards. The bills also provide that some portion of the funds can be used to pay hospitals for uncompensated care for trauma patients. To put these funding levels in perspective, an estimate of the 1986 losses incurred just by Florida's trauma centers totaled $35 million, an amount exceeding the most generous amount that the bills would provide for all states (41). One controversy surrounding this proposed legislation is the extent to which it would require adherence to the ACS standards. Opponents claim both that the standards are too rigid and that it is improper to rely so heavily on a private body to determine the standards.

Questions about the rationale for a federal role in trauma care fall into two related categories, planning and financing. If the benefits of improved trauma care accrue to persons outside of the jurisdiction that must pay for the costs of the improvements, then arguably such care will be underprovided and other jurisdictions should contribute to those costs. Although this externalities argument clearly supports a funding base that is broader than a city or than most counties, the situation with respect to states is less clear. A study (26) of trauma deaths at rural hospitals in the Rocky Mountain states found that 33% of them were nonresidents. A California study (46) of MV deaths in the 1960s found that the figures were 22% for rural areas, but only 6% for urban areas. In terms of the externalities argument, these figures might support only a modest federal subsidy. Nevertheless, citizens likely place a substantial value on knowing that a reasonable level of trauma care is available no matter where in the nation they are.

A different argument stresses the pecuniary costs and benefits of trauma care to federal taxpayers. If a trauma system could prevent 20 deaths a year in a region, the extra taxes received annually by the Treasury would, in a steady state, have a present value (discounted at 6%) of about $1.2 million (assuming a present value of $300,000 in lost wages per person and a 20% federal tax share) (36). Although some of that revenue would be offset by higher federal medical care expenditures for patients covered by Medicare or Medicaid, federal support could still be justified at least as long as that support actually contributed to preventing deaths and not merely to relieving the burden on other payors.

Yet, in any circumstances in which a trauma system represents a good investment for federal taxpayers, it represents an even better deal for society as a whole. Even if we treated foregone earnings as the full measure of the benefits of preventing a death (which is much too low a figure), the federal tax share is only a fraction of the social benefit. And, if the benefits of trauma systems to society outweigh the costs, but state and localities have been slow to establish them, then there is a rationale for a federal role in prodding them into action with planning requirements and funding to implement the plans. Recent federal bills would authorize funds for these activities. A central controversy is the extent to which the bills should mandate that hospitals designated as trauma centers be required to meet ACS standards. The lack of a strong empirical basis for those standards argues against rigid requirements, as does the variety of circumstances in different states. On the other hand, some standards are needed if the exercise is to be meaningful. In addition, if, as described below, reimbursement for trauma is tied to designation as a trauma center, then some standards are required.

Except perhaps in small states, implementation of trauma systems requires organizations at the substate, regional level. Transfer agreements among hospitals must be developed and monitored; prehospital services must be coordinated and provided with medical control; and a quality assurance and assessment process must be established. Sometimes, county EMS programs can provide the organizational framework, but new organizational forms often may be needed. The funding for these organizations should come, at least in part, from states and the federal government.

The financial losses incurred in treating trauma patients can be viewed as part of the larger problem of uncompensated care, much of which is concentrated at particular public and urban hospitals. Measures to address that larger issue are beyond the scope of this paper. However, one can question whether there is any greater reason to relieve hospitals of the burden of uncompensated trauma care than of other uncompensated care. The answer is that the trauma problem is somewhat distinctive in light of the specific public policy objective of concentrating severely injured patients (and, consequently, financial losses) at trauma centers. In assessing financing proposals, several criteria should be kept in mind: the proposal should encourage proper triage; it should provide incentives for hospitals to keep costs down; it should not impose high administrative costs; and it should be perceived as fair, both in its treatment of different hospitals and different types of patients.

The financial burdens on hospitals from trauma care vary depending upon many factors, including the adequacy of the state's Medicaid payments, the availability of other reimbursements for indigent care, the strictness with which the state enforces laws requiring mandatory automobile insurance, the distribution of patients among hospitals, and the general economic and insurance status of the population served by the trauma center. Because the nature of the problems vary, no one solution will address them all.

Suggestions to address the financial issues have taken several forms (15). Because elderly patients comprise only a small percentage of trauma center patients, Medicare's DRGs have not had a major impact on most centers. However, several states, including New York and New Jersey, use DRGs for all payors, and more have begun using DRGs for Medicaid payments. Some private insurers also have moved to prospective payment. Given this growing use, developing appropriate DRGs for trauma is important.

In 1989, New York State introduced five new DRGs for serious trauma, and Medicare has since adopted them. A study at one New York hospital indicated that the new DRGs cut losses from trauma about 25%–50% (26a). Trauma DRGs can be adjusted to compensate more adequately for severe trauma. However, as noted above, adjustments using ISS scores alone will not do a very good job of capturing differences in treatment costs. It may be possible to develop better predictors of length of stay by incorporating other variables, such as age, preexisting conditions, and mechanism of injury. In the meantime, payments for cases with relatively high costs, e.g. blunt trauma with an ISS greater than 14 or 19, could be increased if the patient were treated at a state-designated trauma center. Although the payment per case might not be much more accurate in reflecting the costs of individual patients, the payments would at least go to the right hospitals. This policy also has the attractive feature that it would not provide a perverse incentive for nontrauma centers to keep the more severely injured. (A stricter rule that would further spur better triage would deny any payment for those patients who were treated at nontrauma centers. There are probably too many justifiable reasons for exceptions to this rule to warrant imposing it.)

Beyond DRGs, states could give annual subsidies to designated trauma centers to cover some of their fixed costs. Such an approach would be especially appropriate if a state wished to establish trauma centers in relatively rural areas. Because rural trauma is largely due to MV crashes, reimbursement tends to be relatively good; however, the number of cases is likely to be too small to allow a hospital to cover its fixed costs. In more urbanized areas, as a substitute or supplement, subsidies could be tied to the number of serious trauma patients seen there.

Another suggestion (15) has been to expand Medicaid coverage specifically for victims of major trauma. An ISS threshold would have to be set and the coverage would have to be limited to individuals below some financial threshold.

SUMMARY AND RESEARCH NEEDS

The available evidence suggests that the introduction of trauma systems in urban areas can prevent deaths at a relatively low cost. Although this conclusion is not certain, it seems solid enough to justify support for public policies to facilitate the diffusion of trauma systems. The federal government should require states or regional bodies to designate appropriate hospitals as trauma centers and to mandate the development of transfer agreements among hospitals.

The federal and state governments should develop plans to mitigate the financial losses that trauma centers often will experience and provide funds to establish regional bodies to monitor the performance of trauma systems. The current deemphasis on government planning and controls in favor of competitive behavior among hospitals will not lead to adequate trauma care in the United States. But hortatory planning documents will not suffice either, as they need to be backed up with financial resources and incentives.

Many of the key assumptions behind trauma system planning need to be tested. Planners could do a better job if they knew more about "what works for whom." The ACS (2) acknowledges that its standard calling for a minimum of 350 major trauma cases at a trauma center, based on a minimum of 50 cases a year per surgeon, has no empirical basis in trauma research. Similarly, the notion that major trauma victims have a "golden hour" in which to receive definitive care lacks a strong or precise empirical basis. The concepts of "practice makes perfect" and the golden hour have major implications for the design of trauma systems. A clearer understanding of these issues would put trauma planning on a much firmer basis.

To investigate these and other issues, it would be useful to employ the TRISS method to examine mortality differences among hospitals for different subgroups of patients (e.g. different severity groups, and CNS injuries versus others) in a population-based study, i.e. one not limited only to those admitted to trauma centers. In addition, it would be valuable to carry out before-after studies, using TRISS, in regions where trauma systems are being implemented.

The issue of the impact of potential trauma care changes on head injuries is especially important because these injuries contribute to the great majority of MV deaths. In addition, it would be useful to understand more clearly the level of impairments that those who are saved are left with and how these vary with the quality of trauma care.

The effectiveness and cost of trauma systems in rural areas have not received much attention. Almost certainly, the quality of trauma care is worse for persons injured in rural areas, and the cost per death prevented of improving it is likely to be higher. Yet, until more well-controlled evaluations of different approaches are carried out, the worth of different approaches cannot be assessed.

ACKNOWLEDGMENTS

We would like to thank Ed Hannan, Mike Gilbertson, John Fortune, Jane Murphy, and John Milliren for discussions that helped us develop the ideas presented here and Ellen MacKenzie and Lester Lave for comments on an earlier draft.

Literature Cited

1. Abt Assoc. 1988. *Trauma System Development*. Dep. Transp. Rep. HS 807 257
2. Am. Coll. Surg. 1987. *Hospital and Prehospital Resources for Optimal Care of the Injured Patient*. Chicago: Am. Coll. Surg.
3. Aprahamian, C., Wolferth, C. C., Darin, J. C., McMahon, J., Weitzel De-Veas, C. 1989. Status of trauma center designation. *J. Trauma* 29:566–70
4. Baker, S. P., O'Neil, B., Haddon, W.,

Jr., Long, W. B. 1974. The injury severity score. *J. Trauma* 14:187–96
5. Baxt, W. G., Berry, C. D., Epperson, M. D., Scalzitti, V. 1989. The failure of prehospital trauma prediction rules to classify trauma patients accurately. *Ann. Emerg. Med.* 18:21–28
6. Baxt, W. G., Moody, P. 1987. The impact of advanced prehospital emergency care on the mortality of severely brain-injured patients. *J. Trauma* 27:365–69
7. Becker, D. P., Gade, G. F., Miller, J.

D., 1990. Prognosis after head injury. In *Neurological Surgery* ed. J. R. Youmans. Philadelphia: Saunders. 3rd ed.

8. Boyd, C. R., Tolson, M. S., Copes, W. S. 1987. Evaluating trauma care: The TRISS method. *J. Trauma* 27:370–78

9. Brown, S. T., Foege, W. H., Bender, T. R., Axnick, N. 1990. Injury prevention and control: Prospects for the 1990s. *Annu. Rev. Public Health* 11:251–66

10. Cales, R. H. 1984. Trauma mortality in Orange County: The effect of implementation of a regional trauma system. *Ann. Emerg. Med.* 13:1–10

11. Cales, R. H., Trunkey, D. D. 1985. Preventable trauma deaths. *J. Am. Med. Assoc.* 254:1059–63

12. Campbell, S., Watkins, G., Kreis, D. 1989. Preventable deaths in a self-designated trauma system. *Am. Surg.* 55:478–80

13. Cayten, C. G., Stahl, W. H., Byrne, D., Murphy, J. 1989. *DRG length of stay outliers: MVC vs penetrating injuries.* Presented at Ann. Proc., Assoc. for Adv. Auto. Med., 33rd, Des Plaines, Ill.

14. Certo, T. F., Rogers, F. B., Pilcher, D. B. 1983. Review of care of fatally injured patients in a rural state: Five-year follow-up. *J. Trauma* 23:559–65

14a. Champion, H. R., Copes, W. S., Sacco, W. J., Lawnick, M. M., Grann, D. R., et al. 1990. A new characterization of injury severity. *J. Trauma* 30:539–45

15. Champion, H. R., Mabee, M. S. 1990. *An American Crisis in Trauma Care Reimbursement.* Publ. 3–90, Washington, DC: Wash. Hosp. Cent.

16. Champion, H. R., Sacco, W. J., Hunt, T. K. 1983. Trauma severity scoring to predict mortality. *World J. Surg.* 7:4–11

17. Detmer, D. E., Moylan, J. A., Rose, J., Schulz, R., Wallace, R., et al. 1977. Regional categorization and quality of care in major trauma. *J. Trauma* 17:592–99

18. Eastman, A. B., Lewis, F., Champion, H., Mattox, F. 1987. Regional trauma system design: Critical concepts. *Am. J. Surg.* 154:79–87

19. Fife, D., Barancik, J. I., Chatterjee, B. F., 1984. Northeastern Ohio trauma study: II. Injury rates by age, sex, and cause. *Am. J. Public Health* 74:473–78

20. Fitts, W. T., Lehr, H. B., Bitner, R. L., Spelman, J. W. 1964. An analysis of 950 fatal injuries. *Surgery* 56:663–68

21. Foley, R. W., Harris, L. W., Pilcher, D. B. 1977. Abdominal injuries in motor vehicle accidents: Review of care

of fatally injured patients. *J. Trauma* 17:611–15

22. Frey, C. F., Huelke, D. F., Gikas, P. W. 1969. Resuscitation and survival in motor vehicle accidents. *J. Trauma* 9:292–310

23. Gennarelli, T. A., Champion, H. R., Sacco, W. J., Copes, W. S., Alves, W. M. 1989. Mortality of patients with head injury and extracranial injury treated in trauma centers. *J. Trauma* 29:1193–1202

24. Gertner, H. R., Baker, S. B., Rutherford, R. B., Spitz, W. U. 1972. Evaluation of the management of vehicular injuries secondary to abdominal injury. *J. Trauma* 12:425–31

25. Goldberg, J., Levy, P. S., Morkovin, V., Goldberg, J. B. 1983. Mortality from traumatic injuries. *Med. Care* 21:692–704

26. Houtchens, B. A. 1977. Major trauma in the rural mountain west. *J. Am. Coll. Emerg. Phys.* 6:343–50

26a. Joy, S., Yurt, R. 1990. An all-payor prospect payment system (PPS) based on diagnostic related groups (DRGs): Financial impact on reimbursement for trauma care and approaches to minimizing loss. *J. Trauma* 30:866–73

27. Kane, G., Engelhardt, M. S., Celentano, J., Koenig, W., Yamanaka, J., et al. 1985. Empirical development and evaluation of prehospital trauma triage instruments. *J. Trauma* 25:482–89

28. Kilberg, L., Clemmer, T. P., Clawson, J., Woolley, F. R., Thomas, F. et al. 1988. Effectiveness of implementing a trauma triage system on outcome. *J. Trauma* 28:1493–98

29. Kreis, D. J., Plascencia, G., Augenstein, D., Davis, J. H., Echenique, M. et al. 1986. Preventable trauma deaths: Dade County, Florida. *J. Trauma* 26:649–54

30. Lowe, D. K., Gately, H. L., Goss, J. R., Frey, J. L., Peterson, C. G. 1983. Patterns of death, complication, and error in the management of motor vehicle accident victims: Implications for a regional system of trauma care. *J. Trauma* 23:503–9

31. MacKenzie, E. J., Steinwachs, D. M., Ramzy, A. I., Ashworth, J. W., Shankar, B. 1990. Trauma casemix and hospital payment: The potential for refining DRGs. *Health Serv. Res.* In press

32. Mendeloff, J. M. 1983. Problems in valuing lives. *J. Health Polit. Policy Law* 8:554–81

33. Morris, J. A., Jr., Mackenzie, E. J., Edelstein, S. L., 1990. The effect of pre-existing conditions on mortality in

trauma patients. *J. Am. Med. Assoc.*
263:1942–46
34. Neumann, T. S., Bockman, M. A.,
Moody, P., Dunford, J. V., Griffith, L.
D., et al. 1982. An autopsy study of
traumatic deaths: San Diego 1979. *Am.
J. Surg.* 144:722–27
35. Ramenofsky, M. L., Luterman, A.,
Quindlen, E., Riddick, L., Curreri, P.
W. 1984. Maximum survival in pediatric trauma: The ideal system. *J. Trauma*
24:818–23
36. Rice, D. P., MacKenzie, E. J., and
Assoc. 1989. *Cost of Injury in the
United States: A Report to Congress.*
San Francisco: Inst. Health Aging,
Univ. Calif. and Inj. Prev. Cent., Johns
Hopkins Univ.
37. Rivara, F. P., Maier, R. V., Mueller, B.
A., Luna, G. A., Dicker, B. G. et al.
1989. Evaluation of potentially preventable deaths among pedestrian and bicyclist fatalities. *J. Am. Med. Assoc.*
261:566–70
38. Roy, P. D. 1987. The value of trauma
centres: A methodologic review. *Can. J.
Surg.* 30:17–22
38a. San Diego County. 1985. *Evaluation of
Trauma Care*
39. Schwab, C. W., Young, G., Civil, I.,
Ross, S. E., Talucci, R. et al. 1988.
DRG reimbursement for trauma: The demise of the trauma center. *J. Trauma*
28:939–46
40. Shackford, S. R., Hollingworth-
Fridlund, P., Cooper, G. F., Eastman,
A. B. 1986. The effect of regionalization upon the quality of trauma care as
assessed by concurrent audit before and
after institution of a trauma system: A

preliminary report. *J. Trauma* 26:812–
20
41. State of Florida, Health Care Cost Containment Board. February 1989. *A Study
of Trauma Care Costs in Florida*
42. Teufel, W. L., Trunkey, D. D. 1977.
Trauma centers: A pragmatic approach
to need, cost, and staffing patterns. *J.
Am. Coll. Emerg. Phys.* 6:546–51
43. Trunkey, D. D. 1990. What's wrong
with trauma care? *Bull. Am. Coll. Surg.*
75:10–15
44. Trunkey, D. D., Lim, R. C. 1974. Analysis of 425 consecutive trauma fatalities: An autopsy study. *J. Am. Coll.
Emerg. Phys.* 3:368–71
45. US Congress, Office Technol. Assess.
1989. *Rural Emergency Medical Services—Special Report, OTA-H-445*
Washington, DC: GPO
46. Waller, J. A., Curran, R., Noyes, F.
1964. A preliminary study of urban and
rural fatalities in California. *Calif. Med.*
101:272–76
47. West, J. G. 1982. Validation of autopsy
method for evaluating trauma care.
Arch. Surg. 117:1033–35
48. West, J. G., Cales, R. H., Gazzaniga,
A. B. 1983. Impact of regionalization:
The Orange County experience. *Arch.
Surg.* 118:740–44
49. West, J. G., Trunkey, D. D., Lim, R.
C. 1979. Systems of trauma care: A tale
of two counties. *Arch. Surg.* 114:455–
60
50. West, J. G., Williams, M. J., Trunkey,
D. D., Wolferth, C. C. 1988. Trauma
systems: Current status—future challenges. *J. Am. Med. Assoc.* 259:3597–
3600

Annu. Rev. Publ. Health 1991. 12:425–57

UNDERSTANDING THE EFFECTS OF AGE, PERIOD, AND COHORT ON INCIDENCE AND MORTALITY RATES

Theodore R. Holford

Yale University Medical School, New Haven, Connecticut 06510

KEY WORDS: time trends, vital rates, estimable functions, Poisson regression, lung cancer

INTRODUCTION

Time trend analysis for disease incidence and mortality has a long history in public health. These trends are significant because they can be highly suggestive as to what might be expected in the future and they are an effective approach to understanding disease etiology. A display of summary rates, such as a direct adjusted rate, over time is one approach to the analysis of time trends in disease incidence and mortality. Although this approach has the advantage of simplicity, it suffers from significant limitations; important details in the trends are lost in the averaging process involved in generating a summary rate. In many instances, these details have contributed significantly to the understanding of time trends for disease.

Initial approaches to the detailed analysis of time trends relied on the graphical presentation of age-specific rates and consideration of whether the resulting age patterns were consistent with knowledge about the biology of the disease. Although a visual approach remains an important part of the analysis of time trends, there also are efforts to consider more formally the effect of time through regression analysis. These attempts bring to the fore the limitations that can result from the concept of time trends in epidemiologic data that are strongly related to age.

425

0163-7525/91/0501-0425$02.00

Age plays a role in the etiology of most diseases. If you follow a group of subjects from birth, their risk for disease would vary as the birth cohort aged. Different birth cohorts may have different levels of exposure to a particular risk factor, which might be expected to produce a change in disease incidence for individuals born at a particular time, i.e. a cohort effect. For example, children born during the years when it was not uncommon to prescribe diethylstilbestrol to pregnant women might face a lifetime risk for certain types of cancer that differs from that faced by children born at another time. Not only are factors at the year of birth identified as a cohort effect, but any factor that affects disease incidence that is related to year of birth. Cigarette smoking is a habit that generally is started in the late teens or early twenties. Thus, large changes in smoking habits tend to be changes that depend on a person being of a particular age when there is an increase in the number of individuals starting to smoke. Hence, diseases that are strongly related to cigarette smoking would be expected to produce a pattern with birth cohort, even though there was nothing associated with birth itself that influenced disease risk.

Although factors that are identified with birth cohort might influence time trends in disease incidence, vital statistics usually are reported by year of diagnosis and age. One approach to summarizing time trends is to look at the patterns by the date the disease was diagnosed, i.e. the period. If there are cohort trends, then you also would expect to see some changes when analyzing trends by period. In addition to these indirect effects, there also might be unique period effects that are produced by inducing a similar change in disease risk for all individuals alive at a particular point in time, regardless of age. For instance, a pollutant in the air or the water supply might be expected to produce the same change in disease risk for everyone in the population. Changes in medical technology also might produce such a period effect by reducing the number of diagnoses that are missed or by detecting disease in less severely ill patients, thereby producing an artifact that may not represent an important change in the public's health.

A classic example of the value of considering time trends by period of diagnosis and by birth cohort is found in the study of trends in lung cancer mortality. The incidence of lung cancer for women living in Connecticut could be studied using Korteweg's (23) approach. These data illustrate various approaches for investigating time trends (see Table 1). The age-specific rates are plotted against age in Figure 1, which uses Korteweg's graphical approach to the analysis. To avoid the problem of reading a graph with too many lines, the data only are shown for every other five-year period. Solid lines indicate the age distributions when the data are considered for each of the periods. Interestingly, rates tend to reach a plateau or to even decline in the oldest age groups.

The pattern in the age distribution for lung cancer might seem inconsistent

Table 1 Number of lung cancer cases and incidence rates for women in Connecticut, 1940–1984

	\multicolumn{9}{c}{Period}
Age	1940–4	1945–9	1950–4	1955–9	1960–4	1965–9	1970–4	1975–9	1980–4

Number of Lung Cancer Cases

Age	1940–4	1945–9	1950–4	1955–9	1960–4	1965–9	1970–4	1975–9	1980–4
20–4	1	1	1	0	1	1	2	0	4
25–9	0	2	1	2	1	4	2	2	1
30–4	3	3	3	5	6	5	10	17	8
35–9	4	5	8	13	20	13	29	39	38
40–4	5	6	13	20	36	51	61	85	79
45–9	17	10	21	36	61	81	118	145	118
50–4	10	24	20	34	58	113	200	229	307
55–9	18	22	28	38	72	128	221	332	453
60–4	22	30	38	44	69	121	236	418	561
65–9	14	31	31	59	84	120	236	404	597
70–4	17	29	51	61	85	82	149	322	509
75–9	13	21	29	43	47	76	111	222	314
80–4	6	9	14	32	29	58	64	122	210

Incidence Rate x 100,000

Age	1940–4	1945–9	1950–4	1955–9	1960–4	1965–9	1970–4	1975–9	1980–4
20–4	0.24	0.26	0.27	0.00	0.25	0.19	0.32	0.00	0.59
25–9	0.00	0.48	0.24	0.50	0.25	0.84	0.36	0.33	0.15
30–4	0.81	0.72	0.67	1.12	1.35	1.14	2.17	3.03	1.27
35–9	1.16	1.31	1.88	2.77	4.14	2.87	6.91	8.44	6.68
40–4	1.53	1.74	3.39	4.49	7.47	10.52	13.37	20.43	17.22
45–9	5.42	3.20	6.22	9.12	13.83	16.82	24.05	32.53	28.82
50–4	3.65	8.24	6.34	9.89	15.26	25.69	41.37	48.28	69.86
55–9	8.14	8.61	9.82	12.56	21.97	34.17	52.49	72.83	98.61
60–4	11.43	13.96	15.83	16.63	23.85	38.10	67.17	106.75	130.97
65–9	8.95	17.80	15.54	25.33	32.70	44.83	83.05	125.09	163.36
70–4	15.63	23.59	35.24	34.71	42.47	37.40	63.77	127.21	174.76
75–9	19.29	24.93	30.36	38.06	35.67	48.38	60.33	113.30	142.53
80–4	17.07	21.25	27.08	50.94	38.16	60.74	53.70	87.89	135.70

with the expectation that lung cancer risk, like the risk of epithelial tumors in general, would continue to increase with age. A further analysis of these data evaluates the age distribution by following the same birth cohort as it ages. In this instance, the age distributions would follow the patterns shown by the broken lines in Figure 1. The relationship with age now shows a steady increase for all birth cohorts. In addition, the pattern with cohort is consistent with trends in cigarette smoking, which is now recognized as the leading cause of this disease (11, 44).

A good graphical display of data can expose relationships not evident in a more formal approach to data analysis, such as a regression model. However, because the trends are not always as evident, a formal model is helpful. In

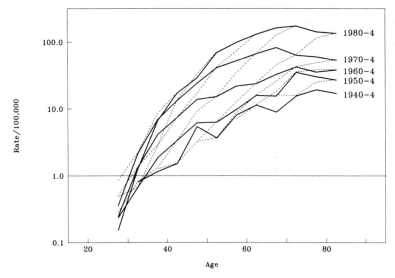

Figure 1   Lung cancer incidence rates for Connecticut women by age (solid lines = constant period, and broken lines = constant cohort).

addition, model fitting yields objective criteria for selecting the best among several alternative descriptions of data and provides a test of whether the observed pattern is real or random.

The emphasis of this discussion is the interpretation of results from fitting regression models to data that include age, birth cohort, and period or year of diagnosis. The details of model fitting are described elsewhere (1, 15, 16, 19, 27), and no specialized programs are necessary. Unfortunately, the results of these analyses can be confusing, and indeed contradictory. Thus, a clear and appropriate set of assumptions must be set out at the beginning.

TIME EFFECTS FOR VITAL RATES

To tackle some of the difficulties in interpreting the results from age-period-cohort (APC) models, it is necessary to have an understanding of the source of the problem, which is the interrelationships among these three factors. In this section, I describe those relationships in some detail and then indicate the effect they will have on models that include all three factors.

Relationship Between Age, Period, and Cohort

There are three time factors that are of interest in the models under consideration: age of the subject at time of diagnosis (a); year (period) in which the disease is diagnosed (p); and year a subject is born (cohort) (c). The bottom part of Table 1 shows the relationship among these factors according to the way in which population based data usually are collected. The columns contain age-specific rates for a period, and the rows are age groups. To follow an individual cohort, traverse down a diagonal line in the table and observe all of the corresponding combinations of a and p. If you know any two of a, p, or c, the third can be determined. For example, persons who died on their 52nd birthday in 1963 were born in 1911. This correspondence among the factors is called a linear dependence. In regression analysis, when regressor variables are linearly dependent, it is not possible to attribute separate effects to each of these factors. In this instance, the dependence is an algebraic relationship in which $c = p - a$.

Intervals and Overlap

When population-based data are tabulated for the calculation of age-specific rates, there is a necessary grouping of time into intervals. The most common practice is to present data in five- or ten-year ranges broken down by age and period. The bottom half of Table 1 shows a typical breakdown that might be used for summary purposes, which uses five-year intervals for both age and period. Because of this somewhat crude measure of age and period, there remains some ambiguity when you try to identify a cohort associated with a particular range for period and age (4). For example, women aged 20–24, when diagonosed in 1945, will have been born sometime from 1920 to 1925; those aged 20–24 in 1949 were born from 1924 to 1929. Hence, the incidence rate in the first row and second column of the table refers to women born from 1920 to 1929, although the length of time a woman might contribute to this rate would vary from five years if born in the middle of the decade, to less than a year if born early or late in the decade. I tabulate the data using equal intervals for age and period, and identify cohorts by the midpoint of the cohort interval for purposes of reference.

Example with Linear Trends

To illustrate the difficulty that arises in the analysis of regression models for the effect of age, period, and cohort, consider a hypothetical example. Suppose that the mean response, μ, is linearly related to age (a), period (p), and cohort (c). It is common for μ to represent the log of an incidence or mortality rate, but it also could represent the rate measured on another scale. Hence,

$$\mu = \beta_0 + \beta_a\, a + \beta_p\, p + \beta_c\, c \qquad\qquad 1.$$

Consider the hypothetical case in which one person has found estimates of the parameters in equation 1 to be

$$\hat{\mu}_1 = -104.00 + 0.20\ a + 0.10\ p - 0.05\ c \qquad\qquad 2.$$

A second investigator, who used the same data, estimated parameters for the identical model by using a different computer program and obtained

$$\hat{\mu}_2 = -104.00 - 0.20\ a + 0.50\ p - 0.45\ c \qquad\qquad 3.$$

The interpretation of these two models differs, because equation 2 suggests that the incidence is increasing with age, whereas equation 3 suggests that it is decreasing. By substituting some typical values of a, p, and c, you can find the fitted values from these two particular models, e.g.

$$-104.00 + 0.20(30) + 0.10(1960) - 0.05(1930) = 1.50$$
$$= -104.00 - 0.20(30) + 0.50(1960) - 0.45(1930)$$

The fitted values for equations 2 and 3 are identical for all possible combinations of age, period, and cohort, as the difference, $\mu_1 - \mu_2$, is a multiple of $(a - p + c)$ and is, therefore, zero.

To understand this apparent paradox better, consider the problem in more detail. By substituting into equation 1 the expression for $c = p - a$, you obtain

$$\hat{\mu} = \beta_0 + [\beta_a - \beta_c]\ a + [\beta_p + \beta_c]\ p \qquad\qquad 4.$$

For a different set of parameters, β'_a, β'_p and β'_c, the fitted values will be identical if $[\beta_a - \beta_c] = [\beta'_a - \beta'_c]$ and $[\beta_p + \beta_c] = [\beta'_p + \beta'_c]$.

Nonidentifiability Problem

The crux of the problem with APC models is that there is no unique set of regression parameters when all three of these factors are in the analysis simultaneously, because these parameters are hopelessly entangled. In the hypothetical example given in equations 2 and 3, you might bring other knowledge to bear on the question, which might indicate that a decline in incidence with age is very unlikely, and contradicts what is known about the biology of the disease. Hence, some parameter estimates may be dismissed out of hand, but many combinations of parameters can fit the data equally well, and honest differences of opinion may arise among investigators.

When bringing outside information to bear on the question of possible parameters, you always should keep in mind that some of what is assumed to be well known about incidence and mortality trends is based on analyses that have not taken alternative explanations into account. These analyses may themselves suffer from the limitations inherent in the interpretation of the APC models. Hence, considerable care must be used when applying this external information.

In the next section, I discuss a more general APC model, which allows for the possibility of curvature in the trends. Although this model is of more general interest, it still suffers from the same nonidentifiability problem. This problem can be resolved by clearly specifying the assumptions used to obtain a solution, or by limiting the summary to results that can be identified. Unfortunately, some current methods are completely arbitrary and only serve to obscure the real limitations in summarizing time trends for disease.

A REGRESSION MODEL FOR THE EFFECT OF TIME

The regression models on which most of this discussion is based involve additive contributions of the three time factors described above. When using mathematical equations to describe relationships, the question of scale or the manner in which the factors affect the rate must be considered. An additive model for rates might be expressed as

$$\lambda_{ij} = \eta + \pi_i + \delta_j$$

where λ_{ij} is the rate, π_i and δ_j are effects due to two factors, and η is a constant that might be interpreted as a base rate. This model, identical to the one used in the analysis of variance, has several limitations for the analysis of rates, including the possibility of negative fitted rates and the empirical finding that this model does not provide a good description for many incidence and mortality rates (33, 36, 37, 43). Multiplicative effects also have received considerable attention in models for disease rates because they have been found to work well in many practical situations. These may be expressed as

$$\lambda_{ij} = H \cdot \Pi_i \cdot \Delta_j$$

Taking the logarithm of both sides gives the additive form in which scientists usually work with this model,

$$\log \lambda_{ij} = \log H + \log \Pi_i + \log \Delta_j$$

The discussion in this section relates to any model that can be formulated as additive effects of the factors.

General Age-Period-Cohort Model

When estimating the effects of age, period, and cohort, you do not want to limit the systematic changes to simple linear trends, as in equation 1. There also may be a degree of curvature for the factor, which often is interesting in its own right. I assume that in a table of rates, age is divided into equally spaced intervals indexed by $i(=1, \ldots ,I)$. Likewise, the period groups, generated by the same interval spacing, are indicated by $j(=1, \ldots ,J)$. Finally, cohort is represented by $k(=1, \ldots ,K)$. Table 1 gives one breakdown of age and period into categories, with the corresponding cohorts shown on the diagonal. The interrelationship among these three factors implies that there is a similar relationship among these indices, as $k=j-i+I$. The general form of the regression model that includes all three factors is given by additive effects for age, period, and cohort,

$$m_{ijk} = \mu + \phi_{ai} + \phi_{pj} + \phi_{ck} + \epsilon_{ijk} \qquad 5.$$

where m_{ijk} represents the observed disease rate, the log rate, or some other transformation of the rate. The other parameters in the model are ϕ_{ai}, ϕ_{pj}, and ϕ_{ck}, which represent age, period, and cohort effects, and ϵ_{ijk} is random error. Additional constraints on the parameters must be made to obtain a solution. One approach is to set $\phi_{a1}=\phi_{p1}=\phi_{c1}=0$, which is the constraint used by computer programs such as GLIM (17). An alternative approach is to require that the sums of the effects be zero,

$$\Sigma_i \phi_{ai} = \Sigma_j \phi_{pj} = \Sigma_k \phi_{ck} = 0 \qquad 6.$$

which are the so-called usual constraints. Unfortunately, forcing the parameters to satisfy these constraints does not entirely resolve the uniqueness problem.

Estimable Functions of the Parameters

A model that included the effects of age, period, and cohort was fitted to the data shown in Table 1. In this instance, a log-linear model for the rates, i.e. a multiplicative model, was fitted to the data by assuming a Poisson distribution for the observed number of lung cancer cases. The particular parameter estimates reported here are maximum likelihood estimates, which were obtained by using the regression package GLIM. Alternative computer programs are also available, e.g. Frome (15).

Table 2 gives three different sets of parameter estimates that were obtained by fitting a model with the same three regressor variables to the data. The differences arise because of the linear dependence among the indices i, j, and k, so that an additional constraint is required if a specific set of parameters is to be obtained. In this instance, the constraints resulted from equating the effects of the first and last levels of cohort, age, and period respectively, constraints that were arbitrarily applied by a computer program based on the order in which the variables were stated. Although the parameters differ

Table 2 Age parameters and slopes from three equivalent age-period-cohort models for the data on lung cancer incidence shown in Table 1

Level	$\phi_{c1} = \phi_{c21}$ Coefficient	Deviations	$\phi_{a1} = \phi_{a13}$ Coefficient	Deviations	$\phi_{p1} = \phi_{p9}$ Coefficient	Deviations
Age						
20–4	−3.5188	−0.6972	−0.8268	−0.6972	−5.0272	−0.6972
25–9	−3.1510	−0.7996	−0.9076	−0.7996	−4.4079	−0.7996
30–4	−2.0521	−0.1711	−0.2574	−0.1711	−3.0577	−0.1711
35–9	−1.1518	0.2590	0.1942	0.2590	−1.9060	0.2590
40–4	−0.4139	0.5267	0.4835	0.5267	−0.9167	0.5267
45–9	0.1235	0.5938	0.5722	0.5938	−0.1279	0.5938
50–4	0.6162	0.6162	0.6162	0.6162	0.6162	0.6162
55–9	1.0075	0.5373	0.5589	0.5373	1.2589	0.5373
60–4	1.3641	0.4236	0.4668	0.4236	1.8669	0.4236
65–9	1.6555	0.2447	0.3095	0.2447	2.4097	0.2447
70–4	1.8191	−0.0620	0.0244	−0.0620	2.8247	−0.0620
75–9	1.8364	−0.5150	−0.4070	−0.5150	3.0933	−0.5150
80–4	1.8653	−0.9563	−0.8268	−0.9563	3.3736	−0.9563
Slopes						
Age	0.4703		0.0216		0.7217	
Period	0.2555		0.7042		0.0041	
Cohort	−0.0200		−0.4687		0.2314	

considerably, each model produces identical fitted values. Nevertheless, there is an underlying structure to these parameter estimates, which can be seen by a closer inspection of the age parameters displayed in Table 2. The overall trends in the age effects for these three analyses are indeed different. Fitting a regression line through these values by using a normalized age index, $[i-(I+1)/2]$, as the regressor variable, I obtain the fitted line $0.4703 \cdot (i-7)$ for the first set of parameters, which was obtained by setting $\phi_{c1} = \phi_{c21}$. Similarly, the second model with $\phi_{a1} = \phi_{a13}$ gave the line $0.0216 \cdot (i-7)$, and the final model with $\phi_{p1} = \phi_{p9}$ gave the line $0.7217 \cdot (i-7)$.

To understand the common features among these parameter estimates, I now remove the overall linear trend and consider the remaining residual, or the curvature. This is accomplished by subtracting the estimated parameter from the fitted line. For the first age group's parameter in column 1, this would be $-3.5188 - 0.4703 \cdot (1-7) = -0.6972$. By repeating this calculation for all age groups in each column of parameter estimates, we notice that the curvature effects are an invariant set of estimates, unlike the overall slopes or linear effects. To represent this more formally, let us represent the age effects using two components,

$$\phi_{ai} = [i - (I+1)/2] \, \beta_a + \gamma_{ai} \qquad\qquad 7.$$

in which β_a is the overall slope or the linear term, and γ_{ai} is the curvature. Similarly, the period and cohort parameters have linear and curvature components, and, in general, curvature remains the same, regardless of the parameterization used, i.e. the curvature is said to be an estimable function of the parameters (20, 35, 41). The slopes, however, are not estimable.

Although the slopes for the various sets of parameters may vary widely, they can only do so in a limited way, as was shown in the first hypothetical example. If the linear parameters for age, period, and cohort are represented by β_a, β_p, and β_c respectively, then

$$x \, \beta_a + y \, \beta_p + (y - x) \, \beta_c \qquad\qquad 8.$$

is estimable where x and y are arbitrary constants (20). For example, by setting x=y=1 you can see that $\beta_a + \beta_p$ is estimable. Notice that in the three sets of parameters for lung cancer shown in Table 2, the sums of the age and period slopes are 0.7258 in all instances. Likewise, x=1 and y=0 demonstrates that $\beta_a - \beta_c$ is estimable. Similarly, you can find other combinations of the slopes that are not affected by arbitrary constraints applied to the parameters.

This result has some practical value because it implies that, although the overall slopes are not confined, they cannot vary independently of each other. If any one of the slopes is fixed at a particular value, then the other two are immediately determined, as well. The three slopes from an arbitrary model can be represented by

$$\begin{aligned}
\beta_a^* &= \beta_a + \nu \qquad\qquad 9.\\
\beta_p^* &= \beta_p - \nu \\
\beta_c^* &= \beta_c + \nu
\end{aligned}$$

where β_a, β_p, and β_c are the true slopes and ν is an unknown indeterminate constant. For example, if you are particularly interested in period trend, it is disconcerting that the true slope might be either increasing or decreasing, depending on the unknown ν. However, β_a also depends on this indeterminant constant; thus, if it is implausible biologically that the rate decreases with age, then the values for ν that make the age slope negative must be implausible, as well. When ν is known to lie within a particular range, then a corresponding range of values also must hold for the period and cohort effects.

The concept of a regression line and residuals about that line is a fundamental idea in evaluating trends in data, which is fairly easy to grasp.

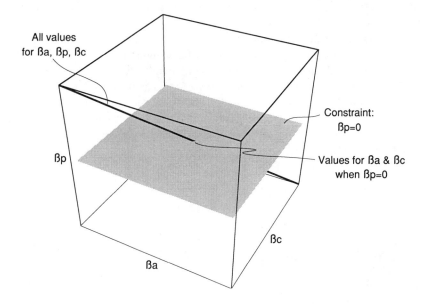

Figure 2   The relationship among the age, period, and cohort slopes, and the specification of a unique set of parameters through a constraint represented by the plane.

Although this concept is not the only way of defining estimable functions of the parameters, it does clarify which aspects of the age-period-cohort model parameters are affected by the limitation, and which are not. In addition, by limiting the difficulty in the general APC model to just three parameters, it is easier to see the interrelationships among the many alternative approaches to this problem that have been suggested in the literature. The slopes for period and cohort are essentially the same as the period and cohort drift parameter described by Clayton & Schifflers (5, 6). The sum of the period and cohort slopes, $\beta_p + \beta_c$, is referred to as the net drift, and the result in equation 8 shows that this is estimable.

Values for the three slopes, β_a^*, β_p^*, and β_c^*, can be represented in a three-dimensional graph, with each slope on one of the axes, as shown in Figure 2. Ideally, the slopes would be identified by a point in the graph, and the statistical problem is to find the best estimate of that point. However, if you vary the unknown quantity ν in equation 9, then you can see that instead of a point, there is a line hanging in the three dimensional graph that represents all slopes that give the identical fit to the data. When a solution is offered to the nonidentifiability problem, the proposal essentially suggests a plane that contains the plausible slope. For example, you might choose a plane that fixes the period slope, β_p^*, as shown in Figure 2. When the plane intersects the line at a point, then this point of intersection uniquely identifies the values for all three slopes.

With this linear and curvature representation you can readily reformulate the parameters by using alternative sets of assumptions to determine how sensitive the results are to a particular assumption. To illustrate how you can find a set of parameters based on another set of constraints by using the estimated functions of the slopes and the individual curvature terms, consider once again the data on lung cancer shown in Table 1. Suppose that you wish to reparameterize the first set of slopes in Table 2, assuming that $\beta_p=0$. Equation 9 implies that

$$\nu = \beta_p - \beta_p{}^* = -0.2555$$

Hence, the corresponding slopes for the other two factors are

$$\beta_a = \beta_a{}^* - \nu = 0.4703 - (-0.2555) = 0.7258$$
$$\beta_c = \beta_c{}^* - \nu = -0.0200 - (-0.2555) = 0.2355$$

If the assumption about the period slope is incorrect, then you have induced a corresponding bias in all of the effects.

Once the particular slope has been identified, the effects for the individual categories can be found by adding together the corresponding linear and curvature components. For instance, the effect for the ith age would be determined by

$$\phi_{ai} = [i - (I+1)/2] \beta_a + \gamma_{ai}$$

where γ_{ai} is the corresponding curvature component. By using our example, the effect for the first age group is estimated by

$$[1 - 7] 0.7258 + (-0.6972) = -5.0520$$

ALTERNATIVE CONSTRAINTS ON MODEL PARAMETERS

The most direct approach for dealing with nonidentifiability is to specify constraints on the model parameters, so that there is no longer a problem with the remaining parameters. I now describe several different constraints that are used with APC models and point out some of the weaknesses in their use.

Two-Factor Models

Perhaps the simplest approach to nonidentifiability is the attempt to avoid it altogether by not considering all three factors simultaneously. When fitting such a two-factor model, the interpretation of the results seems straightforward: The degrees of freedom are one less than the number of levels for the factor, and the regression program will not reveal any difficulty with the resulting parameters. If such a model gives a good fit to the data, or if the excluded factor does not result in a significant deterioration in fit, then there is a certain degree of elegance in its use. However, an examination of the results from limiting the three-factor model to just two factors reveals that there still may be a lingering source of bias in the parameters.

Testing for the period effect by comparing the fit of an APC model with an AC model is itself influenced by the nonidentifiability problem. The null hypothesis that there is no period effect in a model can be written as

$$H_0: \; \phi_{p1} = \phi_{p2} = \ldots = \phi_{pJ} = 0$$

where the usual constraints, $\Sigma \; \phi_{pj} = 0$, imply $(J-1)$ degrees of freedom for the test. Because the slope for period is entangled hopelessly with the age and cohort slopes, there is the loss of one more degree of freedom for the test of a period effect in the presence of age and cohort, i.e. $(J-2)$ degrees of freedom. These $(J-2)$ degrees of freedom for period are really testing whether there is a significant curvature component to the period effects, $H_0: \; \gamma_{p1} = \gamma_{p2} = \ldots = \gamma_{pJ} = 0$.

Tests of age and cohort effects, when the other two factors are included in the model, also are tests of curvature and not the overall slope. It is impossible to test the null hypothesis that the slope is zero, $H_0: \; \beta_p = 0$, when both age and cohort also are included in the model, without knowing the constant ν. Likewise, an AC model cannot escape bias because of the period slope, as the estimates of age and cohort slopes obtained by fitting such a model are really estimates of $\beta_a + \beta_p$ and $\beta_c + \beta_p$, respectively.

It would be surprising if a causal agent that changed over time did so in a strictly linear fashion. Typically, you also would expect to see a certain amount of curvature, which may be detected as either a period or a cohort effect, so that there is certainly some insight that can be gained even from a test of curvature. Day & Charnay (8) have suggested analyzing data from several countries to improve the chances for detecting whether period or cohort is the more important factor. Nevertheless, the possibility exists that there is very little curvature in exposure trends over time, a pattern that may be consistent for the various populations under study. This possibility makes it likely that an important trend would be missed. Hence, an analysis that is limited to the consideration of just two factors is not really a solution to the problem, because the possibility for bias has not been eliminated.

Equate Two or More Effects

A second approach to finding a unique set of parameters is to equate two, rather than all, of the effects for one of the model factors (2, 3, 13), as in the method of dropping a factor. For instance, two adjacent period effects may be set equal to each other because there is reason to believe that no change in period occurred, e.g.

$$\phi_{p1} = \phi_{p2}$$

Clayton & Schifflers (6) suggested a variation on this approach that assumes the mean of the successive differences is zero. In the case of the period effect, this variation implies that the mean of $(\phi_{p2}-\phi_{p1})$, $(\phi_{p3}-\phi_{p2})$ . . . is zero. Such an assumption is equivalent to equating the first and last period effects, $\phi_{p1}=\phi_{pJ}$, which was the constraint applied for the parameters displayed in Table 2, as the last parameter was set to the first for cohort, age, and period in the three respective columns. This constraint is simple to apply. It forces the parameters to return to the original level, which generally would make the parameters similar to those obtained in the following section. Equating the first and last categories is the constraint applied by the regression package GLIM when there is a linear dependence in the factors.

Once you decide to set two of the period effects equal to each other, the remaining parameters can be determined uniquely, and together they will yield a unique slope. A unique slope for period will, in turn, force the age and cohort slopes to be unique, through the result in equation 9, so that the entire APC model is now defined. Similarly you could equate two cohort or age effects, or indeed the difference between any two effects can be set equal to a constant, which results in a unique set of model parameters.

The advantage of this approach to the nonidentifiability problem is that it is simple to understand and apply. In addition, it does not force equality for all of the effects, as is the case when one of the factors is dropped entirely from the model. Unfortunately, there generally is not a sound basis for equating two effects, and it may be based on the reasoning that, "There is no reason to expect a change during these years, therefore they will be assumed to be equal." It often is true that equality of the fourth and fifth cohorts is just as logical as the first and second in a particular situation, and the resulting parameter estimates can vary considerably for these equally plausible assumptions. Because of the remaining ambiguity, this approach leads easily to the kind of dispute that was referred to earlier, in which the trends appear to be different, and there is no way to say which is better by using only the data.

Zero Period Slope

An alternative to the method that equates two of the parameters is a restriction that defines one of the slope parameters directly. For example, you might specify that there is no period slope, $\beta_p=0$ (20). This approach is the immediate generalization of the deletion method; both assume that the overall slope is zero, but the zero slope does not at the same time require that all of the curvature terms be set to zero. It also might be more stable than an assumption that equates just two effects, in that it involves a longer span of time, and more data are involved. However, it is not a solution to the nonidentifiability problem, and it can induce a bias for all three slopes.

Another variation on this approach is to fix the slope over a shorter span of time, rather than the entire span. For example, you might assume that there is no trend with period for 1950–1969, a span of four five-year periods. This variation would avoid some of the lack of stability associated with equating just two periods, which is actually equivalent to setting the slope for just two adjacent periods equal to zero.

Roush et al (36, 37) undertook a systematic study of cancer incidence by using data from the Connecticut Tumor Registry. This analysis focused primarily on the curvature effects for each of the time factors, but in the summary graphs, a period slope of zero was specified, $\beta_p=0$. The rationale for this approach was threefold: there is a strong biological basis for an age effect on cancer, so that if only one factor is unimportant, it is likely to be either period or cohort; empirical results strongly suggested that cohort had a stronger association with incidence than period; and the assumption that $\beta_p=0$, was less restrictive than ignoring the effect of period altogether.

Period and Cohort Drift

Clayton & Schifflers (5, 6) describe an approach to analyzing time trends that considers an overall "drift" with period

$$\mu_{ij} = \mu + \phi_{ai} + j \cdot \beta_p$$

or cohort

$$\mu_{ik} = \mu + \phi_{ai} + k \cdot \beta_c$$

These models are more restrictive than the two-factor models, as the period or cohort effect is forced to be linear. In addition, we cannot distinguish between these two models, as they give an identical fit to the data because of the problem of nonidentifiability. As we now know, two models that produce the same fitted values can produce different parameters, and in this case the age effects, ϕ_{ai}, can differ considerably.

The introduction of the idea of drift led Clayton & Schifflers (6) to suggest a hierarchy of models:

1. Age
2. Age + (Period or Cohort) Drift
3. a. Age + Period
   b. Age + Cohort
4. Age + Period + Cohort

Fundamental to this development is the primacy of the effect of age on disease, so that, as usually would be reasonable, Clayton & Schifflers do not entertain models that exclude age. A significance test that compares the fit of model 2 with either models 3a or 3b, is equivalent to a test for period or cohort curvature that adjusts for age and the corresponding slope. The comparisons between 3b or 3a with 4 give the tests for period adjusted for cohort and vice versa. This approach effectively carries the idea of linear and curvature components of effect down to the level of the two factor model, which can help to clarify the comparison of the adjusted and the unadjusted effects of period and cohort. However, when summarizing the results of an analysis, you are still left with a similar array of choices for the drift parameter, i.e. the slope.

ATTEMPTS TO SOLVE THE NONIDENTIFIABILITY PROBLEM

Many authors seem to offer solutions to the nonidentifiability problem; they give approaches that yield a unique set of parameters without the appearance of adopting arbitrary constraints. In this section I describe two such proposals. Both methods are fairly complex; thus, to really understand their lack of a sound biological foundation, it is necessary to describe them in some detail. The third approach described here considers a nonlinear model, which also introduces another level of complexity into the analysis.

Osmond & Gardner Method

Osmond & Gardner (31) propose a method for analyzing APC models, which I refer to as the OG method. I discuss this method in some detail because it has been used by several investigators. By understanding the details, you will see its limitations, and you also will be able to translate results from this approach into those of any other by using equation 9. By concentrating once again on the slopes, I use equation 9 to express the OG slope for age as

$$\beta_a(OG) = \hat{\beta}_a + \hat{\nu} \qquad\qquad 10.$$

where $\hat{\beta}_a$ is an age slope that has been estimated by using an arbitrary method for fitting the model, and $\hat{\nu}$ is to be estimated. Similarly, the period and cohort slopes are

$$\beta_p(OG) = \hat{\beta}_p - \hat{\nu} \qquad\qquad 11.$$
$$\beta_c(OG) = \hat{\beta}_c + \hat{\nu} \qquad\qquad 12.$$

Because the details for the proposed estimator of ν are complex, I leave a more complete description for the Appendix. The idea is to find an estimator for ν by minimizing the disagreement between the three-factor model and each of the two-factor models. After a careful evaluation, we find that these constraints depend on the number of levels for each of the factors, the parameters from the two-factor models, and the mean squared error from these subset models. These combine to yield parameters that tend to be in closer agreement with the two-factor models, especially those that give a good fit to the data. Although the method has some appeal, there are several points of criticism that can be raised.

A close inspection of the weights used by this method reveals that they do not depend on the underlying biology of the disease. For example, cohort slopes generally are given greater weight than either age or period, simply because there are more cohorts in the typical table of rates. In addition, the use of one over the error mean square as a weight for the corresponding two-factor parameters makes use of a value that cannot be specified a priori. Intuition might suggest that a model with a good fit, i.e. a small mean square error, be given more weight than a model that fits more poorly. However, because the slopes are indeterminant, there is little substantive justification for the weights because they are only dependent on the curvature components.

The mean square error depends on the age distribution of the population under study, which is usually affected by factors other than the disease in question. Two populations might have identical age-specific incidence rates but very different age distributions in the populations, which could alter the mean squared errors and lead to a different set of estimates. These constraints also depend on the results of fitting various subset models, some of which are likely to give a poor fit to the data. It is not clear that a poor fitting model can provide any useful information on the parameter estimates. Finally, the constraints are so complicated that it is difficult to know and understand what is being achieved by their application, even for the very dedicated investigator. Hence, not only does the method have all of the weaknesses inherent in the other arbitrary approaches, but it also is difficult to interpret.

Robertson & Boyle Method

A proposal by Robertson & Boyle (34) for solving the nonidentifiability problem, noted the difficulty with determining unique cohorts in a table of

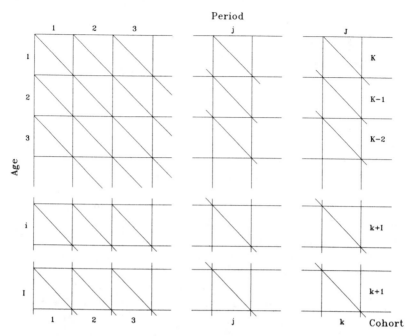

Figure 3   Division of age and period into triangular regions so that cohorts do not overlap.

rates broken down by age and period. They suggested that an exact accounting of age, period, and cohort would result in a unique set of parameters, thus solving the problem. The reason for this optimism is unclear, as the hypothetical examples shown in equations 2 and 3 clearly demonstrate; the problem exists even if time is precisely determined. Hence, we should not be surprised to find that a solution to the problem has once again proven to be elusive (6, 32, 42).

To insure the absence of any overlap for the intervals of age, period, and cohort, this method avoids the typical checkerboard partitioning of time by age and period used in constructing Table 1. Instead, each square of time is divided in half diagonally, as shown in Figure 3, so that we are now dealing with an array of triangles. Horizontal and vertical lines still divide age and period into unique intervals. However, the addition of a diagonal partition has resulted in a refinement that gives a unique, rather than an overlapping, partition of the cohorts.

The index $i(=1, \ldots ,I)$ again is used for the age intervals, and $j(=1, \ldots ,J)$ for the period intervals. The cohorts now are slightly different from before, as nonoverlapping cohorts follow the alternating upper and lower triangles shown along a diagonal in Figure 3. I denoted a particular cohort in this model by k^*. For the two triangles that make up the square for age group i and period j, the cohort indices are

$$k^* = j - i + I \qquad \text{for the lower triangle cohort}$$
$$= j - i + I + 1 \qquad \text{for the upper triangle cohort.}$$

Unlike the earlier representation, the indices i, j, and k^* are not linearly dependent. The rate for all subjects observed in time defined by one of these age-period-cohort triangles is assumed to have a model of the same form as that used earlier, namely

$$\mu_{ijk^*} = \mu + \phi_{ai} + \phi_{pj} + \phi_{ck^*}$$

Because the indices are not linearly dependent, there is no longer a nonidentifiability problem with the parameters. Hence, the slope, as well as the curvature terms, are all uniquely determined.

To apply this method in its original form, you must have information on date of birth for each individual that contributes to the numerator and denominator of the rate for a given triangle. Often, this detailed information is unavailable, as the data may be available only in aggregate, as in Table 1. In these instances, date of birth is effectively missing, and Robertson & Boyle propose a modification of their procedure that incorporates the EM-algorithm (9) for dealing with these missing data, while preserving the uniqueness of their solution.

To understand the weakness of this proposal, it is again sufficient to consider only the slopes for the three factors, because we have established that the curvature components are unique. So that

$$\mu_{ijk} = \beta_0 + i \cdot \beta_a + j \cdot \beta_p + k^* \cdot \beta_c \qquad \qquad 13.$$

and all of the parameters are estimable. The problem is that the indices are not good representations of their respective measures of time. Consider the square corresponding to the ith age group and the jth period shown in Figure 3. If the population under study has ages and periods that are uniformly distributed over the square, then the lower triangle will tend to have individuals that are older than those in the upper triangle, because there are more possible older ages that can occur in the lower triangle, whereas the upper has more younger ages (6). If i represents the mean age index for the square, and if the distribution over the square is uniform, then the mean ages for the two triangles are

Age: $i + \frac{1}{6}$ lower triangle
$i - \frac{1}{6}$ upper triangle

On the average, the difference in age between the upper and lower triangles is one third the width of the age interval. Hence, the use of the same index i to represent age in the two triangles introduces a bias for the regressor in both triangles. There are similar biases for the period and cohort indices

Period:	$j - \frac{1}{6}$	lower triangle
	$j + \frac{1}{6}$	upper triangle
Cohort:	$k - \frac{1}{3} = j - i + 1 - \frac{1}{3}$	lower triangle
	$k + \frac{1}{3} = j - i + 1 + \frac{1}{3}$	upper triangle

If we use the unbiased indices for the triangles, the linear dependence emerges once again in that

$$(\text{age}) - (\text{period}) + (\text{cohort}) - 1 = 0$$

for both the upper and lower triangles. Hence, the linear independence that resulted in a unique set of parameter estimates arose from the use of a biased representation of age, period, and cohort. Unbiased terms lead to the original nonidentifiability problem in which the parameters are not estimable. A solution that results entirely from the use of biased regression parameters is generally biased itself; thus, this method does not offer a practical resolution of the problem.

Nonlinear Models

The difficulty caused by the nonidentifiability problem has led some investigators to consider the use of intrinsically nonlinear models. One example is the model that Moolgavkar et al (29) used,

$$\mu_{ijk} = \mu + \phi_{pj} + \phi_{ck} + \phi_{ai} \cdot \delta_j \qquad\qquad 14.$$

which also was considered by James & Segal (22). In this model, ϕ_{pj} and ϕ_{ck} represent the effects due to period and cohort, respectively. The effect of age, ϕ_{ai}, is included along with a multiplicative factor involving period, δ_j, which can modify the effect of age. Equation 14 is but one example of a nonlinear model for the effect of time. In some instances, a convincing rationale can be given for such a model, based on knowledge about the underlying biology of the disease. Models of this form are especially interesting, because in most situations this model will yield a unique set of parameters, without the use of arbitrary constraints, which leads proponents to prefer this model to the one given in equation 5. However, you should notice that the special case where

$$\delta_j = 1 \text{ for all } j$$

is identical to equation 5, so we should proceed cautiously.

It is well known that intrinsically nonlinear models often have complex regions where the different parameters give nearly identical fitted values to the data, resulting in unstable parameter estimates (see Chapter 10 of Ref. 12, for a more complete discussion of nonlinear regression). Understanding these regions can be difficult, and interpreting the model that yields these single point estimates of the parameters also can be confusing. The conditions for nonunique parameters given above are those that include the log-linear model used in these analyses. When the model in equation 5 gives a good fit to a set of data, the parameters in equation 14 may be near this region where ambiguity in the parameters exist, so that the point estimates of the parameters may be unstable (6, 43).

INVARIANT PARAMETERS FROM THE AGE-PERIOD-COHORT MODEL

Given the severe problems of analyzing time trends in disease incidence and mortality, you might ask whether anything can be gleaned from such data. To ignore time trends is to ignore a tool that historically has provided valuable insights into disease etiology. You cannot ignore or hide the nonidentifiability issue when analyzing trends. Inherent limitations in these analyses can be handled only by confronting the problem and making thoughtful and clearly specified assumptions when summarizing the results. In this section, I describe some approaches that have provided valuable insights into the effects of age, period, and cohort.

Restricting Summary to Estimable Effects

Restricting the summary of results to estimable functions of the parameters has the advantage of being invariant with respect to the particular approach used in obtaining parameter estimates (20). In the strictest sense, this means that most of the attention should focus on the curvature in the trends instead of the overall slope, because the curvatures are estimable and the slopes are not. Kupper et al (24) warn that the curvature terms are of limited utility in isolation from the linear trend. Indeed, without knowledge of the linear component of trend it is impossible to address even the simplest question of whether the trend is increasing or decreasing with one of the time factors. Nevertheless, sometimes the interesting questions can be addressed by simply considering curvature effects.

Tango & Kurashina (43) considered just the curvature effects in a study of age-period-cohort models for mortality from diabetes, ischemic heart disease, liver cirrhosis, and suicide in Japanese men. This analysis showed that men born in the Showa Era (1925–1940) had a risk that was higher than expected when considering the overall trend among men born to surrounding cohorts. The reason for this difference is not immediately clear, but it was thought that a variety of socioeconomic factors could come into play, because most of the adolescent growth for these men occurred during World War II when there was nutritional deprivation. In addition, these men made the largest contribution to the period of rapid economic growth that occurred in Japan during the 1960s, all of which may have had deleterious effects on mortality. By limiting the inference to curvature in the trends, the results are stronger, as the conclusions among different analysts would be likely to agree. In addition, by using a simple and clearly specified approach, an alternative constraint can be applied readily by using the results in equation 9.

To show that a particular cohort departs from the overall trend, Tango & Kurashina suggest evaluating local curvature, defined by the second order differences

$$C_k = \phi_{c,k-1} - 2 \cdot \phi_{c,k} + \phi_{c,k+1}$$

This contrast is estimable and it essentially compares the kth cohort with the cohorts on either side. Because of overlapping cohort intervals, and because local change might occur right on a division point for the cohorts, they also suggest an analysis that basically considers the average of adjacent second order differences, i.e.

$$D_k = (C_k + C_{k+1})/2$$

Forecasting Incidence and Mortality Trends

Forecasting trends in disease is fraught with difficulties because you must make assumptions that cannot be verified until the future has been observed. Nevertheless, it is an exercise that has considerable merit for planning health care needs and prevention strategies, despite the rather spectacular failures that can be cited. In making a forecast that is based on a model, it is most common to assume that the trends of the past will continue into the future. Kupper et al (24) and Clayton & Schifflers (6) warn that this is a very strong assumption, which may well be unwarranted. Nevertheless, it is an assumption that is commonly made in other contexts, and it is one that seems reasonable in the absence of contradictory information. Interestingly, this assumption results in projected rates for which the nonidentifiability problem is irrelevant because the projected rates are estimable (21, 30).

Once again, I demonstrate this property by using a model that only includes linear terms. More complicated models, which include curvature terms, present no new statistical problems, because curvature parameters are estimable. The transformed rate for the ith age, jth period, and kth cohort is

$$\mu_{ijk} = \mu + i \cdot \beta_a + j \cdot \beta_p + k \cdot \beta_c$$

To obtain a forecast, we follow the same cohort in time by increasing the age and the period index by one unit, which gives

$$\mu_{i+1,j+1,k} = \mu + (i+1)\cdot\beta_a + (j+1)\cdot\beta_p + k\cdot\beta_c$$

The resulting change in time is the difference between the two rates,

$$\mu_{i+1,j+1,k} - \mu_{ijk} = \beta_a + \beta_p$$

which is an estimable function of the slopes (see Eq. 8). Hence, a forecast is not entangled hopelessly in nonidentifiability, and it is possible to use the model for projections (21, 30).

Restricted Ranges for Slopes

Yet another approach for using knowledge about the underlying biology of a disease to understand something about the trends involves a restriction on more than one of the time factors. Wickramaratne et al (46) analyzed the effects of age, period, and cohort on risk of major depression in five US communities. Although a specific assumption about the overall trends with period and cohort was not possible, it did seem reasonable to assume that there was not a decreasing trend with either period or cohort, i.e.

$$\beta_p \geq 0 \tag{15.}$$

and

$$\beta_c \geq 0 \tag{16.}$$

Adding β_c to both sides of equation 15 gives

$$\beta_p + \beta_c \geq \beta_c \geq 0$$

Because the sum of the period and cohort slopes, $\beta_p + \beta_c$, is estimable, this effectively puts bounds on the cohort slope, so that it can only vary within this range of values. In a similar way, there are corresponding ranges possible for the period slopes

$$\beta_p + \beta_c \geq \beta_p \geq 0$$

and the age slopes,

$$\beta_a + \beta_p \geq \beta_a \geq \beta_a - \beta_c$$

where the upper and lower values for the inequality are estimable.

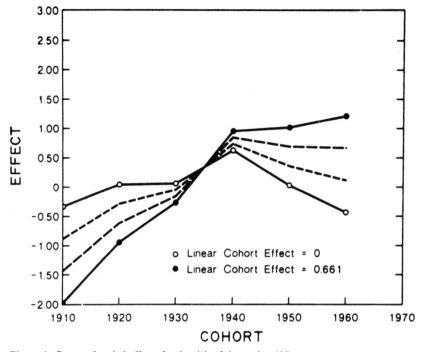

Figure 4   Range of period effects for the risk of depression (46).

To illustrate the information that can be obtained from this approach, consider the cohort effects for the risk of depression in women, given by Wickramaratne et al, and shown in Figure 4. The investigators were particularly interested in the cohort born during 1935–1944, and it is clear from the figure that for this range of possible slopes for the cohort effects, there is still an apparent increase in risk that occurred for those born during this period. Hence, although a precise quantitative statement is not possible, the analysis does qualitatively address a question of scientific interest, while quantifying the uncertainty associated with the aspect of trend that cannot be identified.

INCORPORATING INFORMATION ON KNOWN RISK FACTORS

In the study of time trends for a disease, time itself is not likely to be the causal agent, but instead acts as a surrogate for a causal agent that is changing over time. This suggests that the fitting and interpretation of age-period-cohort models is only a first step in understanding trends, and further analyses should be considered that more directly evaluate the risk factors themselves.

By going beyond this basic model, you can avoid the nonidentifiability problem altogether by considering a more biologically plausible model. Examples of this approach can be found in work on diseases about which there is already some understanding of etiology, e.g. tuberculosis (26), lung cancer (40), bladder cancer (28, 40), pancreatic cancer (28), and breast cancer (18, 29). These attempts have not been entirely successful for several reasons, including the lack of precise information on risk factors, the availability of information only in aggregate form and not by separate subgroups, and the complete absence of population-based exposure data on some known risk factors. However, it does seem desirable to develop models that are more closely motivated by the underlying biology, to achieve a better understanding of the processes that drive the time trends.

INTERACTIONS

One limitation in the type of models considered above is that they assume that the effect of each factor does not depend on the level of the others, i.e. possible interactions among the factors of interest are not considered. The inclusion of interactions in the model often makes the results even more difficult to interpret. This is especially true when you consider the effects of age, period, and cohort because the estimable functions of the interaction parameters can be complicated.

To illustrate some of the difficulty in considering interactions, suppose that we use just the factors age and period in the analysis of a set of age-specific rates. These rates can be completely described by the model

$$\mu_{ij} = \mu + \phi_{ai} + \phi_{pj} + \phi_{ap,ij} \qquad\qquad 17.$$

where ϕ_{ai} is the main effect for age, ϕ_{pj} is the main effect for period, and $\phi_{ap,ij}$ is the interaction between the two factors. This model will fit the table of rates exactly, because there are as many parameters in the model as there are rates; hence, it is called a saturated model.

By looking more closely at the models given in equations 5 and 17, we can see that the only difference between the two is that the first model includes a cohort effect, ϕ_{ck}, and the second an age-period interaction, $\phi_{ap,ij}$. Because the interactions saturate the model that only includes main effects due to age and period, you might think of the cohort effect as a particular type of age-period interaction (25). Similarly, you could describe the period effect as a particular type of age-cohort interaction. Because any model that includes the main effects and the interactions of two of the three time factors will be a saturated model, it follows that general models that include interactions among the three time factors, as well as main effects for all three time factors, also will be saturated. Fienberg & Mason (14) have studied polynomial models for the three time factors, and have indicated which interactions can be identified. The interpretation of interactions in higher order polynomial models is difficult under the best of circumstances, without complicating things still further with the nonidentifiability problem. Hence, considerable care is needed when introducing interactions into these models.

Interactions that involve the comparison of trends in different populations, however, have been successfully applied. An interaction between cohort and geographic region, for example, would suggest that the cohort trends were not the same in the different regions, but these effects cannot be determined in general. Day & Charnay (8) point out that if the age trends are assumed to be equal for the different regions, i.e. there is no interaction between age and region, then the interactions that involve period and cohort can be estimated. A possible rationale for this assumption is that the effect of aging is a biological constant across the regions; thus, the only variation is expected for the period and cohort effects. However, Clayton & Schifflers (6) indicate the danger of this assumption in that differences in exposure to risk factors among the regions may well affect the age parameters, as well. The limitation of this assumption is particularly clear in comparisons between men and women, and not regions. For many diseases, hormonal changes, such as those that occur around menopause, may affect disease incidence, so that it is not reasonable to assume that the age effect is the same for the two groups.

POWER CONSIDERATIONS

It is not uncommon in epidemiological studies to find that cohort effects appear to be more significant statistically than period. For example, in a systematic analysis of time trends in cancer incidence rates in Connecticut, Roush et al (36, 37) found that cohort, more often than period, was the predominate factor for most sites, which might have been caused by some inherent statistical advantage of the cohort factor over the period factor. One difference in the two factors is that cohort has many more degrees of freedom than period. Although additional degrees of freedom increase the likelihood of a good fit, you should remember that there is a corresponding penalty that corrects the p-value. A factor with many degrees of freedom actually may be at a severe disadvantage if the relationship with the response is a relatively simple polynomial. However, the relative power of detecting separate time effects also can be affected by interval overlap for the cohorts, sparse data for early and late cohorts, and the span of time covered.

The problem of interval overlap for the cohorts was described in some detail earlier, and this lack of uniqueness in the cohort intervals can be thought of as an error in classification. When there are errors in the regressor variables, the corresponding parameter estimates generally are biased, which

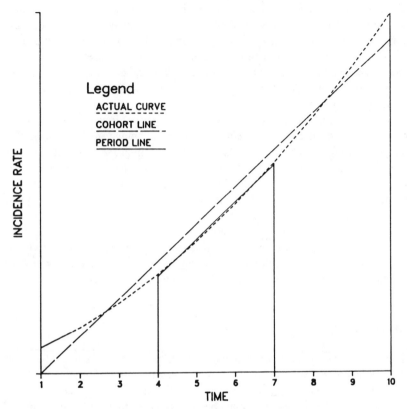

Figure 5   Approximation of a curve with a straight line by using different time spans.

is true even if there is no overall bias in the regressor variables, so that they are correct "on the average." How much this problem influences the ability to detect cohort effects, as compared with period or age effects, is not well understood, but it would certainly tend to wash out relatively short-term trends for cohort.

As we can see in Table 1, the earliest cohorts are represented by the oldest age groups and the latest cohorts are in the youngest age groups, which reduces the precision for early and late birth cohorts. There are fewer actual rates that go into the estimate of an extreme cohort effect, which also effectively reduces the number of cases in these extreme cohorts. Thus, their precision when using Poisson regression is reduced. Because periods generally are represented by all age groups, they would seemingly have a power advantage over cohort in this respect.

However, there are more cohorts that cover a longer span of time, which seems to increase power to detect cohort effects, especially when using relatively simple polynomial models. Consider the graph shown in Figure 5, which displays a curved line with small breaks that represents a particular time trend. If data are only available for the time span from 4–7, then the curve is well approximated by a straight line, which is shown by the solid line. But, when the span of time is much longer, in this case from 1–10, we clearly can see that the straight line is not at all adequate. In general, a longer time span would make it more likely to detect significant curvature than a short span, for the identical curve.

Although period may have the power advantage in terms of the number of observations in all categories, cohort has the advantage in terms of having data over a long time span. You might wonder which factor has the greater overall statistical power for detecting curvature effects. Schymura (38) suggests that the net advantage is in favor of cohort. She has found expressions for the variance of the quadratic and cubic polynomial terms for period and cohort when each rate has the same degree of curvature. In these cases, the cohort variance is always smaller than the period variance, which gives it the greater power to detect statistical significance for the same degree of curvature. This analysis did not consider the more usual case in which rates are estimated with unequal precision, but many calculations suggest that it holds here, as well.

SUMMARY AND CONCLUSION

Time trends for population-based disease rates often are summarized by using direct adjustment by period of diagnosis or death. Similarly, the effect of age often is presented graphically as age-specific rates for a given period of diagnosis. These approaches may be necessary if there is an absence of long-term data, as they provide a natural way for annually updating information when monitoring trends, or they may be a convenient way of summarizing a large amount of data (7, 10, 11, 39, 45). However, these summaries only can adjust for the effect of age in a given period; they implicitly ignore the cohort effect. The effect of cohort is an important factor in understanding time trends for many diseases. Thus, it is not advisable to use data analytic strategies that routinely ignore it.

Another alternative to modeling is to give a graphical presentation of the age-specific rates themselves. As I noted in the introduction, some of the first analyses to identify the effect of cohort on diseases, such as tuberculosis and lung cancer, relied entirely on a graphical analysis. Although graphs certainly are an important part of the interpretation of time trends, it would be a mistake to limit your analysis to impressions of points on a graph. For example, such a perusal would not give an objective indication of the statistical significance of a particular pattern. Regression analysis forces us to recognize a fundamental problem with interpreting time trends in disease rates—a problem that you should remember, even when trying to understand a graphical display of time trends in age-specific rates.

ACKNOWLEDGMENT

This work was supported by National Cancer Institute grant number CA30931.

APPENDIX

The Osmond-Gardner Method

The OG method makes use of parameter estimates that are obtained from each of the three two-factor models determined by dropping either age, period, or cohort from the model. As noted in the text, unique parameter estimates from these two factor models can be readily obtained by fitting a model without the explicit specification of a further constraint. Let the full set of model parameters be represented by the vector $\mathbf{\Psi}' = (\mathbf{\phi}_a', \mathbf{\phi}_p', \mathbf{\phi}_c')$, and the corresponding parameters when period and cohort are dropped from the model are

$$\mathbf{\Psi}_{(p)} = (\mathbf{\phi}_{a(p)}', \mathbf{0}', \mathbf{\phi}_{c(p)}')$$

and

$$\mathbf{\Psi}_{(c)} = (\mathbf{\phi}_{a(c)}', \mathbf{\phi}_{p(c)}', \mathbf{0}')$$

respectively, where the parenthesis, $(\cdot)$, is used to represent a factor that has been dropped from the model. Because age is recognized as such a strong predictor of disease, this method does not ignore its effect entirely, but makes an adjustment by allowing for the age effects when both period and cohort are dropped from the model, $\mathbf{\phi}_{a(pc)}$. This adjustment is accomplished by fitting the model

$$\mu_{ijk} - \phi_{a(pc)i} = \mu + \phi_{pj} + \phi_{ck} \qquad \text{A1.}$$

where $\phi_{a(pc)i}$ is considered a known constant. The age parameters for this so-called period-cohort model are given by $\mathbf{\phi}_{a(a)} = \mathbf{\phi}_{a(pc)}$. The corresponding period and cohort parameters are found by fitting the model described in equation A1, which gives the complete set of regression parameters,

$$\mathbf{\Psi}_{(a)} = (\mathbf{\phi}_{a(a)}', \mathbf{\phi}_{p(a)}', \mathbf{\phi}_{p(a)}')$$

The estimate of ν is obtained through a least squares approach, in which the quantity to be minimized is a weighted sums of squares of all these parameter estimates

$$S_{(a)}/\rho_{(a)} + S_{(p)}/\rho_{(p)} + S_{(c)}/\rho_{(c)}$$

The term $\rho_{(\cdot)}$ represents the mean square error for the model that drops the corresponding factor from the model,

$$S_{(\cdot)} = \Sigma_m [\phi_{(\cdot)m} - \phi_m - h_m \nu]^2 \qquad\qquad A2.$$

and

$$
\begin{aligned}
h_m &= i - (I+1)/2 && \text{for the age parameters} && A3.\\
&= -j + (J+1)/2 && \text{for the period parameters}\\
&= k - (K+1)/2 && \text{for the cohort parameters}
\end{aligned}
$$

Scrutiny of this expression reveals a similarity between this approach for finding an estimate of ν and the method of least squares for finding the slope of a line. From equations A1–A3 it is apparent that,

$$
\begin{aligned}
\hat{\nu} &= \beta_a(OG) - \hat{\beta}_a\\
&= -\beta_p(OG) + \hat{\beta}_p\\
&= \beta_c(OG) - \hat{\beta}_c
\end{aligned}
$$

which suggests that the OG estimate of the indeterminate quanity, $\hat{\nu}$, can be expressed in terms of averages of $(\beta_{a(\cdot)}, -\beta_{b(\cdot)}, \beta_{c(\cdot)})$. Let the slope for factor e with factor f eliminated be represented by $\beta_{e(f)}$, and let the slope from an arbitrary APC model be β_e for e, f=a,p,c. For the model with the fth factor removed, the weighted mean of the slopes is

$$\bar{\beta}_{(f)} = \Sigma_e w_e \cdot \beta_{e(f)} / \Sigma_e w_e$$

where the weights are

$$w_e = \Sigma_m h_m^2$$

and h_m are the constants defined in equation A3 for factor e. These weights depend on the number of levels for a particular factor, so that factors with more levels are given greater weight. Hence, cohort generally is given more weight than either age or period. In a similar manner, the mean slope for the arbitrary APC model is $\bar{\beta}$, which can be expressed as a correspondingly weighted mean. The final step is to combine the mean slopes for the subset

Table A1   Calculation of the Osmond-Gardner constraints for the lung cancer data shown in Table 1

(e)	$\Sigma_m\ h_{m^2}$	A + P + C	Model A + P (C)	A + C (P)	P + C (A)	Osmond-Gardner
β_a	182	0.4703	0.4772	0.7372	0.4901	0.6495
$-\beta_p$	60	-0.2555	-0.3085	0.0000	-0.6815	-0.0763
β_c	770	-0.0200	0.0000	0.2428	-0.2087	0.1592
$\bar{\beta}_{(e)}$		0.0539	0.0675	0.3173	-0.1110	
$\rho_{(e)}$			2.7837	1.3914	334.4624	
Weighted Mean				0.2331		

models, by using as weights the reciprocal of the mean square error for the subset model, $1/\rho_{(f)}$,

$$\bar{\beta}_{(\cdot)} = \Sigma_f\ (1/\rho_{(f)}) \cdot \bar{\beta}_{(f)}\ /\ \Sigma_f\ (1/\rho_{(f)})$$

which gives an estimate of the indeterminate constant

$$\hat{\nu} = \bar{\beta}_{(\cdot)} - \bar{\beta}$$

As an example of the application of this method, consider once again the trends in lung cancer for women living in Connecticut. Suppose you have obtained the slope estimates from the parameters shown in the first column of Table 2, and you wish to summarize these results using the OG method. A summary of the calculations is shown in Table A1. Columns 3–6 give the slope parameters from either the full three-factor model, or one of the three two-factor models, and a weighted mean of these is calculated by using the weights in column 2, $\Sigma_m\ h_m^2$. A weighted average of the means for the two-factor models is then obtained by using $1/\rho_{(f)}$ as the weights, yielding

$$\hat{\nu} = 0.2331 - 0.0539 = 0.1792$$

Hence, the OG-slopes are estimated by

$$\hat{\beta}_a(OG) = 0.4703 + 0.1792 = 0.6495$$
$$\hat{\beta}_p(OG) = 0.2555 - 0.1792 = 0.0763$$
$$\hat{\beta}_c(OG) = -0.0200 + 0.1792 = 0.1592$$

Literature Cited

1. Aitkin, M., Anderson, D., Francis, B., Hinde, J. 1989. *Statistical Modelling in GLIM*. Oxford: Clarendon
2. Barrett, J. C. 1973. Age, time, and cohort factors in mortality from cancer of the cervix. *J. Hyg. Camb.* 71:253–259
3. Barrett, J. C. 1978. The redundancy factor method and bladder cancer mortality. *J. Epidemiol. Community Health* 32:314–16
4. Case, R. A. M. 1956. Cohort analysis of mortality rates as an historical or narrative technique. *Br. J. Prev. Soc. Med.* 10:159–71
5. Clayton, D., Schifflers, E. 1987. Models for temporal variation in cancer rates. I: Age-period and age-cohort models. *Stat. Med.* 6:449–67
6. Clayton, D., Schifflers, E. 1987. Models for temporal variation in cancer rates. II: Age-period-cohort models. *Stat. Med.* 6:469–81
7. Cook, P. J., Doll, R., Fellingham, S. A. 1969. A mathematical model for the age distribution of cancer in man. *Int. J. Cancer* 4:93–112
8. Day, N. E., Charnay, B. 1982. Time trends, cohort effects, and aging as influence on cancer incidence. In *Trends in Cancer Incidence*, ed. K. Magnus, pp. 51–65. Washington, DC: Hemisphere
9. Dempster, A. P., Laird, N. M., Rubin, D. B. 1977. Maximum likelihood from incomplete data via the EM Algorithm. *J. R. Stat. Soc. B* 69:1–38
10. Doll, R., Cook, P. 1967. Summarizing indices for comparison of cancer incidence data. *Int. J. Cancer* 2:269–79
11. Doll, R., Peto, R. 1981. The causes of cancer. *J. Natl. Cancer Inst.* 66:1192–1308
12. Draper, N. R., Smith, H. 1981. *Applied Regression Analysis*, pp. 458–517. New York: Wiley. 2nd ed.
13. Fienberg, S. E., Mason, W. M. 1978. Identification and estimation of age-period-cohort models in the analysis of discrete archival data. In *Sociological Methodology 1979*, ed. K. F. Schuessler, pp. 1–67. San Francisco: Jossey-Bass
14. Fienberg, S. E., Mason, W. M. 1985. Specification and implementation of age, period and cohort models. In *Cohort Analysis in Social Research*, ed. W. M. Mason, S. E. Fienberg, pp. 45–88. New York: Springer-Verlag
15. Frome, E. L. 1983. The analysis of rates using Poisson regression models. *Biometrics* 39:665–75
16. Frome, E. L., Checkoway, H. 1985. Use of Poisson regression models in estimating incidence rates and ratios. *Am. J. Epidemiol.* 121:309–23
17. GLIM Working Party 1987. *The GLIM System, Release 3.77*. Oxford: Numerical Algorithms Group, Ltd.
18. Hahn, R. A., Moolgavkar, S. H. 1989. Nulliparity, decade of first birth, and breast cancer in Connecticut cohorts, 1855 to 1945: An ecological study. *Am. J. Public Health* 79:1503–7
19. Holford, T. R. 1980. The analysis of rates and survivorship using log-linear models. *Biometrics* 36:299–305
20. Holford, T. R. 1983. The estimation of age, period and cohort effects for vital rates. *Biometrics* 39:311–24
21. Holford, T. R. 1985. An alternative approach to statistical age-period-cohort analysis. *J. Clin. Epidemiol.* 38:831–36
22. James, I. R., Segal, M. R. 1982. On a method of mortality analysis incorporating age-year interaction, with application to prostrate cancer mortality. *Biometrics* 38:433–43
23. Korteweg, R. 1951. The age curve in lung cancer. *Br. J. Cancer* 5:21–27
24. Kupper, L. L., Janis, J. M., Karmous, A., Greenberg, B. G. 1985. Statistical age-period-cohort analysis: A review and critique. *J. Chron. Dis.* 38:811–30
25. Kupper, L. L., Janis, J. M., Salama, I. A., Yoshizawa, C. N., Greenberg, B. G. 1983. Age-period-cohort analysis: An illustration of the problems in assessing interaction in one observation per cell data. *Commun. Stat. Theor. Method* 12:2779–2807
26. Mason, W. M., Smith, H. L. 1985. Age-period-cohort analysis and the study of deaths from pulmonary tuberculosis. In *Cohort Analysis in Social Research: Beyond the Identification Problem*, ed. W. M. Mason, S. E. Fienberg, pp. 151–227. New York: Springer-Verlag
27. McCullagh, P., Nelder, J. A. 1989. *Generalized Linear Models*, pp. 193–214. London: Chapman & Hall. 2nd ed.
28. Moolgavkar, S. H., Stevens, R. G. 1981. Smoking and cancers of bladder and pancreas: Risks and temporal trends. *J. Natl. Cancer Inst.* 67:15–23
29. Moolgavkar, S. H., Stevens, R. G., Lee, J. A. H. 1979. Effect of age on incidence of breast cancer in females. *J. Natl. Cancer Inst.* 62:493–501

30. Osmond, C. 1985. Using age, period and cohort models to estimate future mortality rates. *Int. J. Epidemiol.* 14:124–29

31. Osmond, C., Gardner, M. J. 1982. Age period and cohort models applied to cancer mortality rates. *Stat. Med.* 1:245–59

32. Osmond, C., Gardner, M. J. 1989. Age, period, and cohort models: Non-overlapping cohorts don't resolve the identification problem. *Am. J. Epidemiol.* 129:31–35

33. Rewers, M., Stone, R. A., LaPorte, R. E., Drash, A. L., Becker, D. J., et al. 1989. Poisson regression modeling of temporal variation in incidence of childhood insulin-dependent diabetes mellitus in Allegheny County, Pennsylvania, and Wielkopolska, Poland, 1970–1985. *Am. J. Epidemiol.* 129:569–81

34. Robertson, C., Boyle, P. 1986. Age, period, and cohort models: The use of individual records. *Stat. Med.* 5:527–38

35. Rogers, W. L. 1982. Estimable functions of age, period, and cohort effects. *Am. Soc. Rev.* 47:774–96

36. Roush, G. C., Holford, T. R., Schymura, M. J., White, C. 1987. *Cancer Risk and Incidence Trends: The Connecticut Perspective*, pp. 15–26, 467–508. New York: Hemisphere

37. Roush, G. C., Schymura, M. J., Holford, T. R., White, C., Flannery, J. T. 1985. Time period compared to birth cohort in Connecticut incidence rates for twenty-five malignant neoplasms. *J. Natl. Cancer Inst.* 74:779–88

38. Schymura, M. J. 1986. *Age, period and cohort trends in cancer incidence in urban and non-urban Connecticut, 1940–1979*, pp. 54–72. Ph.D. dissertation. Yale Univ.

39. Silverberg, E. 1983. Cancer statistics. *CA* 33:9–25

40. Stevens, R. G., Moolgavkar, S. H. 1979. Estimation of relative risk from vital data: Smoking and cancers of the lung and breast. *J. Natl. Cancer Inst.* 63:1351–57

41. Tango, T. 1985. Statistical model of changes in repeated multivariate measurements associated with the development of disease. *Comput. Stat. Data Anal.* 3:77–88

42. Tango, T. 1988. Statistical modelling of lung cancer and laryngeal cancer incidence in Scotland, 1960–1979. *Am. J. Epidemiol.* 127:677–78

43. Tango, T., Kurashina, S. 1987. Age, period and cohort analysis of trends in mortality from major diseases in Japan, 1955 to 1979: Peculiarity of the cohort born in the early Showa Era. *Stat. Med.* 6:709–26

44. US Public Health Serv. 1979. *Smoking and Health: A Report of the Surgeon General*. Washington, DC: US Dep. Health Educ. Welf., Public Health Serv.

45. Waterhouse, J., Muir, C., Shanmugaratnam, K., Powell, J., eds. 1983. *Cancer Incidence in Five Continents*. Lyon: Int. Agency Res. Against Cancer

46. Wickramaratne, P. J., Weissman, M. M., Leaf, P. J., Holford, T. R. 1989. Age, period and cohort effects on the risk of major depression: Results from five United States communities. *J. Clin. Epidemiol.* 42:333–43

Annu. Rev. Publ. Health 12:459–80

CARCINOGENIC EFFECTS OF MAN-MADE VITREOUS FIBERS

Philip E. Enterline

Department of Biostatistics, Graduate School of Public Health,
University of Pittsburgh, Pittsburgh, Pennsylvania 15261

KEY WORDS: fibrous glass, mineral wool, ceramic fibers, epidemiology, cancer

INTRODUCTION

Man-made vitreous fibers (MMVF) have been produced both in the US and Europe for more than 100 years.[1] These fibers are of considerable interest in terms of their potential human health effects largely because of similarities to asbestos fibers. Concern for health hazards associated with MMVF was accelerated greatly by the appearance of papers, starting in 1972, which proved that fibrous glass, the principle type MMVF, is capable of producing cancer when implanted in the pleura of rats. The papers concluded that it is the geometry of asbestos fibers that produce cancer, rather than their chemical composition (39, 46, 47).

Asbestos is a well established cause of lung cancer and pleural and peritoneal malignant mesothelioma. Some researchers believe that asbestos has its effects on lung tissue because of the lung's inability to phagocytize these fibers (29). When a long, thin asbestos fiber is inhaled, the lung macrophages (the scavenger cells in the lung) engulf a fiber incompletely, and there is an escape of destructive intracellular enzymes to the surrounding tissue from the region where the fiber protrudes from the cells periphery. These enzymes ultimately cause damaged cells and fibrosis, and this scarring probably renders the entrapped pulmonary epithelium more susceptible to malignant

---

[1]MMVF often are referred to as man-made mineral fibers. This technically is incorrect, as a mineral cannot be man made.

0163-7525/91/0505-0459$02.00

transformation. This theory is supported by the observation that respirable asbestos fibers, whose length is less than the diameter of a macrophage, produce little if any fibrosis or lung cancer in animal experiments. There also is some support for this theory from epidemiologic investigations, whereas long, thin fibers can be very effective in producing both fibrosis (52) and respiratory cancer in experimental animals (55). Pleural and peritoneal malignant mesothelioma also is believed to be due to scarring comparable to that which takes place in the lung (29, 48). These cancers apparently occur when an inhaled fiber penetrates the lung and translocates to the pleura or peritoneum. Thus, if MMVF have effects comparable to asbestos, they must be of about the same dimension as asbestos and be capable of producing fibrosis. Although the majority of MMVF are too large to be respirable, all products have some respirable fibers in the size range thought to be important in the initiation of human respiratory cancers (28).

TYPES OF MAN-MADE VITREOUS FIBERS

Currently, there are four commercially important types of MMVF: fibers made from molten magmatic rock; fibers made from molten slag from metallurgical processes, such as iron, steel, or copper production; fibers made from kaolin clay or the oxides of alumina, silicon, or other metals (referred to here as ceramic fibers); and fibers made from glass. There are three main types of glass fibers: ordinary glass wool, continuous filament, and a special purpose fine fiber. The market for each type of fiber differs somewhat because of the particular fiber properties, although there is considerable overlap.

Slag or rock wool fibers primarily are used for high temperature insulation applications and for residential insulation. Rock and slag wool fibers have a high melt temperature. They also can be used to prevent the spread of fires from floor to floor in high-rise buildings. Slag/rock wool fiber in ceiling tile acts as a fire barrier and a sound attenuating material.

Ceramic fibers have very high temperature resistance and are used primarily for high temperature insulation applications, including thermal blankets for industrial furnaces and vacuum formed parts for specialty products with high temperature tolerances. They are a substitute for asbestos in high temperature insulation applications.

Ordinary glass wool products include batts for thermal insulation of commercial and residential structures, granular or loose-fill products for attic insulation, and heavier density products with more board-like characteristics for thermal, as well as acoustical, insulation properties in air handling systems and ceiling systems. Special purpose fine fibers are manufactured for highly specialized applications, such as aerospace insulation, airplane insulation, and sophisticated filtration applications. Continuous filament or textile fiberglass products are used in applications such as reinforced plastics, in which a large fiber diameter is desired for superior reinforcing properties.

PRODUCTION OF MAN-MADE VITREOUS FIBERS

In the United States, the first MMVF were produced in 1870 by using slag from furnaces that had produced iron to cast Union army guns. Commercial production of rock wool began in Indiana in 1897. Commercial fiberglass production did not begin until the mid-1930s, whereas production of ceramic fibers did not begin until the 1950s (48a). Manufacturing facilities usually specialize in one type of fiber, except where rock/slag fibers are produced. A single facility sometimes will alternate between the use of rock and slag or will mix the two.

There currently are over 100 MMVF production facilities throughout the world with a worldwide production of roughly 6 million tons in 1985 (26). This estimate contrasts with worldwide production of asbestos, which peaked at around 4 million tons in 1976. Nearly half of worldwide production of MMVF is in North America, most of which is in the United States where fibrous glass accounts for about 80% of MMVF production. There are 19 plants in the United States that make slag wool fiber, 1 plant that makes rock wool fiber, 40 plants that make glass fibers, and 12 plants that make ceramic fibers (49).

PHYSIOCHEMICAL PROPERTIES OF MAN-MADE VITREOUS FIBERS

Although MMVF generally are thought of as a class of fibers, they differ considerably and should not be considered as a single entity. These fibers may differ in terms of physical properties because of the manner in which the fibers are manufactured and because of the raw materials used. The raw materials also impart a variety of chemical properties to MMVF. In general, MMVF are more soluble than asbestos when exposed to body fluids; however, there are exceptions to this rule. Bellman (5), for example, has shown that there are special glass fibers that are, in fact, less soluble than asbestos. Solubility is related to durability in human body tissues, and fiber durability is probably important in fiber carcinogenesis. Related to durability is the fragility of MMVF. Man-made vitreous fibers have neither a definite chemical composition nor a crystalline structure. They tend to fracture laterally, whereas naturally occurring fibers, like asbestos, are crystalline in structure and tend to fracture longitudinally. This distinction is important, as Assuncao & Corn (1) have shown that with the application of energy, asbestos merely forms thinner and thinner fibers, whereas MMVF become granular. Thus, to the extent that residence time in human tissue has implications for human pathology, most forms of MMVF apparently should have much less potential for producing disease than asbestos fibers.

Another important feature of MMVF is that when used for insulation, they usually contain a binder to give bulk and certain insulating properties. The chemicals used as binders include formaldehyde, which potentially produces cancer. In addition, oils are present on the fibers, which were used primarily as dust suppressants and which could be carcinogenic. Thus, in epidemiologic and experimental investigations of MMVF, any effects observed might be related to some of the chemicals used in the preparation of the fibers. In addition, when evaluating the effects of exposure of workers who produce these fibers, polycyclic aromatic hydrocarbons and other combustion by-products present in the working environment might have some effect on worker health.

LEVELS OF HUMAN EXPOSURE

Exposure levels of MMVF currently are expressed as respirable fibers per cubic centimeter of air (f/cc), and fibers are counted by phase contrast optical microscopy (PCOM). The counting method involves collecting a measured quantity of air through a membrane filter by means of a battery powered sampling pump. The filter is then mounted on a glass slide and made optically transparent with acetone/triactin. The number of respirable fibers in randomly selected areas of filter is counted by using PCOM at magnifications at about 500x. Respirable fibers are those objects longer than 5 μm and narrower than 3 μm with the length/diameter ratio greater than 3 to 1. Essentially, this same method is used to count asbestos fibers. Although fiber concentrations usually are expressed as fibers greater than 5 μm in length and less than 3 μm in diameter per cc of air (f/cc), it is not certain how long a fiber should be to have biologic activity. Although the length of a fiber has little influence on its aerodynamic properties, there is some agreement that fibers longer than 200 μm would be too large to be inhaled (50). In implantation experiments by Stanton et al (46), the optimum fiber length for the production of malignant mesothelioma in rats was greater than 8 μm. The optimum fiber diameter was less than 1.5 μm.

Airborne fiber concentrations are highly dependent on the fiber diameter in a particular product. This relationship is shown in Figure 1. Insulating wool fibers made from rock, slag, or glass have diameters ranging from 2–9 μm; special purpose fine fibers have diameters from .1–3 μm; ceramic fibers have diameters from 1.2–3 μm, which is similar to special purpose fine fibers; and continuous filament glass fibers have diameters ranging from 6–15 μm.

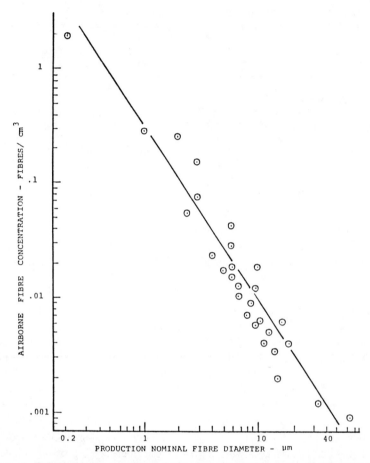

Figure 1   Relationship between measured average exposures, expressed as fibers/cc (determined by phase contrast microscopy), and nominal diameter of fiber manufactured. (Reproduced with permission from Ref. 16.)

In 1990, the Thermal Insulation Manufacturers Association (TIMA), the trade association for MMVF producers, reported fiber concentrations shown in Table 1 to the US National Institute for Occupational Safety and Health (NIOSH) to assist them in proposing new regulatory standards. This report represents sampling during 1985–1989. No data were reported for rock/slag wool products, although fiber concentrations probably would be similar to those shown for glass wool. The current US Occupational Health and Safety Administration's (OSHA) permissible exposure level for asbestos is .2 f/cc. If this were applied to MMVF, MMVF apparently would be above this level in many situations. The fiber concentrations in glass fiber production facilities

Table 1   MMVF fiber concentrations in the US by process[a]

Process	No. of Samples	Mean Fiber Concentration (f/cc)	% less than	
			1 f/cc	3 f/cc
Glass Fiber Production	1569	.39	94.3	97.4
Glass Wool	1032	.11	98.9	99.6
Glass Filament	189	.03	100.0	100.0
Small Diameter Fiber	348	1.42	77.3	89.7
Glass Fiber End Users	443	.25	93.0	99.5
Ceramic Fiber Production	1152	.65	79.2	97.5
Ceramic Fiber End Users	103	1.17	58.2	90.3

[a] from reference 49

shown in Table 1 are somewhat higher than those reported by Esmen et al (16) in a survey of ten US glass fiber production facilities. They are similar, however, to data from European glass wool plants (37) and data from six European rock wool plants (7).

Of particular importance for epidemiological investigations related to cancer are fiber exposure levels in the past, as cancer has a long latent period. For asbestos cancer, the latent period is believed to be 20 years or more. Past exposure has been only investigated for glass and rock/slag wool fibers, because ceramic fibers have been produced too recently to warrant such investigations. Exposure levels for workers who produce glass wool fibers probably have changed very little over time. Although the reduction in the size of fibers produced resulted in higher concentrations of airborne fibers, the addition of dust suppressants and improvements in ventilation in production facilities tended to offset this increase (26). For rock/slag wool, however, past exposures for workers who produce these fibers were probably considerably higher, largely because of a change in the way this material was produced and the absence of dust suppressing agents (36). Esmen et al (17) has estimated that workers exposed to rock/slag wool averaged 1.5 f/cc before 1945 based on dust data for a wool production plant collected in 1935. This estimate was confirmed in an experiment in which a rock/slag wool production process was operated under conditions that existed in the 1940s (8). When mineral oil was used as a dust suppressant, as was believed to be the case in the rock wool production facility upon which Esmen based his exposure estimates, the average concentration was 1.5 f/cc; when not used, the concentration was around 5 f/cc. Thus, although fiber concentrations in glass wool and rock/slag wool plants are now about the same, epidemiologic studies that relate past levels of fiber exposure in production workers to their mortality experience show much higher cumulative levels of

Table 2   Fiber[a] concentrations in ambient air in the Federal Republic of Germany in 1981–1982[b]

| Measuring Site | No. of Samples | f/cc | | | | Size of glass fibres[c] (μm) | |
		Total	Chrysotile	Amphibole	Glass	Median Diameter	Median Length
Duisburg	17	0.041	0.0022	0.0019	0.00050	0.26	2.54
Dortmund	6	0.036	0.0026	0.0019	0.00170	0.25	3.06
Dusseldorf	21	0.027	0.0014	0.0013	0.00040	0.30	3.64
Krahm (rural area)	9	0.012	0.0005	0.0007	0.00004	0.89	2.76

[a] Not reported in this table are fibers classified as quartz, aluminum, iron, rutile, sulphur or others
[b] From reference 24

exposure for mineral wool workers than for glass wool workers. Some users of ordinary glass and rock/slag wool probably have higher exposures than shown in Table 1. Esmen et al (18) reported average exposures exceeding 1 f/cc for workers who insulate attics with rock/slag wool.

Past exposure to MMVF both in the US and in Europe has been low relative to exposure during the production or use of asbestos products. In the principal epidemiologic studies of asbestos products and insulation workers, which identified asbestos as a human carcinogen fiber, exposures were estimated to be 8–12 f/cc over a period of many years. World War II shipyard workers were probably exposed to asbestos at about 2 f/cc (11).

Both asbestos and MMVF are contaminants in ambient air. Table 2 shows that glass fibers can be found in the air in urban areas of Germany. There were, however, roughly 40 times more asbestos than glass fibers present, and the glass fibers seen were relatively short and unlikely to be pathogenic (24). At five locations in California, glass fibers less than 2.5 μm in diameter determined by light microscopic count and by electron microscopic count averaged .00026 f/cc (2). Glass fibers can be found in the lungs of workers who produced these fibers, as well as in the general population, but at a much lower level than asbestos fibers (33).

In many countries, MMVF are regulated only as nuisance dust or in terms of their chrystalline quartz content. In 1977, NIOSH recommended a 3 f/cc permissible exposure limit for glass fiber, but this has not been acted upon by OSHA. In 1988, OSHA announced its intention to regulate fibrous glass dust and mineral wool dust and proposed a permissible exposure level of 5 mg/m^3 for fibrous glass dust and 10 mg/m^3 for mineral wool. Recently, NIOSH requested comments and secondary data relevant to synthetic and natural fibers and probably will produce a new recommended exposure limit. Sweden limits exposures to MMVF to 1 f/cc for a full working day, whereas the United Kingdom recommends 2 f/cc.

EXPERIMENTAL EVIDENCE

Three types of animal experiments have been reported: inhalation, intratracheal injection, and intracavitary injection. Inhalation experiments are preferred over other types, because these best represent the conditions of exposure in humans. Unfortunately, these experiments are time-consuming and expensive, and it is not certain that a suffcient fiber dose reaches the lung to produce tumors. Intratracheal injection is a less expensive way to expose animals and insures that measured doses do reach the animal's lung. If the question is whether MMVF are capable of producing cancer in the lungs of animals, then either method seems appropriate. If the question is whether MMVF are likely to produce cancer given physiologic defenses against the inhalation and retention of fibers and the distribution of fibers when they reach the lung, then inhalation experiments clearly are preferable.

In 1987 the International Agency for Research on Cancer (IARC) examined the animal evidence for the carcinogenicity of MMVF (25). In their report, 14 animal inhalation experiments were reviewed. Of these, 8 involved glass fibers and none were positive; 3 involved rock/slag fibers and none were positive; and 3 involved ceramic fibers of which one was positive (seven tumors in 48 exposed animals and one in 39 control animals) and in another there was one mesothelioma in 50 hamsters. There was little or no evidence of fibrosis in the inhalation studies that involved glass or rock/slag wool fibers, and tissue response was confined to an accumulation of pulmonary macrophages, many of which contained fibers. For ceramic fibers, however, the inhalation studies showed some evidence of fibrosis. Thus, at the time of the IARC review, there was no evidence from animal inhalation studies of a carcinogenic effect of glass, rock, or slag fibers, but some evidence for ceramic fibers. However, even with asbestos, it has not been easy to produce cancer in animal inhalation studies. Despite studies dating as early as 1931, it was not until 1967 that an animal inhalation experiment with asbestos produced clearly positive results (22, 22a). Moreover, in some of the animal studies reviewed by IARC, in which asbestos exposed animals were used as a control, few or no tumors were produced.

Since the 1987 IARC review, there has been an 18-month inhalation study of ceramic fibers in which 36 pleural mesotheliomas were observed in 102 hamsters. Seven lung cancers and three mesotheliomas were observed in a 24-month inhalation study in rats. Fiber used in this experiment generally was less than 3 μm in diameter and 15 μm or more in length (F. J. Rauscher 1990, personal communication). Mean fiber diameter of ceramic fiber currently produced is 1.4 μm, and mean length is 15.8 μm (49). Animal evidence from inhalation studies now appears positive for ceramic fibers.

Some of the earliest experiments with MMVF fibers involved intratracheal

Table 3 Tumor production in animals following intratracheal injection with glass fibers[a]

	No. of Animals	No. of Tumors
Study by Smith et al (45) (female Osborne-Mendel rats)		
Glass Fiber	22	0
Asbestos	25	2
Control	150	0
Study by Feron et al (20) (Syrian golden hamsters)		
Glass Fiber	130	4
Asbestos	112	4
Control	59	0
Study by Pott et al (40) (male Syrian golden hamsters)		
Glass Fiber	274	86
Asbestos	142	18
Control	135	2
Study by Pott et al (41) (female Wistar rats)		
Glass Fiber	34	5
Asbestos	35	15
Control	40	0

[a] adapted from reference 25

injection of glass fibers. The earliest was reported by Gardner in 1942 (21, 22). He concluded that glass fiber is not fibrogenic, nor does it cause other significant reactions in the lung. In 1970, an animal study was reported in which glass fiber (average diameter of 1 μm and a length of 50 μm or less) was administered by intratracheal injection and by inhalation. Neither fibrosis or tumor formation was observed within 24 months (23). Perhaps the most widely quoted intratracheal injection study was reported by Wright and Kushner in 1976 and in 1977 (30, 55). Various types of asbestos and glass fibers were injected intratracheally into groups of 30 guinea pigs. This study showed that all long fibers, whether asbestos or glass, produced some fibrosis, whereas short thin fibers failed to produce any fibrosis. The reaction caused by glass fibers was less pronounced than that produced by asbestos, although it was qualitatively similar. The four intratracheal injection studies reviewed by IARC in 1987 showed mixed results with regard to tumor production with glass fibers (25). Table 3 shows the results of the four studies. Pott et al (40, 41), in two studies, produced many tumors with glass fiber and with asbestos, whereas Smith et al (45) and Feron et al (20) produced few tumors either with glass fiber or with asbestos.

As noted earlier, the experiments that suggested that MMVF might have the same potential for producing cancer as asbestos involved intracavitary implantation (39, 46, 47). The International Agency for Research on Cancer reviewed 27 studies in which MMVF was implanted into the pleura or peritoneum. When glass fibers were used, 10 of 14 produced tumors; when rock wool fibers were used, all three studies reviewed produced tumors; when slag wool fibers were used, one of two studies produced tumors; and when ceramic fibers were used four of eight produced tumors.

Clearly, there are differences in the outcome of apparently similar animal studies, which could be because of differences in the observation periods, difficulty in calculating incidence rates because of a lack of survival data, differences in the fiber size used or in the fiber durability, short exposure periods, differing fiber and dose data, or chance due to small numbers of animals (25). Unfortunately, many studies do not adequately describe the fibers used, and most express dose by weight, rather than as number of fibers, so that the actual fiber exposure is unknown. Type of fiber is undoubtedly of importance. As noted above, there are many types of MMVF fiber of varying size and solubility. A recent unpublished review of all the intratracheal and intracavitary fibrous glass injection studies considered by IARC concluded that positive responses were obtained only when special purpose fine fibers with nominal diameter less than 1 μm were used (49).

The IARC Working Group considered that there was sufficient evidence for the carcinogenicity of glass wool and ceramic fibers in experimental animals, limited evidence for the carcinogenicity of rock wool in experimental animals, and inadequate evidence for the carcinogenicity of slag wool in experimental animals (25).

CARCINOGENIC EFFECTS IN HUMANS

The Metropolitan Life Insurance Company conducted the earliest study of the effects of MMVF on humans, and Carpenter & Spolyar (6) reported the results in 1945. The purpose was to determine whether pneumoconiosis or fibrosis was related to the inhalation of MMVF. Chest x-rays were taken on workers who had been exposed while producing rock and slag wools. No chest abnormalities were observed, except for one case of silicosis that apparently was related to earlier employment. Subsequently, little data on respiratory disease among MMVF workers were reported until the late 1960s, when the oldest and largest fibrous glass plant in the United States was the site of several cross-sectional studies involving chest x-rays and lung function testing. These studies did not suggest any relationship between glass fiber exposure and pulmonary abnormalities (9, 34, 51, 54). In 1983, Weill et al (53) reported on a study of pulmonary disease among workers employed in five fibrous glass and two slag wool plants in the United States. This study found a low category profusion of parenchymal small opacities in some workers and concluded that exposure to fine glass fiber may lead to low level profusion. They concluded that progressive diffuse pulmonary fibrosis associated with exposure to fine fiberglass was unlikely, although it could not be firmly ruled out. No pulmonary function abnormalities were detected in this study.

Cross-sectional studies, which involve taking chest x-rays and pulmonary function testing, are useful for detecting diseases like pneumoconiosis, which persist for a long period of time. They are less useful, however, for studies of diseases like cancer, which are much more acute and have a low prevalence. The best way to determine whether a substance has some effect on cancer in humans is to conduct longitudinal studies that cover long periods of time during which the incidence of cancer can be documented. Such studies usually are retrospective—they cover some past period and examine the mortality experience of a group of workers up to some recent date. In studies of this type, excesses and deficits in mortality usually are expressed as a percentage of an expected death rate based on the mortality experience of some comparison population. This percentage is called a Standardized Mortality Ratio (SMR). It is the ratio of observed to expected deaths usually multiplied by 100 to represent a percentage.

In 1975, the first reported study of this type that related to MMVF was a study of men who had reached age 65 and had retired during 1945–1972 from six plants. The men were engaged mainly in the production of fibrous glass insulation (14). These workers were followed for deaths through 1972 by using company records. Their mortality rates were compared with those of all US men of the same age who lived in the same time periods. The death rate for this cohort was low, with an SMR for all causes of death of only 85. That is, the all-cause death rate was 85% of the death rate that would have been observed had the cohort experienced the same mortality experience as US men living at the same ages during the same time period. There was no excess for any cancer. Also included was a study of men who retired for disability during the same period from the same six plants. The distribution of reasons for disability were compared with disability retirements as reported by the US Social Security Administration for the entire US. The causes of disability were similar in these two groups and did not suggest any important health hazards.

In the 1970s, NIOSH initiated mortality studies of workers from two large MMVF production facilities. One was a study of the mortality experience of men initially employed in 1940–1949 and who had five or more years employment in fibrous glass production, packing, or maintenance by June 1, 1972 (4). Mortality was reported as of June 1, 1972. These workers were from the same plant where workers had been studied with chest x-rays (9, 34, 51, 54). The results were expressed as SMRs, as in the 1975 study described above, with the mortality experience of workers compared with the mortality experience for men living in the United States at the same ages and time periods as the workers under study. There were no important excesses for any cancer and no relationship between respiratory cancer and time since first exposure to MMVF. As noted earlier, if MMVF were a cause of respiratory cancer, one would expect an excess to show up some years after exposure started, a period thought for asbestos to be roughly 20 years. Thus, time since first exposure is important in epidemiological studies of cancer. The NIOSH study was accompanied by an industrial hygiene survey, which showed average fiber concentration in the plant to be .08 f/cc. For fibers examined, the median fiber diameter was 1.8 μm with 85% of the fibers less than 5.3 μm. Median length was 28 μm with 89% less than 50 μm (4).

In one part of the fibrous glass plant, there had been production of special purpose fine fibers. Based on surveys of this and other plants, it was concluded that the concentration of airborne fibers where there was fine fiber production was much higher than in the other areas. To evaluate the potential carcinogenicity of exposure to these fibers, a case-control study was carried out. For each malignant respiratory disease death in the overall study, a control was selected sequentially from an alphabetized list of all members of the study population matched on birthdate, plus or minus six months, and on race and sex. Of the 16 respiratory cancer deaths, four were employed in the section of the plant where fine fibers were believed to have been produced; of the 16 matched controls, none were employed in this area. This relationship was of borderline statistical significance (4). There was a controversy between the research group and the owners of the plant regarding which of the cases and controls were actually exposed to fine fibers and how the analysis should have been done (27). Perhaps as a result, this part of the report was not given wide distribution.

The second NIOSH study was of men who worked a year or more during 1940–1948 in a plant that had produced rock/slag wool (35, 42). This plant was the one studied many years earlier by Metropolitan Life (6). These workers were followed for death through 1974. This plant was selected by the investigators as being one of the oldest rock/slag wool plants in the United States and one which had a sizable workforce. Thus, this plant was perhaps the one most likely to show excesses in cancer and respiratory disease if, in fact, exposure to rock/slag wool fibers had such health effects. There was no excess in all causes of death when compared with US white men, but a slight excess (SMR = 102) for all cancers. This excess was primarily due to digestive cancer, for which the SMR was 130. For respiratory cancer, the SMR was 89. The study provided some evidence of occupationally related digestive cancer, as the SMRs for this condition increased with time since first exposure and with duration of exposure. There were no such trends for lung cancer. As in the study by Bayliss et al (4), this study included the results of an industrial hygiene survey. The overall average fiber level for the plant was .06 f/cc. The fiber diameters ranged from 1.7 μm to 2.7 μm, and lengths ranged from 6.8 μm to 24.8 μm.

By the early 1970s, the US MMVF producing industry became sufficiently concerned about the possible carcinogenic effects of MMVF to commission a large industrial hygiene study and a large mortality study of several plants located in the United States. The industry was represented in this effort by TIMA, a group that has had a long interest in the health of its workers. A total of 17 plants were selected for study, of which six produced rock and/or slag wool, and three produced glass filament. Eight engaged primarily in the production of glass wool, one of which produced only special purpose fine fiber. One of the glass wool plants was the subject of an earlier mortality study by Bayliss et al (4), and one of the rock/slag wool plants was studied by Ness et al (35) and Robinson et al (42). These 17 plants were thought at the time to be among the oldest in the United States. Thus, they represented a workforce that was likely to have had long exposure with ample opportunity for cancer to occur if, in fact, exposure to MMVF is related to cancer. Moreover, the plants were not thought to have ever used asbestos, as asbestos exposure would confound the findings.

Over 17,000 men were identified as having a year or more experience in MMVF production during 1945–1963. In the most recent report on this study, follow-up for deaths was through 1985 and represented nearly a half million person years at risk (31). In calculating expected numbers of deaths, the mortality experience of the male population in the areas where the plants were located was used, rather than the population of the entire US as in earlier studies. This method is believed to be superior because there are geographic variations in mortality probably related to cultural, ethnic, and socioeconomic factors, which probably are reflected in the mortality experience in individual plants. To some extent, the use of local area mortality to calculate expected deaths corrects this variation.

For all of 1946–1985, there were statistically significant excesses in mortality for all causes of death (SMR = 103), all malignant neoplasms (SMR = 110), respiratory cancer (SMR = 120), nonmalignant respiratory disease (SMR = 112), and nephritis and nephrosis (SMR = 146). The elevated death rate for all causes of death in this group of workers was somewhat surprising, as most studies of employed populations show that they are healthier than the general population from which they are drawn. Persons healthy enough to work would not ordinarily include persons in institutions or disabled persons, for example. These groups are likely to have high death rates and they are represented in the general population.

Table 4   Observed (Obs) deaths and SMRs for respiratory cancer, 1946–1985, by production process, plant, and time since first employment: US study

Production Process	Plant	<20 y		20 + y	
		OBS	SMR	OBS	SMR
	Total	14	61.3	70	111.9
Fibrous	2	3	29.1[a]	36	128.1
Glass	5	2	45.8	18	94.4
Filament	16	9	110.6	16	104.0
	Total	60	104.3	280	113.5[a]
Fibrous	1	4	76.8	13	95.4
Glass	4	12	124.9	32	113.8
Wool	6	6	109.2	14	108.2
	9	31	110.6	197	114.5
	10	0	0.0	1	105.8
	11	2	59.6	11	138.7
	14	2	106.1	2	43.8
	15	3	88.4	10	155.4
	Total	15	141.6	58	134.2[a]
Rock/slag	3	3	124.6	13	79.2
Wool	7	2	222.4	5	318.1[a]
	8	2	141.6	4	74.0
	12	4	247.8	8	231.8
	13	1	92.6	5	209.3
	17	3	94.3	23	164.3

[a] p less than .05

Table 4 shows the main findings from the US MMVF workers study as they relate to respiratory cancer. For each of the 17 plants studied, respiratory cancer SMRs less than 20 years since first exposure and 20 years or more since first exposure were found. Numbers of workers studied were small in many plants, and there is considerable variation in SMRs among plants. Only special purpose fine fibers were produced in plant 10. There were only 96 workers studied from this plant. Special purpose fine fibers also were produced occasionally in plants 1, 6, and 9.

For fibrous glass filament and fibrous glass wool plants, SMRs 20 years since first exposure were similar, and for glass wool plants the SMR was statistically significantly elevated. The SMR for rock/slag wool plants was considerably higher than for glass wool plants and was statistically significantly elevated. Although the SMR of 113.3 for fibrous glass wool plants was statistically significant, the magnitude of the excess is not large and could be due to confounding by factors not considered in the study. The SMR of 134.2 for rock/slag wool workers is more likely to be important and, because of its magnitude, is less likely to be due to confounding.

An exposure estimate was made for each worker. Mean worker exposure was estimated to be .351 f/cc for mineral wool workers, .039 for fibrous glass workers (but .292 for workers from the plant that produces special purpose fine fibers), and .009 f/cc for workers producing glass filament (15). These levels for glass fiber exposure are very low when compared with data shown in Table 1. This difference may be because they represent a time weighted exposure of workers across all jobs, many of which had little exposure. On the other hand, exposure levels may have been underestimated in the US study.

In the latest update of the US study, a Poisson regression modeling of SMRs for respiratory cancer was carried out. Several models were tested. In one model, the covariates production process (as shown in Table 4), year of hire, time since first employment, and duration of employment were considered in combination for the total MMVF cohort. None of these factors were found to be statistically significantly related to SMRs for respiratory cancer. Other models, which used other combinations of covariates, including level of fiber exposure, were tested and none were found to be statistically significant. The entire process was repeated, and fibrous glass workers and rock/slag wool workers were examined separately. The only positive result was a statistically significant variability among plants in the rock/slag wool group after other factors (covariates), possibly related to mortality from respiratory cancer, were considered. This result can be seen easily by examining Table 4. Twenty years or more since first exposure, four of the six mineral wool plants had elevated SMRs, and one was statistically significant; two had SMRs that were low.

Another part of the most recent analysis was an examination of respiratory cancer mortality among workers who had exposure to special purpose fine fibers. In an earlier update, there appeared to be a good relationship between SMRs for these workers and time since first exposure. In the latest update, however, this relationship is considerably weaker.

In the latest update of the US study, there were four deaths from malignant pleural mesothelioma, according to information on death certificates. Only two of these deaths were coded to cause of death rubrics, which generally are recognized as being consistent with the diagnosis of malignant pleural mesothelioma. Using deaths coded to these rubrics for the entire United States indicates that two deaths in a cohort of the size studied in the US MMVF study is not a significant excess. Malignant mesothelioma is a feature of asbestos exposure, and the fact that the disease was not in excess in the US study is reassuring.

A study parallel to the one conducted in the United States was initiated in Europe in 1976 and supported by the Joint European Medical Research Board, a registered charity funded by the European MMVF industry (44). This study investigated the mortality of about 21,000 workers from 13 plants

Table 5 Observed (Obs) deaths and SMRs for lung cancer[a] by production process and time since first employment: European and US studies

| Production Process | Study | Time Since First Exposure | | | |
| | | <20 y | | 20 + y | |
		OBS	SMR	OBS	SMR
Fibrous Glass Filament	European	15	115.4	0	—
	U.S.	14	61.3	70	111.9
Fibrous Glass Wool	European	47	95.3	46	111.4
	U.S.	60	104.2	280	113.5[b]
Rock/Slag Wool	European	47	114.4	34	139.9
	U.S.	15	141.6	58	134.2[b]

[a] Respiratory cancer for US
[b] p less than .05

in seven Western European countries. Workers were followed for deaths from the beginning of MMVF production, which ranged from 1933 to 1961, through 1982. Of the total workers studied, about 10,000 were engaged in the production of rock/slag wool, 8000 in glass wool production, and 3500 in continuous glass filament production. In total, there were 364,000 person-years at risk.

For workers with one year or more work experience, the SMR for all causes of death was slightly elevated (SMR = 102), based on a comparison with national death rates in the seven countries where the plants were located. The elevation was statistically significant for all malignant neoplasms (SMR = 109), for lung cancer (SMR = 128), and for violent deaths (SMR = 117). There was one death from malignant mesothelioma, which was not an excess. Table 5 compares data on lung cancer from the European study with data on respiratory cancer (474 out of 497 were lung) from the US study. In this table, local death rates were used to calculate expected deaths for both the US and the European studies.

Agreement between the US and European findings is good for workers 20 years or more since first exposure for fibrous glass wool and rock/slag wool. No deaths in the 20 years or more since first exposure were observed for fibrous glass filament in the European study, although 2.3 were expected. The biggest discrepancy in findings is between rock/slag wool workers less than 20 years since first exposure. The SMR of 141.6 for this group in the US study is puzzling; if mineral wool behaves like asbestos in producing cancer, one would not expect see an excess in such a short period. This elevation in the SMR possibly is due to chance. It also is possible that there was some worker selection for respiratory cancer in the US study, such as a cancer hazard in work before employment in the rock/slag wool industry or habits associated with respiratory cancer, such as cigarette smoking. Twenty years or more since first exposure, SMRs are almost identical for both glass wool and for rock/slag wool workers in the two studies.

In the European study, levels of exposure were not quantified. Rather, "technological phases," which reflected different levels of exposure to fibers at different time periods, were identified. For workers engaged in rock/slag wool production, there was a strong relationship between SMRs for lung cancer and technological phase: an SMR of 257 for workers who were present during the early technological phase when exposure was believed to be the highest; 141 for workers present in the intermediate phase; and 111 for those who worked only in the late phase, when exposure was probably the lowest. Twenty years or more since first exposure, the decreasing trend for lung cancer from the early to the late technological phase was statistically significant. For workers engaged in the production of glass wool, SMRs were much lower and were unrelated to technological phase. As in the American study, there was no relationship between lung cancer and duration of employment. There was, however, some relationship with time since first exposure. Perhaps the most striking feature of the European study was that the lung cancer excess seen for rock/slag wool workers in the early technological phase was predicted based upon their likely level of fiber exposure.

In 1987, the IARC Working Group evaluated the carcinogenic risk of MMVF based upon epidemiologic data (25). The principal mortality data used in the evaluation were an earlier report on the US study (15) and the European study (44), plus a Canadian study of glass wool workers in a single plant, which showed a substantial and statistically significant SMR for lung cancer of 194, 20 years or more since first exposure (43). The Working Group concluded that there is inadequate evidence for the carcinogenicity of glass wool and of glass filament in humans and that there is limited evidence for the carcinogenicity of rock/slag wool in humans. No data were available at that time with regard to carcinogenicity of ceramic fibers to humans.

IARC OVERALL EVALUATION

The overall evaluation of carcinogenicity of MMVF based on experimental, human, and other data was that glass wool is possibly carcinogenic to humans. This overall classification is based mainly on animal data. Glass filaments were considered not classifiable to the carcinogenicity to humans. Rock/slag wool was classified as possibly carcinogenic to humans, with this classification based largely on human evidence. Ceramic fibers were classified as possibly carcinogenic to humans, with this classification based on animal data.

DISCUSSION

Nonasbestos mineral fibers cause cancer in humans, as evidenced by the relationship between the fiber zeolite and mesothelioma in Turkey (3). Also, some MMVF clearly causes cancer in animals. The carcinogenicity of these fibers likely is related to their durability, their dimensions, and the dose of fibers received to target tissue. These factors sometimes are referred to as the three Ds: Dose, Dimension, and Durability. In this regard, MMVF differs widely, with some too large to be respirable and some perhaps more durable than asbestos. Thus, given the right combination of durability and dimension, and a sufficient dose, some MMVF probably present a significant risk to humans. Special purpose fine fibers and ceramic fibers currently are the most likely candidates. These fibers constitute a very small percentage of total MMVF production today. Special purpose fine fibers make up less than 1% of glass fiber production and the current market for ceramic fibers is very small (49). Nearly all MMVF produced are in the form of glass filament and ordinary glass or rock/slag wool.

Glass filament is unlikely to pose a significant cancer hazard to humans, as the diameters of these fibers usually are too large to be respirable, and epidemiologic studies clearly are negative. Epidemiologic data on glass wool fiber workers could be interpreted as negative, but given the respirability and durability of some of these fibers, coupled with the results of animal investigations, they likely pose a small risk where exposures are high.

The epidemiologic data for rock/slag wool workers appears positive. Only the US study estimated fiber exposure. Although this is high (.351 f/cc) for rock/slag wool workers relative to exposure levels for glass wool workers (.039 f/cc), this level of exposure would probably not produce a detectable excess in respiratory cancer even if the fibers were asbestos. At a 1982 meeting in Copenhagen, findings from the US, European, and Canadian studies were presented. McDonald (32) reviewed the combined studies and felt that, given the low exposure levels, a greater excess in lung cancer would not be observed "even if we were dealing with asbestos." In reviewing updated data in 1986, Doll (10) made a similar comment. He felt that the very low fiber counts observed were difficult to associate with any risk, given our knowledge of the effects of chrysotile asbestos, and that the observed risk would suggest that MMVF must be more carcinogenic than chrysotile asbestos. There is nothing about the fibers themselves, however, and there is little in animal experiments that would suggest that these fibers are, indeed, more carcinogenic than asbestos. In fact, just the opposite seems to be the case. In nearly all animal experiments, in which asbestos is used as a control, the tumor incidence in animals exposed to MMVF is considerably lower than in animals exposed to asbestos. Doll has suggested that perhaps the historic exposure estimates used in epidemiologic studies are wrong either for MMVF or for asbestos or both. An important question is whether dust suppressants were used at the times at which workers in the two large epidemiologic studies of MMVF were exposed. In the European study, if dust suppressants were not used, fiber levels could have been 10–26 f/cc. Given that the duration of exposure lasted about two years, the excess observed in slag wool workers in the early technologic phase . . . "lies within the dose-response estimate from other studies on workers exposed to chrysotile asbestos" (44). In the US study, dust suppressants presumedly were used. If they were not, exposure estimates probably are much too low.

Were the excesses observed in rock/slag wool workers possibly caused by something other than MMVF exposure? One explanation is that asbestos was used in rock/slag wool plants, which is the reason for the excess. A study of lung tissue from workers in the US studies shows the presence of amosite asbestos for workers from two rock/slag wool plants—one with a high and one with a low respiratory cancer SMR 20 years or more from first exposure (13, 33). In both the US and the European studies, the respiratory cancer SMR for plants in which asbestos may have been used is about the same as in the plants in which it is believed asbestos was not used. Nevertheless, asbestos exposure in some plants probably made a contribution, but it does not explain all of the excess.

Contaminants other than asbestos in the plants under investigation may have played a role, as some are likely carcinogens. In the European study, however, no evidence could be found to suggest that the use of bitumin or pitch or the use of formaldehyde as a resin binder, all of which have been implicated as carcinogens, had any effect on lung cancer mortality.

There is some evidence that the excess in rock/slag wool workers was due to the use of slag, which was contaminated with some cancer causing agents (12, 31). In the US study, two of the six rock/slag wool plants originally were rock wool plants, and these plants had a low respiratory cancer SMR 20 years or more since first exposure (plants 3 and 8 in Table 4). Many of the workers studied from these plants worked during later periods when slag was used, however, so the low death rates cannot be attributed entirely to the absence of slag exposure. In the European study, however, there were some plants that never used slag; these plants had no excess in lung cancer 20 years or more since first exposure (SMR = 91). In both the US and the European studies, the respiratory cancer SMR was highest in plants in which slag, which was believed to be contaminated with arsenic, was received from copper smelters. Thus, in both the US and the European studies, the use of slag in producing wool may have played a role in the respiratory cancer excess seen. It would be important to study further the possible role of contaminants in slag used to produce MMVF and to determine whether they are incorporated in the fibers themselves or only present in the work environment. Nearly all rock/slag wool currently produced in the US is made from slag.

As Pott (38) pointed out, many questions about MMVF have yet to be answered. The role of surface properties of fibers is unclear. Also, it is not certain how durable a fiber needs to be to initiate the carcinogenic process. How long do fibers have to stay in the bronchial wall or serosa tissue to cause an alteration that can lead to the development of a tumor without the further presence of fibers? Does a longer persistence time lead to a proportionately greater effect? Should the persistence time be longer in humans than in rats?

Over the past few years there has been a trend to the production of smaller diameter MMVF because of their superior insulation and other properties. Moreover, the gradual removal of asbestos from the marketplace has stimulated the production of asbestos substitutes with properties that made asbestos both useful and dangerous. Most MMVF now in production are much less hazardous than asbestos, and some MMVF present no significant cancer hazard. Nevertheless, exposure to MMVF should be regulated in the same manner as exposure to asbestos. As is true for asbestos in many countries, some types of MMVF should be regulated at lower levels than others. Some uniform method is needed to test for the carcinogenicity of MMVF now in use. Even more important, new forms of MMVF should be tested before they are widely produced, and the production of fibers most likely to pose a health hazard should be discouraged.

Literature Cited

1. Assuncao, J., Corn, M. 1975. The effects of milling on diameters and lengths of fibrous glass and chrysotile asbestos fibers. Am. Ind. Hyg. Assoc. J. 36:811–19
2. Balzer, J. L. 1976. Environmental data: airborne concentrations found in various operations. In Occupational Exposure to Fibrous Glass, A Symposium, US Dep. Health, Educ. Welf. HEW Publ. No. (NIOSH) 76–151, pp. 83–89. Washington, DC:HEW
3. Baris, Y. I. 1980. The clinical and radiological aspects of 185 cases of malignant pleural mesothelioma. In Biological Effects of Mineral Fibers, ed. J. C. Wagner, 30:937–47. Lyon, France: IARC Sci. Publ.
4. Bayliss, D., Dement, J., Wagner, J. 1976. Mortality patterns among fibrous glass production workers-provisional report. See Ref. 2, pp. 349–63
5. Bellmann, B., Muhle, H., Pott, F., Konig, H., Kloppel, H., et al. 1987. Persistence of man-made mineral fibres (MMMF) and asbestos in rat lungs. Ann. Occup. Hyg. 31:693–709
6. Carpenter, J. L., Spolyar, L. W. 1945. Negative chest findings in a mineral wool industry. J. Indiana State Med. Assoc. 38:389
7. Cherrie, J., Dodgson, J., Groat, S., Maclaren, W. 1986. Environmental surveys in the European man-made mineral fiber production industry. Scand. J. Work Environ. 12(1):18–25
8. Cherrie, J., Krantz, S., Schneider, T., Ohberg, I., Kamstrup, O., Linander, W. 1987. An experimental simulation of an early rock wool-slag wool production process. Ann. Occup. Hyg. 31(4B):583–93
9. Detreville, R. T. P., Hook, H. L., Morrice, G. 1970. Fibrous glass manufacturing and health: Results of a comprehensive physiological study: Part II. Trans. Ind. Health Found., Pittsburgh. Proc. 35th Annu. Meet., Bull. No. 44:103–11
10. Doll, R. 1987. Symposium on MMMF,

Copenhagen, Oct. 1986: Overview and conclusions. *Ann. Occup. Hyg.* 31:805–19

11. Enterline, P. E. 1981. Proportion of cancer due to exposure to asbestos. *Proc. of the Conf. on the Quantif. of Occup. Cancer, Banbury Rep.* 9: *Quantif. Occup. Cancer.* Cold Spring Harbor, NY: Cold Spring Harbor Lab.

12. Enterline, P. E. 1990. Role of man-made mineral fibers in the causation of cancer. *Br. J. Int. Med.* 47:145–46

13. Enterline, P. E. 1990. Letter to the Editor. *Br. J. Int. Med.* 47:646–47

14. Enterline, P. E., Henderson, V. 1975. Mortality and morbidity experience of retired fibrous glass workers. *Arch. Environ. Health* 30:113–16

15. Enterline, P. E., Marsh, G. M. 1987. Mortality update of a cohort of US man-made mineral fiber workers. *Ann. Occup. Hyg.* 31:625–56

16. Esmen, N., Corn, M., Hammad, Y., Whittier, D., Kotsko, N. 1979. Summary of measurements of employee exposure to airborne dust and fiber in 16 facilities producing man-made mineral fibers. *Am. Ind. Hyg. Assoc.* 40:108–17

17. Esmen, N. A., Hammad, Y., Corn, M., Whittier, D., Kotsko, N., et al. 1978. Exposure of employees to man-made mineral fibers. *Environ. Res.* 15:265–78

18. Esmen, N. A., Sheehan, M. J., Corn, M., Engel, M., Kotsko, N. 1982. Exposure of employees to man made vitreous fibers. Installation of insulation materials. *Environ. Res.* 28:386–98

19. Deleted in proof

20. Feron, V. J., Scherrenberg, P. M., Immel, H. R., Spit, B. J. 1985. Pulmonary response of hamsters to fibrous glass: chronic effects of repeated intratracheal instillation with or without benzo (a)pyrene. *Carcinogenesis* 6:1495–99

21. Gardner, L. U. 1942. Ann. Rep. Saranac Lab. Study Tuberculosis

22. Gross, P., Braun, D. C. 1984. *Toxic and Biomedical Effects of Fibers,* p. 154. Park Ridge, NJ: Noyes

22a. Gross, P., deTreville, R. T. P., Tolker, E. B., Kaschak, M., Babyak, M. A., et al. 1967. Experimental asbestosis. The development of lung cancer in rats with pulmonary deposits of chrysotile asbestos dust. *Arch. Environ. Health* 15:343–55

23. Gross, P., Kaschak, M., Tolker, E. B., Babyak, M. A., deTreville, R. T. P. 1970. The pulmonary reaction to high concentrations of fibrous glass dust. *Arch. Environ. Health* 20:696–704

24. Hohr, D. 1985. Investigations by transmission electron microscopy of fibrous particles in ambient air (Ger.). *Staub. Reinhalt. Luft* 45:171–74

25. IARC. 1988. *IARC Monogr. Evaluation of the Carcinogenic Risk of Chemicals to Humans,* Vol. 43: *Man-made Mineral Fibers and Radon.* Lyon, France: IARC

26. Int. Programme Chem. Saf.-WHO. 1988. Environmental health criteria 77-Man-made mineral fibres. Geneva: WHO

27. Konzen, J. L. 1976. Rebuttal on the mortality patterns among fibrous glass workers by D. Bayliss et al. *Natl. Tech. Inf. Serv.,* No. BP-257-784, Mar. 16

28. Konzen, J. L. 1980. *Man-made vitreous fibers and health.* Presented at Natl. Workshop on Substit. for Asbestos, US Environ. Prot. Agency and US Consum. Prod. Saf. Comm., July 14–16

29. Kuschner, M. 1987. The effects of MMMF on animal systems. *Ann. Occup. Hyg.* 38:791–97

30. Kuschner, M., Wright, G. W. 1976. The effects of intratracheal instillation of glass fiber of varying size in guinea-pigs. See Ref. 2, pp. 151–68

31. Marsh, G. M., Enterline, P. E. 1990. Mortality among a cohort of US man-made mineral fiber workers: 1985 follow-up. *J. Occup. Med* 32:594–604

32. McDonald, J. C. 1984. Peer review: mortality of workers exposed to MMMF-current evidence and future research. In *Biological Effects of Man-Made Mineral Fibers,* pp. 369–80. *Proc. WHO/IARC Conf.* Copenhagen: WHO Reg. Off. Eur.

33. McDonald, J. C., Case, B. W., Enterline, P. E., Henderson, V., McDonald, A. D., et al. 1990. Lung dust analysis in the assessment of past exposure of man-made mineral fiber workers. *Ann. Occup. Hyg.* 34:427–41

34. Nasr, A. N. M., Dtichek, T., Scholtens, P. A. 1971. The prevalence of radiographic abnormalities in the chests of fiber glass workers. *J. Occup. Med.* 13:371–76

35. Ness, G. O., Dement, J. M., Waxweiler, R. J. 1979. A preliminary report of the mortality patterns and occupational exposures of a cohort of mineral wool production workers. In *Dusts and Diseases,* ed. R. A. Lemen, J. M. Dement, pp. 233–49. Park Forest, Ill: Pathotox

36. Ohberg, I. 1987. Technological development of the mineral wool industry in Europe. *Ann. Occup. Hyg.* 31(4B):529–45

37. Ottery, J., Cherrie, J. W., Dodgson, J., Harrison, G. E. 1984. A summary report

on environmental conditions in 13 European MMMF plants. See Ref. 32, pp. 83–117

38. Pott, F. 1987. Problems in defining carcinogenic fibers. *Ann. Occup. Hyg.* 31(4B):799–802

39. Pott, F., Huth, F., Friedrichs, K. H. 1974. Tumorigenic effect of fibrous dusts in experimental animals. *Environ. Health Perspect.* 9:313–15

40. Pott, F., Ziem, U., Mohr, U. 1984. Lung carcinomas and mesotheliomas following intratracheal instillation of glass fibres and asbestos. In *Proc. of the 6th Int. Pneumoconiosis Conf.*, pp. 746–56. Bochum, Germany, Sept. 20–23, 1983, Vol. 2. Geneva: Int. Labour Off.

41. Pott, F., Ziem, U., Reiffer, F.-J., Huth, F., Ernest, H., Mohr, U. 1987. Carcinogenicity studies of fibres, metal compounds, and some other dusts in rats. *Exp. Pathol.* 32:129–52

42. Robinson, C. F., Dement, J. M., Ness, G. O., Waxweiler, R. J. 1982. Mortality patterns of rock and slag mineral wool production workers: An epidemiological and environmental study. *Br. J. Ind. Med.* 39:45–53

43. Shannon, H. S., Jamieson, E., Julian, J. A., Muir, D. C. F., Walsch, C. 1987. Mortality experience of glass fiber workers: extended follow-up. *Ann. Occup. Hyg.* 31:657–62

44. Simonato, L., Fletcher, A. C., Cherrie, J., Andersen, A., Bertazzi, P., et al. 1987. European historical cohort study: extension of the follow-up. *Ann. Occup. Hyg.* 31:603–23

45. Smith, D. M., Ortiz, L. W., Archuletea, R. F., Johnson, N. F. 1987. Long-term health effects in hamsters and rats exposed chronically to man-made vitreous fibers. *Ann. Occup. Hyg.* 31:731–54

46. Stanton, M. F., Layard, M., Tegeris, A., Miller, E., May, M., et al. 1977.

47. Stanton, M. F., Wrench, C. 1972. Mechanisms of mesothelioma induction with asbestos and fibrous glass. *J. Natl. Cancer Inst.* 48:797–821

48. Suzuki, Y., Kohyama, N. 1984. Malignant mesothelioma induced by asbestos and zeolite in the mouse peritoneal cavity. *Environ. Res.* 35:277–92

48a. Thermal Insulation Manuf. Assoc. 1980. *Facts About Man-Made Vitreous Fibers.* 7 Kirby Plaza, Mt. Kisco, NY

49. Thermal Insulation Manuf. Assoc. 1990. *Health and Safety Aspects of Man-Made Vitreous Fibers.* Stamford, Conn: TIMA

50. Timbrell, V. 1976. Aerodynamic considerations and other aspects of glass fiber. See Ref. 2, pp. 33–50

51. Utidjian, H. M. D., Detreville, R. T. P. 1970. Fibrous glass manufacturing and health: report of an epidemiological study. Parts I and II. *Proc. 35th Annu. Meet. Ind. Health Found., Pittsburgh*

52. Vorwald, A. J., Durkan, T. M., Pratt, P. C. 1951. Experimental studies of asbestosis. *Arch. Ind. Hyg.* 3:1–43

53. Weill, H., Hughes, J. M., Hammad, Y. Y., Glindmeyer, H. W., Sharon, G., et al. 1983. Respiratory health in workers exposed to man-made vitreous fibers. *Am. Rev. Respir. Dis.* 28:104–12

54. Wright, G. W. 1968. Airborne fibrous glass particles: chest roentgenograms of persons with prolonged exposure. *Arch. Environ. Health* 21:175–81

55. Wright, G. W., Kuschner, M. 1977. The influence of varying lengths of glass and asbestos fibres on tissue response in guinea pigs. In *Inhaled Particles*, Part 1, ed. W. H. Walton, 4:455–72. Oxford: Pergammon

Carcinogenicity of fibrous glass: pleural response in the rat in relation to fiber dimension. *J. Natl. Cancer Inst.* 58: 587–603

Annu. Rev. Publ. Health. 1991. 12:481–518

THE 20-YEAR EXPERIMENT: ACCOUNTING FOR, EXPLAINING, AND EVALUATING HEALTH CARE COST CONTAINMENT IN CANADA AND THE UNITED STATES

Robert G. Evans, Morris L. Barer, and Clyde Hertzman

Departments of Economics and Health Care and Epidemiology, University of British Columbia, Vancouver, British Columbia, Canada V6T 1Z6

KEY WORDS: North America, health services delivery, health care costs

Cost Control—In Which Direction and by Whom?

Since the late 1960s, concerns over the escalating costs of health care have been expressed with increasing vigor on both sides of the Canada-United States border. This is in sharp contrast with the previous 20 years, during which the principal policy concern was to "meet needs" by finding ways to expand the flow of resources into health care. In retrospect, the turning point in Canada was marked by the 1970 publication *Task Force Reports on the Costs of Health Care* (22). The 1970 Annual Report of the Economic Council of Canada (36) also expressed concern about the cost trends of the 1960s. "Cost Containment" became part of the American health agenda, at least rhetorically, at about the same time. As we attempt to assess the effects of efforts at containment, it is important to remember that before about 1970 no one was really trying. It is only since that time that policies can be said to have "succeeded" or "failed."

Perhaps even more important, not everyone is trying to contain costs now. By accounting definition, the costs of health care (total expenditures) are

481

0163-7525/91/0501-0481$02.00

identically equal to the total incomes earned from its provision. Cost containment is income containment. Those whose incomes, career aspirations, and professional selfexpression are targeted for limitation will always resist. When they are able to organize, and when their incomes are, on average, substantial, the resistance becomes very powerful.

The identity of expenditures and incomes holds no matter how the delivery and payment process may be organized—public or private, centralized or decentralized. Resistance will emerge in any system, independently of any relationship between the level of provision of health care and the needs, however defined, of the population served. Those who would argue that the almost universally expressed concern over "cost explosions" represents a real consensus are being at best naive, at worst deceptive. The objective of containment can only be pursued through conflict between those whose incomes are derived from the provision of care and those who pay for it.

Different forms of organization make this conflict more or less overt or implicit, determine who is drawn into the struggle and how, and influence the terms of the conflict and the balance between gainers and losers (45). Such differences matter; like any conflict within a society, health care finance is not a "zero-sum game." Some structures and processes for managing the opposition of interests may be unambiguously better than others, for (almost) all concerned.

Those of us who ultimately use and pay for care are really not seeking cost minimization, but a balance among multiple objectives: affordability, acceptability, comprehensiveness, effectiveness. "Cost-[containment] alone is an absurd aim. At the limit, an obsession with it drives one inexorably to the zero point . . . " (29). The growing emphasis on containment is rooted in the belief that present systems are not yielding "value for money," that equal or greater benefits of health and satisfaction could be had for lower (or at least less rapidly rising) overall outlays.

Thus, lessons as to the relative success of alternative approaches to cost containment, from the North American (or any other) experience, have to be drawn in the overall context of relative system performance. Successful cost containment must not simply contain costs. Moreover, in that context, clear-cut conflicts of economic interest are inevitably (and often deliberately) intertwined with complex, ambiguous, and sometimes heart-rending questions of social choice.

Canada in a North American Context: Divergent Paths to Different Places

This said, the contrast in aggregate experience on the two sides of the border is dramatic and startling. As shown in Figures 1 and 2, the pattern of growth in aggregate expenditures relative to national income, for both total health care and hospital and medical care, was virtually identical before the 1970s. When both countries wanted to expand, both did so. When both attempted to limit the expansion, Canada was successful. The United States was not. Figures 1 and 2 form the backdrop to all subsequent analysis of cost containment in North America, as research has focused on the components, causes, and consequences of this divergence.

The basic structure of the discussion is now well known from a multitude of papers and articles in the academic, trade, and popular press, official reports and hearings, conferences and conventions, and private conversations. Canada and the United States are as similar as any pair of countries on the globe. They share a common language, have closely interlinked economies and communications media, and have strong similarities of cultural and historical experience and geographic setting. For the last quarter century, however, they have had very different systems for financing hospital and medical care.

In Canada, each of the ten provinces runs a public insurance program, financed from general tax revenue, which pays for "all medically necessary"

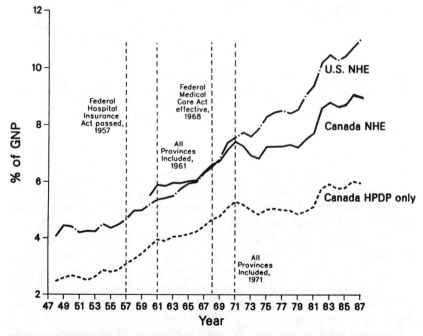

Figure 1   Total health expenditure as share of GNP in Canada and the US, 1948–1987 (HPDP = hospitals, physicians, dentists, and prescription drugs). (Assembled at the Health Policy Research Unit, University of British Columbia, from estimates prepared by staff of the Health Information Division, Health and Welfare Canada, and of the Office of National Cost Estimates, US Health Care Financing Administration.)

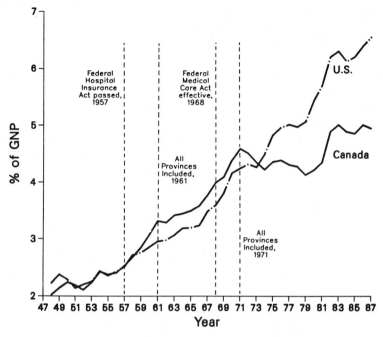

Figure 2   Hospital and physician expenditure as share of GNP in Canada and the US, 1948–1987. (Assembled at the Health Policy Research Unit, University of British Columbia, from estimates prepared by staff of the Health Information Division, Health and Welfare Canada, and of the Office of National Cost Estimates, US Health Care Financing Administration.)

care for all its residents. Physicians are reimbursed according to a periodically negotiated fee schedule, uniform within each province, and hospitals receive an annual global budget. Extra-billing is not permitted, and the patient is not financially involved; there are no point-of-service charges. No correspondingly compact description of health care finance in the United States is possible, but its general features are widely known.

In the late 1960s, when the payment systems began most clearly to diverge, the organization of the delivery of care was also quite similar on both sides of the border. This similarity was reflected in cost performance over the preceding two decades. Since then, there have been substantial changes in the United States, largely in response to pressures created by changes in the financing system.

The result has been a large-scale social experiment, in which each country serves as a quasicontrol against which to identify the impact of policy measures adopted by the other. If we had done what the Americans (Canadians) did, then our experience would have been like theirs—in some presumably connected dimension—accordingly the difference in our experience represents the effect of our policies. The lessons available are thus powerfully extended beyond those which can be inferred from within a single jurisdiction.

Most obviously, the striking differences in cost growth shown in Figures 1 and 2 correlate closely with the Canadian extension of universal public coverage from hospital to physicians' care, and the change in policy emphasis from expansion to containment. *Prima facie* this suggests a causal relationship, and has led many students of health care (including ourselves) to conclude that cost containment in Canada has been not merely a correlate, but a consequence of universal public funding. Sole-source funding, through agencies with the incentives and authority to establish control, appears to be the critical element for cost containment. More generally, as Marmor emphasizes, the "political markets" in which public policy is determined may be balanced or imbalanced (41, 73). The seemingly inevitable escalation of health care costs occurs in an imbalanced market in which the beneficiaries are organized and concentrated, while the losers are not. Concentrating the financing process in one budget balances the interests involved, and enables those interested in control to be more effectively represented.

Interpreting Divergence: The Politics of Comparative Policy Analysis

The validity of the quasicontrolled experiment depends upon the adequacy of the control. If the two countries were identical in all respects, except for their modes of funding of hospital and medical services, then presumably a Canadian system transplanted to the United States would function just as it does in Canada, and conversely. In reality, of course, the comparison is inevitably imperfect. If the countries were identical, after all, how did they come to adopt different funding systems in the first place?

One must be careful, however, to distinguish between other factors, in addition to funding processes, which might bear upon the relative performance of the two health care systems, and those much more general political and cultural differences, which lie behind the evolution of the different funding systems themselves. Whether one could transplant a Canadian-style funding system to the United States, and what the result of such an effort might look like, is a different question from that of identifying the specific features of the two systems that have led to their divergent cost performance.

Current explorations, mostly within the United States itself, of partial or wholesale Canadian system duplication have begun to reveal some deep-rooted political, philosophical, and cultural differences in the two societies, which represent real barriers to importation. But such differences, particularly those of political institutions and culture, do not in themselves invalidate otherwise strong conclusions about the effects of funding processes. Cost differences may be entirely attributable to differences in systems of funding health care, yet politics and culture may underlie the choice of systems, thereby circumscribing the possible means with which to close the cost gap.

The other relevant factors, and the degree to which they differ, are matters for judgment and debate. Since the end of 1988, however, the academic discussion has become entangled with major issues on the domestic American political agenda. The general recognition in the United States that the competitive, market-oriented health care policies of the 1980s have been no more successful than the regulatory policies of the 1970s—if anything, perhaps less so—has led to a remarkable resurgence of interest in foreign models, and in Canada in particular.[1]

The inevitable result has been a polarization of the discussion. Those with an economic, political, or ideological stake in the status quo argue that the two countries are so different in critical respects that the Canadian experience is irrelevant. Those most acutely disturbed by the present American situation downplay the differences in their enthusiasm for an alternative system that has actually been extensively field-tested and appears to work significantly better. Somewhere in between are those analysts [Enthoven (38), Rodwin (76)] who concede the gross inadequacy of the present situation, but believe that it may be possible to build upon strengths in the American environment so as to create a health care system superior to Canadian or Western European models, and *a fortiori* superior to the form those models might take when transplanted into the American environment. Indeed, the peculiar political structure of the United States does raise serious and complex questions as to how a universal public insurance program could be implemented and administered, even if a strong consensus could be reached on its desirability (46).

But, the clash of economic and ideological interests is not restricted to the relevance of the Canadian experience. It spills over into the comparative analysis of the two systems, and the judgments about whether one or the other does work better. Those American individuals and organizations whose interests would be threatened by such imports have reacted in a perfectly

[1]A good argument can be made that these labels were as much rhetoric as substance. American advocates of competition in health care can claim with some justice that their policies have never seriously been tried. But, with equal justice, Marmor has referred to the regulators of the 1970s as "scared of their own shadows"—in the United States, serious regulation was never tried either. In fact, one could argue that competition in the 1980s in the United States has been more highly regulated than regulation in the 1970s. In any case, a policy that cannot be implemented is still a failed policy.

predictable and understandable way through what can be described, depending upon one's point of view, as either informational or smear campaigns.[2]

A particularly blatant example was the American Medical Association's (AMA) 1989 fund-raising letter to its members: "We need your support now. We need your help to continue reaching millions of Americans. We must tell them the facts about the hidden dangers in a Canadian-type health care system—before it's too late." The alleged hidden dangers all stem from the comparative success of the Canadian system in containing costs, and thereby underfunding health care—or at least physicians' incomes.

On the other hand, spokespersons for the American insurance industry have claimed that the Canadian health care system has not been more successful in containing costs, which if true would make the concerns of the AMA somewhat less clear. Because the message of Figures 1 and 2 is fundamental to the rest of this paper, these arguments deserve detailed consideration at this point.

But Is Canada Real? The Politics of Denial

The major theme is that comparisons based on shares of the Gross National Product (GNP) are invalid, because they reflect trends both in health care and in overall economic growth. Comparisons of per capita spending trends are offered as a superior indicator of relative success in cost containment. In particular, it has been alleged that the divergence in share of GNP spent on health care after 1970 results, not from slower growth in health care costs in Canada, but from faster growth in GNP (47).

Such an experience would still be unusual, because the conventional wisdom among students of international health cost comparisons is that the income elasticity of health spending is greater than unity. As a general tendency, leaving aside short-term effects of the business cycle, nations with higher per capita incomes spend a larger, not a smaller, share on health. Why then would the Canadian share *fall* with rising incomes?

But the real situation is much simpler. The apparently much more rapid growth in the Canadian economy is largely an illusion, a result of a higher overall inflation rate (45). If one adjusts for differences in inflation, the growth in real output per capita has been similar in the two economies over the post-1970 period. Between 1970 and 1984, the annual average rate of growth in constant dollar GNP was 2.16% in Canada, and 1.73% in the US.

---

[2]A more subtle blocking tactic, which has the strength of recruiting the research community in an exercise that is more legitimate from their perspective is the discovery that other countries— the 1990 favorite is Germany—are in some crucial respects more similar to the United States. Changes in American health policy should then wait upon more detailed study of circumstances in those countries.

An annual advantage of 0.42% is nowhere near large enough to explain the discrepancies in Figures 1 and 2. Indeed, a principal reason for using the GNP as a denominator is to adjust for such inflation differentials. Per capita comparisons, on the other hand, are very sensitive to the exchange rates used for currency conversion, which have been subject to large fluctuations over this period.

The key point, however, is that the national accounts of the two countries do not show large differences in per capita growth rates over the relevant period. On the other hand, studies of long-term trends in productivity in the Organization for Economic Cooperation and Development (OECD) nations do show a significant growth advantage for Canada (59, 63). But, these comparisons of output per worker, which are adjusted for changes in capital stock, participation rates, terms of trade, etc., are not equivalent to measures of overall economic capacity.

Furthermore, such data also show an advantage for Canada in the pre-1971 period. The convergence hypothesis, which these data support, postulates that other industrialized countries are slowly catching up to the leader in output per worker—the US—but the catch-up process was at work long before 1971. Figures 1 and 2 show that Canadian and US experience was parallel before 1971 and diverged afterwards; the break point cannot be explained by long-run productivity trends.

Finally, the divergence in costs after 1971 shows up most prominently in the components of health expenditure covered by the Canadian public plans: hospitals, physicians, and prepayment and administration. For example, from 1971 to 1985, Canadian physicians' share of national income rose by only 3%, from 1.31% to 1.35%. Dentists, not covered by the public plans, increased their share by 35%, from 0.33% to 0.47%. No similar divergence is shown in the US data. The share of the three covered sectors rose in total by 5% over this period, whereas that of the uncovered sectors rose by 40%. A denominator effect should not be so selective (23, 24).

Moreover, the mechanisms whereby these results were achieved are known. A significant contributor has been the more effective price controls in Canada; but these have been the subject of yet another form of confusion. Comparative data on health sector price trends, compiled by the OECD, appear to show little difference between Canada and the United States, and these, too, have been quoted in the American debate. But the OECD analysts compiled these price indexes to be consistent with Consumer Price Indexes, so they excluded services provided through public plans (30)! They thus describe trends in the absence of public control, not in its presence.

After demolition of the major theme—that no containment occurred—there remains a minor theme, that the effect was real but temporary and unsustainable.[3] This draws on arguments by clinicians in the US, that containment is ultimately impossible. Figures 1 and 2 show a substantial containment effect immediately after the introduction of Medicare, followed by more rapid increases in costs in the late 1970s, and a big jump in 1982 that cannot wholly be attributed to the 1982 recession.

Does this pattern reflect a one-time containment effect? As emphasized above, cost containment involves real professional and economic costs for powerful groups in society. The consequent conflict is a permanent feature of a contained system. In the early 1970s, payers had the upper hand in most provinces in Canada. But in the late 1970s, shifts in institutional structure, combined with new provider strategies, changed the balance of forces, and escalation resumed. The 1980s saw the adoption of more radical strategies by payers, and the ratio has been relatively stable since 1982, in the 8.5%–9% range.

There has been a slow upward creep towards 9%, which might be interpreted as weakened control. But, the share of total health expenditure accounted for by the components covered by the public plans—hospitals, physicians, and (most of) prepayment and administration—has fallen. Consequently, their share of GNP has been steady at 5% from 1982 to 1987. The escalation has occurred in components of cost not covered by universal provincial plans.

Furthermore, the cycle of pressure and control unfolds differently in different provinces. Prosperity in Western Canada—oil—led to more relaxed payer attitudes in the late 1970s, followed by much tougher measures in those provinces after the recession of 1982. In the mid-1980s, Ontario increased its spending considerably, only to put on the brakes in the late 1980s. Quebec, for many reasons, has applied tougher controls for more than a decade.

In general, health care costs are constantly tending to explode, and the effectiveness of administrative controls fluctuates with the economic and electoral cycles. The long-term trend, however, shows a substantial degree of control combined with periodic slippage, and there is no reason to expect that pattern to change. The long-run trends, which are frequently identified as undermining cost control—population aging and technological advance—turn out on closer inspection to be sustainable within current constraints (40).

This rather long diversion illustrates the principal effect of the "anti-Canada" campaigns. A great deal of time and energy is expended to get back

---

[3]Some such arguments are based on comparisons over time periods that reach back into the 1960s, when the Canadian Medicare plans covering physicians were not in effect, and the thrust of public policy was still expansion, not containment. Figures 1 and 2 clearly show the policy turning point; the selective choice of time periods for comparison is always a potential source of confusion.

to the starting point. The irony is that the extraction of understanding from the joint North American experience has become increasingly difficult, in direct response to the increasing political relevance of that understanding.

Expanding the Comparative Horizon: North America in International Context

The inferences from the North American experience can be significantly strengthened, however, by broadening one's focus to include the developed countries of Western Europe, Japan, and the South Pacific (72). All have some form of universal coverage, through public or highly regulated quasipublic agencies that either deliver care directly, or pay those who do.[4] Some rely on a single national agency, e.g. the British National Health Service, others have single agencies within each region responsible for providing (Sweden) or paying for (Canada) care. Still others have a small (France) or large (Germany, Japan) number of not-for-profit insurance agencies, but the policies and processes of agencies are tightly regulated and coordinated by government.

Since the late 1970s or early 1980s, virtually all these countries have stabilized their spending on health care (as a share of national income), and some (Denmark, New Zealand, Sweden) have even lowered it (80). The United States is an outlier, by a wide margin. It is also the only nation without a universal funding system. The inference is thus powerfully reinforced that universality, in combination with the development of single source funding and bilateral financial interests and powers, are the conditions for cost containment.

Both are necessary. Universality without single source funding and bilateral negotiations over budgets leads to uncontrolled cost escalation; single source funding without universality leads not to cost control, but to the transfer of costs to other parties (42). But, universality may be the primary factor. Canadian and Western European experience has shown the development of both mandates and mechanisms for cost control, and the concentration over time of funding sources, within the framework of universal systems. Single source funding systems in the absence of universality, such as Medicare in the United States, have resulted not in cost containment but in the transfer of costs from the government budget to those of private insurers and individuals.

---

[4]Some countries also have a small private sector, which overlaps with (the United Kingdom) or substitutes for (Germany) public coverage. The key difference from the United States is that such private systems enroll a small minority (10% or less) of wealthy and generally healthy citizens. Only in the United States are the *low income* (and generally less healthy) citizens partitioned off from the mainstream system.

In the broader international context, Canada is far from being a model of economy. As Figure 3 shows, Canada has the second most expensive health care system in the world, though it is not far above several of the major European nations. If cost control were the only objective, both Canada and the United States should be looking at the United Kingdom or Japan, not studying each other. Thus, the relevance of a focus on North America turns on the exploration of the context in which, and methods by which, cost containment has or has not been achieved, and the balance struck between containment and other health system objectives. Cost containment per se, though it may be surprising to Americans, seems at least during the 1980s to have been the normal experience of developed nations.

Causes and Consequences of Divergence

The research agenda of those studying the North American experience has been dominated by comparisons of aggregate costs and utilization and by the exploration of the effects of particular institutions and processes on these relatively more measurable features—the extended footnotes, as it were, to Figures 1 and 2. Before summarizing the findings of these studies, however, it seems logical to consider the payoff, the benefits in a broad sense, of the two health care systems to the populations that they purport to serve.

Here we distinguish two classes of evidence. One may study the accessibility and acceptability of the different forms of health care, and their associated cost containment processes and outcomes: Are people happy with the way their needs are met? Or, one may try to measure the actual health status of different populations, and the extent to which this might be attributable to

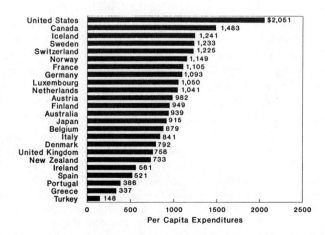

Figure 3   Per capita health spending, 1987 (Source: OECD, Health Data Bank, from Ref. 80).

their respective health care systems: Do the systems work? The data on either dimension of system outcome or effect are not extensive, but are growing; these issues can also be addressed indirectly through some of the data on utilization and cost.

Finally, behind the patterns of cost, utilization, effect, and satisfaction at any point in time are a series of previous decisions about capital formation— the development of numbers and types of physical facilities, skilled personnel, and technological know-how. Today's problems and opportunities largely are the result of capital decisions made years, or even decades, ago. Correspondingly, current investments in buildings and equipment, trained manpower, and research and development have powerful dynamic effects (7).

The relationship among these subcomponents of capital formation is complex, with important elements of both complementarity and substitution. Taken together, however, they have extremely important implications for future trends in access, utilization, and costs and for the sustainability of present patterns. Indeed, on both sides of the border it appears that long-term capital development strategies have been inconsistent with the sustainability of short- and long-term cost containment objectives, and research clearly pointing this out has had little effect.

Spending and Satisfaction: Are the Customers Happy?

Cross-border polling data on individuals' attitudes to their health care systems cast a very interesting light on the North American experience (16, 17). Canadians report a much higher level of satisfaction with their health care system than Americans do; most Americans polled (89%) believe that their system requires fundamental changes or complete restructuring.[5] Indeed, presented with a capsule description of the Canadian system, a substantial majority of Americans (61% in 1988, 66% in 1990) stated that they would prefer that approach to their own system. Only 3% of Canadians expressed a preference for the American way.

These findings confirm Canadian domestic polls, which in turn are reflected in political behavior. Universal health insurance is by far the most popular public program in the country. All the major pieces of federal legislation on which it is based - the Hospital Insurance and Diagnostic Services Act of 1957, the Medical Care Act of 1966, and the Canada Health Act of 1984, were passed unanimously by the federal House of Commons.

---

[5]A majority of those polled expressed satisfaction with their own care. This was true in each of the three systems (17), although many more Americans than Britons or Canadians expressed some degree of dissatisfaction with personal care. Most people in most places have, rightly or wrongly, a considerable degree of confidence in the providers who care for them. But this confidence is distinct from their views about the overall system of health care funding and delivery. American physicians, however, seem predominantly satisfied with their system (58).

Such all-party support is unique to health care and emphasizes the severe political consequences of being perceived as "against Medicare." There is no serious public constituency that is overtly against the present system; those who seek to undermine it do so by expressing general support while recommending specific "improvements."

The simple inference is that cost control is compatible with a high degree of popular support, maintained over decades. Conversely, a high level of spending does not necessarily yield satisfaction ("money can't buy me love"), which is good news for cost containers. A successful control program need not generate a public backlash, and is even consistent with a high level of maintained satisfaction with the overall system.

But, the reality is a bit more complex. The ten-country Harris polls reported by Blendon et al (16) show a consistent positive relationship between per capita spending on health care and expressed level of public satisfaction with health care. The outstanding exception is the United States, where spending is highest and satisfaction lowest. Among universal systems, tighter cost containment may well result in lower levels of satisfaction, a finding again consistent with domestic Canadian polls, which show high levels of support for increased health spending, relative to other potential uses of public funds.

Attempting to draw inferences from the North American experience alone, then, may be misleading insofar as it involves comparing a relatively high cost, but "normal," European-style system (Canada) with a system that has no parallels in the developed world and a uniquely unfavorable combination of costs and satisfaction (the United States). The lesson for the United States might be that a switch to any sort of universal system, if it could be made, could lead to lower cost and increased public support; the lesson for Canada is that when one already has a universal program, there may be a trade-off between cost control and public satisfaction. Countries such as the United Kingdom and Japan, with strong centralized political systems, seem to be able to maintain a tighter grip on costs and to tolerate greater public unhappiness; a wealthier and more decentralized nation may not have this option.[6]

Accessibility: Whose Care is Controlled?

The Canadian system is accessible, as well as acceptable. North American experience suggests that the one follows from the other. As noted, the entire Canadian population is covered "on equal terms and conditions" as the federal

[6]An important distinction emerges from the findings of Blendon et al (16). Controversy over health care finance is universal, which suggests that it results from attempts (successful or otherwise) to control costs, regardless of the actual level of spending. This is predictable, as expenditure control is by definition income control. But it is remarkable that, underlying the public controversy fed by well-defined interest groups, the level of satisfaction of the citizenry is apparently linked to the level of expenditure.

legislation states for all medically necessary hospital and medical care and without direct charge. In the United States, somewhere between 30 and 40 million persons have no insurance coverage, perhaps as many again have coverage wholly inadequate to deal with any serious illness or injury, and most of the population are at risk of some significant financial outlay in the event of illness or injury.[7] Such outlays bear most heavily on those at lower incomes. In consequence, a significant psychological cost of the American funding system is the uncertainty it creates for those with fragile health and fragile finances (2, 86).

Interestingly, polls also indicate that within the United States, dissatisfaction with the health care system is correlated with the experience of out-of-pocket costs (16). This finding suggests that American advocates of increased out-of-pocket charges to contain costs can expect further deterioration in public satisfaction, considerable resistance, and, from the experience of other countries, little or no prospect of success. Direct charges are neither necessary nor sufficient for cost control, and other systems do not rely on them. Some countries, e.g. Canada, Germany, and the United Kingdom, have none. Others, e.g. France and Japan, impose small charges on some of the population; but, there is no apparent relation between such policies and the levels or trends in costs. Only in the United States, again an outlier, are such charges taken seriously as cost containment mechanisms, in the context of largely private insurance.[8]

[7]The continuing efforts to refine the estimates of the number of uninsured Americans appear to us (admittedly outsiders) as pointless and perhaps counterproductive. No one suggests that the number is not so high as to represent a major public issue; what difference does it make whether the number is 30 million or 40 million? To take up scarce research capability and policy attention refining within this range seems to be as wasteful and irresponsible as ordering diagnostic tests that one knows will have no bearing on therapy.

[8]Interestingly, the strongest support for direct charges to patients, both in the United States and out, seems to come from two professional groups—physicians, and economists with a strong ideological commitment to market mechanisms. The former argue that such charges are needed to increase the flow of resources into underfunded health care systems; the latter that they will limit or reverse the growth of costs. Both cannot be right; both groups, however, stand to benefit from such policies.

The benefit to physicians is direct—direct charges to patients undermine efforts by payers to control fees and/or total budgets. Canadian medical spokespersons refer to extra-billing as a "safety valve" to protect physicians against successful cost (income) control. This view, which is consistent with the Canadian and, we believe, European experience (8, 88) is a direct contradiction of the simple-minded economic hypotheses, which link higher direct charges to lower utilization and costs. Nevertheless, policies based upon such hypotheses, whether they are right or wrong, provide professional scope (and employment) for economists skilled in manipulating the intellectual apparatus of supply and demand.

If a surgeon sees every health problem as a surgical diagnosis, then a neoclassical economist sees every human relationsip as a market.

The removal of financial barriers did appear to have a significant effect on patterns of access to health care in Canada. In the early and mid-1970s, several studies were done of the distribution of use of services under universal medical or hospital care coverage (10, 14, 18, 20, 37, 71). The conclusions were consistent; universal coverage resulted in a redistribution of utilization of care from more to less well off individuals, and essentially eliminated income gradients in use.

The establishment of targeted public programs, Medicare and Medicaid, in the United States also had a significant positive effect on access for disadvantaged groups, if not (as the Canadian law requires) on "equal terms and conditions." The difference appears to be that subsequent efforts to contain costs have been applied more stringently in those programs, which has resulted in growing differentials in access. In addition, partial and categorical programs inevitably leave a large pool of under- and uninsured.

Universal Coverage and Cost Containment: Mutual Interdependence

Current proposals to incorporate these groups into the insurance system, e.g. the Pepper Commission, seem to be stonewalled because of their cost implications. Yet, the purported cost implications of such proposals are directly related to the financing system within which the coverage extension would take place. The additional costs of the Pepper Commission proposals could be funded out of the savings represented by the difference between Canada and the United States in health care administrative costs alone. The excessive overhead cost of a pluralistic system of piecemeal and partial coverage—the incomes of administrators, accountants, actuaries, salesmen, lawyers, even economists—exceeds the additional cost of actually providing the currently uninsured with care, in a universal system.

The linkage between universality and cost containment is a two-way street. Failure to achieve universality in the early 1970s has left the United States as the only country unable to contain its costs. Now, politically unacceptable costs or choices appear to make it impossible in the 1990s to extend the present system universally. The great irony here is that cost concerns appear to be the impediment to American movement on universality. Yet, most other developed societies have achieved cost containment, in more or less acceptable ways, because of that very characteristic of their health care financing systems.

Extending coverage, in the absence of any other changes, will indeed have major cost implications. If one is unable or unwilling to take advantage of the potential for cost control in universal coverage, extending coverage becomes simply an add-on to a system without any inherent cost control mechanisms. And the increases in costs will simultaneously be increases in provider incomes. It is thus no coincidence that the AMA supports allegedly universal access through piecemeal extension, while bitterly opposing a universal insurance system (83). But they are not the only providers involved.

Confusion over the linkage between universal coverage, access, and cost containment has led to suggestions in the United States that successful cost control would inevitably require "rationing" of care, which would in turn bear most heavily on vulnerable groups in the population—the elderly or those living in remote regions. The experience of other countries with universal systems has been exactly the opposite. There was a shift of access from higher to lower income persons when universal medical insurance was introduced in Quebec (37). More recent studies in Canada and Australia have shown general growth in the utilization of physicians' services, with much more rapid increases by the elderly population (11, 12, 54). Acute care hospital utilization in Canada has fallen overall, but (age-adjusted, per capita) use by the elderly has fallen less, or has actually increased, depending on the measures used (44, 64).

The geographic distribution of physicians' services remains a contentious issue in Canada, as in many other countries. But, there is no evidence that it is growing more unbalanced (54). Residents in nonmetropolitan areas actually make more use of hospital space, and while they use fewer physicians' services, their access is growing roughly in parallel with that in metropolitan areas. Within the universal programs, a variety of different policies have been tried to encourage physicians to locate outside the metropolitan areas (5). Thus, rather than being a source of further inequality, the universal system provides additional policy levers to try to alleviate the natural tendency for health care providers to concentrate in metropolitan areas.

Indeed, aggregate patterns of physician utilization show remarkably similar trends on both sides of the border, despite major differences in the payment systems, reflecting the parallel growth in physician supply (8). The distribution of care may be different, however; in the United States, lack of insurance coverage, and resultant high out-of-pocket costs, do have a significant effect upon utilization and health for some parts of the population (e.g. 19, 31, 55). The global approaches to cost containment employed in Canada and the European nations apparently facilitate greater equity of access, which is harder to maintain, or in any case has not been maintained, south of the border.

Whether that equity means only that access has been impeded for everyone, the allegation that cost containment in Canada (and presumably *a fortiori* everywhere else in the developed world) has been associated with "rationing" of effective services and thus threats to health and happiness, which would be unacceptable to Canadians if they knew what was happening,[9] raises additional issues of research and evaluation that are best deferred until the discussion of comparative analyses of utilization and costs. First, however, we consider some of the available comparative data on population health status.

Cost Containment and the Health of Populations: What Price Savings?

A health care system cannot be judged simply through a popularity contest. Access is a means to an end, not an end in itself; well-functioning systems deny access to inappropriate or harmful care. Although the linkage is much weaker than most people imagine, societies provide and fund health care for the same reason that individuals seek it and use it. They anticipate some corresponding benefits in terms of improved health. Most of the political conflict over health spending is couched explicitly, though usually inaccurately, in terms of threats to health from inadequate, "underfunded" care. If not enough is spent, people will die, or at least suffer as a result of remediable but unremedied conditions. The British refer to "shroud-waving."

Does cost containment have a cost in terms of health? Are Canadians healthier because their access to care is unimpeded by financial barriers, or are Americans healthier because they spend more on care? And, which Canadians/Americans? The American without insurance? The Canadian without a coronary artery bypass graft? Most of these difficult questions (whom to count, how to weight and aggregate people), are moot because so little is known, in any country, about either the health status of the population or the effectiveness of health care interventions, let alone the connection between the two. One might have hoped that successful cost containment would have been associated with a rapid expansion of such knowledge, because when less is spent it is more important to spend effectively. One would be disappointed.

On the crude macro-indicators of health status, Canada looks better than the United States. Life expectancies at birth are greater; at 73.3 and 80.2 years, Canadian males and females were, by 1987, living on average 1.7 and 1.6 years longer than their US counterparts (92). Moreover, the Canadian data continue to improve, whereas female life expectancy at age 65 in the United

[9]Or at least would be unacceptable to Americans. Because the Canadian health care system is already more expensive than any other in the world outside the United States, this claim can only represent another version of the assumption that everyone else is out of step but Uncle Sam (1). So why are Americans so dissatisfied, and others not?

States has not increased for a decade (48).[10] But, one should not too quickly attribute the Canadian advantage to universal insurance. Life expectancies have been rising faster in Canada for the last 40 years, contemporaneous with, rather than subsequent to, the province-by-province phasing in of universal insurance coverage (84).

Infant death rates, which may be more sensitive to health care, also look better north of the border. Indeed, American infant mortality rates for the late 1980s (10.1 deaths per 1000 live births in 1987) are above any of the countries of Western Europe, and begin to approach those in the former East Bloc countries. Canada, at 7.3 deaths per 1000 births, is roughly in the middle of the range of Western European countries.[11]

The poorer American performance on such gross measures does not, of course, lead to any necessary inferences about the relative effectiveness of different health care systems. It is conceivable that American health care contributes at least as much to the health of its population as does care in Canada and Western Europe, but that other features of American society make the task much more difficult. For example, the US averages may be pulled down by a substantial underclass of poor, and poorly educated, members of minority groups, with very severe health problems, who are less prominent in more homogeneous societies.

Members of an underclass do not come identified as such in statistical tabulations. One can, however, address this point indirectly by comparing regions and subpopulations. The province of British Columbia and the state of Washington are quite similar economically, socially, and geographically; the latter excludes the underclasses of the urban Northeast and the rural Southeast. Yet, male and female life expectancies in British Columbia (total population) exceed those of their counterparts in the white population of Washington by between 1.5 and 2 years. The gap is very similar to the national differences, and has grown by about one half a year between 1975 and 1985 (65).

---

[10]Fries (48) interprets this stability as supportive of a biological limit to the life span. But it is not obvious how this interpretation can be reconciled with the observation that ten other countries show longer female life expectancies than the United States. Japanese females have an advantage of more than three years (92).

[11]The comparison with the countries of Eastern Europe is instructive. Some critics of the Canadian health care system point out that universal insurance is a hollow boast if a system is so inadequately funded or so badly organized that its nominal beneficiaries cannot get adequate or appropriate care at all. Unquestionably, this is a possibility, and it may have some relevance in the formerly socialist countries of Eastern Europe, which have combined rhetorically free access to care with inadequate health care systems. Their aggregate measures of health status are both low and deteriorating (60). But, the criticism clearly has no relevance to Canada, where health indicators are, as in most of the Western European countries, above those of the United States and improving.

This suggests that the aggregate differences apply to the mainstream populations in each country; they are not simply an artifact that results from adding in a disadvantaged subgroup unique to the United States. One cannot conclude from these differences that the US health care system is less effective overall. But one can say two things.

First, the aggregate data definitely do not show any disadvantage to Canada from its lower health spending. Such data are a weak test, but they do provide some opportunity for the "hidden dangers" of universal public health insurance to show themselves in premature mortality. They have not done so.

Second, suppose that one accepts the hypothesis that Americans really do buy more health improvement with their additional spending, but that other features of American society place them at a greater disadvantage, which is only partly compensated by more or better care. It would seem to follow that American *health* policy might be more effective if resources were diverted from the present, uniquely high level of spending on health care, to identify and address some of the other determinants of health which, *ex hypothesi*, place Americans at such a disadvantage. If they spent less on health care, Americans might be healthier, depending, of course, on how the saved resources were used, and by whom.

Although there is no evidence that (relatively) successful cost containment has had a negative effect on health status in Canada, it is intriguing to note that Canadian aggregate mortality data are inferior to those of Japan, by almost the same (large) margins as they surpass those of the United States. And this despite much lower levels of health care spending in Japan and a Japanese health care system described by one external observer as "an anachronism" (62, 74, 80). These observations underscore the inadequacy of current knowledge of the determinants of population health status and demolish the simple-minded assumption of a direct linkage between health care spending and health outcomes.

Moreover, although the removal of financial barriers to health care in Canada appears to have equalized access, it has not equalized health status across socioeconomic classes (88, 89). The finding of socioeconomic gradients in health status is general across developed nations; no form of organization of health care services has eliminated these (35). There is, however, some evidence beginning to emerge that the time lags required to influence such gradients may be much longer than previously appreciated—at least decades—so it may be too soon to tell (13).

Recent data on Canadian infant death rates can be read either way. The social class gradient has narrowed sharply between 1971 and 1986; a gap of 9.8 deaths per 1000 live births between top and bottom income quintiles in 1971 has been reduced to 4.8 in 1986 (88). On the other hand, the ratio of infant mortality rates in the lowest income quintile to that in the highest has

500 EVANS, BARER & HERTZMAN

fallen by only 14.1%. from 1.96 to 1.82. For male babies, the ratio has remained unchanged at 2 to 1, which suggests a constant proportionate risk factor—low income—operating on a falling base rate. Still, the ratio has fallen by one-third for low income female babies, and when one looks at the gradient across income quintiles, rather than just the ratio of highest to lowest, infant mortality rates among the intermediate income quintiles are clearly converging to those of the highest in relative, as well as absolute, terms.

Moreover, data are emerging that show specific health effects of inadequate access to care among subsets of the American population. Failure to contain costs may be harmful to health, insofar as it leads to program cutbacks that bear differentially on marginal or vulnerable groups. To the extent that this is so, an important lesson is that containment pressures that are broadly distributed, are less threatening to health than those which are selective in their impact. The providers of care, when confronted with globally constrained resources, may make allocation decisions that more closely correspond to the needs of patients.

But do they, in fact? Research on variations in medical practice patterns now extends across many nations, with different systems of health care delivery and levels and patterns of funding (3). Several such studies have been done in Canada (77). As in the United States, these studies show large variations in procedural and utilization rates among regions, hospitals, and physicians, which cannot be attributed to any identifiable differences in patient needs (see, e.g. 54). Cost containment does not lead to therapeutic convergence. On the other hand, Chassin et al (26) and Leape et al (67) in the United States have found no support for the assumption that variations in use rates correlate with variations in appropriateness; if they do not, then the presence or absence of practice variations in Canada cannot in itself tell us about the relative prevalence of inappropriate use.

But, when resources are constrained, do the outcomes for particular patients deteriorate? This is the rhetorical cutting edge—the patients who "die on the waiting list" or suffer noisily or in silence. And when they are cared for, do limitations on facilities or technology result in worse outcomes? If, in the United States, those without resources cannot get into the queue at all, this may be small comfort to the Canadian (or German or Englishman) whose prospects for timely and effective care have shrunk with the budget.

Very little research has been done that directly compares patient outcomes across the border, although this is beginning to change. A recent paper compares postsurgical mortality for selected procedures in Manitoba with that in New England (78). For certain high-risk procedures, the New Englanders have better outcomes; for medium and low risk the advantage is with Manitoba. Overall, there is not a lot to choose between the two systems. Certainly there is no support for an argument that the much lower cost of hospital care in

Manitoba is "killing patients." But, are patients perhaps not reaching the hospital at all? Or, going in the other direction, are costs of care perhaps not as different between the two systems as the data displayed in Figures 1 and 2 would suggest? This question, finally, leads into the discussion of the aggregate cost and utilization data, which are both extensive and widely published.

So Where Are the Canadian Savings, and Why Aren't Americans Healthier?

The differential in overall health expenditures, which has emerged since 1971, resolves into three components: costs of prepayment and administration, payments to physicians, and expenditures on hospitals (6, 40, 45). These components correspond to the areas covered by the Canadian public insurance programs.

CANADIANS PROVIDE CARE; AMERICANS SHUFFLE PAPER   Most striking of all is the large gap that has emerged over the last 30 years in prepayment and administration costs (Figure 4). In 1960, these costs were similar (as a

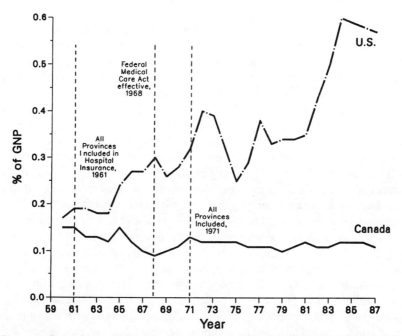

Figure 4 Costs of prepayment and administration as share of GNP in Canada and the US, 1960–1987. (Assembled at the Health Policy Research Unit, University of British Columbia, from estimates prepared by staff of the Health Information Division, Health and Welfare Canada, and of the Office of National Cost Estimates, US Health Care Financing Administration.)

share of national income) in both countries; by now they are between five and six times higher in the United States. The growing complexity of the American health care system, and particularly the more and more elaborate processes being adopted to contain costs, have been associated with a growth in administrative expenses, which has no international parallel.

Cost containment, Canadian-style, does not appear to have large overhead costs; American-style efforts now absorb at least one half a percentage point of national income—tens of billions of dollars—over and above the costs of actually providing care. These expenses are the revenues of American insurance companies, which would disappear in a Canadian-style system. Not surprisingly, the Health Insurance Association of America is critical of the Canadian approach.

The prepayment and administration expenses reported in the health expenditure statistics of each country refer only to the costs of running the agencies responsible for administering the payment process. They do not include administrative costs borne by the providers of care, which have also grown rapidly in the United States in response to the increasing complexity of the payment system. These costs are included in the reported expenditures on the services of the providers themselves—hospitals, physicians, nursing homes. Yet further costs are borne by beneficiaries or their agents. The time and trouble required of patients seeking reimbursement, or corporate outlays on benefits administration, are also much greater in the United States, but are not recorded in any of the comparative data. Thus, the gap shown in Figure 4 significantly understates the true difference in overhead costs.

Such excessive overhead could perhaps be justified if it yielded benefits in the form of a better-managed, more efficient and effective health care system, and/or greater levels of public satisfaction. Under the circumstances, however, it appears to be pure waste motion. It is hard to see how this component of the Canada/United States expenditure gap could have any connection to health outcomes. Indeed, the extra cost may lower the quality of care, if the administrative burden on providers not only increases their financial outlays, but reduces the time and energy they have available to care for patients.

In the case of administrative costs, the connection between accounting for the divergence and explaining it is close. A single payment agency, which covers the whole population and reimburses all providers either on a single fee schedule (physicians) or global budgets (hospitals), can dispense with many of the administrative functions of private insurers. Once a public decision has been made to cover the whole population, on equal terms, such activities as marketing, rate-making, and determining eligibility and coverage in a wilderness of differing contracts, are superfluous. The distinction between accounting and explaining is more important, however, for the other two components, which is where much recent research has been focused.

TRENDS IN PHYSICIANS' FEES: PAYING LESS FOR MORE IN CANADA   The gap in expenditures on physicians' services corresponds to different rates of escalation of fees (6, 8, 49). Over the last 20 years, Canadian physicians' fees have risen at about the same rate as the general price level; in the United States, they have risen considerably faster (as they did in Canada before 1971). The concern by American analysts that bargained fee constraints would simply result in increased billing activity and higher apparent utilization (51) has been found to have some validity (8, 49), but the bargaining process and appropriately structured fee schedules can place limits on this response. Nevertheless, some of the Canadian provinces are beginning to impose various forms of quantity caps, as well. Quebec, with the tightest limits on fee escalation, has the longest experience with such caps (8, 27, 69).

In this area, the Canadian experience and understanding seems to parallel closely that of the American Physician Payment Review Commission (53). Cost containment requires the establishment of uniform fee schedules and elimination of extra-billing by physicians (in American terms, mandatory assignment).[12] From the providers' perspective, extra-billing serves as a "safety valve" whereby they can keep fees escalating more rapidly than the negotiated rates, and keep political pressure on payers to increase those rates. Consistent with this view, fees have risen much more rapidly in Ontario and Alberta, where extra-billing was permitted until 1986, than in Quebec, where it was eliminated in 1970.

The relatively limited research on extra-billing also suggests that it is primarily a way around price controls (90). The optimal situation for the provider is to divert efforts to contain costs into efforts to transfer costs among multiple payers, while permitting the overall cost to escalate (42).

As this discussion suggests, there has been no empirical support for the conventional, positively-sloped supply curve of economic theory. Cost containment through fee restraint leads, at least in the short run, to upward pressure on output, not withdrawal of services. Indeed, the provinces that have imposed caps on overall billing volumes, Quebec and more recently British Columbia, have had the tightest controls on fees. Cost containment might conceivably lead to long run reductions in supply if it discouraged entry to, or encouraged exit from, the profession. This, however, is not happening anywhere in Canada.

---

[12]In the United States, physician billing above scheduled rates or screens is often referred to as "balance billing," which implies that the fee demanded by the individual practitioner is in some sense the "real" bill, and any difference between that and the amount paid by the reimbursing agency is the balance to be paid by someone—usually the patient. Insofar as the reimbursing agency may be attempting to contain costs by restricting the escalation of fees, this language embodies an explicit rejection of the legitimacy of that attempt.

The availability of physicians is high and rising rapidly, although the surge in American production in the last decade has not been matched. By the end of 1990, there will be about 62,000 physicians in Canada, or about 435 persons per physician. The supply is growing, on average, about 2% per year faster than the population (25), and all provinces are struggling with the expenditure implications.[13] In the United States, from 1976 to 1986, physician supply grew on average 3% faster than the population; this rate of growth implies fewer than 400 persons per American physician after 1990 (85).

Canadian physicians are neither abandoning the field, nor working less hard, in response to the less rapid growth of fees.[14] Accordingly, Canadians are not receiving fewer medical services as a result of (relative) cost containment; they may, in fact, be receiving more. But, they pay less (through the tax system) per service. It is not obvious, a priori, why this form of containment should be any more threatening to their health than the reduction in costs of insurance administration.

Interestingly, the long-run picture may be changing in the United States, where applications to medical schools are falling; there are now about 1.7 applicants per place. In Canada, the ratio is still over 4.0 (79). Although the form of containment adopted in Canada has not discouraged entry, it is at least possible that the radical changes in health care delivery and finance in the United States have had this result. But the difference in medical school fees, which are only about $2000 per year in Canada, may also play a role.

WHAT HAPPENS IN HOSPITALS? PLENTY, BUT WITH WHAT EFFECT?   The third component of the cost differential, outlays on hospital care, has been the focus of considerable recent cross-border comparative research. Studies by Detsky et al (32, 33) in Ontario have demonstrated not only the effectiveness of the global budget mechanism in containing costs, but also the selective impact of that constraint on intensity of servicing, i.e. costs per capita or per patient day after adjustment for changes in wages and other input prices. Barer & Evans (6) found similar results from a national data set; the rate of increase of real resources in the hospital sector has been slower in

---

[13]The threat that large numbers of physicians would leave for the United States was part of the original bargaining over Medicare in the 1960s, and arose again in fee bargaining in the 1970s. But, the numbers of out-migrants have never been large (except just after the Viet Nam war), and the threat has long lost its credibility. The "flight of Canadian physicians" is now an American creation, for internal consumption only.

[14]At some level of fee restraint, such responses would undoubtedly be observed. But medicine is still the highest paid occupation in Canada, and the numbers are still climbing as fast as training capacity permits. Physicians in other countries [e.g. Israel (9)] fare relatively much less well economically than their Canadian counterparts, yet there is no shortage of individuals eager to practice medicine.

Canada than in the United States. Newhouse et al (75), after examining data on the over-65 population in selected provinces/states and adjusting for case-mix and length of stay, reached the same conclusion: Differences in intensity of service per patient-day account for most of the difference in per capita costs.

Rates of admission to hospital are very similar in the two countries, about 145 per 1000 population in Canada (64) and about 140 in the United States (34). Patient-days per capita are substantially higher in Canada, about 2000 days per 1000 population, compared with 900 in the United States (52). After adjustment for the high proportion of long-stay patients in Canadian hospitals, the Canadian rate for patients in short-stay units only is about 1250 per 1000 population.[15]

Acute care hospitals in Canada operate at considerably higher average occupancy rates, between 80% and 85%, compared with about 65%–70% in the United States. Thus, the claims in the United States that the Canadian system experiences more crowding, rescheduling of elective surgery, and waiting lists, have some validity. But this is a reflection of more hospital-intensive styles of health care practice, not fewer facilities.

In both countries, efforts to contain hospital costs have been associated with reductions in utilization for acute care patients over the last two decades. But, the mechanisms have been different. The US Prospective Payment System and various forms of private managed care have encouraged hospitals to shorten stays and to provide more care on an outpatient basis. Hospital utilization has dropped, though costs appear to have been transferred from one setting to another, rather than reduced (50). In Canada, there has been a significant expansion of extended care hospitalization in acute care hospitals, which has effectively reduced acute care capacity without actually closing beds (44, 64). Thus, a simple comparison of intensity of servicing in the form of costs per patient-day, adjusted for input prices, would be incomplete and potentially misleading because the mix of patient-days in Canadian hospitals has shifted so much more towards extended care in the last 20 years.

Another important source of difference in hospital costs is the administrative superstructure within the hospital itself. The complexities of the American payment system require a major administrative effort within hospitals to handle the paper flow and the accounting. To the extent, then, that American efforts to contain costs have increased the complexity of the funding and administrative system, they have, in fact, added to costs, but diverted resources away from patient care. A simple comparison of trends in intensity of

---

[15]Reported hospitalization rates differ markedly from one province to another, largely because of differences in the organization of long-term care systems and in the use of hospitals by extended care patients. Long-term care is not part of the federal-provincial insurance program, and so is not standardized across provinces. Interprovincial differences in acute care use are less pronounced, though real.

servicing in Canada and the United States will thus include in the latter the increased services of accountants, public relations specialists, marketers, and administrators who are on the hospital payroll or otherwise part of its budget. But one would be surprised to find that these increased services were associated with increases in patient satisfaction or improved outcomes.

Back-of-the-envelope calculations suggest that these extra administration costs, included as hospital expenditures, are in the tens of billions (61). Expert opinion of hospital administrators with experience on both sides of the border is supportive. Several research studies are currently under way in this area. Katz & Schwendiman (66) have reported a comparison of British Columbia and Washington State, which shows that administrative overhead (in 1988) made up 18.3% of hospital budgets north of the border, compared with 30.3% south of it. Remarkably, according to their admittedly tentative data, this discrepancy accounts for about three quarters of the total difference in hospital spending. They report per capita hospital spending in British Columbia (adjusted to US dollars) as 80.5% of the Washington level; but net of administrative expenditure the ratio is 94.4%.

If this finding is valid and generalizes, it implies that over 10% of American hospital costs are, from the Canadian perspective, waste motion. Moreover, because there is little difference in hospital spending on patient care, there is no obvious reason to expect any difference in patient outcomes. (Hospital spending in British Columbia tends to run below the Canadian national average by about 5%.)

More sharply focused studies of particular procedures on both sides of the border have shown differences in rates of performance for a small set of high profile interventions—cardiac bypass surgery, lens implants, and certain orthopedic procedures—but not differences overall—not for cardiac surgery in total, for example (4). New high technology diagnostic equipment—magnetic resonance imaging, CAT and PET scanners—is also less widely available per capita, though those in Canada may be more heavily used. The Canadian form of cost containment appears to slow the rate of growth of new and expensive procedures, relative to that in the United States, a sort of institutionalized foot-dragging.

Whether this is good or bad for the health of patients is difficult to say; it definitely cannot be assumed a priori that Canadians are necessarily at a disadvantage. On the one hand, the discrepancy between the availability of new facilities and procedures in Canada, compared with the United States right next door, creates great political pressures for expansion that often spill into the media. They feed the eternal provider complaint of "underfunding," as the doctors in the world's second most expensive system compare their facilities with those in the most.

On the other hand, American researchers find evidence of significant overprovision of specific procedures in the American system (e.g. 26), which suggests that Canadian patients may be better off with a more conservative approach.[16] Furthermore, delay is not necessarily bad; mortality and complication rates tend to fall as experience is gained with new procedures. Such rates also fall with increased volume of throughput, which implies that restraining the number of facilities (and practitioners), and thus concentrating cases, can have further beneficial effects (28, 70).

In general, however, the particular procedures, which become foci of political and media attention in Canada and which are seized upon by defenders of the status quo in the United States to illustrate Canadian inadequacies, do not represent major parts of the Canadian health care budget. They become issues because of the *way* in which costs are contained—global restraints—but not *because* costs are contained. The annual increase in payments to general practitioners in a Canadian province would be large enough to double the payments not only for coronary artery bypass surgery, but for all cardiac surgery, with money left over. The political struggles are between payers who want to fund new priorities at the expense of old, and providers who feel that health priorities are, or should be, indefinitely expansible.

Capital Formation and Cost Control: Creating Income Claimants

Lying behind this struggle over social priorities, however, are long-run policies with respect to capital investment in the health care sector. Such capital takes three forms: buildings and equipment, human resources, and new technological know-how (7). As noted above, Canadian policies that have been reasonably successful in achieving cost containment year by year have not been backed up by long-run policies of capital acquisition and deployment, which assist and sustain those constraints. Quite the contrary, for two of the three components of capital, policy has militated against cost containment. Research and analysis pointing out this discrepancy has had little or no impact on either side of the border.

PHYSICIAN MANPOWER: FAULTY FORECASTS HAVE LONG-TERM CONSEQUENCES   Most apparent have been the mismatches between cost containment and manpower training. The 1964 Report of the Royal Commission on Health Services (21), which was the fundamental policy document that led to the extension of public insurance coverage from hospitals to physicians'

---

[16]A sad irony from the American experience is provided by a Los Angeles study, which shows a strong positive relationship between rates of cesarian section (after adjustment for other predisposing factors) and income of mother (actually average income of census tract of residence) (55, 82). Although this reveals a close connection between income and access, which has no counterpart in the Canadian system, the rate among upper income mothers was well above that judged appropriate by experts. The lower income patients had on average worse access—at least lower utilization—but may have had better care. More is not necessarily better.

services, included estimates of needs for health personnel, particularly physicians, and recommended a substantial expansion in training facilities. The expansion took place over the subsequent decade. But, the population forecasts on which these estimates were based were made just before the collapse of fertility rates in the mid-1960s; thus, for the early 1990s, the forecasts were too high by about 10 million, or more than 30%.

By the early 1970s, it was apparent that a major demographic transition had occurred, and that the long-run population of Canada was going to be much lower than previously expected. Medical training places, however, were not scaled back. Hence the steady rise of 2% per year in the physician to population ratio. Thus, there is a head-on collision between the income aspirations of an ever-increasing physician supply and the cost containment objectives of governments.

This collision also projects into the hospital domain. Constraints on hospital budgets and capital spending have meant that, on average, physicians face a steadily falling stock of hospital facilities and personnel available to serve their patients (6). In simple terms, the bed to doctor ratio is falling as a result of the increase in physician supply, and this is perceived by physicians as an increasingly severe shortage of beds. On a per capita basis, they are wrong, but for each of them individually, the perception is correct.

PHYSICIAN SURPLUSES, NURSE SHORTAGES   The rising number of physicians per bed has led to increasing pressure to put patients through hospital beds at a more rapid rate, a pressure greatly exacerbated by the shift over the last two decades of large numbers of hospital beds from acute to extended care. Lengths of stay in acute care have fallen sharply, which puts growing pressure on nursing staffs. The acuity or severity of patients increases in response to the increased intensity of interventions to which they are exposed, and the lower intensity "late days of stay" are now more commonly spent at home. At the same time, the fertility collapse of the 1960s has within the last decade dramatically reduced the pool of 20-year-old women from which nurses have traditionally been recruited, and the range of other occupational opportunities for women has greatly expanded. A chronic shortage of nurses is the inevitable result.

Cost containment mechanisms interact with these human resource problems in several ways. First, the increased supply of physicians means that costs continue to climb even if fees are contained, because the volume of billings expands along with the numbers of physicians. There is no evidence of saturation, of falling physician workloads in response to increased supply. This situation leads directly to government attempts to place caps on overall outlays, which would imply falling average incomes per physician (in real or purchasing-power terms). The inevitable result is an increase in political tension and conflict.

But secondly, the asymmetry of fee-for-service reimbursement for physicians and global budgets for hospitals enables physicians to have effective first call on health budgets by adjusting their billing behavior. In the absence of volume caps, fee-for-service payments are still open-ended. Thus, it is difficult to reallocate funds from paying physicians, who are clearly not in shortage, to paying nurses, who are. Hospitals find it harder to compete, in an ever more competitive female labor market, even as the increased pressure for access from an increased physician supply continues to raise nursing workloads and stress levels.

The mismatch problem is apparently less severe in the United States, partly because the cost containment efforts have not been successful, and partly because a greater proportion of care has migrated out of the hospital, which reduces the demand for bed space and nursing personnel. Overall costs have continued to climb, and physician incomes have expanded to support the increasing physician workforce, without requiring a complementary increase in hospital personnel.

Nevertheless, the steady increase in physician supply in the United States has created exactly the same dilemma for cost containment: What will all the physicians do? Average physician incomes in the United States have been maintained in the face of steadily rising numbers, by a combination of price increases at rates exceeding inflation and increasing billing opportunities. Successful containment, if it is ever achieved, must close off both those avenues. Either physician average incomes, or their numbers, or both, must grow less rapidly, if at all.

This proposition is not dependent upon the position that one takes on the politically loaded question of whether there is a physician surplus in Canada, the United States, or anywhere else. Surplus is a normative word, which draws in a complex of ideological commitments and economic interests. But, whether or not one feels able to use the word, it is simply elementary arithmetic that a steady increase in physician supply, relative to the population, must result in either a corresponding increase in the proportion of national income made over to physicians or a fall in the relative income of physicians.

Those who argue that physicians are not in surplus generally take the position that, for various reasons, more services are or will be needed (56, 57), and/or that as long as additional physicians are keeping busy, then by definition they must be needed (81). Health expenditures should accordingly be further increased, not contained. Unfortunately, this style of argument is inherently circular and serves to justify the status quo whatever the level of physician supply or its rate of increase.

As documented by Lomas et al (68), exactly the same arguments have been used in Ontario, principally by representatives of medical schools, for nearly 25 years, during which time the physician to population ratio has risen by about 60%. Contrary to widespread belief, the aging of the population has a very small effect upon the needs for physicians' services (91). Nevertheless, physician workloads have not declined, and curtailing the rate of increase has, throughout that period, been regarded as premature by the medical schools.

It would not be the least of many ironies in this field if American efforts to contain costs, although unsuccessful in the short run, have made the practice of medicine so unattractive that the number of new applicants continues to fall, to a point that current training places cannot be filled, while those who do enter choose salary over fee-for-service, at lower incomes. These trends, which are current in America, have no Canadian counterparts. If continued long enough, they will reduce the cost pressures from physician supply. On the other hand, the more successful short-run containment in Canada has occurred in ways which have not discouraged new entry to medicine, and thus result in ever more upward pressure on expenditures in the long run![17]

CAPACITY AND KNOW-HOW: IF WE CAN, WE MUST!   Moving away from personnel, the control of physical capital has been more successful in Canada, through a combination of constraints on fee schedule structures and dual budgeting in hospitals. Hospital budgets reimburse operating costs only; capital allocations are controlled separately. Because physicians are rarely reimbursed through the fee schedule for the technical component of costs of major diagnostic and therapeutic equipment, they do not set up facilities outside hospitals. Thus, proliferation of physical capital has been better controlled in Canada, which has made a substantial contribution to the overall control of costs. A large part of the political controversy arises from the difference between controlled physical capital and uncontrolled human capital, the latter regarding the former as a shortage.

But, all forms of health capital appear to be subject to Roemer's Law— capacity attracts use. For the long run, this process appears to be most troubling with respect to technological capital or know-how. Extensive public and private efforts are devoted to the development of new diagnostic and therapeutic maneuvers, particularly in the United States, but the Canadian activity is negligible only by comparison. In principle, the new interventions based on such new knowledge could either raise or lower health care costs; in practice, there has been a pronounced bias toward upward pressure. A consideration of the economic incentives bearing on the research industry itself clarifies the sources of this bias (39).

As in the case of physician manpower, therefore, we find a great deal of effort being put into a form of capital formation, which may be in direct conflict with the objective of cost containment. A frequent American criticism

---

[17]Worse still, Canada and the United States each accept the accreditation of the other's medical schools. Thus, American schools with empty places could top up with Canadians, who could then return home to accelerate the increase in the Canadian supply.

of the Canadian health care system has been the limitations placed on the development and proliferation of new technologies in the process of containing costs. If the health care system is viewed, like defense, as a major forcing bed for the development of new technological capabilities, it is hard to see how one can simultaneously control the costs of that system. Nor is it so much the costs of development—research budgets per se—that create problems. The Canadian health care system comes under severe pressure from increased professional and patient expectations, which result from new developments in the United States or Germany.

A possible response might be a much more active program of technology assessment to screen and manage the introduction of new technologies. In fact, the most active such program in the world is clearly in the United States; Canada has done little or nothing in this area. The implication is that, heretofore, there has been neither a necessary nor a sufficient linkage between technological assessment, or the broader study of procedural appropriateness, and cost containment. We are, therefore, dubious that major initiatives in this area will contribute to cost containment, however meritorious they may be in themselves in improving the effectiveness of care (7, 43).

What Can We Learn? What Have We Learned? What's Next?

To date, the most effective control instruments have been relatively blunt—overall budgetary constraints—not combined with close examination of the effectiveness of the services provided or foregone. The ever increasing pressures from technical advance and expanding human capital may change this generalization; Canada, like the European countries, is expressing increased interest in technological assessment and quality assurance, but it is too soon to say if this interest will have significant policy impact.

This experience emphasizes that cost containment is fundamentally a political problem, not a technical one. It has not been achieved through sophisticated incentive systems to modify the behavior of providers or patients, or equally sophisticated analyses of the effects of particular services in particular circumstances—neither economists nor clinical epidemiologists have played critical roles. Containment is in essence a remarkably simple process. One constructs a payment system in which all expenditures flow through one budget, and then one places that budget in the hands of an agency with the political authority and motivation to limit its growth.

Some countries, such as Canada, Sweden, and the United Kingdom, do this explicitly. Australia, Germany, and Japan achieve the same result by imposing a detailed control structure on a nominally decentralized system. But the control structure must be comprehensive, authoritative, and binding—and it is. One way or another, the total amount of money flowing to the health care system, from whatever source, is directly constrained.

Those subject to such controls can be expected to work hard both to increase the flow of resources through the controlled channel, and to open up other channels not subject to the overall limitation—hence the widespread physician enthusiasm for direct billing of patients. Thus, cost containment is an on-going political struggle, in every system, surrounded by more or less political sound and fury depending upon the local political culture. In Canada or France, there may be much public posturing. In Japan, there may be quiet struggles behind the scenes. But, there is no "technical fix" to resolve fundamental conflicts of interest, entangled as they are with fundamental questions of public choice and values.

The inevitability of this permanent struggle, however, should not distract one from the fact that different systems really are different. Access to care, and the financial consequences, are fundamentally different in Canada and the United States. Canadians do not have to fear for their financial health should they become ill, and they do not. Nor do they have to go through the administrative complexities—the "hassle factor" of the American system. Being ill, in pain, and frightened, is enough of a trial without adding the extra burdens of effort and cost, or so Canadians believe. And, with some minor qualifications, so do the citizens of most other developed countries. Individual Americans may also agree; that would explain why they are so much less satisfied with the system they have.

The United States, as Abel-Smith (1) emphasizes, is the "odd man out." It serves as the bad example for all other western industrialized democracies—exemplary of what could happen if one succumbed to the pressures for reintroduction of privatization, pluralism, prices, and the forces of what have never been more than pseudomarkets. Zombie-like, these intellectually dead arguments refuse to rest in peace. The United States also stands alone in its steadfast unwillingness to embrace the notion of universal coverage on (roughly) equal terms and conditions.

The fact that these two American aspects of "going it alone" are inextricably intertwined does not yet seem to have penetrated a sufficiently large American constituency to harness forces for change. The cost control record is dismal; the un- and underinsured are an embarrassment; public dissatisfaction with the system is widespread. Experiences elsewhere (not just in Canada) suggest several alternative variations on a common theme. What are the impediments?

Certainly a large part of the American intransigence has to do with powerful forces who would have much to lose, not from universality alone, but from universality combined with cost control. The AMA and the Health Insurance Association of America (e.g. 87) are acting rationally in mounting anti-Canadian campaigns. One can only point out, again and again, that Canada has the second most expensive health care system in the world, that if Canada is really so bad then the rest of the industrialized world is in even rougher shape; that it is Americans, not Canadians or Britons, who are acutely dissatisfied with their system; that it is Americans whose costs are out of control, and who are embarrassed by their medical under-class.

There is, however, another source of resistance to cost containment. In a pluralistic system, some persons are much more vulnerable than others. Attempts to control overall costs without also widening the safety net of insurance may, and typically do, fall most heavily on those whose needs are greatest and resources least, precisely because they are least able to defend themselves. Even in a system that they believe to be overfunded, citizens who are concerned about the condition of the most vulnerable may fear with good reason that it is the most needed services, not the least needed, which will be limited. Universal coverage thus not only provides the means for cost control, but may contribute to the mobilization of will.

In the final analysis, cost containment cannot depend on selling the idea to all threatened or interested parties. The key is overall budgetary control, through a combination of control of the amount of capital that represents the claims on incomes, and control of the income levels received by the owners of that capital. Responding to threatened interest groups, like research on ways of identifying and eliminating ineffective care, is a possible means of developing a constituency of support for such a structure. Better information on the efficiency of alternative interventions or forms of organization may indicate how best to allocate resources "within the globe." But, such studies will not ensure that the expenditure target is hit. Without exogenously set and enforced limits, they will be the bullet forever chasing the moving target.

Exactly how such global constraints can be crafted in the American political and administrative environment is not clear. Certainly, outsiders have no particular advantage in offering advice. What does seem clear, however, is that American health policy is frozen into a "catch-22" situation in which cost control is impossible in the absence of a universal funding system, and universal coverage is impossible because it is believed to be too costly!

The understanding that this is a false paradox is slowly spreading among payers and providers alike. Furthermore, general public support for a government-financed, national health care system has grown during the 1980s; nearly three quarters of the American public now favor some such plan (15). But, the views behind such support are not as strongly held as in other countries; moreover the very multiplicity of options serves to paralyse decision. Any one alternative may be preferred to the status quo, but which should be enacted?

Canadian experience points toward decentralization under federal standards, with primary administrative and financial authority at the provincial level—for constitutional reasons, that was always the only real choice. There is a growing interest in some form of subprovincial regionalization of priority-setting, albeit within clear and binding provincial guidelines. Such regions might have populations of between 50,000 and 1 or 2 million. But American traditions and structures favor national authority, which creates programs tens or hundreds of times larger than those in Canada. No one knows if Canadian models could work at such a scale. On the other hand, many Americans seem to have serious doubts about the adequacy of state administrations for such a task, and the largest state is as large as Canada itself.

Finally, the confusion between taxes and other forms of payment seems to undermine political will. Any universal system will require greater tax revenues. The accompanying potential for control of overall costs will, if realized, permit even larger reductions in private insurance premiums and out-of-pocket payments. That is what has occurred in Canada and Western Europe. But Americans seem so resistant to taxes (15), that they do not see the trade-off. Alternatively, they may not believe that their governments are capable of achieving control. Every other country may have established such control, but the average American does not know this. Moreover, any tax-supported national program will inevitably redistribute the costs of care from lower to higher income persons, and Americans seem to be much less willing than Canadians or Europeans to support such implicit income redistribution.

Under these circumstances it seems unlikely that a sufficiently powerful political constituency can be mobilized to break the deadlock, unless or until the pain inflicted by the present system becomes much more widespread, and most of the competing pluralistic approaches are found to be financially, as well as intellectually, bankrupt.

ACKNOWLEDGMENT

The authors would like particularly to thank (and implicate) T. R. Marmor, whose intellectual influence is pervasive, for detailed comments on an earlier draft. They would also like to acknowledge the support of the National Health Research and Development Program and the Canadian Institute for Advanced Research.

Literature Cited

1. Abel-Smith, B. 1985. Who is the odd man out: the experience of Western Europe in containing the costs of health care. *Milb. Mem. Fund Q./Health Soc.* 63(1):1–17
2. Am. Assoc. Retired Pers. 1989. *Access to Health Care: An Analysis of Recent Polling Data*. Res. Data Resour. Dep. Polling Rep. Inc. Washington, DC: Am. Assoc. Retired Pers.
3. Andersen, T. F., Mooney, G., eds. 1990. *The Challenges of Medical Practice Variations*. London: MacMillan

4. Anderson, G. M., Newhouse, J. P., Roos, L. L. 1989. Hospital care for elderly patients with diseases of the circulatory system: a comparison of hospital use in the United States and Canada. *N. Engl. J. Med.* 321(21):1443–48
5. Barer, M. L. 1988. Regulating physician supply: the evolution of British Columbia's Bill 41. *J. Health Polit. Policy Law* 13(1):1–25
6. Barer, M. L., Evans, R. G. 1986. Riding north on a south-bound horse? Expenditures, prices, utilization and in-

comes in the Canadian health care system. In *Medicare at Maturity: Achievements, Lessons and Challenges*, ed. R. G. Evans, G. L. Stoddart, pp. 53–163. Calgary: Univ. Calgary Press, Banff Cent. Sch. Manage.

7. Barer, M. L., Evans, R. G. 1990. *Reflections on the Financing of Hospital Capital: A Canadian Perspective.* HPRU 90:17D, Health Policy Res. Unit. Vancouver: Univ. B.C.

8. Barer, M. L., Evans, R. G., Labelle, R. 1988. Fee controls as cost control: tales from the frozen north. *Milb. Q.* 66(1):1–64

9. Barer, M. L., Gafni, A., Lomas, J. 1989. Accommodating rapid growth in physician supply: lessons from Israel, warnings for Canada. *Int. J. Health Serv.* 19(1):95–115

10. Barer, M. L., Manga, P., Shillington, E. R., Siegel, G. C. 1982. *Income Class and Hospital Use in Ontario.* Toronto: Ont. Econ. Counc.

11. Barer, M. L., Nicoll, M., Diesendorf, M., Harvey, R. 1990. From Medibank to Medicare: trends in Australian medical care costs and use, 1976–1986. *Community Health Stud.* (Aust.) 14(1):8–18

12. Barer, M. L., Pulcins, I. R., Evans, R. G. Hertzman, C., Lomas, J., et al. 1989. Trends in use of medical services by the elderly in British Columbia. *Can. Med. Assoc. J.* 141(1):39–45

13. Barker, W. P., Osmond, O., 1987. Inequalities in health in Britain: specific explanations in three Lancashire towns. *Br. Med. J.* 294:749–52

14. Beck, R. G. 1973. Economic class and access to physician services under public medical care insurance. *Int. J. Health Serv.* 3:341–55

15. Blendon, R. J., Donelan, K. 1990. The public and the emerging debate over national health insurance. *N. Engl. J. Med.* 323(3):208–12

16. Blendon, R. J., Leitman, R., Morrison, I., Donelan, K. 1990. Satisfaction with health systems in ten nations. *Health Aff.* 9(2):185–92

17. Blendon, R. J., Taylor, H. 1989. Views on health care: public opinion in three nations. *Health Aff.* 8(1):149–57

18. Boulet, J. A., Henderson, D. W. 1979. *Distributional and Redistributional Aspects of Government Health Insurance Programs in Canada.* Ottawa: Econ. Counc. Can.

19. Braveman, P., Oliva, G., Miller, M. G. Reiter, R., Egerter, S., et al. 1989. Adverse outcomes and lack of health insurance among newborns in an eight-county area of California, 1982–1986. *N. Engl. J. Med.* 321(8):508–12

20. Broyles, R. W., et al. 1983. The use of physician services under a national health insurance scheme. *Med. Care* 21:1037–54

21. Canada. 1964. *Report.* R. Comm. Health Serv. (Hall Comm.). Ottawa: Queen's Printer

22. Canada, Health Welf. Can. 1970. *Task Force Reports on the Cost of Health Services in Canada, Vols. 1–3.* Comm. Costs Health Serv. Ottawa: Inf. Can.

23. Canada, Health Welfare Can. 1979. *National Health Expenditures in Canada, 1960–1975.* Ottawa: Health Welf. Can.

24. Canada, Health Welfare Can. 1987. *National Health Expenditures in Canada, 1975–1985.* Ottawa: Health Welf. Can.

25. Canada, Health Welf. Can. 1990. *Health Personnel in Canada, 1988.* Ottawa: Health Welf. Can.

26. Chassin, M. R., Kosecoff, J., Park, R. E., Winslow, C. M., Kahn, K. L., et al. 1987. Does inappropriate use explain geographic variations in the use of health care services? A study of three procedures. *J. Am. Med. Assoc.* 258:2533–37

27. Contandriopoulos, A-P. 1986. Cost containment through payment mechanisms: the Quebec experience. *J. Public Health Policy* 7(2):244–38

28. Cromwell, J., Mitchell, J. B., Stason, W. B. 1990. Learning by doing in CABG surgery. *Med. Care* 28(1):6–18

29. Culyer, A. J. 1988. *Health Care Expenditures in Canada: Myth and Reality, Past and Future.* Can. Tax Paper No. 82. Toronto: Can. Tax Found.

30. Culyer, A. J. 1989. Cost containment in Europe. *Health Care Financ. Rev,* Annu. Suppl.:21–32

31. Davis, K., Rowland, D. 1983. Uninsured and underserved: inequities in health care in the United States. *Milb. Mem. Fund Q./Health Soc.* 61(2):149–76

32. Detsky, A., O'Rourke, K., Naylor, C. D., Stacy, S. R., Kitchens, J. M. 1990. Containing Ontario's hospital costs under universal insurance in the 1980s: what was the record? *Can. Med. Assoc. J.* 142(6):565–72

33. Detsky, A., Stacey, S. R., Bombardier, C. 1983. The effectiveness of a regulatory strategy in containing hospital costs: the Ontario experience, 1967–1981. *N. Engl. J. Med.* 309:151–59

34. Donham, C. S., Maple, B. T. 1989.

Health care indicators. *Health Care Financ. Rev.* 11(2):117–36

35. Dutton, D. B., Levine, S. 1989. Socioeconomic status and health: overview, methodological critique, and reformulation. In *Pathways to Health: The Role of Social Factors,* ed. J. P. Bunker, D. S. Gomby, B. H. Kehrer. Menlo Park, Calif: Kaiser Fam. Found.

36. Econ. Counc. Can. 1970. *Patterns of Growth. Seventh Annual Review.* Ottawa: Queen's Printer

37. Enterline, P. E. 1973. The distribution of medical services before and after 'free' medical care—the Quebec experience. *N. Engl. J. Med.* 289:1174–78

38. Enthoven, A. C. 1989. Towards a model system for the financing and delivery of health care in the United States. In *Changing America's Health Care System: Proposals for Legislative Action,* ed. S. Leader, M. Moon, pp. 21–42. Washington, DC: Am. Assoc. Retired Pers.

39. Evans, R. G. 1984. *Strained Mercy: The Economics of Canadian Health Care.* Toronto: Butterworths

40. Evans, R. G. 1986. Finding the levers, finding the courage: lessons for cost containment in North America. *J. Health Polit. Policy Law* 11(4):585–615

41. Evans, R. G. 1990 forthcoming. Life and death, money and power: the politics of health care finance. In *Health Politics and Policy,* ed. T. J. Litman, L. S. Robins. Albany, NY: Delmar. 2nd ed.

42. Evans, R. G. 1990. Tension, compression, and shear: directions, stresses, and outcomes of health care cost control. *J. Health Polit. Policy Law* 15(1):101–28

43. Evans, R. G. 1990 The dog in the nighttime: medical practice variations and health policy. In *The Challenges of Medical Practice Variations,* ed. T. F. Anderson, G. Mooney, pp. 117–52. London: MacMillan

44. Evans, R. G., Barer, M. L., Hertzman, C., Anderson, G. M., Pulcins, I. R., Lomas, J. 1989. The long goodbye: the great transformation of the British Columbia hospital system. *Health Serv. Res.* 24(4):435–59

45. Evans, R. G., Lomas, J., Barer, M. L., Labelle, R. J., Fooks, C., et al. 1989. Controlling health expenditures—the Canadian reality. *N. Engl. J. Med.* 320(9):571–77

46. Feder, J., Holahan, J., Marmor, T. R. 1980. *National Health Insurance: Conflicting Goals and Policy Choices.* Washington, DC: Urban Inst.

47. Feder, J., Scanlon, W., Clark, J. 1987. Canada's health care system (Letter to the Editor). *N. Engl. J. Med.* 317: 320

48. Fries, J. F. 1989. The compression of morbidity: near or far? *Milb. Q.* 67(2): 208–32

49. Fuchs, V. R., Hahn, J. S. 1990. How does Canada do it? A comparison of expenditures for physicians' services in the United States and Canada. *N. Engl. J. Med.* 323(13):884–90

50. Gabel, J., Jajich-Toth, C., de Lissovoy, G., Rice, T., Cohen, H. 1988. The changing world of group health insurance. *Health Aff.* 7(3):48–65

51. Gabel, J., Rice, T. 1985. Reducing public expenditures for physician services: the price of paying less. *J. Health Polit. Policy Law* 9:595

52. Gagnon, M., Mix, P. 1989. Hospital statistics—preliminary annual hospital statistics 1987–88 and list of Canadian hospitals 1988. *Health Rep. 1989* 1(1):113–17, Can. Cent. Health Inf. Stat. Can. Cat. #82–003 Qly, Ottawa: Ministry Supply Serv.

53. Ginsburg, P. B., LeRoy, L. B., Hammons, G. T. 1990. Medicare: physician payment reform. *Health Aff.* 9(1):178–88

54. Gormley, M., Barer, M., Melia, P., Helston, D. 1990. *The Growth in Use of Health Services 1977/78 to 1985/86.* Regina: Sask. Health

55. Gould, J. B., Davey, B., Stafford, R. S. 1989. Socioeconomic differences in rates of cesarian section. *N. Engl. J. Med.* 321(4):233–39

56. Hanft, R. S. 1987. Commentary: the need for more physicians. *Health Aff.* 6(2):69–71

57. Harris, J. E. 1986. How many doctors are enough? *Health Aff.* 5(4):73–83

58. Harris, L. 1987. *Inside America,* pp. 200–5. New York: Vintage

59. Helliwell, J. F., Chung, A. 1990. *Globalization, Convergence, and the Prospects of Economic Growth.* Killam Mem. Lect., Dalhousie Univ., Oct. 12, 1989. Disc. Paper #90–06, Dep. Econ. Vancouver: Univ. B. C.

60. Hertzman, C. 1990. *Poland: Health and Environment in the Context of Socioeconomic Decline.* HPRU 90:2D, Health Policy Res. Unit. Vancouver: Univ. B.C.

61. Himmelstein, D.U., Woolhandler, S. 1986. Cost without benefit: administrative waste in US health care. *N. Engl. J. Med.* 314:441–45

62. Iglehart, J. 1988. Japan's medical care

system—part two. *N. Engl. J. Med.* 319(17):1166–72

63. International comparisons of productivity levels and trends of eleven OECD countries. 1990. *Int. Prod. J.* Spr:67–87

64. Kanigan, M., Mix, P. 1989. Surgical procedures and treatments—historical trends and recent data characteristics. *Health Rep. 1989* 1(1):81–96, Can. Cent. Health Inf. Stat. Can. Cat. #82–003 Qly, Ottawa: Ministry Supply Serv.

65. Katz, A., McCarry, M. 1989. *A Tale of Two Systems: A Comparative Study of the British Columbia and Washington State Health Care Systems and Their Effects on Access, Costs, and Health.* Report 1 of ser. Health Policy Anal. Program, Sch. Public Health. Seattle: Univ. Wash.

66. Katz, A., Schwendiman, M. 1990. *Paying the Price: Health Care Spending by Businesses in British Columbia and Washington State.* Report 2 of ser. Health Policy Anal. Program, Sch. Public Health. Seattle: Univ. Wash.

67. Leape, L., Park, R. E., Solomon, D. H., Chassin, M. R., Kosecoff, J., Brook, R. H. 1990. Does inappropriate use explain small-area variations in the use of health care services? *J. Am. Med. Assoc.* 263(5):669–72

68. Lomas, J., Barer, M. L., Stoddart, G. L. 1985. *Physician Manpower Planning: Lessons from the Macdonald Report.* Ont. Econ. Counc. Disc. Paper Ser., Toronto: Ont. Econ. Counc.

69. Lomas, J., Fooks, C., Rice, T., Labelle, R. J. 1989. Paying physicians in Canada: minding our Ps and Qs. *Health Aff.* 8(1):80–102

70. Luft, H. S., Bunker, J. P., Enthoven, A. C. 1979. Should operations be regionalized? An empirical study of the relation between surgical volume and mortality. *N. Engl. J. Med.* 301:64

71. Manga, P. 1978. *The Income Distribution Effect of Medical Insurance in Ontario.* Toronto: Ont. Econ. Counc.

72. Marmor, T. R., Bridges, A., Hoffman, W. L. 1983. Comparative politics and health policies: notes on benefits, costs, limits. In *Political Analysis and American Medical Care,* ed. T. R. Marmor, pp. 45–57. New York: Cambridge Univ. Press

73. Marmor, T. R., Wittman, D. A., Heagy, T. C. 1976. The politics of medical inflation. *J. Health Polit. Policy Law* 1:69–84

74. Marmot, M., Smith, G. D., 1989. Why are the Japanese living longer? *Br. Med. J.* 299:1547–51

75. Newhouse, J. P., Anderson, G. M., Roos, L. L. 1988. Hospital spending in the United States and Canada: a comparison. *Health Aff.* 7(5):6–16

76. Rodwin, V. G. 1987. American exceptionalism in the health sector: the advantages of 'backwardness' in learning from abroad. *Med. Care Rev.* 44:119–54

77. Roos, L. L., Brazauskas, R., Cohen, M., Sharp, S. M. 1990. Variations in outcomes research. In *The Challenges of Medical Practice Variations,* ed. T. F. Anderson, G. Mooney, pp. 36–58. London: MacMillan

78. Roos, L. L., Fisher, E. S., Sharp, S. M., Newhouse, J. P., Anderson, G. M., Bubolz, T. A. 1990. Postsurgical mortality in Manitoba and New England. *J. Am. Med. Assoc.* 263(18):2453–58

79. Ryten, E. 1989. Trends in the demand for medical education in Canada. *Forum* 22(2):1–8

80. Schieber, G. J., Poullier, J-P. 1989. International health care expenditure trends: 1987. *Health Aff.* 8(3):169–77

81. Schwartz, W. B., Mendelson, D. N. 1990. No evidence of an emerging physician surplus: an analysis of change in physicians' workload and income. *J. Am. Med. Assoc.* 263(4):557–60

82. Stafford, R. S. 1990. Cesarian section use and source of payment: an analysis of California hospital discharge abstracts. *Am. J. Public Health* 80(3):313–15

83. Todd, J. S. 1989. It is time for universal access, not universal insurance. *N. Engl. J. Med.* 321(1):46–47

84. United Nations. 1982. *Levels and Trends of Mortality Since 1950.* New York: United Nations

85. US House Represent. Comm. Ways and Means. 1989. *Background Material and Data on Programs within the Jurisdiction of the Committee on Ways and Means.* WMCP 101-4, Washington, DC: GPO

86. US Natl. Cent. Health Serv. Res. 1987. *A Summary of Expenditures and Sources of Payment for Personal Health Care Service from the National Medical Care Expenditure Survey.* Data Preview #24, Natl. Health Care Expend. Study. Washington, DC: DHHS(PHS)NCHSR

87. Vancouver Sun. 1990. US insurers argue against Medicare. June 26, A5

88. Wilkins, R., Adams, O., Brancker, A. M. 1990. Changes in mortality by income in urban Canada from 1971 to 1986. *Health Rep. 1989* 1(2):137–74,

Can. Cent. Health Inf. Stat. Can., Cat. #82–003 Qly, Ottawa: Ministry Supply Serv.

89. Wolfson, M., Rowe, G., Gentleman, J. F., Tomiak, M. 1990. *Earnings and Death—Effects Over a Quarter Century.* Intern. Doc. #5B, Program Popul. Health, Can. Inst. Adv. Res. Vancouver: Univ. B.C.

90. Wolfson, A. D., Tuohy, C. J. 1980. *Opting Out of Medicare: Private Medical Markets in Ontario.* Ont. Econ. Counc. Res. Study #19. Toronto: Univ. Toronto Press

91. Woods, Gordon Manage. Consult. 1984. *Investigation of the Impact of Demographic Change on the Health Care System in Canada: Final Report.* Prepared for Task Force Alloc. Health Care Resour. Ottawa: Can. Med. Assoc.

92. World Health Organ. 1989. *1989 World Health Statistics Annual.* Geneva: WHO

Annu. Rev. Publ. Health. 1991. 12:519–41

CHILDHOOD PRECURSORS OF HIGH BLOOD PRESSURE AND ELEVATED CHOLESTEROL

D. R. Labarthe, M. Eissa, and C. Varas

The Southwest Center for Prevention Research, School of Public Health, The University of Texas Health Science Center, Houston, Texas

KEY WORDS: epidemiology, cross-sectional studies, longitudinal studies, tracking, growth and development

INTRODUCTION

For several decades, high blood pressure and elevated cholesterol have been established as risk factors for atherosclerosis and, thus, for most cardiovascular morbidity and mortality of industrialized countries. More recently, developing countries are recognizing the public health burden of high blood pressure and elevated cholesterol, as a result of demographic changes, which have seen increasing proportions of populations reach the sixth decade of life and beyond, and social and behavioral changes, which have fostered the development of the risk factors (12). Thus, the consequences of high blood pressure and elevated cholesterol, in addition to cigarette smoking and other factors, now constitute a global public health problem.

The causes of coronary heart disease and other complications of atherosclerosis and hypertensive disease must be sought earlier in life than the age range in which these events become especially common, i.e. at age 40 and older. The theoretical foundation for this concept is reinforced strongly by pathological evidence, including that from postmortem examinations of young military casualties. These examinations show that the vascular lesions of atherosclerosis commonly are present in the coronary arteries and aorta before age 20 (see, for example, Ref. 40). Geographically widespread evidence that aortic

519

and coronary atherosclerosis already may be extensive by age 20 has been summarized in an Expert Committee Report from the World Health Organization (WHO) (66). McGill (39) speculated that the prevention of atherosclerosis and its complications requires intervention before age 20.

In the US and elsewhere, epidemiologic studies of children, especially school-age populations, which concern the risk factors for the adult manifestations of atherosclerosis and hypertension, have become common, especially since the early 1970s. The National Heart and Lung Institute provided a special impetus to such studies in the US by establishing two Specialized Centers of Research in Atherosclerosis, which focused primarily upon children: the Bogalusa (Louisiana) Heart Study and the Muscatine (Iowa) Study. The Institute established two other centers that included childhood components: the Miami (Florida) Study and the Rochester (Minnesota) Study.

These and other investigations have generated a large body of evidence on epidemiologic and other aspects of the major risk factors—prominently blood pressure and cholesterol—in childhood. Current data have led to optimism about the potential for prevention of adult cardiovascular diseases through intervention in childhood (68).

It is timely, then, to review the lines of established epidemiologic evidence regarding the early development of these two major risk factors for adult cardiovascular diseases around the world. We begin this discussion with attention to several underlying issues common to both blood pressure and cholesterol, which is useful background for examining each of these risk factors separately. Then, we will present observational studies, both cross-sectional and longitudinal, and intervention studies for blood pressure and cholesterol. Finally, we will consider the implications of the evidence with respect to theory, practice, and further research.

ISSUES COMMON TO BLOOD PRESSURE AND CHOLESTEROL IN CHILDHOOD

Importance of the Risk Factors in Childhood

Among the many uses of epidemiology, three are particularly relevant here: understanding of natural history, determining the potential for prevention, and predicting the future course of disease processes.

NATURAL HISTORY   As noted above, atherosclerosis is very gradual in its development, with progression from the first or second decade of life to the appearance of clinical manifestations decades later (39). A comprehensive understanding of natural history must begin well before age 20. Ideally, both genetic and environmental factors, and their interactions, should be investigated from conception through the overt appearance of atherosclerosis and its complications. However, such prospective observation of individuals over periods of several decades would be a formidable logistical task. Further, at the end of such a period of follow-up, the earliest observations from decades before may have little relevance to current circumstances.

Accordingly, studies have adopted much more limited objectives. Evidence on the early development of both blood pressure and cholesterol is typically limited to ages before adulthood, without linkage to observations separately reported among adults. We will note some important exceptions.

PREVENTION   Determination of the potential for prevention, as distinct from scientific understanding alone, is another impetus to investigation of blood pressure and cholesterol in childhood. Concepts of prevention have been developed, which are specifically applicable to these risk factors during childhood.

The strategy of primary prevention of coronary heart disease during adulthood, had been characterized as comprising the "high-risk approach" and the "population approach," terms adopted by WHO (66) for concepts that Rose (49) had initially put forward. The objective of the high-risk approach is to identify those individuals at the upper extreme of risk with respect to blood pressure or cholesterol levels (or other factors) and to intervene aggressively to reverse the indicated risks. The objective of the population approach, based on the wide distribution of excess risk over a range of less extreme values of the risk factors, is to intervene in the population at large thereby shifting the whole distribution to reduce average risk. An important feature of primary prevention, by either approach, is that it addresses already-established risk factors, at either the individual or the population level.

An alternative strategy has been described, which Strasser (54) termed "primordial prevention," or prevention of the development of the risk factors themselves. The concept of primordial prevention depends implicitly on the potential for effective intervention in advance of the progression of blood pressure, cholesterol concentration, or other risk factors to undesirable levels.

Both high-risk and population approaches can be applied to primordial prevention by analogy to primary prevention. A high-risk approach is feasible if one can identify those individuals at highest risk of progression from desirable to undesirable levels of the risk factors, such as those with relatively high values of blood pressure or a family history of lipid abnormalities. A population approach to primordial prevention is possible if the conditions known to produce high risk, such as a dietary pattern related to high levels of blood cholesterol, are absent. Based on current knowledge of the natural history of blood pressure and cholesterol, primordial prevention must begin in childhood.

PREDICTING THE COURSE OF THE DISEASE PROCESS   As we noted earlier, demographic and social changes in developing countries have led or may lead atherosclerosis and its complications to become equally important as causes of morbidity and mortality in the developing world as they are in industrialized countries. In light of the evidence we will review, can predictions about the future course of cardiovascular diseases be made with confidence at this time, if we consider what is known about these risk factors in childhood? We will address this question in the conclusions.

The Context of "Childhood"

From the perspective of the epidemiology and prevention of cardiovascular diseases, how is "childhood" defined by age and in the specification of the population of interest? In the present context, childhood refers inclusively to the period from birth to early adulthood. Lower and upper age boundaries, respectively, might be taken as birth and age 24, the upper limit of "youth," according to WHO (68). Relatively few observations are available among newborns and infants, however, and the same is true beyond high school age. For practical purposes, most studies are of age groups within the typical school-age population, approximately 6–18 years of age. For convenience, we will use the term childhood in this broader sense (ages 6–18), except where specific reference is needed to a particular period, such as adolescence, or a stated age group.

Studies of risk factors in childhood are often, and not surprisingly, based on school populations. Such populations are readily defined, are typically enumerated in advance for administrative purposes, and may be exceptionally accessible. The disadvantages include the unsuitability of some school environments and schedules for the requirements of data collection, the commonly reduced participation rates among older students, and the inability to reach the "drop-out" population.

Despite these limitations, many investigators have utilized such settings satisfactorily. In addition, interventions not involving the school may be unlikely to have much influence. Thus, studies of these risk factors in childhood generally are studies of school-age populations, in the school environment. The context of the family and other social institutions often is lacking, and the preschool, postschool, and school drop-out populations often are unstudied.

Several other aspects about childhood require mention, including the universal, and biologically defining, characteristic of childhood: growth and physical maturation. Countless physiologic, metabolic, and other processes in childhood are fundamental background to the study of any specific biologic phenomenon during this period of life.

Second, we must understand the dynamics of these developmental processes, or their variations in times of onset and rates of progression. Whatever changes occur during childhood in blood pressure and cholesterol levels, for example, they are concomitants of an increase in height (or length), which is about threefold from birth to age 20, but which is strikingly nonuniform in rate, as indicated by the well-recognized adolescent growth spurt (58). Meanwhile, weight may increase fifteenfold or more, also at rates that vary throughout childhood.

Third, a consequence of these prior considerations is that specificity of classification of study subjects by age should be much narrower in childhood than in adulthood. Even one-year age groups can represent marked heterogeneity in degrees of growth and maturation. Any reservation on this point will yield quickly to Tanner's graphic representation of three boys of identical birthdate whose appearances are those of child, boy, and man (58). Specificity by sex also is necessary, although particular characteristics differ greatly in the ages at which this differentiation appears.

Fourth, the common practice of conducting discrete studies of childhood on the one hand and adulthood on the other prevents continuity of observations, which corresponds to continuity of the developmental processes that are the object of study. Few studies directly link evidence concerning blood pressure or cholesterol in childhood with that in adulthood, and a gap in observations remains between late school age and midadulthood.

Finally, the title of this review implies attention to serial measurements of blood pressure or cholesterol, which begin in childhood and extend into adulthood. For both of these risk factors, values considered to be undesirable in adulthood also may occur within childhood. Therefore, interest in serial observations arises within childhood and not only between childhood and later periods of life.

Predictions From Observations in Childhood

Prediction of subsequent observations from those on a given occasion can be based on any of several epidemiologic approaches. Most common is the use of cross-sectional surveys, in which multiple age groups are observed. For example, an approximation to the future blood pressure levels of present 6-year-olds is given by the average levels observed in successively older age groups, examined in the same survey. Such data, though not strictly predictive, often are taken implicitly as indicating the age patterns to be expected in the same or similar populations at times subsequent to the original survey.

Studies in which the prediction of risk factor levels is addressed formally often are termed "tracking" studies. Tracking refers to the degree of continuity among successive observations of a measured attribute in individual subjects. Indices of tracking may be based either on the absolute values of the measurement, such as correlation coefficients between paired observations over time, or on relative values, such as percentile ranks among individuals measured in which subjects often are categorized in decile or quintile groups. In the case of such relative values, the focus of analysis often is on the group at the highest level of the distribution on initial observation and on whether such ranking persists during remeasurement over intervals of months or years.

Another approach to investigation is to monitor serial observations in individual subjects, by repeating measurements on several occasions over a period of several years, and to present the actual values at successive ages (separately by sex) as they develop. By analogy to the familiar process of monitoring height and weight changes in the care of infants and children, we refer to this approach as the development of "growth curves" for the risk factors, in contrast to the tracking studies described above.

For both blood pressure and cholesterol, the discussion that follows will emphasize the natural history of their development in childhood, including cross-sectional surveys, longitudinal studies of both tracking and growth, and those aspects of intervention studies most relevant to the question of precursors in childhood of high blood pressure and elevated cholesterol.

BLOOD PRESSURE

A Note on Measurement

Blood pressure in epidemiologic studies and in the context of public health is defined on the basis of indirect, rather than intra-arterial, measurements and is expressed in units of millimeters of mercury (mmHg). Measurements are made in relation to the auscultatory phenomena, termed the Korotkoff sounds, which correspond to systolic and fourth- and fifth-phase diastolic pressure. These phenomena and the techniques of measurement are described in standard references (18, 59). Inferences based on any one study or set of measurement conditions must be qualified by the possibility of systematic differences in measurement. Despite such qualifications, however, many aspects of the epidemiology of blood pressure have been observed consistently and have provided a sound basis for biological understanding (67).

Natural History

CROSS-SECTIONAL SURVEYS   When we compare those cross-sectional surveys of blood pressure that have especially broad age coverage within the period of childhood, their similarities in general form and in age-specific mean values between populations are striking. They also are greater than are the similarities found in comparing such surveys among adults (5, 32).

By examining such data closely, after pooling survey data from many childhood populations, we find consistently upward changes in systolic blood pressure levels that clearly increase in slope for boys and girls after about age 12. For girls, the slopes level off and actually reverse in trend in the late teens; for boys, the steeper teenage slope continues until apparently stabilizing without further immediate increase at about age 18 (Figure 1) (5). Systolic pressures of 100 mmHg at age 6 for both boys and girls thus reach mean values of about 122 and 111 mmHg, respectively, at age 18.

For diastolic pressures, fourth- and fifth-phase measurements tend to be reported from different studies; relatively few reports contain both types of diastolic readings in a single population. The patterns observed for fourth-phase diastolic pressure in both boys and girls are similar to those found for systolic pressure (Figure 2). However, for the fifth-phase readings (Figure 3), the age gradient is less distinct between boys and girls and does not show the decrease observed for girls in systolic and fourth-phase diastolic pressure. For fourth-phase readings, the mean values increase from 63 to 72 mmHg for boys and from 64 to 67 mmHg for girls, from age 6 to 18. Corresponding values for fifth-phase readings are 59–72 and 60–72 mmHg, in the different sets of populations for which these measurements were reported. (Within any single population, the mean values for fifth-phase diastolic pressure are necessarily lower than those for fourth-phase pressure.)

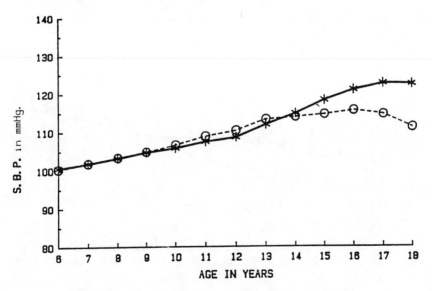

Figure 1 Pooled values, all qualifying studies. Means of SBP by age and sex.
*—*Males; - -O- -Females

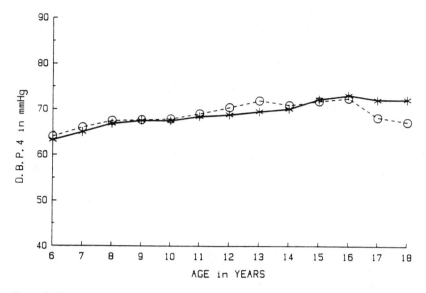

Figure 2 Pooled values, all qualifying studies. Means of DBP4 by age and sex.
*—*Males; - -O- -Females

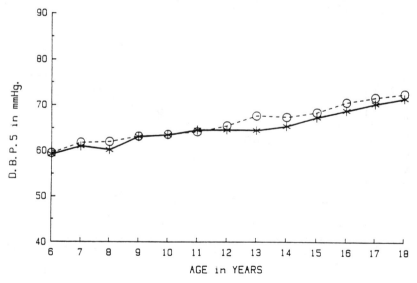

Figure 3 Pooled values, all qualifying studies. Means of DBP5 by age and sex.
*—*Males; - -O- -Females

When cross-sectional surveys are compared among populations, the extremes of the age-specific mean values by sex are within about 5% of the pooled age-specific mean value for systolic pressure. The range is somewhat wider, about 7% above and below the pooled mean values, for age-specific mean values of fourth-phase diastolic pressure. Results for fifth-phase diastolic pressure are similar, if one population with exceptionally low values is excluded (32).

These and other observations from cross-sectional studies suggest that the three measures of blood pressure commonly recorded, systolic, fourth-phase, and fifth-phase diastolic pressure, reflect different aspects of hemodynamic or circulatory development. They should, therefore, be distinguished whenever possible. Reference should be made specifically to one or another measure, not simply to "blood pressure." In addition, the close resemblance among populations in age-specific mean values of blood pressure, especially systolic, implies that the different environmental circumstances of different populations, and even genetic differences, may have limited bearing on the early age pattern in the development of this risk factor.

Whether, for example, racial differences occur in the early development of blood pressure remains unclear. Cross-sectional surveys in adults demonstrate consistently higher mean values of systolic and diastolic pressure in blacks than in whites in the US, but corresponding comparisons in black and white children and adolescents are mixed (2, 3, 47, 48). In addition, dietary influences, such as sodium or salt intake, have been studied with inconsistent results. For example, Schachter et al (50) found significant correlations between sodium intake and systolic pressure among infants, but the correlation was positive in whites and negative in blacks. Ellison et al (14) found no significant associations between blood pressure and either urinary sodium excretion or a ratio of this value to caloric intake (a measure of "saltiness" of the diet).

LONGITUDINAL STUDIES: TRACKING   In an extensive review, Szklo (57) summarized nine studies of tracking of blood pressure. Through 1988, we found 39 such reports, although in several cases—especially the Bogalusa Heart Study and the Muscatine Study in the US—several reports have come from a single investigation, so that altogether 26 studies are represented. Often these reports have provided only summary statistical results for an entire study population, which comprise a wide range of ages. The most informative reports give results specific for much narrower age strata, ideally by single year of age or less. Of the 39 reports, 18 (corresponding to 12 studies) provided data for groups no broader than three years in age at first observation.

Meaningful conclusions can be drawn from these selected studies, but several points concerning the design and methods of these studies require comment. These investigations were undertaken independently and were not intended for formal comparison. Major differences are found among the designs of these studies. For example, with respect to the age selection of subjects, in some studies a single age cohort was followed for examination at successive ages; in others, successive cohorts were observed so that different subjects were represented at different ages. Other differences among studies include the frequency of examination and overall duration of follow-up, the procedures for blood pressure measurement, and the definitions and criteria for tracking. Nevertheless, we can draw some consistent impression from this evidence.

Some resemblance to later systolic blood pressure readings within individual subjects is detectable from about six months of age. Such temporal consistency is established somewhat later for diastolic pressure and remains weaker than for systolic pressure; the distinction between fourth- and fifth-phase diastolic pressure in these respects is unclear. The strength of tracking correlations for observations over a fixed time interval, such as one year, tends to increase with increasing age at first examination, from late infancy to adolescence. There may be some sex differences in the strength of these correlations, but such results are inconsistent. Determinants of the strength of tracking correlations or of persistence in high ranks in the blood pressure distribution may differ at different ages or stages of maturation, but conclusions at this level of detail cannot be supported convincingly from the available data. Factors that contribute to the prediction of later blood pressure levels from previous ones are primarily measures of change in weight, skinfold thickness, ponderosity, or other indicators of increasing adiposity; family history of high blood pressure also may contribute (33, 35, 36).

Overall, these observations strongly suggest that the progressive increase of blood pressure with age, which occurs on average in the childhood population, may be partly determined by very early influences. However, the strength of these influences and the timing of their operation remain unclear.

LONGITUDINAL STUDIES: GROWTH OF BLOOD PRESSURE   The studies just reviewed, which report on various measures of tracking, do not provide data suitable for investigating the growth of blood pressure in a manner analogous to growth curves for height and weight discussed above. The studies in which the early development of blood pressure can be addressed in this way are those that present the absolute values of systolic and diastolic blood pressure for individuals observed over the course of several years' follow-up. We have identified only three such studies that are appropriately sex-specific, and two others in which the longitudinal data for boys and girls are combined (R. Jiles and D. R. Labarthe 1988, unpublished). These studies are limited in both the age ranges observed and the numbers of occasions of observation within each age cohort. They also differ in other aspects of the design. Only one report provides sex-specific data of this kind below age 11.

From these reports we can conclude for systolic pressure that increasing mean values generally were observed at successive years, from age 7 to 18 for both boys and girls, with a continuing increase to age 20, but not in every population. This age pattern, based on cohort studies, generally conforms with expectations from the cross-sectional studies reviewed above. Fourth-phase diastolic pressures declined or showed little change after age 11 in girls, whereas they increased from about age 16 to 18 for boys. Changes in fifth-phase diastolic pressure were inconsistent for girls; for boys, there were increases from about age 13 or 14 to age 18, with mixed directions of further change to age 20.

These longitudinal studies do not provide the desired growth curves, but do point to the potential value of such studies, especially those designed and monitored to assure comparable observations in multiple populations.

These observations of natural history, from both cross-sectional and longitudinal studies, strongly suggest that to understand and control the development of blood pressure as a risk factor for coronary heart disease, and to prevent the emergence of high blood pressure at levels that require treatment for a great many adults, the changes that occur throughout childhood and adolescence must be considered. The acceleration in blood pressure change with age, most clearly evident in the large-scale survey data, approximately coincides with the adolescent growth spurt. Patterns of change in blood pressure in relation to the dynamics of change in body mass index throughout childhood also have been demonstrated (33). The interrelations of risk factor development in childhood and adolescence, with the complex processes of growth and maturation, require special attention that has no direct parallel in adulthood.

INTERVENTION STUDIES   Intervention studies and statements of intervention policy contribute to the discussion of the precursors of high blood pressure and elevated cholesterol by indicating views of investigators and policy makers about the importance of possible precursors. The formal experience with intervention on blood pressure during childhood and adolescence is reflected in several reports, reviewed more fully elsewhere (33). Most relevant here is the choice of intervention in these studies, as they reflect views of possible causes of high blood pressure or, more generally, determinants of blood pressure levels in the population at large. Eleven of these reports concern children with persistently high percentile ranks of blood pressure or with obesity, positive family history of hypertension, or other special characteristics. Of 13 distinct studies, 14 concern more general populations of children, not selected with respect to prior blood pressure levels or other personal attributes.

In the group of 11 studies, in high risk children, physical activity was most common as a mode of intervention (6 studies), followed by diet (4), drugs (4), sodium or potassium intake (1), and muscle relaxation (1) (combinations of these were used in some of the 11 studies). Except for drug therapy, each of the other interventions used suggests the view of the investigators that limited physical activity, inappropriate dietary patterns, or undue neuromuscular tension contribute as determinants of the high blood pressure levels observed.

The intervention in the 14 studies in general populations was most often educational, either with multiple components (11 studies) or restricted to sodium or potassium intake (3), diet more generally (2), or physical activity (2). Again, diet and physical activity were targeted for intervention, which indicates a view that these factors are important as determinants of blood pressure levels in childhood.

The results of the intervention studies described here were inconsistent with respect to the occurrence of blood pressure change, the apparent response of systolic vs. diastolic pressure, and in boys vs. girls. There were some positive effects (systolic or diastolic blood pressure reduction in boys or in girls) in several of the studies, but taken together the results do not provide clear evidence of blood pressure-lowering effects. For example, experimental reduction of sodium intake resulted in relatively lower blood pressure in infants (27), but not in adolescents (10). However, young adults described as having "mildly elevated blood pressure" experienced reduction in pressure not with sodium restriction alone, but only in combination with potassium supplementation (23).

It is difficult to draw firm conclusions from these studies as to the effectiveness of these interventions on change in blood pressure and, therefore, to find experimental confirmation of the role of these factors as precursors of high blood pressure. There may be many reasons why true benefit may not have been detectable in these studies, however. We will address this issue in the conclusions of this review.

To illustrate an approach to intervention policy concerning blood pressure in childhood, the Report of the Second Task Force on Blood Pressure in Children (59) provides a particularly detailed example. This Report, prepared under the auspices of the National Heart, Lung, and Blood Institute of the National Institutes of Health, updated a similar report published ten years earlier. The update revised the reference percentile values of blood pressure by age and sex. It also proposed allowances for differences in growth in the interpretation of blood pressure levels observed in examining children.

Significantly, the Second Task Force introduced a qualification to the earlier classification scheme by noting that children who are at the upper extreme of height or lean body mass, as well as that of systolic or diastolic pressure, for their respective age-sex groups should be considered to have normal blood pressure. This provision recognizes the strong relation between blood pressure and growth and avoids misclassification as abnormal of those children whose blood pressure levels reflect growth beyond that of their age-sex peers.

Obesity is addressed differently by the Task Force. In the absence of obesity, persistent readings at or above the ninety-fifth percentile indicate the need for diagnostic evaluation and possible treatment. If obesity is present and the blood pressure readings are at or above the ninetieth percentile, weight control is advocated as the first step of treatment. This recommendation reflects the view that relatively high blood pressure values may be caused by obesity and may be expected to respond to its reduction.

The individuals identified for intervention under the Task Force recommendations, from birth to age 16, are those whose values are high only in relation to their age-sex peers, not in absolute terms. (Only at age 16 do the numerical criteria reach the values, such as a diastolic pressure of 90 mmHg or greater, which would be considered in adulthood as warranting intervention.) The rationale for this approach is based on tracking, with the implication that those individuals most at risk of future hypertension are those who are highest in rank at the ages before hypertension, in absolute terms, appears. In the Task Force scheme, the most important precursor of high blood pressure is the percentile rank of systolic or diastolic blood pressure at the moment. The Task Force recognizes height and lean body mass as determinants of blood pressure that explain high values on presumed nonpathological bases during childhood and adolescence. This concept, if valid, evidently does not apply to adults, in whom height appears unrelated to blood pressure levels except for an inverse relation after adjustment for weight or body mass index (13). Harlan et al (24) observed that lean body mass decreases with age, whereas mean values of blood pressure continue to increase. The Task Force treats obesity, however, as a precursor and determinant whose reversal may be beneficial in reducing relatively high blood pressure levels. This concept appears to hold in adulthood also, although it leaves unexplained the occurrence of high blood pressure among the nonobese.

CHOLESTEROL

Natural History

CROSS-SECTIONAL SURVEYS   Reported surveys of blood cholesterol levels in childhood are similar in some respects to those of blood pressure. However, there are differences in the nature of the observations for these two risk factors. For cholesterol, the collected population surveys (34) indicate patterns of variation by age, which differ among populations. When the age range from 6 to 18 years is considered, a striking curvilinear pattern appears, which is characterized by a prominent inverse change in the early teens; preteen levels are reached again by the late teens (B. O'Brien et al 1988, unpublished). Populations differ, however, in the ages at which the pre-adolescent peaks and the minimum adolescent values occur. Therefore, pooling of values among surveys in the manner shown above for blood pressure surveys would obscure this otherwise consistent pattern. Strobl & Widhalm (55) give a more detailed discussion of the age patterns of several lipid fractions.

Several investigators have compared age-specific mean values of total cholesterol between populations (Figure 4) (34). Between-population differences as great as 60 mg/dl have been demonstrated clearly in some of these comparisons, some of which indicate parallel differences in measures of growth and of diet (30, 70). Racial comparisons, for example those between black and white children, often, but not invariably, have been reported as showing higher mean levels of total cholesterol in blacks (4, 8, 9, 29, 42, 48, 65). Our own review (34) indicated that in the Health and Nutrition Examination Survey of 1971–1974 the age-specific mean values for cholesterol were similar between blacks and whites, although blacks more often had higher values in other studies. Higher levels of HDL cholesterol have been observed in black children than in whites (4, 41).

Familial studies of cholesterol and other blood lipids have consistently indicated familial aggregation, both within and between generations. Such results have been found in studies of absolute values of cholesterol or other lipids, or in the presence of hyperlipidemia or overt atherosclerosis, such as

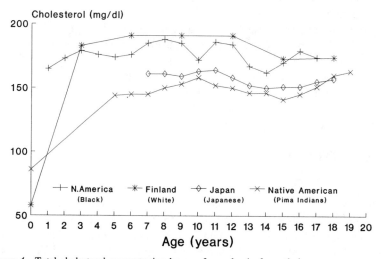

Figure 4 Total cholesterol concentration by age for males in four ethnic groups.

the occurrence of myocardial infarction in a young parent (7, 19, 21, 26, 28, 38, 43, 46, 51). Recent studies have addressed several of the lipoprotein fractions, some of which appear to be more specific markers of familial resemblance than is total cholesterol or the cholesterol components of the lipoproteins (6, 31, 53, 69).

Lipoprotein (a) has been investigated in family studies and has been found to interact importantly with other markers of lipid phenotypes, and it is a topic of current and proposed studies (52; Boerwinkle 1990, personal communication). Studies of the heritability of lipid components have been reported but have not been consistent. These inconsistencies perhaps reflect differences in methods between investigations (15, 25, 63, 64).

LONGITUDINAL STUDIES: TRACKING   As was done for blood pressure, we may examine throughout childhood and adolescence longitudinal data concerning blood cholesterol, from the perspectives of both tracking and absolute longitudinal change. Fewer such longitudinal studies are available than for blood pressure. There are 17 identified reports of tracking, which represent nine different studies, including seven reports from the Bogalusa Heart Study and three from the Muscatine Study. In only nine of these reports were data analyzed for age intervals as narrow as three years. Conclusions can best be drawn from this limited subset of the reports.

Significant correlations among serial measurements for total cholesterol and for low-density lipoprotein cholesterol appear most consistently at about six months of age, although weaker relations are evident when 1-week-old or even cord blood samples are used to determine the baseline reference value (11, 16, 20, 56). For high-density lipoprotein cholesterol and triglycerides, such a pattern is not established until at least one year of age. Those individuals who remain in high percentile ranks for various lipid fractions may tend to have positive family histories of diabetes mellitus or clinical coronary heart disease, especially on the paternal side, and greater personal increases in weight or measures of adiposity, than those who do not remain in high ranks. It is difficult to reach more specific conclusions, with broad applicability, about the tracking of total cholesterol levels during this period of life, from the data reported thus far.

Prediction of early adult lipid levels was attempted in the Muscatine Study. Participants were classified according to their percentile ranks for cholesterol at selected ages (from 9–10 to 17–18 years, at the extremes) and their observed risks of ranking above the ninetieth percentile value at ages 20–25 or 26–30 (37). The increases in risks from the lowest to the highest baseline percentile ranks, in accordance with the model used, were from 0% to 10% for the zero to sixtieth percentiles to about 40% for the ninety-ninth percentile, largely irrespective of age at the reference examination. This increase was true for both males and females and in relation to the values at follow-up for either the age group of the early twenties or the later twenties. The only apparent major exception (whether significantly different from the other patterns was not addressed in the report) was that for men, ranking below or above the ninetieth percentile at age 20–25 was better predicted from reference examinations at age 17–18 than from examinations at earlier ages. The basis for these particular variations in the age- and sex-specific patterns of tracking for total cholesterol is not apparent.

LONGITUDINAL STUDIES: GROWTH OF CHOLESTEROL VALUES   As was found for blood pressure, far fewer reports present the information necessary to describe growth of cholesterol than to describe its tracking (M. Eissa and D. R. Labarthe 1989, unpublished data). Only three reports have given age-intervals and sex-specific absolute values for total cholesterol over three or more years, and differences in such aspects of study design as age structure of the populations and their follow-up make coverage of the period of childhood and adolescence seriously incomplete. Taken together, these few studies do indicate a decrease in total cholesterol in the early teenage years, which is consistent with the cross-sectional patterns of cholesterol values by age for both boys and girls. No continuous longitudinal curve of cholesterol values by age can be constructed, however.

These population data on blood cholesterol concentrations, taken from both cross-sectional and longitudinal studies, have many limitations. Nonetheless, they indicate that mean values decrease transiently in temporal relation to puberty, that marked population differences do occur within childhood, and that subsequent values are somewhat predictable from observations at earlier ages. If the potential for effective control of progression in cholesterol values from childhood into adulthood is to be fully realized, further understanding of this natural history will be an essential intermediate step.

INTERVENTION

We have identified 36 studies that concern experience with intervention to reduce cholesterol levels in childhood; 23 in subjects with elevated cholesterol values, and 13 in general populations not selected on the basis of known cholesterol values. The intervention methods used in the first group of studies were based on diet in seven studies, drug intervention in four, and a combination of diet and drugs in seven others; various treatments were used in the remaining five studies, including one with surgical treatment (partial ileal bypass). Aggressive treatment was more commonly used in these intervention studies than in those that addressed blood pressure, and dietary patterns were often the main or a prominent adjunctive treatment. These studies thus reflect a view that dietary patterns are an important determinant of elevated cholesterol values in childhood.

In the studies of unselected populations, the interventions were dietary in six instances, educational programs in five, and physical activity in three. Again, behavioral factors, including diet and physical activity, are prominent, as in the intervention studies on blood pressure in childhood.

In most, but not all of the first group of studies, the authors reported some decrease in blood cholesterol from baseline values. They attributed this decrease to the intervention, but many of those studies were uncontrolled. In the latter group, evidence of benefit was found in one half of the studies. Overall, these studies on cholesterol levels have failed to provide strong experimental evidence to support the causal contribution of diet and physical activity to the determination of the observed values. Some of the reasons for possible false negative results are addressed in the conclusions.

For blood cholesterol, formal recommendations for intervention, until recently, have been much less detailed than those for blood pressure. These recommendations also have reflected conflicting views on the importance of family history as a factor in identifying high risk of elevated cholesterol values.

The most extensive recommendations published to date are those found in the American Health Foundation monograph on blood lipids in children (69). These recommendations depart from the previous view that cholesterol screening in children should be limited to those with a positive family history of overt coronary heart disease or hyperlipidemia. The emphasis of intervention is on dietary patterns, with the goals of reduction of excess body weight toward the ideal and alteration of diet composition to conform to prescribed proportions of calories from specific constituents. These recommendations also indicate that dietary factors are the most important modifiable determinants of blood cholesterol values in childhood and, hence, precursors of elevated cholesterol early in life.

INTERACTIONS AMONG THE RISK FACTORS

This review has specifically focused on blood pressure and cholesterol levels as they occur in childhood and adolescence; other factors related either to the risk of atherosclerosis or to the development of these two of the major risk factors have been addressed incidentally. There is evidence of interaction among these factors, however, which should not be overlooked. For example, smoking, using oral contraceptives, and drinking alcohol during adolescence have been studied, as they relate to either blood pressure or lipid levels in this same period of life (1, 17, 22, 45, 60–62). Smoking is inversely associated with levels of systolic blood pressure, oral contraceptive use is directly associated with systolic blood pressure and cholesterol levels, and alcohol (not yet studied to our knowledge in relation to either blood pressure or total cholesterol in childhood and adolescence) may be directly associated with HDL cholesterol levels. In other possible interactions among these several factors, current evidence is either lacking or inconsistent.

CONCLUSIONS

Theory

The theoretical basis for understanding the development of atherosclerosis as a gradual process with onset well before age 20 is supported by the evidence concerning the early natural history of two of its main predictors, blood pressure and cholesterol. Indications of relations between these risk factors and possible determinants of the levels of these factors themselves, such as dietary pattern, weight changes, physical activity pattern, and family history, add to the plausibility of important biological connections among these phenomena.

The evidence concerning blood pressure and that concerning cholesterol differ in possibly important respects, however. Blood pressure levels are similar among different populations for corresponding age-sex groups, whereas marked differences are found for cholesterol. Blood pressure levels, which in absolute terms equal those warranting treatment in adulthood, are infrequent below age 16; for cholesterol, values warranting treatment by adult standards are recognized early in childhood before a decrease in levels, on average, in the early teenage years. Thus, relations between these two risk factors and the underlying processes of growth and maturation cannot be identical. Even for the different measures of blood pressure (systolic, fourth- and fifth-phase diastolic), there are sufficient differences in the patterns and timing of their changes with age that they cannot relate in the same way to those processes. Thus, although the general concept that adult levels of blood pressure and cholesterol have important precursors in childhood is reinforced by the evidence considered here, we are far from a complete theoretical formulation of the relations involved.

Practice

Practice and policy statements, which concern intervention to modify the development of blood pressure and cholesterol, center mainly on general patterns of diet and physical activity, with intermediate goals of modifying weight, or weight gain, or body composition. Height and lean body mass are proposed as adjusting factors in the interpretation of blood pressure measurements, but obesity or overweight are regarded as targets of intervention to reduce both blood pressure and cholesterol levels. On the basis of current knowledge, these approaches appear sound, with potential benefit and little or no risk of harm when properly implemented. In contrast to the patterns of behavior concerning diet and physical activity, which are prevalent in the population at large, thus constituting de facto policies, the practices and policies reflected here are preferable at least until further evidence is obtained.

Research

The chief implication for research on the early natural history of atherosclerosis and its major risk factors is that the leads from previous studies, cross-sectional and longitudinal, should be pursued vigorously. Population comparisons are revealing and may be more productive in the future with deliberate planning and collaboration to enhance the value of the comparisons. Longitudinal studies should be conducted with greater intensity, longer duration, and increased numbers of observations within narrow age ranges. Ideally, the comparative and longitudinal approaches will be combined, and cohort studies will be compared in diverse population settings, including different racial groups. Further understanding of interactions among the major risk factors and related behaviors and other attributes also is an important objective of future research in this area.

With respect to intervention studies, the limited conviction on the efficacy of the attempted interventions requires careful evaluation. The expected changes in blood pressure or cholesterol are age- and sex-dependent and appear to be closely related to growth, maturation, and body composition. Especially for systolic blood pressure, the possibility that intrinsic factors related to growth are dominant influences suggests that modifications in diet or physical activity are likely to be very modest and might not have consistent measurable effects. The design of intervention studies to date, including only very short-term evaluation, may have been inappropriate to detect true beneficial effects of these approaches. Therefore, future research should be closely linked with newer insights from observational studies, such as those suggested above.

The third area cited in the opening section of this review was predicting the course of the disease process. This area of inquiry is posed as a challenge to our present knowledge and assumptions about any disease process. Can we today predict the course of development of blood pressure or cholesterol in childhood and the long-term implications of these developments in any population? If, as with the weather, today is the best guide to tomorrow, we should expect no improvement in the rates at which high blood pressure and elevated cholesterol appear in the US population, unless effective intervention were implemented broadly. Accordingly, the frequency of blood pressure and cholesterol levels in the population that require individual treatment would not be expected to diminish. The possibility that the available interventions on diet and physical activity might be effective and in no way harmful justifies their application in settings where long-term monitoring can be conducted to assess their effects. Coupled with improving understanding of the natural history of these risk factors in childhood, such knowledge about the effectiveness of interventions could lead to more serious attempts to predict the future course of this process from the viewpoint of public health practice. A test of our research progress in the coming decade will be to reassess our readiness to undertake such predictions at the end of this period.

ACKNOWLEDGMENT

The authors wish to acknowledge the contributions of Drs. Ge Donker and Jo Anne Grunbaum to the review of familial aspects of blood lipids in children and the interaction among risk factors, respectively, and the support of the Centers for Disease Control, R48-CCR602176–02.

Literature Cited

1. Anderson, L. B., Henckel, P., Saltin, B. 1989. Risk factors for cardiovascular disease in 16–19-year-old teenagers. *J. Int. Med.* 225:157–63
2. Baranowski, T., Tsong, Y., Henske, J., Dunn, K. J., Hooks, P. 1988. Ethnic variation in blood pressure among preadolescent children. *Pediatr. Res.* 23:270–74
3. Baron, A. E., Freyer, B., Fixler, D. E. 1986. Longitudinal blood pressures in blacks, whites, and Mexican Americans during adolescence and early adulthood. *Am. J. Epidemiol.* 123(5):809–17
4. Berenson, G. S., Webber, L. S., Srinivasan, S. R., Cresanta, J. L., Frank, G., Farris, R. 1984. Black-White contrasts as determinants of cardiovascular risk in childhood: Precursors of coronary artery and primary hypertensive diseases. *Am. Heart J.* 108(3):672–82
5. Brotons, C., Singh, P., Nishio, T., Labarthe, D. R. 1990. Blood pressure by age in childhood and adolescence: A review of 129 studies worldwide. *Int. J. Epidemiol.* 18(4):824–29
6. Brunzell, J. D., Sniderman, A. D., Albers, J. J., Kwiterovich, P. O., Jr. 1984. Apolipoproteins B and A-1 in coronary artery disease in humans. *Arteriosclerosis* 4:79–83
7. Chase, G. A., Kwiterovich, P. O., Bachorik, P. S. 1979. The Columbia Population Study II. Familial aggregation of plasma cholesterol and triglycerides. *Johns Hopkins Med. J.* 145:150–60

8. Christensen, B. L., Glueck, C. H., Kwiterovich, P., Degroot, I., Chase, G., et al. 1980. Plasma cholesterol and triglyceride distributions in 13,665 children and adolescents: the Prevalence Study of the Lipid Research Clinics Program. *Pediatr. Res.* 14:194–202
9. Christensen, B. L., Stallones, R. A., Isull, W., Jr., Gotto, A. M., Taunton, D. 1981. Cardiovascular risk factors in a tri-ethnic population: Houston, Texas 1972–1975. *J. Chron. Dis.* 34:105–18
10. Cooper, R., Van Horn, L., Liu, K., Trevisan, M., Nanas, S., et al. 1984. A randomized trial on the effect of decreased dietary sodium intake on blood pressure in adolescents. *J. Hypertension* 2:361–66
11. Darmady, J. M., Fosbrooke, A., Lloyd, J. K. 1972. Prospective study of serum cholesterol levels during first year of life. *Br. Med. J.* 2:685–88
12. Dodu, S. R. A. 1988. Emergence of cardiovascular diseases in developing countries. *Cardiology* 75:56–64
13. Dyer, A. R., Elliott, P., Shipley, M. 1990. Body mass index versus height and weight in relation to blood pressure. *Am. J. Epidemiol.* 131:589–96
14. Ellison, C. R., Sosenko, J. M., Harper, G. P., Gibbons, L., Pratter, F. E., Miettinen, O. S. 1980. Obesity, sodium intake, and blood pressure in adolescents. *Hypertension* 2(Suppl. 1):78–82
15. Feinleib, M., Garrison, R. J., Fabsitz, R., Christian, J. C., Hrubec, Z., et al. 1977. The NHLBI twin study of car-

diovascular disease risk factors: methodology and summary of results. *Am. J. Epidemiol.* 106:284–95

16. Freedman, D. S., Srinivasan, S. R., Cresanta, J. L., Webber, L. S., Berenson, G. S. 1987b. Cardiovascular disease risk factors from birth to seven years of age: The Bogalusa Heart Study. IV. Serum lipids and lipoproteins. *Pediatrics* 5(Suppl. 80):789–96

17. Freedman, D. S., Srinivasan, S. R., Shear, C. L., Webber, L. S., Chiang, Y. K., Berenson, G. S. 1987a. Correlates of high density lipoprotein cholesterol and apolipoprotein A-1 levels in children: The Bogalusa Heart Study. *Arteriosclerosis* 7:354–360

18. Frohlich, E. D., Grim, C., Labarthe, D. R., Maxwell, M. H., Perloff, D., Weidman, W. H. 1988. Recommendations for human blood pressure determination by sphygmomanometers. Report of a Special Task Force Appointed by the Steering Committee, American Heart Association. *Circulation* 77(2):501A–14A

19. Garrison, R. J., Castelli, W. P., Feinleib, M., Kannel, W. B., Havlik, R. J., et al. 1979. The association of total cholesterol, triglycerides and plasma lipoprotein cholesterol levels in first degree relatives and spouse pairs. *Am. J. Epidemiol.* 110:313–21

20. Ginsburg, B. E., Zetterstrom, R. 1980. Serum cholesterol concentration in early infancy. *Acta Pediatr. Scand.* 69:581–85

21. Glueck, C. J., Fallat, R. W., Tsang, R., Buncher, C. R. 1974. Hyperlipidemia in progeny of parents with myocardial infarction before age 50. *Am. J. Dis. Child.* 127:70–75

22. Glueck, C. J., Heiss, G., Morrison, J. A., Khoury, P., Moore, M. 1981. Alcohol intake, cigarette smoking and plasma lipids and lipoproteins in 12–19-year-old children. *Circulation* 64:III48–III56

23. Grobbee, D. E., Hofman, A., Roetlandt, J. T., Boomsma, F., Schalekamp, M. A., Valkenburg, H. A. 1987. Sodium restriction and potassium supplementation in young people with mildly elevated blood pressure. *J. Hypertens.* 5:115–19

24. Harlan, W. R., Hull, A. L., Schmouder, R. L., Landis, J. R., Thompson, F. E., Larkin, F. A. 1984. Blood pressure and nutrition in adults. The National Health and Nutrition Examination Survey. *Am. J. Epidemiol.* 120:17–28

25. Heiberg, A. 1974. The heritability of serum lipoprotein and lipid concentrations. *Clin. Genet.* 6:307–16

26. Hennekens, C. H., Jesse, M. J., Klein, B. E., Gourley, J. E., Blumenthal, S. 1976. Cholcstcrol among children of men with myocardial infarction. *Pediatrics* 58:(2):211–17

27. Hofman, A., Haeebroek, A., Valkenburg, H. A. 1983. A randomized trial of sodium intake and blood pressure in newborn infants. *J. Am. Med. Assoc.* 250:370–73

28. Johnson, B. L., Frederick, F. H., Kjelsberg, M. O. 1965. Distributions and familial studies of blood pressure and serum cholesterol levels in a total community—Tecumseh, Michigan. *J. Chron. Dis.* 18:147–60

29. Khoury, P., Morrison, J. A., Kelly, K., Mellies, M. J., Glueck, C. J. 1981. Studies of blood pressure in hyperlipidemic school children. *Arteriosclerosis* 1(4):280–86

30. Knuiman, J. T., Westerbrink, S., van der Heyden, L., Hermus, R. J. J., Hautvask, J. G. H. J. 1983. Determinants of total and high density lipoprotein cholesterol in boys from Finland, the Netherlands, Italy, the Philippines and Ghana with special reference to diet. *Hum. Nutr.* 37C.237–54

31. Kukita, H., Hiwada, K., Kokuba, T. 1984. Serum apolipoproteins A-I, A-II, and B-levels and their discriminative values in relatives of parents with coronary artery disease. *Atherosclerosis* 51:261–67

32. Labarthe, D. R., Brotons, C., Singh, P., Nishio, T. 1989. Epidemiology of blood pressure in childhood, an international perspective. *Semin. Nephrol.* 9(3):287–95

33. Labarthe, D. R., Mueller, W. H., Eissa, M. 1991a. Blood pressure and obesity in childhood and adolescence: Epidemiologic aspects. *Ann. Epidemiol.* In press

34. Labarthe, D. R., O'Brien, B., Dunn, K. 1991b. International comparisons of plasma cholesterol and lipoproteins. *Ann. NY Acad. Sci.* In press

35. Lauer, R. M., Anderson, A. R., Beaglehole, R., Burns, T. L. 1984a. Factors related to tracking of blood pressure in children. US National Center for Health Statistics Health examination Surveys Cycles II and III. *Hypertension* 6:307–14

36. Lauer, R. M., Clarke, W. R., Beaglehole, R. 1984b. Level, trend, and variability of blood pressure during childhood: The Muscatine Study. *Circulation* 69:242–49

37. Lauer, R. M., Lee, J., Clark, W. 1988. Factors affecting the relationship between childhood and adult cholesterol

levels: The Muscatine Study. *Pediatrics* 82:309–18

38. Lee, J., Lauer, R. M., Clarke, W. R. 1986. Lipoproteins in the progeny of young men with coronary heart disease: children with increased risk. *Pediatrics* 78(2):330–37

39. McGill, H. C., Jr. 1980. Morphologic development of atherosclerotic plaque. In *Childhood Prevention of Atherosclerosis and Hypertension,* ed. R. M. Lauer, R. B. Shekelle, pp. 41–49. New York: Raven

40. McNamara, J. J., Molot, M. A., Stremple, J. F., Cutting, R. T. 1971. Coronary artery disease in combat casualties in Vietnam. *J. Am. Med. Assoc.* 216:1185–87

41. Morrison, J. A., deGroot, I., Kelly, K. A., Mellies, M. J., Khoury, P., et al. 1979a. Black-White differences in plasma lipoproteins in Cincinnati schoolchildren (one-to-one pair matched by total plasma cholesterol, sex, and age). *Metabolism* 28(3):241–45

42. Morrison, J. A., Glueck, C. J. 1981. Pediatric risk factors for adult coronary heart disease: Primary atherosclerosis prevention. *Cardiovasc. Rev. Rep.* 2(12):1269–81

43. Morrison, J. A., Kelly, K., Horvitz, R., Khoury, P., Laskarzewski, P. M., et al. 1983a. Parent-offspring and sibling lipid and lipoprotein associations during and after sharing of household environments: The Princenton School Family Study. *Metabolism* 31(2):158–66

44. Morrison, J. A., Kelly, K., Mellies, M. J., deGroot, I., Glueck, C. J. 1978. Parent-child associations at upper and lower ranges of plasma-cholesterol and triglycerides. *Pediatrics* 62:468–77

45. Morrison, J. A., Kelly, K. A., Mellies, M. J., deGroot, I., Khoury, P., et al. 1979b. Cigarette smoking, alcohol intake, and oral contraceptives: Relationships to lipids and lipoproteins in adolescent school-children. *Metabolism* 28:1166–70

46. Morrison, J. A., Namboodiri, K., Green, P., Martin, J., Glueck, C. J. 1983b. Familial aggregation of lipids and lipoproteins and early identification of dyslipoproteinemia. *J. Am. Med. Assoc.* 250(14):1860–68

47. Reed, W. L. 1981. Racial differences in blood pressure levels of adolescents. *Am. J. Public Health.* 71:1165–67

48. Resnicow, K., Morley-Kotchen, J., Wynder, E. 1989. Plasma cholesterol levels of 6585 children in the United States: Results of the Know Your Body Screening in Five States. *Pediatrics* 84:969–76

49. Rose, G. 1981. Strategy of prevention: Lessons from cardiovascular disease. *Br. Med. J.* 282:1847–51

50. Schachter, J., Kuller, L. H., Perkins, J. M., Radyn, M. E. 1979. Infant blood pressure and heart rate: Relation to ethnic group (Black or White), nutrition and electrolyte intake. *Am. J. Epidemiol.* 110:205–18

51. Schrott, H. G., Clarke, W. R., Wiebe, D. A., Connor, W. E., Lauer, R. M. 1979. Increased coronary mortality in relatives of hypercholesterolemic school children: The Muscatine Study. *Circulation* 59(2):330–26

52. Seed, M., Hoppichler, F., Reaveley, D., McCarthy, S., Thompson, G. R., et al. 1990. Relation of serum lipoprotein (a) concentration and apolipoprotein (a) phenotype to CHD in patients with familial hypercholesterolemia. *N. Engl. J. Med.* 322:1494–99

53. Sniderman, A., Teng, B., Genest, J., Cianflone, K., Wacholder, S., Kwiterovich, P. 1985. Familial aggregation and early expression of hyperapobetalipoproteinemia. *Am. J. Cardiol.* 55:291–95

54. Strasser, T. 1978. Reflections on cardiovascular diseases. *Interdiscip. Sci. Rev.* 3:225–30

55. Strobl, W., Widhalm, K. 1985. The natural history of serum lipids and lipoproteins during childhood. In *Detection and Treatment of Lipid and Lipoprotein Disorders of Childhood,* ed. K. Widhalm, H. Naito, pp. 101–21. New York: Liss

56. Strobl, W., Widhalm, K., Kostnerg, G., Pollak, A. 1983. Serum apolipoproteins and lipoproteins during the first week of life. *Acta Pediatr. Scand.* 72:505–9

57. Szklo, M. 1979. Epidemiological patterns of blood pressure in children. *Epidemiol. Rev.* 1:143–69

58. Tanner, J. M. 1978. *Foetus into Man: Physical Growth from Conception to Maturity.* London: Openbooks. 250 pp.

59. Task Force on Blood Pressure Control in Children. 1987. Report of the Second Task Force on Blood Pressure Control in Children—1987. *Pediatrics* 79:1–25

60. Voors, A. W., Srinivasan, S. R., Hunter, S. M., Webber, L. S., Sklov, M. C., Berenson, G. S. 1982. Smoking, oral contraceptives, and serum lipid and lipoprotein levels in youths. *Prev. Med.* 15:352–62

61. Wallace, R. B., Tamir, I., Heiss, G., Rifkind, B. M., Christensen, B., Glueck, C. J. 1979. Plasma lipids,

lipoproteins, and blood pressure in female adolescents using oral contraceptives. *J. Pediatr.* 95:1055–59

62. Webber, L. S., Hunter, S. M., Baugh, J. G., Srinivasan, S. R., Sklov, M. C., Berenson, G. S. 1982. The interaction of cigarette smoking, oral contraceptive use, and cardiovascular risk factor variables in children: The Bogalusa Heart Study. *Am. J. Public Health* 72:266–74

63. Weinberg, R., Avet, L. M., Gardner, M. J. 1974. Estimates of the heritability of serum lipoprotin and lipid concentrations. *Clin. Genet.* 6:307–16

64. Weinberg, R., Webber, L. S., Berenson, G. S. 1982. Hereditary and environmental influences on cardiovascular risk factors for children. The Bogalusa Heart Study. *Am. J. Epidemiol.* 116:(3):385–93

65. Wheeler, R., Marcus, A. C., Cullen, J. W., Konugres, E. 1983. Baseline chronic disease risk factors in a racially heterogenous elementary school popula-tion: the "Know Your Body" program, Los Angeles. *Prev. Med.* 12:569–87

66. WHO Tech. Rep. Ser., No. 678. 1982. Prevention of coronary heart disease: Report of a WHO Expert Committee. Geneva: WHO

67. WHO Tech. Rep. Ser., No. 715. 1985. Blood pressure studies in children. Geneva: WHO

68. WHO Tech. Rep. Ser., No. 792. 1990. Prevention in childhood and youth of adult cardiovascular diseases: Time for action. Geneva: WHO

69. Wynder, E. L., Berenson, G. S., Strong, W. B., Williams, C., eds. 1989. An American Health Foundation monograph. Coronary artery disease prevention: Cholesterol, a pediatric perspective. *Prev. Med.* 18:323–409

70. Wynder, E. L., Williams, C. L., Laakso, K. Levenstein, M. 1981. Screening for risk factors for chronic disease in children from fifteen countries. *Prev. Med.* 10:121–32

Annu. Rev. Publ. Health 1991. 12:543–66

UPPER-EXTREMITY MUSCULOSKELETAL DISORDERS OF OCCUPATIONAL ORIGIN

Fredric Gerr, Richard Letz, and Philip J. Landrigan

Division of Occupational and Environmental Medicine, Department of Community Medicine, The Mount Sinai School of Medicine, New York, NY 10029

KEY WORDS: occupational disease, carpal tunnel syndrome, tendinitis, hand-arm vibration syndrome, ergonomics

INTRODUCTION

A large literature, relating upper-extremity musculoskeletal disorders to occupational factors, has evolved over the past 100 years. Such disorders have been considered endemic in certain industries, such as meat processing and packing. They also have been reported to occur with high frequency in other trades, such as construction, clerical work, forestry, product fabrication, garment production, health care, underground mining, and the arts (15, 20, 28, 31, 39, 68, 73, 75, 82). In the Bureau of Labor Statistics category "disorders associated with repeated trauma," upper-extremity musculoskeletal disorders are included, for reporting purposes, with other conditions associated with repeated motion, pressure, or vibration, such as noise-induced hearing loss. For this reason, precise estimates of the prevalence of these disorders are not available. It is nevertheless suggestive that, in 1988, the most recent year for which statistics are available, disorders associated with repeated trauma accounted for 48% of all reported occupational diseases (87), a substantial increase from 18% reported in 1982. Upper-extremity musculoskeletal disorders account for the majority of these reports (63).

Occupational epidemiologic studies of upper-extremity musculoskeletal disorders, including tendinitis and carpal tunnel syndrome (CTS), have variously reported etiologic associations with repetitive motion, hand force, awk-

543

0163-7525/91/0501-0543$02.00

ward posture, insufficient frequency of rest breaks, exposure to vibration, and job content or "psychosocial" factors. However, much of the literature examining the relations of upper-extremity musculoskeletal health outcomes to these occupational factors has been flawed. Few studies have employed either rigorous assessments of exposure or well-defined objective measures of outcomes. Consequently, the work-relatedness of many upper-extremity disorders remains controversial.

In this review we shall critically evaluate the scientific evidence that relates occupational factors to musculoskeletal disorders of the upper extremities. Specifically, we shall (a) discuss methodological issues, (b) define the terminology used in this field and address ambiguities, (c) discuss the problems of diagnosis and etiologic attribution that are posed by poorly defined clinical entities characterized by pain and occupational disability, (d) review the literature relating musculoskeletal disorders to use of video display terminals (VDTs), (e) draw conclusions regarding the work-relatedness of these disorders, and (f) present recommendations for further research.

BACKGROUND

The 1971 United States Health Interview Survey estimated that over 18 million noninstitutionalized adults, aged 25–74, suffered from musculoskeletal impairment, and that 2,440,000 of those cases involved the upper extremity or shoulder (22, 45). In 1981, the direct economic cost associated with upper-extremity disorders in the United States was estimated to be over $22 billion (52). Although many of the musculoskeletal disorders identified in large surveys of Americans were due to nonoccupational factors, occupationally related disorders, especially those affecting the upper extremities, are becoming recognized as significant contributors to the overall prevalence of musculoskeletal disease.

The relationship between work and painful musculoskeletal disorders was first described by Ramazzini over 200 years ago:

"... certain violent and irregular motions and unnatural postures of the body, by reason of which the natural structure of the vital machine is so impaired that serious diseases gradually develop therefrom." (70, p. 15)

The National Institute for Occupational Safety and Health (NIOSH) recently has designated occupationally related musculoskeletal disorders as one of the five leading categories of occupational diseases and injuries (15).

Widespread "outbreaks" of upper-extremity musculoskeletal pain have been reported in Japan and Australia over the past two decades. As many as 28% of workers in some departments of a large Australian telecommunications company were affected over a five year period (42). Anecdotal reports suggest the existence of similar problems in certain industries in the United States. For example, a recent NIOSH Health Hazard Evaluation at a large daily newspaper in the northeast United States found that 40% of the participating employees reported having experienced "symptoms compatible with upper-extremity cumulative trauma disorders" during the year preceding the evaluation (61).

Interest in these disorders has emerged recently in the lay press. Record fines levied by the United States Occupational Safety and Health Administration for violations of health and safety regulations intended to prevent occupational musculoskeletal disorders have been major news stories (2, 41), as have special features, such as the *New York Newsday* story "Repetitive Strain Injury May Be Occupational Disease of the '90s" (72).

The peer-reviewed medical literature is rich with studies that attempt to relate occupational factors to musculoskeletal disorders. The affected tissues include the tendons, tendon sheaths, muscles, nerves, bursae, and blood vessels (64). Musculoskeletal disorders that are commonly described in the literature as related or potentially related to occupational factors are listed in Table 1.

Table 1   Musculoskeletal disorders and associated occupational factors reported in the literature

Upper-Extremity Disorder	Occupational Factors
Carpal tunnel syndrome	force [14, 16, 59, 78, 85] repetition [8, 14, 16, 29, 78] awkward posture [16, 27, 55, 56, 86] vibration [16, 29] mechanical stress [86]
Tendinitis	force [5, 53, 91] repetition [5, 51, 53, 71, 91] awkward posture [53, 91] insufficient rest [69]
Epicondylitis	unaccustomed forceful movement [49] repetition [49] forceful grip [79] repeated supination/pronation [79, 88]
Shoulder/neck disorders	overhead work [1] static muscle load [38, 39, 89]
Hand-arm vibration syndrome	segmental vibration [10, 18, 19, 33, 40, 60]
Arm pain in office workers	use of video display terminals [47, 61, 73, 80, 82] psychosocial or workplace organizational factors [72, 82, 87]

Authors of recent reviews (7, 17, 29, 39, 57, 64, 84) have attempted to evaluate and summarize the literature regarding these disorders. These reviews reflect a growing consensus that occupational factors can place workers at increased risk for the development of upper-extremity musculoskeletal disorders. Authors repeatedly note, however, that much of the epidemiologic evidence for the work-relatedness of these disorders is of poor quality. The evidence often consists of little more than case series of affected industrial workers. Few studies have been reported in which rigorous assessment has been made either of exposure or of well-defined health outcomes. This relative lack of sound epidemiologic evidence has led some authors to question the validity of the notion that occupational factors can cause musculoskeletal disorders of the upper extremities (37).

REVIEW OF TERMINOLOGY

The nomenclature describing upper-extremity musculoskeletal disorders of occupational origin is confusing and internally inconsistent. Some terms refer to well-defined clinical entities (i.e. CTS, tendinitis, and hand-arm vibration syndrome), whereas others are vague or inclusive of a wide variety of less well-defined soft tissue disorders (i.e. repetition strain injury). For the purpose of clarity, we will provide a brief review of the terminology used in the literature. Critical evaluation of studies relating occupational exposures to soft tissue disorders will follow.

CARPAL TUNNEL SYNDROME   This syndrome is characterized by neuritic symptoms, such as pain, paresthesias, and numbness in the cutaneous distribution of the median nerve. It is universally accepted that CTS is the clinical concomitant of compression of the median nerve as it passes through the carpal canal in the wrist. Physical signs include diminished sensibility to vibration and light touch in the cutaneous distribution of the median nerve, as well as abnormal two-point discrimination. Thenar muscle weakness and atrophy, as well as Phalen's sign (reproduction of hand symptoms following one minute of wrist flexion) or Tinel's sign (electric shock sensation radiating into the hand upon tapping the wrist), are classic findings in CTS. Electrodiagnostic studies are currently the "gold standard" for the evaluation of suspected CTS. Typical findings include prolongation of the distal motor latency of the median nerve, slowing of median sensory conduction velocity across the wrist, and denervation of the abductor pollicis brevis muscle (46, 83). Clinical signs and symptoms are not fully diagnostic of CTS. At this time, the best evidence for the sensitivity of clinical examination by a neurologist for the diagnosis of this syndrome is 84% with a specificity of 72% (44). The sensitivity and specificity of Tinel's sign were 0.60 and

0.67, respectively, and of Phalen's sign 0.75 and 0.47, respectively (44). Other studies of the sensitivity and specificity of these tests for the detection of CTS have found similar results (24, 32). At this time, most authorities agree that a combination of characteristic symptoms, signs, and electrodiagnostic findings is the most valid means of diagnosing this syndrome (23, 46, 65, 74, 81).

TENDINITIS   Tendinitis and tenosynovitis refer to inflammation of the tendon and tendon sheath, respectively. Both are associated with painful impairment of motion involving the tendon. Tendon swelling, as well as crepitations, can be found on physical examination (13, p. 119). Tenosynovitis can progress to stenosing tenosynovitis, characterized by narrowing of the tendon sheath (48) and triggering movements of the digits ("trigger finger"). Although the most commonly affected tendons include the dorsal extensors of the wrist, the extensor carpi ulnaris, and the long abductor and short extensor of the thumb (de Quervain's disease) (13, p. 119), any muscle-tendon unit of the extremities can be affected (48). Some authors distinguish tendinitis from peritendinitis, which refers to inflammation of the muscle tendon junction and adjacent muscle tissue. The diagnosis is based on the presence of pain on palpation of the tendon, pain localized to the tendon on resisted movement, crepitations on palpation over the tendon, or the presence of warm, swollen tendons on palpation.

HAND-ARM VIBRATION SYNDROME   This disorder of blood vessels and peripheral nerves is caused typically by use of hand-held vibrating tools (60). It also has been referred to as white finger, vibration white finger, occupational Raynaud's disease, and vibration syndrome (18). These terms all refer to a clinically and epidemiologically distinct disease entity. The vascular component of the disorder is characterized clinically by cold-induced vasospasm, indistinguishable from Raynaud's disease, and pathologically by hypertrophy of the medial muscular layer of the digital arterial wall and by perivascular fibrosis (60). The neurological component is characterized clinically by abnormal sensory and motor function and likely involves both nerve fibers and mechanoreceptors (66). Some controversy exists regarding the diagnostic distinction between the neurological component of hand-arm vibration syndrome and CTS, because both diffuse neuropathy and focal slowing of median nerve sensory conduction velocity at the wrist have been found in symptomatic workers using vibrating tools (19).

CUMULATIVE TRAUMA DISORDER   This term has been used commonly in the United States. Its origins can be found in Tichauer's classic review, in which he stated: ". . . industrial health care must consider a different kind of impairment caused insidiously over lengthy periods of time by gradual, cumulative, and often imperceptible overstrain of minute body elements." (86, p. 63) Armstrong (4) has defined cumulative trauma disorders as: "Those disorders of the muscles, tendons, nerves, and blood vessels that are caused, precipitated, or aggravataed by repeated exertions or movements of the body." Armstrong explicitly stated that the term cumulative trauma disorder is not meant to serve as a diagnosis, but that rather it refers to a class of disorders "with similar characteristics" including pathogenesis; documented relationship to exposure; chronicity of onset and response to treatment; symptoms that are often poorly localized, nonspecific, and episodic; and association with multiple occupational and nonoccupational factors (4). Armstrong noted a tendency for cumulative trauma disorders to be underreported and recommended the use of epidemiologic methods to isolate jobs, tools, areas, plants, or industries with excessive risk.

REPETITION STRAIN INJURY   This term was popularized in Australia during the 1970s and 1980s when an apparent epidemic of diffuse arm pain was noted among a variety of occupational groups, including both those traditionally considered to be at risk for occupationally related musculoskeletal disorders, such as assembly line workers, and those previously thought to be at lower risk, such as clerical workers. The term was best defined by the Worksafe Australia—National Occupational Health and Safety Commission document "Repetition Strain Injury (RSI): A Report and Model Code of Practice":

> Repetition Strain Injury (RSI), also known as Occupational Overuse Syndrome, is a collective term for a range of conditions characterized by discomfort or persistent pain in muscles, tendons, and other soft tissues, with or without physical manifestations. Repetition Strain Injury is usually caused or aggravated by work, and is associated with repetitive movement, sustained or constrained postures and/or forceful movements. Psycho-social factors, including stress in the working environment, may be important in the development of Repetition Strain Injury. Some conditions which fall within the scope of Repetition Strain Injury are well-defined and understood medically, but many are not, and the basis for their cause and development is yet to be determined. It occurs among workers performing tasks involving either frequent repetitive and/or forceful movements of the limbs or the maintenance of fixed postures for prolonged periods, e.g., process workers, keyboard operators, and machinists. (62, p. 7)

The report acknowledged that the majority of cases were not well defined, and that the most notable feature of these cases was the reporting of upper extremity or neck pain.

OCCUPATIONAL CERVICOBRACHIAL DISORDERS   This term refers to disorders of the neck and shoulder that have been related by some authors to occupational factors (38, 39, 89). Waris (89) has reviewed these disorders and included cervical syndrome, tension neck syndrome, humeral tendinitis, and thoracic outlet syndrome in this category. Cervical syndrome results from degenerative changes in the cervical spine. Tension neck syndrome, also referred to in the literature as tension myalgia, has been defined as a complex of pain, tenderness, and stiffness of muscles, coupled with the physical finding of muscle spasm. Humeral tendinitis refers to both supraspinous and bicipital tendinitis. Thoracic outlet syndrome is the result of neurovascular compression at the superior thoracic outlet. The term occupational cervico-brachial disorder was used extensively in Japan to describe an epidemic of work related shoulder and neck pain (54).

OVERUSE SYNDROME   Overuse syndrome was characterized by Dennett & Fry (25) as "a musculoskeletal disorder characterized by pain, tenderness, and often functional loss in muscle groups and ligaments subjected to heavy or unaccustomed use." Fry (30) noted that pain is the predominant symptom and may occur in the hand and wrist area, forearm, elbow, shoulder area, scapular area, and neck. In addition, he described the possibility of sensory loss that can "mimic other conditions" (30, p. 728) and indicated that the disorder could arise bilaterally, even in the absence of symmetrical loading. Physical examination is positive for the condition when the patient experiences tenderness on palpation of the affected muscles, joints, and ligaments. Puffer & Zachazewski (67) provided a similar description of overuse syndrome.

REGIONAL MUSCULOSKELETAL ILLNESS   This term has been championed by Hadler (36). He believes that the hypothesis that upper-extremity disorders are caused by occupational factors is unsubstantiated empirically. He argues that upper-extremity symptoms (the "predicament" of arm pain) are common. In addition, although he notes that discomfort of the upper extremities can be associated with occupational factors, he insists that upper-extremity musculoskeletal disorders that are characterized by a "dystrophic, atrophic, or overtly inflammatory state" (37, p. 39) have not been associated etiologically with work. He claims that the discomfort experienced by workers is best considered a form of "fatigue" (35) or "soreness" (37), rather than a workplace-induced musculoskeletal disorder.

Summary and Recommendations

One of the major impediments to diagnostic clarity and etiologic understanding of upper-extremity musculoskeletal disorders is widespread use of confusing and inconsistent terminology. A variety of terms have been introduced in the literature to allow reference to a heterogeneous group of upper-extremity musculoskeletal disorders that have in common an apparent increase in prevalence under certain occupational conditions. These terms include cumulative trauma disorder, repetition strain injury, occupational cervico-brachial disorder, and overuse syndrome. Despite the fact that some investigators have stated that these terms are synonymous, critical review of the literature fails to support this concept.

Another problem is that the terms repetition strain injury, cumulative trauma disorder, and occupational overuse imply etiology. There is not, however, substantial evidence that these disorders arise from cumulative trauma or that repetitive strain is the critical exposure. Indeed, the studies by Silverstein and colleagues (5, 77, 78), reviewed below, fail to show an increase in the prevalence these disorders with increasing work duration. The cross-sectional design of their studies may preclude observation of an exposure-response relationship as a result of survival bias or the effects of changing of job activities with increasing tenure; nevertheless, the available data certainly do not yet support the concept of "cumulative trauma."

If an all-inclusive term is required, the terms "musculoskeletal disorders of occupational origin" and "soft tissue disorders of occupational origin" seem more descriptive and should be applied to nonarticular musculoskeletal, vascular, and neurologic disorders for which significant elevations in risk are associated with occupational factors. For most applications, however, well-defined entities (i.e. CTS or tendinitis) should be used when attempting to relate occupational factors to musculoskeletal health outcomes. The term "upper-extremity pain syndrome" is recommended for those patients with upper-extremity pain who have symptoms that are not consistent with conventional diagnostic categories and normal physical examinations and physiological studies. Collective terms, such as RSI, are not diagnoses and should not be used in such cases.

EPIDEMIOLOGIC EVIDENCE FOR WORK RELATEDNESS

We review here the evidence for a causal relationship between workplace exposures and upper-extremity musculoskeletal disorders. We will summarize and critique the most rigorous studies aimed at testing the hypothesis that occupational exposures are causally associated with upper-extremity musculoskeletal disorders. In addition, we survey the voluminous literature that describes and characterizes the hand-arm vibration syndrome, a well-studied disorder caused by exposure to high frequency vibration. Finally, we will examine two poorly characterized disorders of the upper extremities, RSI and musculoskeletal discomfort among VDT users. For the purpose of this review, we have divided these disorders into "well-defined" and "poorly defined" categories.

Well-Defined Disorders

Carpal tunnel syndrome, tendinitis, and hand-arm vibration syndrome are the musculoskeletal disorders of the upper extremities that have most convincingly been associated with occupational factors. Well-defined disorders other than these, such as cervical radiculopathy, supraspinatus (rotator cuff) tendinitis, and epicondylitis, have been described in the orthopedic, rheumatologic, and occupational medicine literature, but at this time have not been so clearly associated with work.

CARPAL TUNNEL SYNDROME AND TENDINITIS   Stock (84) has provided the most rigorous review of the literature to date that relates occupational exposures to upper-extremity musculoskeletal disorders. She performed an exhaustive literature search followed by critical evaluation and metaanalysis of those published studies that met well-defined criteria, including adequate definition of the study population; inclusion of an appropriate comparison group; appropriate measures of exposure; use of well-defined musculoskeletal endpoints that included objective physical signs of disease in addition to the presence of symptoms; and appropriate study design consisting of either case-control, cross-sectional, longitudinal cohort, or randomized controlled trial. She did not include studies of the hand-arm vibration syndrome. Of the 54 potentially relevant studies initially identified, Stock found that only five published papers and one Ph.D. thesis (5, 53, 59, 76, 77, 78) met the a priori criteria for inclusion. Stock then applied a series of validity tests to these studies and concluded that one of the initially identified papers on occupational CTS (59) should be excluded from the analysis because assessments of exposure in it were seriously flawed. The earliest of the four remaining published papers describes a study of Finnish assembly line packers in a food processing plant (53). The three remaining published papers were based on Silverstein's Ph.D. thesis (76) (see Table 2). We examine these four papers in some detail and also refer the reader to Stock's analysis (84).

Luopajarvi et al (53) performed an extensive upper-extremity evaluation on 152 female assembly line packers in a food processing plant and 133 female department store workers (excluding cashiers). Exposure assessment was not as rigorous as that employed by Silverstein and colleagues (described below), and was provided in the form of semiquantitative descriptions of the occupational tasks performed by both workers and referents. However, determination of health outcomes was rigorous and included assessment of both subjective symptomatology and physical examination findings. Waris et al (90) described in detail the methods used to diagnose neck and limb disorders. Their review retains considerable utility today. The major finding of the study was that "muscle-tendon syndrome," i.e. both tenosynovitis and peritendinitis of the hand and wrist flexors and extensors, was found in 56% of the assembly

Table 2 Exemplary papers relating workplace ergonomic factors to upper-extremity musculo-skeletal disorders

Publication	Outcome(s)	Study population
Luopajarvi et al [49]	Tendinitis, tenosynovitis	163 female assembly line packers in a food production factory and 143 department store workers (excluding cashiers)
Silverstein et al [70]	Hand-wrist cumulative trauma disorders: tendinitis, tenosynovitis, de Quervains disease, trigger finger, carpal tunnel syndrome, Guyon tunnel syndrome, digital neuritis	574 active industrial workers in 6 plants performing 35 "jobs": electronics assembly, major appliance manufacturing, investment casting of turbine engine blades, apparel sewing, ductile iron foundry, bearing manufacturing
Silverstein et al [71]	Carpal tunnel syndrome	Same as above plus a second bearing manufacturing plant, for a total of 652 workers performing 39 "jobs"
Armstrong et al [5]	Tendinitis (subset of above disorders)	Same as above

line packers, compared with 14% of the department store workers. The authors concluded that this highly statistically significant excess disease in the process workers was due to occupational factors, including rapidity of the work, extremes of posture, static muscle loading, and high hand forces.

In the first of their papers, Silverstein and colleagues (77) investigated the association between two occupational factors—force and repetition—and tendon-related disorders (tendinitis, tenosynovitis, de Quervain's disease, and trigger finger) and peripheral nerve entrapments (CTS, Guyon tunnel syndrome, and digital neuritis). Measures of exposure included assessment of hand forces by use of surface electromyography and of repetitiveness by videotaping the work process on a sample of the 574 study participants. The video system also allowed evaluation of postural factors, such as wrist deviation and type of grasp. Jobs involving exposure to vibration were noted. General criteria for the diagnosis of musculoskeletal outcomes required that on interview subjects have symptoms of pain, numbness, or tingling; symptoms lasting more than one week or occurring more than 20 times in the previous year or both; no evidence of acute traumatic onset; no related systemic diseases; and onset since working on the current job. On physical examination, subjects were required to have the characteristic signs of muscle, tendon, or peripheral nerve lesions, although these were not specified in the paper. On both history and physical examination, 51 subjects had a condition that met the criteria for the upper-extremity disorders of interest. Men and women were not evenly distributed in exposure categories (high-force low-repetition, low-force high-repetition, and high-force high-repetition). In addition, there were differences in the distributions of exposure group and sex between plants. For example, there were, surprisingly, no women in the low-force low-repetition category in two of six plants, and no men in the high-force high-repetition category in two plants. To control for these potentially confounding effects, Mantel-Haenszel χ-square and logistic regressions analyses were performed. In particular, most analyses included adjustment for plant, which had a strong and inconsistent effect on the magnitude of the estimated odds ratios. For example, in analyses comparing high-force high-repetition men with low-force low-repetition men, the crude odds ratio was 27.1 and the plant-adjusted odds ratio was 4.9, whereas in corresponding analyses for both sexes combined the crude odds ratio was 17.2 and the plant-adjusted odds ratio was 30.3. The authors concluded that high force and high rates of repetition were positively associated with the musculoskeletal outcomes studied and that the combination of the two exposures increased the magnitude of the association more than either factor alone.

Silverstein et al (78) also investigated the association of the occupational factors force and repetition specifically with CTS. Methods were identical to those in the previous paper, except that data were included from a seventh industrial plant and the only outcome for which analyses were reported was CTS. Carpal tunnel syndrome was diagnosed when symptoms of pain, numbness, or tingling were present in the distribution of the median nerve and had occurred more than 20 times or had lasted more than one week during the previous year. A history of nocturnal exacerbation also was required. On physical examination, either Phalen's or Tinel's sign were required. Competing diagnoses, such as cervical radiculopathy, were identified on physical examination, and subjects with those diagnoses were excluded from the analysis. Twenty-five (3.8%) subjects met the criteria for classification as having CTS by history alone; 14 (2.1%) met the criteria by both history and physical examination. For those classified as CTS-positive by both history and physical examination, the crude odds ratio between high-force high-repetition and low-force low-repetition groups was 8.4, and the plant-adjusted odds ratio was 14.3. Odds ratios for high-force low-repetition and for low-force high-repetition groups relative to low-force low-repetition groups were not significantly greater than one, which indicated that force and repetition were synergistic risk factors for CTS.

Analyses associating upper-extremity tendinitis with force and repetition were reported as part of another paper published by Armstrong et al (5). The

29 cases of tendinitis reported are the same 29 cases of tendon-related disorders reported by Silverstein et al (77). A job-adjusted odds ratio for the development of tendinitis of 29.4 was reported for the high-force high-repetition group compared with the low-force low-repetition group. A crude odds ratio of 16.6 can be calculated from the data provided. Gender-specific odds ratios were not included, as they were in the two other published reports from essentially the same study, in which confounding by gender was suggested.

HAND-ARM VIBRATION SYNDROME   This disorder, characterized by episodes of Raynaud-like vasospasm, as well as numbness and tingling of the fingers, results from exposure to hand-arm vibration (10, 18, 19, 33, 60). In the United States, Alice Hamilton first noted the condition among rock drillers (40). The United States Public Health Service estimates that 1.45 million American workers are at risk for this disorder (60). Occupations in which a high prevalence of disease has been found include grinders, forestry workers who use gasoline powered chain saws, and rock drillers. The occupational factor common to all affected populations is the use of tools that allow transmission of high frequency vibration to the hand and arm. Although objective measures of abnormal function are now becoming available, the current consensus staging system (10, 33) is based solely on symptoms of disease. This staging scheme allows for independent assessment of the severity of the vascular and neurological components of the syndrome, as they can occur independently of each other and can be of differing severity. The recent NIOSH document "Criteria for a Recommended Standard-Occupational Exposure to Hand-Arm Vibration" (60) recommends use of the staging scheme for surveillance of workers. Additionally, it recommends medical removal of workers with advanced stages as the primary method of protecting workers from this disorder.

A differential diagnostic issue of concern is the potential overlap in signs and symptoms between the hand-arm vibration syndrome and idiopathic CTS (18, 28). Although focal slowing of median nerve conduction velocity at the wrist suggestive of CTS has been described in vibration-exposed workers, a diffuse nerve and receptor pathology also is common in these workers (60, 66) and provides the basis for differentiating the two entities. It is unlikely, therefore, that the sensorineural symptoms prevalent among vibration-exposed workers are the result of vibration-induced CTS, as some authors propose (28).

Armstrong et al (6) have suggested that the chronic nerve disorder associated with use of vibrating power tools is due to focal nerve compression secondary to the high hand forces required by their use, as opposed to a direct neuropathic contribution of segmental hand-arm vibration. Indeed, because the two exposures—force and vibration—often occur concomitantly, separation of the effects of each is difficult. Nevertheless, a growing literature clearly indicates that vibration is etiologic in the development of both a vasospastic disorder of the upper extremity and a diffuse distal neuropathy. The neuropathy associated with vibration has been characterized both clinically and electrophysiologically (9, 11, 19, 60) and is unlike the focal nerve compression, i.e. CTS, that has been associated with the occupational factors force and repetition.

CRITIQUE   The studies by Silverstein and colleagues are the best epidemiologic evaluations to date of the relationship between musculoskeletal disorders of the upper-extremity and occupational factors. They applied explicit operational definitions of health outcomes, including physical examination findings. The large sample size allowed powerful statistical tests on the results, and exposure characterization efforts were exemplary. The use of videotaped analysis of the work cycle to assess the repetitiveness of work and deviations of the joints (postural factors), as well as the use of electromyographic analysis of muscle activity to assess the force used by the subject, have greatly improved the validity of assessment of exposure. These methods of exposure assessment are, however, cumbersome and have been used to quantify exposures among only a small sample of the exposed population. For the future, the development of valid and more readily applicable measures of exposure will be valuable when performing large occupational epidemiologic studies.

Although the work of Silverstein and colleagues has shown that force and repetition are significant risk factors for tendinitis and CTS, their results suggest that other, unmeasured exposures or factors contribute to the development of these disorders. Specifically, the fact that the estimated odds ratios in analyses reported by Silverstein and colleagues changed substantially when they were plant-adjusted, implies that something differentially distributed among the plants not attributable to force and repetition category, gender, age, or current job tenure was associated with the outcomes being investigated. Although posture variables are often mentioned as risk factors for tendinitis and CTS, they were not found to be significantly associated with these outcomes in this study. The authors also noted that vibration was a confounder in this study, but they did not suggest that it was the exposure responsible for the plant effect. Inclusion of a plant effect to account for systematic effects of unmeasured variables improves the fit of the statistical model to the data observed in this particular study and reduces the statistical error to allow more powerful tests of the significance of other effects in the model (e.g. exposure category). However, inclusion of a plant effect in the statistical model may result in biasing the estimates of the other parameters in the model. Furthermore, plant effects have no utility as predictor variables outside the study in which they are used, and odds ratios derived from models employing them should not be used to estimate risk in other exposure situations.

In the interest of rigorous definition of outcomes, all-inclusive terms, such as cumulative trauma disorder, should be avoided. As Silverstein and colleagues have done in recent published papers, outcomes should be restricted to individual clinical entities, such as CTS and tendinitis. To avoid misclassification of health outcome in future studies, researchers should employ quantitative, objective methods. For example, it is unclear how well, on clinical grounds alone, Silverstein et al were able to distinguish CTS from other nerve compression disorders, such as cervical radiculopathy, thoracic outlet syndrome, and pronator teres syndrome, which can cause similar symptoms and physical findings. The state-of-the-art for the diagnosis of CTS is electrodiagnostic evaluation coupled with appropriate signs and symptoms (23, 32, 44, 74, 81). Epidemiologic studies should employ, and the NIOSH surveillance case definition of CTS (16) should be modified to include, electrodiagnostic verification of median nerve disease at the wrist for all "cases." Unfortunately, electrodiagnostic studies are painful, and their administration requires a skilled technician and sophisticated equipment. Of great priority in this field is the development of nonaversive, noninvasive, objective methods for the identification and assessment of severity of entrapment neuropathies and other peripheral nerve disease.

Methods of objective assessment of exposure and health outcome are not as well established for hand-arm vibration syndrome as they are for tendinitis and CTS. Objective verification of the disease is needed, however, as the currently accepted staging system is based on symptoms. Specifically, objective, quantitative measures of both neurologic and vascular dysfunction must be validated and employed in worker surveillance programs. Regarding vibration exposure, substantial variability in measurements and interpretations of tool accelerations has led NIOSH to question their utility in disease prevention and to recommend that worker protection be based on disease surveillance (60). The utility of this worker protection strategy needs to be evaluated formally and compared with strategies that do not require overt disease as evidence of potentially dangerous exposure.

Finally, improvements in characterization of both outcomes and exposures need to be employed in prospective epidemiologic studies to overcome inherent limitations of the cross-sectional study design.

Poorly Defined Disorders

The previous section on well-defined disorders summarized the current knowledge regarding the work-relatedness of a group of musculoskeletal disorders (CTS, tendinitis, and hand-arm vibration syndrome) that are widely recognized as distinct clinical entities. A growing literature, much of which has emerged over the past decade from Australia, indicates that some workers also may be at risk for the development of upper-extremity problems that do not fit conventional medical categories and are controversial even regarding their existence. A marked increase in the diagnosis of repetition strain injury in Australia has had tremendous impact on both the practice of medicine and on the compensation system in that country. Unfortunately, little descriptive or analytic epidemiology is available to clarify issues of etiology or even to allow precise definitions of the disorder.

A related area of great current interest is that of the musculoskeletal effects reported to be associated with VDT use. Many of the workers in Australia diagnosed as having RSI were VDT operators. Considerable interest has emerged in the United States and elsewhere regarding this issue. Several municipalities, including New York City, have introduced legislation intended to protect VDT users from a variety of potentially adverse effects, including musculoskeletal disorders. The question is highly relevant as the estimated number of VDTs in use in the United States alone now exceeds 70 million (21).

REPETITION STRAIN INJURY   Although descriptive epidemiology from Australia is incomplete, there have been indications that an apparent dramatic increase in the incidence of this disorder occurred there in the 1970s and 1980s. For example, reports of musculoskeletal diseases to compensation authorities in New South Wales, Australia, increased from 980 cases in 1978 to 4490 cases in 1983 (62). The most recent evidence indicates that the incidence of RSI peaked in 1985 and has since been decreasing rapidly (34, 43). Telecom Australia, a large telecommunications company, reported that 284 cases per 1000 clerical workers and 343 cases per 1000 telephonists occurred from 1981 to 1985 (42). The average duration of absence from work was 24 days. A marked decline in the incidence of RSI cases has occurred at Telecom since the peak of 600 new cases in the last quarter of 1984 to fewer than 25 new cases in the last quarter of 1988, a number almost identical to that for early 1981 (43).

The poorly defined nature of this disorder caused considerable controversy in Australia, and a variety of competing theories regarding its genesis have been published. Deves & Spillane (26) have reviewed four perspectives on the occurrence of this disorder:

1. Medical model: Workers are afflicted with a diagnosable physical condition that is causally related to the occupational ergonomic conditions.
2. Psychiatric model: Workers are afflicted with a conversion or a somatization disorder. Sufferers experience pain in the absence of organic disease.

3. Malingering model: Workers are not afflicted with either organic or psychiatric disorders. Rather, they are deliberately falsifying symptoms to achieve material benefits.
4. Patienthood model: Workers are part of a broad movement that provides "a convenient and socially acceptable medium through which discontent about the nature and conditions of work can be communicated symbolically, thereby facilitating personal coping."

Because both the existence and the work-relatedness of the condition have been questioned, McDermott (48) wrote of RSI: "There is no agreement concerning the cause; the pathology is unknown; the clinical features are diffuse; there are no useful diagnostic investigations; and the prognosis is uncertain." More recently, Hocking (43) has reported "The Royal Australasian College of Physicians has stated that the epidemic was not related to any injury as a result of work practices."

Many of the Australian workers who experienced work-related, upper-extremity pain failed to respond to conventional therapeutics, such as abstinence from occupational exposure, physical therapy, and anti-inflammatory medication (58). Pain often was incapacitating and out of proportion to physical findings. Many sufferers remained unable to return to employment for prolonged periods of time (42, 57).

Despite the lack of a unifying pathophysiological model for RSI, Browne et al (12) proposed a clinical staging system. Stage 1 disease is characterized by aching and tiredness of the affected limb, which occurs during the work shift and resolves overnight and on days off work. Physical signs are not present. Stage 2 symptoms are more intense during the workshift than are those of Stage 1, and fail to resolve overnight. Physical signs may be present. Stage 3 disease is characterized by aching, fatigue, and weakness, which are present at rest and occur following nonrepetitive movements. Physical signs are present. This stage of disease may persist for months or years. Browne et al provided no guidance regarding the specific physical signs that might be present.

MUSCULOSKELETAL DISCOMFORT AMONG VDT OPERATORS   An issue of particular interest in the Australian experience was that a large proportion of symptomatic workers were employed in jobs that required the use of video display equipped data entry or word processing terminals (42, 58, 62). Experience at our occupational medicine clinic and information from representatives of both management and organized labor (50) indicate that a sharp rise in the frequency of reporting of soft tissue pain by VDT operators is occurring in the United States. Studies in the United States and elsewhere have attempted to relate symptoms of musculoskeletal discomfort to the use of VDTs, as well as to work organizational factors. We will discuss the largest of these studies.

In the earliest of these studies Smith et al (80) used a questionnaire to assess the frequency of musculoskeletal and other symptoms among clerical and professional workers who used VDTs and among nonusers. The VDT-exposed clerical workers were employed as data entry clerks, data retrieval clerks, classified advertising clerks, circulation and distribution clerks, and telephone inquiry clerks. Their work was described as highly regimented, with little operator control. The clerical nonusers were employed in jobs "identical to those of the clerical VDT operators, except that they did not use the VDT in performing their task. Their working conditions were almost identical to those of the clerical VDT operators" (80, p. 390). The professional VDT users were mainly reporters, editors, copy editors, and printers who had greater control over the structure of their workday. Clerical VDT users reported significantly more upper-extremity musculoskeletal discomfort than did either professionals who used VDTs or nonusers. Professionals using VDTs did not report more upper-extremity musculoskeletal discomfort than the nonusers. The response rate was low (less than 50%), and no measures of risk (e.g. odds ratio or relative risk) were presented. Formal ergonomic evaluations of workstations were not reported, and other exposure parameters, such as the number of hours per day spent typing or typing speed, were not described. In addition to reporting the most musculoskeletal discomfort, clerical workers also reported the highest stress levels, followed by the controls and professional VDT operators. Smith et al concluded that "there must be other factors beyond the physical presence of the VDT that contribute to the health complaints and stress level of the clerical operators. One such factor may be job content." Smith et al mention rigid work practices, high production standards, constant pressure for performance, absence of operator control, and little identification with and satisfaction from the end product of their work activities as contributory to the elevation in health complaints seen in the clerical VDT operators compared to professionals using VDTs.

Knave et al (47) performed a study of subjective symptoms and discomfort among 400 VDT operators and 150 referents in Sweden. Only those employees using VDTs more than five hours per day were eligible for inclusion in the exposed group. Little information was provided regarding the work tasks of the referents, and Knave et al used a questionnaire to measure both exposure and outcome. Musculoskeletal complaints were more common among the VDT operators than they were among the referents, but the differences were not statistically significant. When "complaint scores" were calculated for different anatomic regions, significant differences were observed between VDT operators and non-VDT users for the shoulder and back regions but not for hand, forearm, elbow, upper arm, and neck. There were reporting differences between men and women. Measures of risk were not presented. The authors concluded that VDT operators may possibly suffer from more musculoskeletal discomfort in their shoulders, neck, and back than do non-VDT users.

In a cross-sectional study, Rossignol et al (73) used a questionnaire to assess health outcomes among 1545 clerical workers. Subjects were employed in banking, communications, computer and data processing services, hospitals, public utilities, and civil service. Among all VDT users, the prevalence of musculoskeletal cases (any workers who reported experiencing one or more adverse musculoskeletal condition "almost always" or who missed work because of one of these conditions) increased with increasing average daily use of the VDT. Specifically, relative to nonusers, the prevalence ratios were 0.9 (90% CI 0.7–1.1) for subjects who used VDTs 0.5–3 hours per day, 1.2 (0.9–1.5) for the 4–6 hour per day group, and 1.8 (1.4–2.2) for the group that worked 7 or more hours per day. The authors considered this finding to be evidence for a dose-effect relationship. When stratified by specific musculoskeletal complaint, the prevalence of both neck and shoulder discomfort increased monotonically with increasing daily VDT use. The relationship between arm or hand pain and VDT use was not, however, so clear. The authors recommended restricting VDT use to three hours or less to decrease the frequency of discomfort and prevent any associated "chronic effects."

Stellman et al (82) performed a cross-sectional study of 1032 female office workers. They used a questionnaire to assess the relationship between office work, including the use of VDTs, and the development of a variety of health outcomes, including musculoskeletal symptoms. They used the occupational categories of part-day typist, full-day typist, part-day VDT user, full-day VDT user, and clerk. The factors measured included job characteristics, such as decision-making latitude and ability to learn new things on the job; characteristics of the physical environment, such as work station adjustability; visual and musculoskeletal symptoms; and job satisfaction. Full-day VDT users reported significantly more overall musculoskeletal discomfort than the other groups. Musculoskeletal symptom prevalence averaged over all exposure groups ranged from 10% to 30%, depending upon the specific anatomic regions. Full-day VDT users reported the highest levels of discomfort of the exposure groups for all musculoskeletal symptoms (hand cramps, arm and wrist pain, neck and shoulder pain, and back pain). Part-day VDT users did not report significantly different levels of musculoskeletal discomfort from nonusers. Interestingly, full-day VDT users had the lowest levels of job satisfaction in four of five such categories in the study and also complained of more discomfort related to their workstations. Stellman et al concluded that "automated office technology is associated with an increase in stressful working conditions and lower job satisfaction" and recommended integration of computer and noncomputer tasks as a strategy for reducing "the potentially stressful aspects of these jobs." They did not discuss the possibility that VDT workstations were selectively introduced into jobs that were more stressful or allowed less control over the work-process. Although their data are consistent with the idea that office technology increases the risk of musculoskeletal complaints, other explanations in which VDTs are markers for the real etiology of the health outcomes (i.e. stressful work) also are viable.

A NIOSH Health Hazard Evaluation (61) at a large daily newspaper also used a questionnaire to evaluate the relationship between work-related factors and symptoms of upper-extremity and neck discomfort in 834 employees, including reporters, editors, and classified advertisement salespersons. Of the group, 331 (40%) reported "symptoms consistent with upper-extremity cumulative trauma disorders" during the year preceding the study. Odds ratios estimated by using logistic regression techniques were 2.5 (95% CI 1.0–5.6) for hand/wrist symptoms and 4.1 (1.8–9.4) for shoulder symptoms among self-reported "fast" typists relative to nontypists. Odds ratios for the variable employment as a reporter/writer were 2.4 (1.6–3.4) for hand/wrist symptoms and 2.5 (1.5–4.0) for elbow/forearm symptoms. Percentage of time spent typing was significantly associated with elbow-forearm symptoms among those typing more than 80% of the time (OR = 2.8, 95% CI = 1.4–2.7) and neck symptoms for those typing 60%–79% of the time (OR = 2.2; 1.0–5.4), as well as for those typing 80%–100% of the time (OR = 2.8; 1.4–5.4). They concluded that a hazard for upper-extremity cumulative trauma disorders was present at the facility.

RECOMMENDATIONS   The Australian epidemic of an apparently work-related upper-extremity pain syndrome that often is incapacitating and refractory to conventional therapy is of great concern. The disorder was diagnosed among industrial, clerical, and other populations. The diagnosis became so prevalent that it nearly caused collapse of the worker compensation system (26). Since 1985, a decrease in the incidence of RSI, almost as dramatic as the increase from 1981 to 1985, has occurred in some job categories (34, 43), but not in others (34). No consensus has emerged in Australia regarding the etiologies, pathogenesis, treatment, or prevention of this entity. Growing factionalization has arisen during the debate, with claims of fraud at one end of the spectrum and of profound medical epidemic at the other. Currently, there is growing acecdotal evidence that local epidemics of a similar poorly defined upper-extremity pain syndrome are becoming common in the United States. Given the potentially large number of workers at risk, an epidemic in the United States analogous to the one in Australia would have enormous impact on the public's health, the medical community, the compensation system, and the economy. The occupational medicine community should, therefore, demand high quality epidemiologic and clinical studies of this disorder.

Given the proliferation of VDTs in the workplace and current concern regarding their safety, it is remarkable that virtually no data are available regarding the prevalence of objectively verified musculoskeletal disorders among VDT users. Several large studies have found significant elevations of musculoskeletal discomfort among VDT operators and suggest that soft tissue disorders are associated with their use. Large, well-conducted studies that utilize well-defined objective measures of exposure and outcome are desperately needed to clarify these relationships.

CONCLUSIONS AND RECOMMENDATIONS

1. A consistent and well-defined nomenclature must be developed by consensus and used when describing work-related musculoskeletal disorders of the upper extremity and neck. To clarify the confusion in nomenclature, we suggest that an international panel of experts be assembled to recommend standard terminology for these disorders.

2. All-inclusive terms, such as repetition strain injury, cumulative trauma disorder, and occupational overuse syndrome, should be avoided. If such a term is required, we recommend musculoskeletal disorders of occupational origin. Occupational disease reporting systems should not utilize all-inclusive terminology. Specifically, we recommend that the US Bureau of Labor Statistics abandon the category "disorders associated with repeated trauma," which currently includes noise-induced hearing loss, hand-arm vibration syndrome, CTS, and tendinitis, and tabulate each of these distinct clinical entities separately.

3. Carpal tunnel syndrome, tendinitis and hand-arm vibration syndrome are etiologically related to occupational exposures. Sound epidemiologic studies utilizing quantitative measures of exposure and objective assessment of musculoskeletal outcomes have consistently found increased risks of these disorders in subjects who perform repetitive and forceful work, or who are exposed to hand-arm vibration.

4. Evidence for the work-relatedness of other musculoskeletal disorders of the upper extremities, such as epicondylitis, cervical radiculopathy, and thoracic outlet syndrome, is currently incomplete, although the available data often are suggestive of an occupational etiology.

5. Objective measures of musculoskeletal health outcome must be developed, validated, and used. The presence of pain alone is not necessarily synonymous with the presence of tissue damage or diagnosable soft tissue disorders. Of great priority in this field is the development of nonaversive, noninvasive, objective methods for the identification and assessment of severity of entrapment neuropathies and other peripheral nerve disease.

6. Measures of exposure should be explicit and quantified. Additional research to identify critical exposures, other than force, repetition, and vibration, must be performed. For the future, the development of valid and more readily applicable measures of exposure will be valuable when performing large epidemiologic studies of workers.

7. Clinical and epidemiological studies of the diffuse pain syndrome called "repetition strain injury" must be performed to clarify the extent and etiology of this problem. In particular, studies that include objective evaluation of musculoskeletal outcomes must be performed on VDT operators, the group in which this condition is most commonly described. In the absence of meaningful information about the entity labeled RSI, an unfortunate repetition of the Australian experience could occur in the United States.

SUMMARY

Sufficient evidence is available at this time to conclude that several well-defined soft-tissue disorders of the upper extremities are etiologically related to occupational factors. These disorders include tendinitis of the hand and wrist, CTS, and hand-arm vibration syndrome. Force, repetition, and vibration have been established as risk factors in the etiology of these disorders. Evidence exists that other, poorly understood factors also may contribute to etiology. At this time no firm guidelines can be established regarding maximum no-effect exposure levels. We agree, however, with Armstrong (3): "Although there are no standards for excessively repetitive or forceful work, common sense dictates that these tasks be minimized to the extent possible." Tool and job redesign may be required in many situations to accomplish these goals. In addition to appropriate reductions in risk factors, medical surveillance is required and will allow greater appreciation of the extent of this growing problem, as well as ongoing assessment of the efficacy of preventive intervention.

ACKNOWLEDGMENTS

Partial support was provided by NIOSH (K01-OH00098-01) and the National Institute of Environmental Health Sciences (P30-ES00938). The assistance of Drs. Christopher N. Gray and Ann Williamson in obtaining information from Australia is gratefully acknowledged.

Literature Cited

1. Anderson, J. A. D. 1984. Shoulder pain and tension neck and their relation to work. *Scand. J. Work Environ. Health* 10:435–42
2. Applebome, P. 1989. Worker injuries rise in poultry industry as business booms. *NY Times* Nov. 6:10
3. Armstrong, T. J. 1986. Ergonomics and cumulative trauma disorders. *Hand Clin.* 2:553–65
4. Armstrong, T. J. 1990. Introduction to occupational disorders of the upper extremities. In *Occupational Disorders of the Upper Extremities*. Ann Arbor, Mich: Cent. Occup. Health Saf. Eng.
5. Armstrong, T. J., Fine, L. J., Goldstein, S. A., Lifshitz, Y. R., Silverstein, B. A. 1987. Ergonomic considerations in hand and wrist tendinitis. *J. Hand Surg.* 12A[2 Pt 2]:830–37
6. Armstrong, T. J., Fine, L. F., Radwin, R. G., Silverstein, B. A. 1987. Ergonomics and the effects of vibration in hand-intensive work. *Scand. J. Work Environ. Health* 13:286–89
7. Armstrong, T. J., Silverstein, B. A. 1987. Upper extremity pain in the workplace-role of usage in causality. In *Clinical Concepts in Regional Musculoskeletal Illness*, ed. N. Hadler, 19:333–54. Orlando: Grune & Stratton
8. Birkbeck, M. Q., Beer, T. C. 1975. Occupation in relation to the carpal tunnel syndrome. *Rheumatol. and Rehabil.* 14:218–21
9. Brammer, A. J., Pyykko, I. 1987. Vibration-induced neuropathy. Detection by nerve conduction measurements. *Scand. J. Work. Environ. Health* 13:317–22
10. Brammer, A. J., Taylor, W., Lundborg, G. 1987. Sensorineural stages of the hand-arm vibration syndrome. *Scand. J. Work Environ. Health* 13:279–83
11. Brammer,. A. J., Taylor, W., Piercy, J. E. 1986. Assessing the severity of the neurological component of the hand-arm vibration syndrome. *Scand. J. Work Environ. Health* 12:428–31
12. Browne, C. D., Nolan, B. M., Faithfull, D. K. 1984. Occupational repetition strain injuries. *Med. J. Aust.* 140:329–32
13. Cailliet, R. 1982. *Hand Pain and Impairment.* Philadelphia: Davis. 3rd ed.
14. Carragee, E. J., Hentz, V. R. 1988. Repetitive trauma and nerve compression. *Orthop. Clin. North Am.* 19(1):157–164
15. Cent. Dis. Control. 1983. Musculo-skeletal injuries. *Morbid. Mortal. Wkly. Rep.* 32:485–89
16. Cent. Dis. Control. 1989. Occupational disease surveillance: Carpal tunnel syndrome. *Morbid. Mortal. Wkly. Rep.* 38:485–89
17. Chatterjee, D. S. 1987. Repetitive strain injury—a recent review. *J. Soc. Occup. Med.* 37:100–5
18. Cherniack, M. G. 1990. Raynaud's phenomenon of occupational origin. *Arch. Int. Med.* 150:519–22
19. Cherniack, M. G., Letz, R., Gerr, F., Brammer, A., Pace, P. 1990. Detailed assessment of neurological function in symptomatic shipyard workers. *Br. J. Ind. Med.* 47:566–72
20. Clever, L. H., Omenn, G. S. 1988. Hazards for health care workers. *Annu. Rev. Public Health* 9:273–303
21. Counc. Sci. Aff. 1987. Health Effects of Video Display Terminals. *J. Am. Med. Assoc.* 257:1508–12
22. Cunningham, L. S., Kelsey, J. L. 1984. Epidemiology of musculoskeletal impairments and associated disability. *Am. J. Public Health* 74:574–79
23. Dawson, D. M., Hallett, M., Millender, L. H. 1983. *Entrapment Neuropathies,* pp. 5–59. Boston: Little, Brown
24. de Krom, M. C. T. F. M., Knipschild, P. G., Kester, A. D. M. 1990. Efficacy of provocative tests for diagnosis of carpal tunnel syndrome. *Lancet* 335:393–95
25. Dennett, X., Fry, H. J. H. 1988. Overuse syndrome: A muscle biopsy study. *Lancet* 1:905–8
26. Deves, L., Spillane, R. 1989. Occupational health, stress and work organization in Australia. *Int. J. Health Serv.* 19:351–63
27. Duncan, K. H., Lewis, R. C., Foreman, K. A., Nordyke, M. D. 1987. Treatment of carpal tunnel syndrome by members of the American Society for Surgery of the Hand: Results of a questionnaire. *J. Hand Surg.* 12A:384–91
28. Farkkila, M., Pyykko, I., Jantti, V., Aatola, S., Starck, J., Korhonen, O. 1988. Forestry workers exposed to vibration: a neurological study. *Br. J. Ind. Med.* 45:188–92
29. Feldman, R. G., Goldman, R., Keyserling, W. M. 1983. Peripheral nerve entrapment syndromes. *Am. J. Ind. Med.* 4:661–68
30. Fry, H. J. H. 1986. Physical signs in the hand and wrist seen in the overuse injury syndrome of the upper limb. *Aust. NZ J. Surg.* 56:47–49

31. Fry, H. J. H. 1986. Overuse syndrome in musicians: Prevention and management. *Lancet* 2:728–31

32. Gellman, H., Gelberman, R. H., Tan, A. M., Botte, M. J. 1986. Carpal tunnel syndrome, an evaluation of the provocative diagnostic tests. *J. Bone Joint Surg.* 68A:735–37

33. Gemme, G., Pyykko, I., Taylor, W., Pelmear, P. L. 1987. The Stockholm Workshop scale for the classification of cold-induced Raynaud's phenomenon in the hand-arm vibration syndrome (revision of the Taylor-Pelmear scale). *Scand. J. Work Environ. Health* 13:275–78

34. Gun, R. T. 1990. The incidence and distribution of RSI in South Australia 1980–81 to 1986–87. *Med. J. Aust.* 143:376–80

35. Hadler, N. M. 1986. Industrial rheumatology. *Med. J. Aust.* 144:191–95

36. Hadler, N. M. ed. 1987. *Clinical Concepts in Regional Musculoskeletal Illness.* Orlando: Grune & Stratton

37. Hadler, N. M. 1990. Cumulative trauma disorders: An iatrogenic concept. *J. Occup. Med.* 32:38–41

38. Hagberg, M. 1984. Occupational musculoskeletal stress and disorders of the neck and shoulder: a review of possible pathophysiology. *Int. Arch. Occup. Environ. Health* 53:269–78

39. Hagberg, M., Wegman, D. H. 1987. Prevalence rates and odds ratios of shoulder-neck diseases in different occupational groups. *Br. J. Ind. Med.* 44:602–10

40. Hamilton, A. 1918. *A Study of Spastic Anemia of the Hands of Stone Cutters.* Washington, DC: US Bur. Labor Stat.

41. Hershey, R. D. 1988. Meatpacker fined a record amount on plant injuries. *NY Times* Oct. 29:1

42. Hocking, B. 1987. Epidemiological aspects of "repetition strain injury" in Telecom Australia. *Med. J. Aust.* 147:218–22

43. Hocking, B. 1989. "Repetition strain injury" in Telecom Australia. *Med. J. Aust.* 150:724

44. Katz, J. N., Larson, M. G., Sabra, A., Krarup, C., Stirrat, C. R., et al. 1990. The carpal tunnel syndrome: diagnostic utility of the history and physical examination findings. *Ann. Int. Med.* 112:321–27

45. Kelsey, J. L. 1982. *Epidemiology of Musculoskeletal Disorders,* pp. 3–11. Oxford: Oxford Univ. Press

46. Kimura, J. 1989. *Electrodiagnosis in Diseases of Nerve and Muscle: Principles and Practice.* Philadelphia: Davis. 2nd ed.

47. Knave, B. G., Wibom, R. I., Voss, M., Hedstrom, L. D., Bergqvist, U. O. V. 1985. Work with video display terminals among office employees: 1. Subjective symptoms and discomfort. *Scand. J. Work Environ. Health* 11:457–66

48. Kurppa, K., Waris, P., Rokkanen, P. 1979. Peritendinitis and tenosynovitis. *Scand J. Work Environ. Health* 5(Suppl. 3):19–24

49. Kurppa, K., Waris, P., Rokkanen, P. 1979. Tennis elbow—lateral elbow pain syndrome. *Scand. J. Work Environ. Health* 5(Suppl.3):15–18

50. Levin, S., Mendels, P. 1990. Labor/management case study at Newsday: addressing repetitive strain injuries. *Occupational Disorders of the Upper Extremities.* Ann Arbor, Mich: Univ. Mich. Cent. Occup. Health and Saf. Eng.

51. Lipscomb, P. R. 1944. Chronic nonspecific tenosynovitis and peritendinitis. *Surg. Clin. North Am.* 24:780–94

52. Louis, D. S. 1987. Cumulative trauma disorders. *J. Hand Surg.* 12A(2 pt. 2):823–25

53. Luopajarvi, T., Kuorinka, I., Virolainen, M., Holmberg, M. 1979. Prevalence of tenosynovitis and other injuries of the upper extremities in repetitive work. *Scand. J. Work Environ. Health* 5(Suppl.3):48–55

54. Maeda, K., Horiguchi, S., Hosokawa, M. 1982. History of the studies on occupational cervicobrachial disorder in Japan and remaining problems. *J. Hum. Ergol.* 11:17–29

55. Margolis, W., Kraus, J. F. 1987. The prevalence of carpal tunnel syndrome symptoms in female supermarket checkers. *J. Occup. Med.* 29:953–56

56. Masear, V. R., Hayes, J. M., Hyde, A. G. 1986. An industrial cause of carpal tunnel syndrome. *J. Hand Surg.* 11A:222–27

57. McDermott, F. T. 1986. Repetitive strain injury: a review of current understanding. *Med. J. Aust.* 144:196–200

58. Miller, M. H., Topliss, D. J. 1988. Chronic upper limb pain syndrome (repetitive strain injury) in the Australian workforce: A systematic cross sectional rheumatological study of 229 patients. *J. Rheumatol.* 15:1705–12

59. Nathan, P. A., Meadows, K. D., Doyle, L. S. 1988. Occupation as a risk factor for impaired sensory conduction of the median nerve at the carpal tunnel. *J. Hand Surg.* 13B:167–70

60. Natl. Inst. Occup. Saf. Health. 1989. *Criteria for a Recommended Standard: Occupational Exposure to Hand-Arm Vibration.* US Dep. Health Hum. Serv. Cent. Dis. Control

61. Natl. Inst. Occup. Saf. Health. 1990. *Health Hazard Evaluation Report, Newsday, Inc.* HETA 89-250-2046

62. Natl. Occup. Health Saf. Comm. 1986. *Repetition Strain Injury (RSI): A Report and Model Code of Practice.* Canberra, Aust: Aust. Gov. Publ. Serv.

63. Natl. Saf. Counc. 1989. *Accident Facts: 1989 Edition,* p. 47. Chicago: Natl. Saf. Counc.

64. Parniapour, M., Norden, M., Skovron, M. L., Frankel, V. H. 1990. Environmentally induced disorders of the musculoskeletal system. *Med. Clin. North Am.* 74:347–59

65. Phalen, G. S. 1966. The carpal tunnel syndrome. *J. Bone Joint Surg.* 48A: 211–28

66. Piercy, A. J., Brammer, A. J., Nohara, S., Nakamura, H., Auger, P. L., et al. Assessment of peripheral neuropathies by mechanoreceptor-specific vibrotactile thresholds. *J. Acoust. Soc. Am.* 87 (Suppl. 1):S78 (abstr.)

67. Puffer, J. C., Zachazewski, J. E. 1988. Management of overuse injuries. *Am. Fam. Phys.* 38:225–32

68. Punnett, L., Robbins, J. M., Wegman, D. H., Keyserling, W. M. 1985. Soft tissue disorders in the upper limbs of female garment workers. *Scand. J. Work Environ. Health* 11:417–25

69. Putz-Anderson, V. 1988. *Cumulative Trauma Disorders: A Manual for Musculoskeletal Diseases of the Upper Limbs.* London: Taylor & Francis

70. Ramazzini, B. 1940. *De Morbis Artificum Diatriba.* Transl. W. C. Wright, p. 15. Chicago: Univ. Chicago Press

71. Reed, J. V., Harcourt, A. K. 1943. Tenosynovitis—An industrial disability. *Am. J. Surg.* 62:392–96

72. Roel, R. E. 1989. Workers' disease of the '90s—Adding injury to efficiency. *NY Newsday* Apr. 30:8

73. Rossignol, A. M., Morse, E. P., Summers, M. S., Pagnotto, L. D. 1987. Video display terminal use and reported health symptoms among Massachusetts clerical workers. *J. Occup. Med.* 29:112–18

74. Sandzen, S. C. 1981. Carpal tunnel syndrome. *Am. Fam. Phys.* 24:190–204

75. Sauter, S. L., Gottlieb, M. S., Jones, K. C., Dodson, V. N., Rohrer, K. M. 1983. Job and health implications of VDT use: Initial results of the Wisconsin NIOSH study. *Commun. ACM* 26:284–94

76. Silverstein, B. 1985. *The prevalence of upper extremity cumulative trauma disorders in industry.* Ph.D. Thesis. Univ. Mich., Ann Arbor

77. Silverstein, B. A., Fine, L. J., Armstrong, T. J. 1986. Hand wrist cumulative trauma disorders in industry. *Br. J. Ind. Med.* 43:779–84

78. Silverstein, B. A., Fine, L. J., Armstrong, T. J. 1987. Occupational factors and carpal tunnel syndrome. *Am. J. Ind. Med.* 11:343–58

79. Sinclair, A. 1965. Tennis elbow in industry. *Br. J. Ind. Med.* 22:144–48

80. Smith, M. J., Cohen, B. G. F., Stammerjohn, L. W. 1981. An investigation of health complaints and job stress in video display operations. *Hum. Factors* 23:387–400

81. Spinner, R. J., Bachman, J. W., Amadio, P. C. 1989. The many faces of carpal tunnel syndrome. *Mayo Clin. Proc.* 64:829–36

82. Stellman, J., Klitzman, S., Gordon, G. C., Snow, B. R. 1987. Work environment and the well-being of clerical and VDT workers. *J. Occup, Behav.* 8:95–114

83. Stevens, J. C. 1987. AAEE Minimonograph #26: The electrodiagnosis of carpal tunnel syndrome. *Muscle Nerve* 10:99–113

84. Stock, S. R. 1990. Workplace ergonomic factors and the development of musculoskeletal disorders of the neck and upper limbs: A meta-analysis. *Am. J. Ind. Med.* 19:87–107

85. Tanzer, R. C. 1959. The carpal tunnel syndrome: A clinical and anatomical study. *J. Bone Joint Surg.* 41A:626–34

86. Tichauer, E. R. 1966. Some aspects of stress on forearm and hand in industry. *J. Occup. Med.* 8:63–71

87. US Dep. Labor. 1989. *Bureau of Labor Statistics News.* Washington, DC, Nov. 15

88. Viikari-Juntura, E. 1984. Tenosynovitis, peritendinitis and the tennis elbow syndrome. *Scand. J. Work Environ. Health* 10:443–49

89. Waris, P. 1979. Occupational cervicobrachial syndromes. *Scand. J. Work Environ. Health* 5(Suppl. 3):3–14

90. Waris, P., Kuorinka, I., Kurppa, K., Luoparjavi, T. Virolainen, M., et al. 1979. Epidemiologic screening of occupational neck and upper limb disorders—methods and criteria. *Scand. J. Work Environ. Heath* 5(Suppl. 3):25–28

91. Welch, R. 1972. The causes of tenosynovitis in industry. *Int. Med.* 41(10):16–19

SUBJECT INDEX

CUMULATIVE INDEXES

CONTRIBUTING AUTHORS, VOLUMES 1–12

CHAPTER TITLES, VOLUMES 1–12

EPIDEMIOLOGY/BIOSTATISTICS

ANNUAL REVIEWS INC.

A NONPROFIT SCIENTIFIC PUBLISHER

4139 El Camino Way
P.O. Box 10139
Palo Alto, CA 94303-0897 • USA

ORDER FORM
ORDER TOLL FREE **1-800-523-8635** (except California)
FAX: 415-855-9815

Annual Reviews Inc. publications may be ordered directly from our office; through booksellers and subscription agents, worldwide; and through participating professional societies. Prices subject to change without notice.   ARI Federal I.D. #94-1156476

- **Individuals:** Prepayment required on new accounts by check or money order (in U.S. dollars, check drawn on U.S. bank) or charge to credit card — American Express, VISA, MasterCard.
- **Institutional buyers:** Please include purchase order.
- **Students:** $10.00 discount from retail price, per volume. Prepayment required. Proof of student status must be provided (photocopy of student I.D. or signature of department secretary is acceptable). Students must send orders direct to Annual Reviews. Orders received through bookstores and institutions requesting student rates will be returned. You may order at the Student Rate for a maximum of 3 years.
- **Professional Society Members:** Members of professional societies that have a contractual arrangement with Annual Reviews may order books through their society at a reduced rate. Check with your society for information.
- **Toll Free Telephone orders:** Call 1-800-523-8635 (except from California) for orders paid by credit card or purchase order and customer service calls only. California customers and all other business calls use 415-493-4400 (not toll free). Hours: 8:00 AM to 4:00 PM, Monday-Friday, Pacific Time. **Written confirmation** is required on purchase orders from universities before shipment.
- **FAX: 415-855-9815   Telex: 910-290-0275**
- **We do not ship on approval.**

Regular orders: Please list below the volumes you wish to order by volume number.
Standing orders: New volume in the series will be sent to you automatically each year upon publication. Cancellation may be made at any time. Please indicate volume number to begin standing order.
Prepublication orders: Volumes not yet published will be shipped in month and year indicated.
California orders: Add applicable sales tax. **Canada:** Add GST tax.
Postage paid (4th class bookrate/surface mail) **by Annual Reviews Inc.** UPS domestic ground service available (except Alaska and Hawaii) at $2.00 extra per book. Airmail postage or UPS air service also available at prevailing costs. UPS must have street address. P.O. Box, APO or FPO not acceptable.

ANNUAL REVIEWS SERIES		Prices postpaid, per volume USA & Canada / elsewhere		Regular Order Please Send	Standing Order Begin With
		Until 12-31-90	After 1-1-91	Vol. Number:	Vol. Number:
Annual Review of ANTHROPOLOGY					
Vols. 1-16	(1972-1987)	$31.00/$35.00	$33.00/$38.00		
Vols. 17-18	(1988-1989)	$35.00/$39.00	$37.00/$42.00		
Vol. 19	(1990)	$39.00/$43.00	$41.00/$46.00		
Vol. 20	(avail. Oct. 1991)	$41.00/$46.00	$41.00/$46.00	Vol(s). _____	Vol. _____
Annual Review of ASTRONOMY AND ASTROPHYSICS					
Vols. 1, 5-14	(1963, 1967-1976)				
16-20	(1978-1982)	$31.00/$35.00	$33.00/$38.00		
Vols. 21-27	(1983-1989)	$47.00/$51.00	$49.00/$54.00		
Vol. 28	(1990)	$51.00/$55.00	$53.00/$58.00		
Vol. 29	(avail. Sept. 1991)	$53.00/$58.00	$53.00/$58.00	Vol(s). _____	Vol. _____
Annual Review of BIOCHEMISTRY					
Vols. 30-34, 36-56	(1961-1965, 1967-1987) ..	$33.00/$37.00	$35.00/$40.00		
Vols. 57-58	(1988-1989)	$35.00/$39.00	$37.00/$42.00		
Vol. 59	(1990)	$39.00/$44.00	$41.00/$47.00		
Vol. 60	(avail. July 1991)	$41.00/$47.00	$41.00/$47.00	Vol(s). _____	Vol. _____
Annual Review of BIOPHYSICS AND BIOPHYSICAL CHEMISTRY					
Vols. 1-11	(1972-1982)	$31.00/$35.00	$33.00/$38.00		
Vols. 12-18	(1983-1989)	$49.00/$53.00	$51.00/$56.00		
Vol. 19	(1990)	$53.00/$57.00	$55.00/$60.00		
Vol. 20	(avail. June 1991)	$55.00/$60.00	$55.00/$60.00	Vol(s). _____	Vol. _____

ANNUAL REVIEWS SERIES	Prices postpaid, per volume USA & Canada / elsewhere		Regular Order Please Send	Standing Order Begin With
	Until 12-31-90	After 1-1-91	Vol. Number:	Vol. Number:

Annual Review of CELL BIOLOGY

Vols. 1-3	(1985-1987)	$31.00/$35.00	$33.00/$38.00			
Vols. 4-5	(1988-1989)	$35.00/$39.00	$37.00/$42.00			
Vol. 6	(1990)	$39.00/$43.00	$41.00/$46.00			
Vol. 7	(avail. Nov. 1991)	$41.00/$46.00	$41.00/$46.00	Vol(s). _____	Vol. _____

Annual Review of COMPUTER SCIENCE

Vols. 1-2	(1986-1987)	$39.00/$43.00	$41.00/$46.00			
Vols. 3-4	(1988, 1989-1990)	$45.00/$49.00	$47.00/$52.00	Vol(s). _____	Vol. _____

Series suspended until further notice. SPECIAL OFFER: Volumes 1-4 are available at the special promotional price of $100.00 USA & Canada / $115.00 elsewhere, when all 4 volumes are purchased at one time. Orders at the special price must be prepaid.

Annual Review of EARTH AND PLANETARY SCIENCES

Vols. 1-10	(1973-1982)	$31.00/$35.00	$33.00/$38.00			
Vols. 11-17	(1983-1989)	$49.00/$53.00	$51.00/$56.00			
Vol. 18	(1990)	$53.00/$57.00	$55.00/$60.00			
Vol. 19	(avail. May 1991)	$55.00/$60.00	$55.00/$60.00	Vol(s). _____	Vol. _____

Annual Review of ECOLOGY AND SYSTEMATICS

Vols. 2-18	(1971-1987)	$31.00/$35.00	$33.00/$38.00			
Vols. 19-20	(1988-1989)	$34.00/$38.00	$36.00/$41.00			
Vol. 21	(1990)	$38.00/$42.00	$40.00/$45.00			
Vol. 22	(avail. Nov. 1991)	$40.00/$45.00	$40.00/$45.00	Vol(s). _____	Vol. _____

Annual Review of ENERGY

Vols. 1-7	(1976-1982)	$31.00/$35.00	$33.00/$38.00			
Vols. 8-14	(1983-1989)	$58.00/$62.00	$60.00/$65.00			
Vol. 15	(1990)	$62.00/$66.00	$64.00/$69.00			
Vol. 16	(avail. Oct. 1991)	$64.00/$69.00	$64.00/$69.00	Vol(s). _____	Vol. _____

Annual Review of ENTOMOLOGY

Vols. 10-16, 18	(1965-1971, 1973)					
20-32	(1975-1987)	$31.00/$35.00	$33.00/$38.00			
Vols. 33-34	(1988-1989)	$34.00/$38.00	$36.00/$41.00			
Vol. 35	(1990)	$38.00/$42.00	$40.00/$45.00			
Vol. 36	(avail. Jan. 1991)	$40.00/$45.00	$40.00/$45.00	Vol(s). _____	Vol. _____

Annual Review of FLUID MECHANICS

Vols. 2-4, 7	(1970-1972, 1975)					
9-19	(1977-1987)	$32.00/$36.00	$34.00/$39.00			
Vols. 20-21	(1988-1989)	$34.00/$38.00	$36.00/$41.00			
Vol. 22	(1990)	$38.00/$42.00	$40.00/$45.00			
Vol. 23	(avail. Jan. 1991)	$40.00/$45.00	$40.00/$45.00	Vol(s). _____	Vol. _____

Annual Review of GENETICS

Vols. 1-21	(1967-1987)	$31.00/$35.00	$33.00/$38.00			
Vols. 22-23	(1988-1989)	$34.00/$38.00	$36.00/$41.00			
Vol. 24	(1990)	$38.00/$42.00	$40.00/$45.00			
Vol. 25	(avail. Dec. 1991)	$40.00/$45.00	$40.00/$45.00	Vol(s). _____	Vol. _____

Annual Review of IMMUNOLOGY

Vols. 1-5	(1983-1987)	$31.00/$35.00	$33.00/$38.00			
Vols. 6-7	(1988-1989)	$34.00/$38.00	$36.00/$41.00			
Vol. 8	(1990)	$38.00/$42.00	$40.00/$45.00			
Vol. 9	(avail. April 1991)	$41.00/$46.00	$41.00/$46.00	Vol(s). _____	Vol. _____

Annual Review of MATERIALS SCIENCE

Vols. 1, 3-12	(1971, 1973-1982)	$31.00/$35.00	$33.00/$38.00			
Vols. 13-19	(1983-1989)	$66.00/$70.00	$68.00/$73.00			
Vol. 20	(1990)	$70.00/$74.00	$72.00/$77.00			
Vol. 21	(avail. Aug. 1991)	$72.00/$77.00	$72.00/$77.00	Vol(s). _____	Vol. _____